The **BIOMEDICAL ENGINEERING** Series
Series Editor Michael R. Neuman

Foot and Ankle Motion Analysis

CLINICAL TREATMENT AND TECHNOLOGY

Biomedical Engineering Series

Edited by Michael R. Neuman

Published Titles

Electromagnetic Analysis and Design in Magnetic Resonance Imaging, Jianming Jin

Endogenous and Exogenous Regulation and Control of Physiological Systems, Robert B. Northrop

Artificial Neural Networks in Cancer Diagnosis, Prognosis, and Treatment, Raouf N.G. Naguib and Gajanan V. Sherbet

Medical Image Registration, Joseph V. Hajnal, Derek Hill, and David J. Hawkes

Introduction to Dynamic Modeling of Neuro-Sensory Systems, Robert B. Northrop

Noninvasive Instrumentation and Measurement in Medical Diagnosis, Robert B. Northrop

Handbook of Neuroprosthetic Methods, Warren E. Finn and Peter G. LoPresti

Signals and Systems Analysis in Biomedical Engineering, Robert B. Northrop

Angiography and Plaque Imaging: Advanced Segmentation Techniques, Jasjit S. Suri and Swamy Laxminarayan

Analysis and Application of Analog Electronic Circuits to Biomedical Instrumentation, Robert B. Northrop

Biomedical Image Analysis, Rangaraj M. Rangayyan

An Introduction to Biomaterials, Scott A. Guelcher and Jeffrey O. Hollinger

Foot and Ankle Motion Analysis: Clinical Treatment and Technology, Gerald F. Harris, Peter A. Smith, Richard M. Marks

The **BIOMEDICAL ENGINEERING** Series
Series Editor Michael R. Neuman

Foot and Ankle Motion Analysis

CLINICAL TREATMENT AND TECHNOLOGY

Edited by
Gerald F. Harris
Peter A. Smith
Richard M. Marks

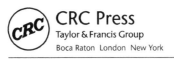

CRC Press
Taylor & Francis Group
Boca Raton London New York

CRC Press is an imprint of the
Taylor & Francis Group, an **informa** business

CRC Press
Taylor & Francis Group
6000 Broken Sound Parkway NW, Suite 300
Boca Raton, FL 33487-2742

First issued in paperback 2019

© 2008 by Taylor & Francis Group, LLC
CRC Press is an imprint of Taylor & Francis Group, an Informa business

No claim to original U.S. Government works

ISBN-13: 978-0-8493-3971-4 (hbk)
ISBN-13: 978-0-367-38873-7 (pbk)

Library of Congress Cataloging-in-Publication Data

Foot ankle motion analysis : clinical treatment and technology / editors, Gerald F. Harris, Peter A. Smith, and Richard M. Marks.
    p. ; cm. -- (Biomedical engineering)
  Includes bibliographical references and index.
  ISBN-13: 978-0-8493-3971-4 (hardcover : alk. paper)
  ISBN-10: 0-8493-3971-5 (hardcover : alk. paper)
  1. Foot--Abnormalities. 2. Ankle--Abnormalities. 3. Gait disorders. I. Harris, Gerald F. II. Smith, Peter A., 1959- III. Marks, Richard M. IV. Title. V. Series: Biomedical engineering series (Boca Raton, Fla.)
  [DNLM: 1. Foot--physiology. 2. Ankle--physiology. 3. Ankle Joint--physiology. 4. Foot Deformities--diagnosis. 5. Gait--physiology. WE 880 F6872 2006]

RD781.F585 2006
617.5'85--dc22
                                         2006102262

Visit the Taylor & Francis Web site at
http://www.taylorandfrancis.com

and the CRC Press Web site at
http://www.crcpress.com

Dedication

This book is dedicated to
Mercy Home for Boys and Girls, Chicago, IL
Dr. Alan Garrigues Smith and Joyce Schlemmer Smith
the Marks Family

Preface

Many adults and children are diagnosed annually with foot and ankle disorders, pathologies, and deformities that are extremely challenging to evaluate and treat. Systems capable of providing accurate and reliable methods for quantitative assessment of these patients have been sought for years. Only recently have technical advances and medical needs begun to merge in order to afford a solid basis for assessment of dynamic foot and ankle pathology. Inevitable results of this merger include better methods of pretreatment planning, surgical and rehabilitative care, and posttreatment follow-up.

This text began with a one-day workshop on foot and ankle motion analysis sponsored by Shriners Hospitals for Children and the National Institutes of Health (NIH). The workshop was conducted on November 15th, 2003 at the Natcher Conference Center in Bethesda, MD. The workshop included national and international researchers from the orthopedic, rehabilitation, engineering, academic, medical-industrial, and clinical disciplines. It focused on clinical needs and scientific advances, with an emphasis on applications, limitations, and problems to be solved. Through the support of Shriners Hospitals, NIH, a host of contributors, and collaboration of the keynote speakers, this work was planned for publication.

The purpose of this book is to: (1) identify clinical needs that can be served by current and emerging technologies, (2) educate readers about recent and anticipated technical advances, and (3) document solid achievements within the technical and clinical communities.

Part 1 of the text presents clinical applications and opportunities in foot and ankle motion analysis. It has been written to convey basic as well as advanced concepts regarding pediatric (Section A) and adult (Section B) applications.

Part 2 of the text presents technological developments and emerging opportunities in foot and ankle motion analysis and is written from a more quantitative perspective. Foot and ankle modeling concepts are described and include seminal developments as well as modern applications and more novel approaches (Section C). Technical advances and emerging horizons related to mechanical paradigms, imaging, kinetics, robotics and simulation, triplanar force sensing, and other exciting technologies are included. Sources of available support for future research and development are described and addressed in the final section of the text (Section E).

The pediatric gait experience with human motion analysis over the past 40 years demonstrates how engineering and clinical synergy have improved medical treatment. In the management of children with cerebral palsy, surgeons now perform several necessary operations under the same anesthesia, thus greatly reducing cost, pain, and inconvenience. Clinical and research applications in human motion analysis have resulted in the development of new approaches to functional assessment and longer-term follow-up. As a result, children in gait analysis–supported environments are receiving fewer and better surgeries. This text provides a basis for expanding these contributions to the broader community of foot and ankle patients, both adult and pediatric.

Contributors to this text have graciously agreed to return all royalties to the Shriners Hospitals for Children.

Editors

Gerald F. Harris, Ph.D., P.E., received the B.S.M.E. degree from the U.S. Naval Academy in 1972 and the Ph.D. degree in biomedical engineering from Marquette University, Milwaukee, WI, in 1981. From 1981 to 1987, he was director of the Biomedical and Biomechanics Research Laboratories at Shriners Hospital, Chicago, IL. In 1987, he joined the biomedical engineering faculty at Marquette University, and in 1989 was appointed director of research in the Department of Orthopedic Surgery at the Medical College of Wisconsin. He currently serves as the director of the Orthopedic and Rehabilitation Engineering Center (OREC) at Marquette University and the Medical College of Wisconsin. His research interests include rehabilitation engineering, orthopedic biomechanics (pediatric and adult), and human motion analysis.

Peter A. Smith, M.D., received a B.S. degree from Stanford University in 1980 and an M.D. degree from New York University in 1984. He completed a residency in orthopedic surgery at the University of Chicago in 1989 and a fellowship in pediatric orthopedics at Newington Children's Hospital in 1990. He has served as an attending orthopedic surgeon at Shriners Hospital for Children, Chicago, since 1990, where he is director of the Osteogenesis Imperfecta Clinic and comedical director of the Motion Analysis Laboratory. He is an associate professor, Department of Orthopedic Surgery, at Rush University Medical Center and an adjunct associate professor of biomedical engineering at OREC at Marquette University and the Medical College of Wisconsin. He participates actively in the teaching programs of orthopedic residents at these institutions and at the University of Illinois and Loyola University in Chicago. Dr. Smith's chief clinical interests are in the orthopedic care of children with neuromuscular disorders such as cerebral palsy and skeletal disorders such as osteogenesis imperfecta.

Richard M. Marks, M.D., received a B.S. degree from Haverford College in 1982 and the M.D. degree in 1988 from Jefferson Medical College, in Philadelphia, PA. He completed an orthopedic surgery research fellowship at Pennsylvania Hospital, Philadelphia, PA, in 1989, and his orthopedic surgery residency in 1994. He completed his orthopedic surgery foot and ankle fellowship from the Union Memorial Hospital, Baltimore, MD, in 1995, and served as an assistant professor of orthopedic surgery at Dartmouth Medical School, Hanover, NH, from 1995 to 1998. He currently is an associate professor of orthopedic surgery at the Medical College of Wisconsin, Milwaukee, WI, where he serves as the director of the Division of Foot and Ankle Surgery.

Contributors

Faruk S. Abuzzahab, M.D., Ph.D.
Marquette University
Milwaukee, Wisconsin
Medical College of Wisconsin
Milwaukee, Wisconsin

Ziad O. Abu-Faraj, Ph.D.
Department of Biomedical Engineering
American University of Science and
  Technology
Beirut, Lebanon

Jeffrey D. Ackman, M.D.
Shriners Hospitals for Children
Chicago, Illinois

Michael Aiona, M.D.
Shriners Hospital for Children
Portland, Oregon

Jason P. Anderson, M.S.
Shriners Hospitals for Children
Greenville, South Carolina

Kelly M. Baker, M.S.
Marquette University
Milwaukee, Wisconsin

Scott A. Banks, Ph.D.
University of Florida
Gainesville, Florida
The BioMotion Foundation
Palm Beach, Florida

Brian S. Baum, M.S.
Baylor University Medical Center
Dallas, Texas

James W. Brodsky, M.D.
Baylor University Medical Center
University of Texas Southwestern
  Medical School
Dallas, Texas

Frank L. Buczek, Ph.D.
Shriners Hospital for Children
Erie, Pennsylvania

Dudley S. Childress, Ph.D.
McCormick School of Engineering
  and Applied Science
Northwestern University
Evanston, Illinois
Northwestern University Feinberg
  School of Medicine
Chicago, Illinois
Jesse Brown VA Medical Center
Chicago, Illinois

Lisa M. Christopher
Shriners Hospitals for Children
Greenville, South Carolina

Chris Church, P.T.
Gait Analysis Laboratory
Alfred I. duPont Hospital for Children
Wilmington, Delaware

Scott Coleman, M.Sc.
Gait Analysis Laboratory
Alfred I. duPont Hospital for Children
Wilmington, Delaware

Kevin M. Cooney, P.T.
Shriners Hospital for Children
Erie, Pennsylvania

Jon R. Davids, M.D.
Shriners Hospitals for Children
Greenville, South Carolina

Roy B. Davis, Ph.D., P.E.
Shriners Hospitals for Children
Greenville, South Carolina

Robin Dorociak, B.S.
Shriners Hospital for Children
Portland, Oregon

Alberto Esquenazi, M.D.
MossRehab Hospital
Philadelphia, Pennsylvania

Anne Gottstein Frea, M.D.
Medical College of Wisconsin
Milwaukee, Wisconsin

Steven A. Gard, Ph.D.
Northwestern University Feinberg
  School of Medicine
Chicago, Illinois
McCormick School of Engineering
  and Applied Science
Northwestern University
Evanston, Illinois
Jesse Brown VA Medical Center
Chicago, Illinois

Claudia Giacomozzi, Ph.D.
Instituto Superiore di Sanita
Rome, Italy

Adam N. Graf, M.S.
Shriners Hospital for Children
Chicago, Illinois

Brian J. Hafner, Ph.D.
University of Washington
Seattle, Washington, D.C.

Andrew H. Hansen, Ph.D.
Northwestern University Feinberg
  School of Medicine
Chicago, Illinois

Diana K. Hansen, B.A.
Mayo Clinic
Rochester, Minnesota

Marian Harrington, Ph.D.
Oxford University
Oxford, United Kingdom

Gerald F. Harris, Ph.D., P.E.
Marquette University
Orthopedic and Rehabilitation
  Engineering Center (OREC)
Marquette University and Medical
  College of Wisconsin
Milwaukee, Wisconsin
Shriners Hospital for Children
Chicago, Illinois

Sahar Hassani, M.S.
Shriners Hospital for Children
Chicago, Illinois

John Henley, Ph.D.
Gait Analysis Laboratory
Alfred I. duPont Hospital for Children
Wilmington, Delaware

David Hudson, Ph.D.
University of Delaware
Newark, Delaware

Eugene G. Jameson, M.S.
Shriners Hospitals for Children
Greenville, South Carolina

Michael D. Jenders, B.S.
Orthopedic and Rehabilitation
  Engineering Center (OREC)
Marquette University and Medical
  College of Wisconsin
Milwaukee, Wisconsin

Dean C. Jeutter, Ph.D., P.E.
Marquette University
Milwaukee, Wisconsin

Jeffrey E. Johnson, M.D.
Washington University School
  of Medicine
St. Louis, Missouri

Kenton R. Kaufman, Ph.D., P.E.
Mayo Clinic
Rochester, Minnesota

Lauren Kersetter, P.T.
Gait Analysis Laboratory
Alfred I. duPont Hospital for Children
Wilmington, Delaware

Hameed Khan, Ph.D.
National Institutes of Health
Bethesda, Maryland

Michael Khazzam, M.D.
Medical College of Wisconsin
Milwaukee, Wisconsin

Steven M. Kidder, M.S.
Marquette University
Medical College of Wisconsin
Milwaukee, Wisconsin

Harold P. Kitaoka, M.D.
Mayo Clinic
Rochester, Minnesota

John P. Klein, Ph.D.
Graduate School of Biomedical
  Sciences
Medical College of Wisconsin
Milwaukee, Wisconsin

Stephen S. Klos, M.D.
Medical College of Wisconsin
Milwaukee, Wisconsin

Brian R. Kotajarvi. P.T.
Mayo Clinic
Rochester, Minnesota

Joseph Krzak, P.T., P.C.S.
Shriners Hospital for Children
Chicago, Illinois

Ken N. Kuo, M.D.
Shriners Hospital for Children
Rush University Medical Center
Chicago, Illinois

William R. Ledoux, Ph.D.
VA Puget Sound Health Care System
Department of Mechanical Engineering
University of Washington
Seattle, Washington

Nancy Lennon, P.T.
Gait Analysis Laboratory
Alfred I. duPont Hospital for Children
Wilmington, Delaware

Gregory S. Lewis
Pennsylvania State University
University Park, Pennsylvania

Xue-Cheng Liu, Ph.D., M.D.
Musculoskeletal Functional
  Assessment Center
Children's Hospital of Wisconsin
Medical College of Wisconsin
Milwaukee, Wisconsin

Jason T. Long, M.S.
Medical College of Wisconsin
Milwaukee, Wisconsin

Lucy Lu, Ph.D.
Graduate School of Biomedical
  Sciences
Medical College of Wisconsin
Milwaukee, Wisconsin

Velio Macellari, Ph.D.
Instituto Superiore di Sanita
Rome, Italy

Bruce A. MacWilliams, Ph.D.
Shriners Hospital for Children,
  Intermountain
University of Utah
Salt Lake City, Utah

Dragomir C. Marinkovich, M.S.
Marquette University
Milwaukee, Wisconsin

Richard M. Marks, M.D.
Medical College of Wisconsin
Milwaukee, Wisconsin

Kristen Maskala, M.D.
Medical College of Wisconsin
Milwaukee, Wisconsin

Brian Mattingly, M.S.
University of Louisville
Louisville, Kentucky

Emily J. Miller, M.S.
Marquette University
Milwaukee, Wisconsin

Freeman Miller, M.D.
Gait Analysis Laboratory
Alfred I. duPont Hospital for Children
Wilmington, Delaware

Duane A. Morrow, M.S.
Mayo Clinic
Rochester, Minnesota

Kelly A. Myers, M.S.
Marquette University
Milwaukee, Wisconsin

Mary Nagai, M.D., Ph.D.
Gait Analysis Laboratory
Alfred I. duPont Hospital for Children
Wilmington, Delaware

Molly Nichols, M.P.T.
Shriners Hospital for Children
Portland, Oregon

James C. Otis, Ph.D.
Lenox Hill Hospital
New York, New York

Steven J. Piazza, Ph.D.
Pennsylvania State University
University Park, Pennsylvania
Pennsylvania State University
Hershey, Pennsylvania

David Pienkowski, Ph.D.
University of Kentucky
Lexington, Kentucky

Rosemary Pierce, P.T.
Shriners Hospital for Children
Portland, Oregon

Michael S. Pinzur, M.D.
Loyola University Medical Center
Maywood, Illinois

Fabian E. Pollo, Ph.D.
Baylor University Medical
  Center
Dallas, Texas

Louis A. Quatrano, Ph.D.
National Center for Medical
  Rehabilitation Research
National Institute of Child Health
  and Human Development
National Institutes of Health
Bethesda, Maryland

Kathy Reiners
Shriners Hospital for Children
Chicago, Illinois

James Richards, Ph.D.
University of Delaware
Newark, Delaware

Christopher Roche, M.S.
Exactech, Inc.
Gainesville, Florida

Benjamin M. Rogozinski, D.P.T.
Shriners Hospitals for Children
Greenville, South Carolina

Jae-Young Roh, M.D.
Shriners Hospital for Children
Chicago, Illinois

Eric S. Rohr, M.S.
Orthopedic and Rehabilitation
  Engineering Center (OREC)
Marquette University and Medical
  College of Wisconsin
Milwaukee, Wisconsin

Adam Rozumalski, M.S.
Gillette Children's Specialty Healthcare
St. Paul, Minnesota

James O. Sanders, M.D.
Shriners Hospital for Children
Erie, Pennsylvania

Jeffrey P. Schwab, M.D.
Medical College of Wisconsin
Milwaukee, Wisconsin

Joseph Schwab, M.D.
Medical College of Wisconsin
Milwaukee, Wisconsin

Michael H. Schwartz, Ph.D.
Gillette Children's Specialty
  Healthcare
St. Paul, Minnesota
University of Minnesota
Minneapolis, Minnesota

Andrea R. Seisler, M.S.
National Institutes of Health
Physical Disabilities Branch
Bethesda, Maryland

Neil A. Sharkey, Ph.D.
Pennsylvania State University
University Park, Pennsylvania

Frances T. Sheehan, Ph.D.
National Institutes of Health
Physical Disabilities Branch
Bethesda, Maryland
University of Maryland
School of Medicine
Baltimore, Maryland

Karen Lohmann Siegel, P.T., M.A.
National Institutes of Health
Physical Disabilities Branch
Bethesda, Maryland

Peter A. Smith, M.D.
Shriners Hospital for Children
Chicago, Illinois
Marquette University
Milwaukee, Wisconsin
Rush-Presbyterian-St. Luke's Medical
  Center
Chicago, Illinois

Robert Stango, Ph.D., P.E.
Marquette University
Milwaukee, Wisconsin

Julie Stebbins, Ph.D.
Oxford Gait Laboratory
Oxford University
Oxford, United Kingdom

Vishwas Talwalkar, M.D.
Shriners Hospital for Children
Lexington, Kentucky

Tim Theologis, Ph.D., M.D.
Oxford Gait Laboratory
Oxford University
Oxford, United Kingdom

Susan Sienko Thomas, M.A.
Shriners Hospitals for Children
Portland, Oregon

John G. Thometz, M.D.
Medical College of Wisconsin
Milwaukee, Wisconsin

Nicky Thompson, M.S.
Oxford Gait Laboratory
Oxford University
Oxford, United Kingdom

Chester Tylkowski, M.D.
Shriners Hospital for Children
Lexington, Kentucky

Matthew R. Walker, M.S.
Shriners Hospital for Children
Erie, Pennsylvania

Mei Wang, Ph.D.
Orthopedic and Rehabilitation
  Engineering Center (OREC)
Marquette University and Medical
  College of Wisconsin
Milwaukee, Wisconsin

Walter J. Whatley, Ph.D.
Composite Products Operation (CPO)
SPARTA, Inc.
San Diego, California

Moreno White, M.S.
Composite Products
  Operation (CPO)
SPARTA, Inc.
San Diego, California

J.D. Yamokoski, Ph.D.
University of Florida
Gainesville, Florida

Linping Zhao, Ph.D.
Shriners Hospital for Children
Chicago, Illinois

Acknowledgments

It is with grateful appreciation that we thank all those who have helped make this book possible. In particular, we express our gratitude to the Shriners Hospitals for Children, not only for the financial support of the workshop, from which this work resulted, but even more for the kindness and philanthropy extended freely to children and young adults throughout the world. We especially thank K. Anne Yadley and Elwood W. Speckmann, former Corporate Directors of Research for Shriners Hospitals, for their continued help and assistance. We are thankful to Newton C. McCollough and Peter F. Armstrong, former and current Directors of Medical Affairs, respectively, at Shriners, for their vision in establishing and maintaining a quantitative motion analysis culture within the Shriners Hospitals system. Without their insight, none of this work would have been possible. We are deeply grateful to NIH for supporting the workshop, which proved to be so essential in forwarding this work. Sincere thanks are extended to Louis Quatrano, Ph.D., Steven Stanhope, Ph.D., and Jill Jordano at NIH for their special concern, assistance, and encouragement.

Special thanks are extended to the staff at Shriners Hospital, Chicago, for their unending devotion and care in supporting both the workshop and the text. We want to thank the Chairman of the Board of Governors at the Chicago Shriners Hospital, Robert Kuehn, for the warm welcome and friendly introductions offered on behalf of Shriners to all workshop attendees. Of special note are the efforts of Sahar Hassani, M.S., Kathy Reiners, and Charlene Johnson. Sahar provided continuous assistance in planning the workshop, scheduling attendees, and coordinating the meeting. Kathy helped us keep the project on schedule while Charlene was never too busy to help out.

The text consists of two parts, one clinical and the other technical. We extend our sincere thanks to all the workshop keynote speakers and chapter authors, engineers, physicians, and health care professionals who have contributed to the book's synergism. Profound gratitude is also extended to our cadre of external reviewers who provided independent critiques and constructive feedback to the authors. We are especially grateful to Karl Canseco and Mary Ellen Ness for their insightful clinical suggestions and to Karla Bustamante, Ph.D., Jason Long, M.S., and Brooke Slavens, M.S., for their technical expertise and insight.

Michael Slaughter, editor, and Jill Jurgensen, project coordinator, from CRC/Taylor & Francis were gracious and accommodating in helping us prepare the text and providing editorial help and assistance with the project.

Michael Jenders was invaluable in bringing the book to fruition. Our many thanks go to Mike for his excellent insight and long hours of meticulous work.

Finally, we thank the graduate and undergraduate students in the Biomedical Engineering Department at Marquette University who helped us improve the workshop with their ideas and suggestions. We also thank the Marquette students in the BIEN-231 class (Musculoskeletal Biomechanics II) who attended and participated in the workshop. Finally, we thank Kelly Ann Myers, M.S., who provided not only a key chapter on a pediatric foot model but also the text cover design.

Table of Contents

1 Foot and Ankle Motion Analysis: Evolutionary Perspectives and Introduction

Gerald F. Harris and Michael D. Jenders

CONTENTS

1.1 HISTORICAL PERSPECTIVE

The study of human motion has been conducted for thousands of years. Records ascribe studies of ritualistic postures and motions used by Taoist priests in the practice of *Cong Fou* as early as 1000 B.C.[1] Hipprocrates, in his book *On Articulations*, describes the relationship between motion and muscle.[1] An appreciation for foot temporal and stride parameters including step duration and step length was offered as early as 1836 by the Weber brothers in their scientific approach to gait mechanics.[2] Foot motion study has since captivated clinicians and researchers for well over a century. In 1872, Eadweard Muybridge, the well-known photographer and cinematographer, studied motion through a series of cameras triggered sequentially to describe the actions of animals and humans.[3] In 1879, Etienne Marey used a specialized shoe pressure system to evaluate cadence.[2] These early and profound contributions have been amplified and complemented by a continuous stream of technological advances and clinical applications over the years. Today, modern technology allows the rapid and accurate analysis of joint angles, angular velocities and angular accelerations (kinematic analysis), ground reaction forces, joint forces, moments and powers (kinetic analysis); electromyographic (EMG) activities, energy cost and consumption; and plantar foot pressures.

For whole-body gait, these analyses have clinical utility in pretreatment assessment, surgical planning, and postoperative follow-up. Gait analysis allows evaluation of abnormalities at multiple joints and resulting multilevel concurrent treatment. It provides a means to differentiate primary conditions from secondary compensations and a means for following quantitative treatment results. Foot and ankle motion analysis is now approaching a similar level of utility. Foot and ankle motion, however, requires specialized systems to track the small segments including, but not limited to, the hallux, forefoot, hindfoot, and tibia/fibula. The increased sophistication of cameras, processing hardware and software, and instrumentation has enabled this "new technology" to progress to the current threshold of clinical application.

1.2 INTRODUCTION TO THE TEXT

1.2.1 PART 1: CLINICAL APPLICATIONS AND OPPORTUNITIES

Part 1 of the text presents clinical applications and opportunities in foot and ankle motion analysis. It has been written to convey basic as well as advanced concepts. The first of two sections (Section A) offers unique insights into pediatric clinical applications. A wide spectrum of children's foot deformities, ranging from congenital to neuromuscular, are presented and discussed in the context of segmental analysis. A detailed review of the pathology and treatment of congenital clubfoot deformity includes results from both standard gait analysis and segmental foot analysis. Another study of a large population of children with treated clubfoot provides a unique perspective on radiographic and plantar pressure findings. Limitations associated with two-dimensional (2D) radiographic imaging are addressed in a clinical presentation of three-dimensional (3D) magnetic resonance imaging (MRI) models of normal and surgically treated clubfeet. The natural history of dynamic foot and ankle deformities in children with cerebral palsy (CP) is documented through plantar pressure assessment, while an insole technique is used to better understand the effects of subtalar arthrodesis in treating pediatric planovalgus foot deformity. Motion assessment is utilized in a clinical study of chemodenervation (botulinum toxin A) and casting to study reductions in dynamic equinus in children with spastic CP. The dynamics of the equinovarus foot are further presented in a study of EMG and clinical outcomes. Walker usage to reduce lower extremity loading is investigated in a clinical study of spastic diplegic gait in children. Perspectives on posture, balance, and responses to dynamic perturbation are provided in a novel comparative study including children with diplegic CP.

1.2.1.1 Section A

Smith et al. (Chapter 2) offer the perspective of a pediatric orthopaedic surgeon in a presentation of several important examples of pediatric foot deformities, which are suitable for study with 3D foot and ankle motion analysis. Foot motion and biomechanical models in terms of clinical significance are discussed. Important findings regarding normal foot and ankle motion are provided in the context of segmental contributions to the overall patterns. With this basis, a series of selected pediatric orthopaedic conditions are presented, where motion analysis is applied. Specific cases are presented for equinus foot deformity, planovalgus foot deformity, varus foot deformity (equinovarus and cavovarus), clubfoot, severe flatfoot deformity, and tarsal coalition. Application of current technologies to combine assessment of motion, forces, and pressures is highlighted.

Khazzam et al. (Chapter 3) review the pathology and treatment of congenital clubfoot deformity. Results from detailed analysis of patients evaluated at long-term follow-up of surgical correction are described. Both standard gait analysis and segmental foot and ankle motion analysis methods are employed. Congenital clubfoot pathoanatomy is discussed and characterized by four basic deformities (cavus, adductus, varus, and equinus). With regard to analysis, clinical and radiographic assessment methods are presented, along with a discussion of treatment options, both nonoperative and surgical. A case study format is used to offer insight into temporal/stride and kinematic results secondary to surgical clubfoot correction. Summary results from a whole-body gait study of 17 subjects following posteromedial soft tissue releases are also presented. Advanced segmental foot analysis is suggested to assess treatment outcomes and for timing of treatment interventions.

Liu and Thometz (Chapter 4) provide valuable insight regarding complete subtalar release for idiopathic clubfoot deformity. The detailed study reviews findings in a population of 17 children treated by complete subtalar release, who were examined by radiography, physical examination, and plantar pressure assessment. Several insole assessments were also included. A series of 68 pediatric controls provided comparative data for the analysis. Findings included significant quantitative differences in specific regions of the foot. The greatest differences in peak pressure loading between clubfeet and normal feet were in the midfoot and hallux regions. Five pressure patterns are identified and described in the clinical study. A detailed case report is used to highlight application of the analysis for treatment. Combined surgical procedures, which are supported by the quantitative analytical approach, in tandem with clinical examination and radiography, are suggested.

Three-dimensional modeling of normal and surgically treated clubfeet is addressed by Talwalkar et al. (Chapter 5). Traditional radiographic angular measurements are noted to be limited in accuracy and precision and not well correlated to clinical outcomes. The inability of 2D radiography to adequately represent the complex structure of the foot is stressed. Alternatives include computed tomography (CT), which provides excellent imaging but requires more exposure than plane radiography. CT also faces limitations in imaging cartilage in the skeletally immature. The ability of MRI to model bony and cartilaginous structures without ionizing radiation is highlighted and noted to be well suited for pediatric applications including clubfoot. Joint surface modeling and congruity assessment are additional advantages of MRI technology. Results from studies of seven adolescents with unilateral clubfoot deformity are presented. Image reconstruction, geometric modeling, and morphological parameters are described. Results are presented from this clinical study, which offers new 3D quantitative information. The method is suggested to follow the growing foot as it is influenced by pathology and/or treatment.

Church et al. (Chapter 6) investigates dynamic foot pressures in the early evolution of foot deformities in children with CP. The lack of agreement in current literature is addressed, regarding the nonsurgical and surgical treatment of foot and ankle deformities in these children. A sparsity of information regarding the natural history of foot and ankle deformities is also cited. The prospective study documents the natural history of dynamic foot and ankle deformities of young children with CP using gait analysis technology. Subjects included ten typically developing 2-yr-olds and 51 children with CP. Thirty-five subjects with CP completed a 6-month follow-up, and 19 completed a 1-yr follow-up. Subjects had a wide variety of baseline function. Children with spastic hemiplegia, diplegia, and quadriplegia, who were able to ambulate with or without an assistive device, were included. Findings from the longitudinal study demonstrated that dynamic foot pressure patterns are still evolving in typically developing 2-yr-old children. Findings from the study also reveal that the presence of valgus foot position is quite prevalent in both typically developing new walkers and young children with CP. Highlights of strategies to correlate motor function, spasticity, range of motion, and other factors are provided as further research is indicated.

Abu-Faraj et al. (Chapter 7) offer an insight into event-related alterations in plantar pressure distribution resulting from subtalar arthrodesis (fusion) for the treatment of planovalgus foot deformity in individuals with CP. Multistep dynamic plantar pressures are studied in hemiplegic and diplegic children and adolescents. A group of subjects with planovalgus foot deformity secondary to spastic CP was evaluated preoperatively and following subtalar arthrodesis for rehabilitation of the foot deformity. The study provides an objective description of plantar foot dynamics for an increased understanding of surgical intervention and rehabilitative treatment of this disorder. The work employs a unique Holter-type, portable, microprocessor-based, inshoe, plantar pressure data acquisition system to record dynamic plantar pressures. The system allows real-time recording of both pressure and temporal-distance gait parameters for up to 2 hr during normal daily activities. Twelve children and adolescents with planovalgus foot deformity secondary to spastic CP were evaluated. Alterations in plantar pressures following foot surgery showed statistically significant increases in pressure metrics at the lateral midfoot and lateral metatarsal head. Significant alterations were not observed at the remaining plantar locations, although subtalar fusion resulted in noticeable decreases in mean peak pressures at the calcaneus, medial midfoot, medial metatarsal head, and hallux.

Sienko-Thomas and Ackman (Chapter 8) provide a detailed history of chemodenervation studies and motion assessment. Also provided are results from the authors' own multicenter study comparing the efficacy of botulinum toxin A alone, casting alone, and the combination of botulinum toxin A with casting. The study focuses on the reduction of dynamic equinus during gait in children with spastic CP. Botulinum toxin A alone was found to provide no improvement in ankle kinematics, velocity, and stride length. Casting together with botulinum toxin A was found to be effective in the short and long term. Ankle kinematics and kinetics, passive ankle range of motion, and Tardieu scale scores were utilized to determine the efficacy of treatment.

The chapter includes case examples of botulinum treatment with muscle length modeling that demonstrates different findings before and after treatment. It is noted that while some treatments such as botulinum toxin A appear to impact the dynamic component of muscle length rather than fixed, the combination of botulinum toxin A and casting may address both the fixed and dynamic components of equinus gait, leading to greater improvement in both clinical and dynamic outcome measures.

EMG analysis and clinical outcomes are assessed by Aiona et al. (Chapter 9) in studies of the equinovarus foot. This work specifically addresses patients with CP who have neuromuscular deficits and a variety of bone and joint deformities. The multiplanar aspects of eqinovarus consisting of ankle inversion at the subtalar joint and ankle equinus are examined. An imbalance of forces across these two joints is recognized as responsible for the deformity. Foot pathomechanics are examined, including both stance and swing phase abnormalities. The biomechanical influences of foot position on the moment arms of the anterior tibialis and posterior tibialis about the subtalar joint axis are discussed. The clinical impact of the equinovarus foot is described, including abnormal plantar pressure distribution, resultant pain, and callus formation. The chapter details an extensive study of equinovarus foot deformity, pre- and post-op in 26 ambulatory patients with CP. Three different surgical procedures are included. Quantitative results are obtained from 3D gait analysis and EMG assessment, including posterior tibialis activity. Following presentation and comparison of the study results, this chapter goes on to propose the continued refinement of accurate kinematic foot models with the ultimate goal of improved treatment outcomes.

Baker et al. (Chapter 10) present unique clinical results from controlled studies of walker-assisted gait in children with spastic diplegic CP. The work recognizes a fundamental difficulty in prescribing walkers for ambulatory assistance. The two most commonly prescribed walkers are the anterior and posterior walkers. This study examines, in detail, usage biomechanics during clinical assessment with each of these walker types. The anterior walker is pushed forward, positioned, and then stepped into. In contrast, the posterior walker is pulled behind the subject, after steppage away from the walker. The two walking patterns create different body positioning and affect the overall gait pattern. There is some controversy as to which walker type is more effective and best matched to the user. The chapter presents lower extremity kinematic results from a comparative study of anterior and posterior walker usage. Results from 11 children with spastic diplegic CP are presented. Gait temporal and stride parameters are also analyzed and differences between the two walker types are highlighted. Results indicated that all lower extremity joints showed a flexion bias with walker usage. The pelvis demonstrated a double bump pattern while hip motion lacked a dynamic range of extension. Knee motion lacked a loading response and ankle motion displayed diminished ranges in all three rockers. Work continues to examine the kinematics in a larger population and to include the effects on the upper extremities, resulting from walker usage. The inclusion of standard outcomes measures is also recommended for future study.

Graf et al. (Chapter 11) employ a unique set of quantitative parameters to examine responses to perturbations of standing balance during translations and rotations about the ankle joint. Included are specific examples from children with

CP, both with and without lower extremity bracing. The study recognizes that children with neuromuscular disorders such as CP often have poor directional specificity with antagonists activating before agonists, delayed onset of muscle activity, poor sequencing of muscle synergies, muscle coactivation, and a decreased ability to generate sufficient forces. As a result, deficiencies present in muscle synergies associated with ankle, hip, and stepping strategies. The range of motion at the foot and ankle is also diminished. The effect of these conditions is to adversely affect standing postural stability and responses to perturbation. The objective of the study was to use a balance assessment protocol to analyze sway energy and other postural metrics in a small group of children with diplegic CP who used articulated ankle foot orthoses (AAFOs). Results include tests from a series of normal children for comparison. The study examines ten nondisabled children with comparisons to children with diplegic CP. Among the findings reported are details regarding weight symmetry, latency in response times, strength of active response (amplitude scaling), a composite motor control test response (which assesses motor system recovery), and an adaptation test (which assesses ability to minimize sway). While lower extremity bracing has been shown to be useful for gait impairments, there is controversy regarding the effects on balance deficits, with mixed findings on overall functional gains. The assessment strategy presented in this chapter is recommended for further study and application.

1.2.1.2 Section B

Section B of the text presents a series of chapters on adult clinical applications. A hallmark of this section is a unique series of clinical investigations of adult foot and ankle pathologies. Gait analysis in PTTD is used to examine a series of patients tested pre- and postoperatively. Chapter 12 offers a quantitative characterization of segmental foot analysis that is considered essential to the study. Another adult foot study provides detailed information from pre- and postoperative assessment of patients with hallux valgus. The study notes that further inclusion of EMG and plantar pressure assessment could lead to improved surgical timing, footwear prescription, and rehabilitation. Hallux rigidus is presented in a study of surgical intervention. Analysis of hallux motion in a series of cases shows improved positioning and range postoperatively. Effective treatment of rheumatoid forefoot deformity is investigated in another study that combines 3D gait metrics with radiographic and clinical assessment tools. The rigid, single-body foot segment incorporated in most lower extremity gait models is shown to be insufficient in a study of patients with ankle arthritis. Chapter 16 offers a paradigm for applying segmental foot analysis techniques to evaluate patients suffering from ankle arthritis before and after treatment. A prospective study is presented, which investigates the hypothesis that total ankle arthroplasty is effective in improving objective parameters of gait in patients with unilateral tibiotalar arthritis. Patients are reported to demonstrate improvements in sagittal range of motion of the ankle following total ankle arthroplasty. In another study, dynamic poly-EMG in gait analysis for the assessment of equinovarus is investigated for a muscle-specific treatment approach to identify specific muscles producing the deformity. Diabetic foot challenges are reviewed with regard to the pathophysiology responsible for the development of foot ulcers. The biomechanical complexities of diabetic foot loading are explored in another chapter, with an overview of neuropathic foot ulcers. The relationship of foot structure to plantar pressures and ulceration and aberrant loading (normal and shear) is discussed. Finally, the Jones fracture of the fifth metatarsal (5th MT) is investigated as a common osseous foot injury that frequently requires surgical treatment.

Marks et al. (Chapter 12) present a detailed analysis of segmental foot motion in a prospective study of PTTD. This study extends beyond previous evaluations of radiographic and clinical results to include the temporal, stride, and kinematic effects of intervention. Traditional kinematic techniques that are suitable for monitoring more proximal joints are not sufficient for describing the complex interrelationships between the ankle, subtalar, and transverse tarsal joints. Results from 27 preoperative and 12 postoperative adults are analyzed, in addition to 25 adult controls. The segmental motion-tracking technique is referenced to a radiographic indexing technique, which is described. Significant temporal and kinematic changes are noted and described in this extensive study. Recommendations regarding clinical impact and further technical implementation are included.

The pathoanatomy of hallux valgus is described by Frea et al. (Chapter 13) in a study of pre- and postoperative gait analysis. Clinical symptoms revealed on physical exam include a lateral deviation of the hallux phalanx, often with impingement of the lesser toes, and a prominence of the medial eminence. Associated deformities include metatarsus primus varus, pronation of the hallux, and second toe hammering. Case examples demonstrate applications of 3D motion analysis to evaluate intervention. The study notes that additional work could lead to additional improvements in treatment, timing of surgical intervention, prescription of modified footwear, and rehabilitation methods following surgery. Integrated EMG and plantar pressure measures as well as functional assessment are recommended.

Schwab et al. (Chapter 14) present work done to quantify foot and ankle segmental motion in patients with hallux rigidus. It is noted that there are few studies of quantified foot and ankle motion in hallux rigidus populations. Case examples are presented in which multisegmental foot and ankle kinematics and temporal-spatial data were obtained using the Milwaukee foot model (MFM). The quantitative analyses found improved walking speeds postoperatively, due to increases in both stride length and cadence. Analysis of hallux motion found improved positioning and range of motion postoperatively. Surgery also served to shift the motion patterns of other foot segments into a more normal range, as evidenced by the sagittal plane differences between pre- and postoperative patterns.

A study of pre- and postoperative gait analysis of the rheumatoid forefoot is provided by Maskala et al. (Chapter 15). They note that while there are many procedures described for the correction of the rheumatoid forefoot deformity, very few offer critical quantitative data. Results are presented from tests of nine independent ambulators with pain and deformity of the forefoot and documented rheumatoid arthritis. Postoperatively, the hindfoot tended to be less dorsiflexed and in a more inverted position. The forefoot was more commonly in a varus position at heel strike, while the hallux tended to assume a less valgus position. At toe-off, the hindfoot tended to be more dorsiflexed, more inverted, and more externally rotated. Also at toe-off, the forefoot was in a more varus position, while the hallux tended to be less dorsiflexed and in less valgus. The tibia was more externally rotated at toe-off and more internally rotated at heel strike. At current follow-up, it appears that forefoot correction consisting of first metatarsal phalangeal (MTP) fusion, lesser metatarsal head resection, and lesser hammertoe correction, with or without extensor hallucis longus lengthening, provides satisfactory outcomes when assessed radiographically, subjectively, and with 3D MFM gait analysis.

Khazzam et al. (Chapter 16) offer a paradigm for applying motion analysis techniques to patients suffering from ankle arthritis before and after treatment. Included is a brief description of ankle anatomy, followed by a review of ankle arthritis and its treatment options. Motion analysis case studies from two patients are presented to clarify the clinical efficacy and usefulness of multisegmental foot and ankle gait analysis. The study found a decrease in temporal-spatial parameters preoperatively, which was noted to improve following surgery. Kinematically, subjects had similar triplanar motion alterations preoperatively. Postoperatively, it appears that subjects' motion was better and that the mode of treatment (fusion or total ankle replacement) did not impact the magnitude of improvement. Of note, the subject that received a total ankle replacement demonstrated greater improvement in range of motion of the hindfoot in the coronal plane. Additional study of a larger patient population is recommended.

Brodsky et al. (Chapter 17) report on gait analysis after total ankle arthroplasty. The chapter notes that total ankle arthroplasty has undergone a renaissance during the past decade. The second generation of ankle replacement prostheses appears to be more successful in providing pain relief for arthritic conditions, while maintaining at least some of the function of the ankle joint. The prospective gait analysis study was performed on 49 patients who were enrolled in a Food and Drug Administration (FDA) clinical trial of the Scandinavian Total Ankle Replacement (STAR). Patients were recruited on a consecutive basis as they presented to the clinic and met the inclusion requirements. Three-dimensional gait analysis was performed between 1 and 2 weeks prior to the ankle replacement surgery and then again at 1 yr after surgery. These tests were again repeated on successive anniversaries of the original surgery up to 5 yr thereafter. The study unequivocally demonstrated improvement in sagittal range of motion of the ankle following total ankle arthroplasty. The difference was statistically significant. The most important unanswered question raised by the study regards the source of the patient's improved gait, i.e., pain relief vs. biomechanical change. The use of segmental motion analysis of the foot and ankle is noted to hold important promise to help address this question.

Alberto Esquenazi (Chapter 18) discusses dynamic, poly-EMG in gait analysis for the assessment of equinovarus foot deformity. The chapter notes that the objectives of dynamic poly-EMG and gait analysis are to assess muscle activity patterns, select specific muscles that may be contributing to the deformity and those that may be playing a compensatory role, and predict the functional behavior after treatment intervention. A method for applying both surface and wire electrodes is described. Surface electrodes are placed over the superficial leg muscles while bipolar wire electrodes are inserted into the deeper leg muscles. Nine muscle-tendon units crossing the ankle are commonly included in the clinical protocol. Detailed findings that support the use of dynamic poly-EMG as a component of instrumented gait analysis are presented.

Michael Pinzur (Chapter 19) notes that over 60,000 lower extremity amputations are performed yearly on the 16 to 18 million individuals with diabetes in the U.S.. Three to four percent of these diabetic individuals will have a foot ulcer at any point in time, and 15% will develop a foot ulcer or foot infection at some point in their lifetime. The development of a foot ulcer in individuals with diabetes is currently appreciated as the risk-associated marker for lower extremity amputation. The pathophysiology of diabetes-associated foot ulcers is discussed and risk factors are identified. Identification of sensory peripheral neuropathy highlights the associated presence of both motor and vasomotor peripheral neuropathies. The greatest challenge to the bioengineering community may be in evaluating the actual forces that lead to tissue breakdown, with shear being the most difficult force to measure.

Diabetic foot biomechanics are discussed by William Ledoux (Chapter 20) in a detailed review of the effects of diabetes on soft tissue characteristics, gait patterns, joint range of motion, ground reaction forces, and foot deformities. The chapter also addresses how foot structure relates to plantar pressure and ulceration, and how aberrant loading (normal and shear) is related to plantar ulceration. It is noted that research has shown that changes in sensory perception due to peripheral neuropathy could cause changes in gait patterns. Peripheral vascular disease, peripheral neuropathy (sensory, motor and autonomic), foot deformity, and aberrant soft tissue loading are all considered to be important etiologic considerations in the development of diabetic neuropathic foot ulcers. The chapter notes that studies have shown retrospectively and prospectively that high peak plantar pressure is associated with plantar ulceration. Recent work has found that it is also important to consider the location of the plantar pressure when assessing how pressure is related to ulcer occurrence. High shear stress is thought to play a role in plantar ulcer development, but the evidence is not as direct as with peak pressure.

Rohr et al. (Chapter 21) examine Jones fractures in a rigorous finite element analysis study. The Jones fracture of the 5th MT of the human foot is one of the most common osseous foot injuries and frequently requires surgical treatment. This particular fracture of the foot occurs during running and sports activities such as recreational basketball. Improved understanding of the biomechanics of the 5th MT is needed to better manage clinical treatment. In this study, a finite element model (FEM) of the 5th MT has been developed by integrating subject-specific structural data from MRI scans and kinematics and kinetics from motion analysis. A systematic approach was used to investigate the effects of muscle and ground reaction forces on the 5th MT stress distribution. Results confirm stress concentrations at the site of the Jones fracture in the proximal metadiaphyseal portion of the 5th MT. Also demonstrated is the prominent effect of the peroneus brevis muscle in producing high stress. Findings of this study support precautionary measures and load control as part of an integrated rehabilitation program for this frequent foot injury.

1.2.2 PART 2: TECHNICAL DEVELOPMENTS AND EMERGING OPPORTUNITIES

Part 2 of the text presents technological advances and identifies emerging opportunities in the area of foot and ankle motion analysis. Content includes quantitative analysis and data interpretation, validation, and testing. Section C focuses on various modeling approaches for the foot and ankle, including seminal developments and more novel work. A variety of exciting technologies in the area of foot and ankle are also included (Section D) in the areas of virtual markers (VMs), joint axis location, imaging, kinetics, triaxial force sensing, prosthetics, and robotic applications. The final chapter in Part 2 (Section E) discusses funding opportunities available for foot and ankle research.

1.2.2.1 Section C

Kidder et al. (Chapter 22) present pioneering work in the development and validation of a system for the analysis of foot and ankle gait kinematics. Prior to this work, the foot was typically modeled as a single, rigid body, neglecting the articulations of the foot segments. A system is presented, which allows for the precise tracking of foot and ankle segments during the stance and swing phases of gait. A four-segment, rigid body model is used to describe the motion of the tibia, hindfoot, forefoot, and hallux segments. Radiographs are used to position reflective markers in relation to the underlying bony anatomy. Testing and assessment of the system are outlined. A five-camera Vicon motion analysis system was used to collect and process foot and ankle motion data from a single adult subject. Results were compared with normalized data from previous work. Plans for clinical application and further improvement of the model are identified.

A similar, multisegment kinematic model is presented by Myers et al. (Chapter 23) for the assessment of the pediatric foot and ankle. Prior to the development of this model, no pediatric foot and ankle models demonstrated sufficient accuracy and clinical viability. The model includes four rigid body segments: the tibia/fibula, hindfoot, forefoot, and hallux. A series of Euler rotations is used to compute relative angles between segments. The first rotation is in the sagittal plane, to provide the highest accuracy in the plane of most clinical interest. A validation protocol for the model is presented, incorporating linear and angular testing. The study population included three normal children between the ages of 6 and 11. A 15-camera Vicon system was used to capture motion data, and a Biodex System 3 was used to generate defined angular motions. Data from the pediatric model were compared to those from an established adult model (MFM), with comparable results.

In Chapter 24, another foot model, the Oxford Foot Model, is presented by Stebbins et al. for the measurement of foot kinematics over an entire gait cycle and plantar pressure in children. An adult Oxford model was modified for application in children with foot deformity, as in CP. Five variations on the model were each tested to determine the most appropriate system for the measurement of intersegmental foot motion in both normal and pathologic (i.e., CP) conditions. Another aim of the work was the development of a reliable, automated plantar pressure measurement system that could be applied in the presence of pediatric foot deformity. Fifteen healthy children aged 6 to 14 were instrumented with reflective markers on the dominant foot, as well as a conventional marker set on their lower extremities. A 12-camera Vicon system was used to capture motion data, and data were also collected from a piezoresistive pressure platform mounted to and synchronized with an Advanced

Mechanical Technology, Inc. (AMTI) force plate. Results showed that the system provided a reliable measure of motion data compared to previously validated adult models, as well as for the measurement of localized forces under the sole.

Davis et al. (Chapter 25) outline the design, development, and evaluation of a multisegment foot model specifically designed to accommodate the primary clinical population, children with CP, at Shriners Hospital for Children, Greenville, SC. Because of the difficulties arising from marker spacing and deformities in this population, several needs were paramount. The model was designed as a two-segment model (forefoot and hindfoot) that would accommodate children and be flexible enough to accommodate significant deformity. The model was also designed to eliminate the need for radiographic analysis and camera repositioning; this was important to allow for integration into a whole-body gait analysis and to streamline the clinical visit process. The Shriners Hospitals for Children Greenville (SHCG) foot model includes several technical markers, significantly reducing the responsibilities of the clinician during data collection. The model has some congruity with the long-established single-segment model, and testing results are favorable. The chapter also presents possible improvements and future directions regarding this model.

The work discussed by Henley et al. (Chapter 26) centers around the assessment of the clinical practicality of a multisegment foot and ankle model. Specifically, the chapter describes a multicenter study in which the reliability of placing markers on a variety of specific anatomical landmarks was assessed. Marker reliability was assessed with 14 adult and 8 pediatric feet. To construct the desired four-segment foot and ankle model, 11 reflective markers were placed at anatomical landmarks. Custom plaster molds were created for each subject and mounted to the floor to insure that the feet remained in the exact same position relative to the camera volume. Marker positions were recorded with an eight-camera system. The subject moved around the room before a second set of data was taken. Marker variations between trials, applications, and different clinicians were measured via deviation ranges and intraclass correlation coefficients (ICCs). The second part of the analysis examined the effects of marker variation on foot kinematic data. Results showed good reliability of marker placement by a single clinician, but poor reliability between multiple clinicians. The study stresses the importance of the clinician's sense of foot anatomy on the resultant kinematic data of the motion analysis.

Kaufman et al. (Chapter 27) divide the leg into three functional segments — the lower leg, hindfoot, and forefoot — for characterization of foot kinematics with a three-body, rigid segment model. A total of 11 reflective markers were placed on anatomical landmarks to define the three-segment model. Motion data were captured via a ten-camera real-time system, and a Eulerian angle system was used to define joint rotations. Data were collected from ten normal subjects aged 31 ± 6 yr. The resultant data agreed well with those from other studies in adults, and hindfoot motion and sagittal plane ankle motion data agreed well with other investigators' results. In general, results agreed with those of Kidder et al. (Chapter 22).

Dragomir Marinkovich (Chapter 28) reports on a pilot study on a spatial linkage model of the ankle complex. Recent technological advances have improved the accuracy and validity of foot and ankle motion analysis. However, current multisegment models are similar in their inability to track the motion of the talus — the common component of the ankle and subtalar joints. Foot pathologies can cause irregular talar loading and motion; thus, knowledge of talar motion would benefit treatment and diagnosis of such pathologies. The proposed model was developed to predict subtalar motion on the basis of the motions of other foot segments. A revolute joint is used to model the ankle joint, and a spatial linkage mechanism is proposed for the subtalar joint based on key anatomical structures and ligaments of the ankle complex. A cadaveric study was used to collect data for creation of the model, to compare the marker based motions to the actual movements of the ankle and subtalar joints. A Biodex 3 apparatus was used to apply known rotations to the ankle joint; motion was tracked via a 15-camera Vicon system and 12 markers placed on the foot, 9 incorporated from the MFM and 3 redundant markers. Results of the spatial linkage model show that the proposed model agrees with observations that the subtalar axis is not fixed during motion. The author proposes further study and refinement before the model is clinically useful.

Walker et al. (Chapter 29) propose a multisegment foot model specific to the assessment of foot biomechanics in dynamic hindfoot varus (DHV). DHV is commonly presented in children with hemiplegic CP and patients of any age with stroke or brain trauma. Surgical correction typically focuses on overactive or out-of-phase tibialis anterior (TA) or tibialis posterior (TP) muscles. Difficulties in diagnosis arise when DHV is presented along with concurrent activity of these muscles. A nonradiographic, anatomical model incorporating the shank, hindfoot, and midfoot was proposed to determine individual contributions of the TA and TP to the varus deformity. For the feasitility study, five children with DHV and neurological impairment and six children with no apparent deformity or neurological impairment (normals) were tested. Two different Vicon systems were used to capture motion data, and patients were instrumented with fine-wire EMG, bilaterally, over the rectus femoris, vastus medialis, semitendinosis, tibialis anterior, and gastrocnemius muscles, and into the belly of the TP on the involved side. The foot model incorporated Cardan angles by Euler decomposition to describe intersegmental articulations. The multisegment kinematic model was able to differentiate between the normals and the affected population. EMG and kinematic data were not able to diagnose the relative contributions of the TA and TP to the varus deformity, however. The chapter provides future direction for the improvement of this methodology.

1.2.2.2 Section D

Schwartz and Rozumalsk (Chapter 30) discuss the application and utility of VMs relative to foot and ankle motion analysis. Physical markers (PMs) form the basis of technical coordinate systems (TCS) in motion analysis. The PMs are affixed to external landmarks for tracking of the underlying anatomy. Usage of PMs has been validated numerous times in research settings and clinical motion analysis laboratories. At times, it is desirable to track motion of points that cannot accommodate PMs, for example, the plantar surface of the foot or certain joint centers. In these cases, VMs indirectly track these points relative to the TCS. The authors assess the accuracy of VMs with a Monte-Carlo simulation, with particular emphasis on foot and ankle, also covering the use of VMs to create virtual shapes (VS). The results of this analysis support the use of VMs and VS in advanced foot and ankle models to provide modeling capabilities in areas where conventional marker placement is not practical. The additional processing time required for these virtual segments is low, and the accuracy can be very high, provided the corresponding PMs are accurately placed.

Piazza and Lewis (Chapter 31) introduce advanced research into the determination of subject-specific ankle joint axes from relevant foot motion data. Errors in joint definitions can have profound, deleterious effects on gait analysis results. Piazza introduces a "functional" method, whereby joint axes and centers are determined from measured joint rotations rather than their relative position to bony landmarks. The knee and hip joints have simple mechanical analogs, making functional determinations of these joint axes straightforward and accurate. The inherent complexity of the ankle joint, with the talocrural and subtalar joints functioning like successive nonparallel hinges, as well as the inaccessibility of the talus to external marking, makes this more difficult. Two promising approaches to functional modeling of the ankle are presented, including a numerical optimization determination of the two joint axes from distal and proximal segmental motion, and a two-axis approximation of the subtalar joint alone. Methods are evaluated with a cadaver model, in which motion of the tibia, talus, and calcaneus were measured directly with markers mounted in the bone. Preliminary results are presented and further direction discussed. Generic joint models have limited clinical utility due to the dynamic variability of joint location and articulation between subjects, and this work has exciting potential to increase the accuracy and validity of motion analysis of the ankle joint.

Yamokoski and Banks (Chapter 32) report on the use of radiography for 3D measurement of skeletal motion, in particular relating to the ankle joint. Over the past 10 to 15 yr, it has become possible for accurate measurement of human motion by dynamic radiography. Traditionally, this approach has been used to assess the kinematics of the major weight-bearing joints — the hip and knee. The intricate motions of the small bones of the ankle present a challenge. Marker-based motion capture has given some insight into ankle kinematics; however, it is susceptible to surface motion, distorting the underlying bony articulations. Ideally, application of dynamic radiography would allow for an alternative accurate, noninvasive technique. The current state of the art is presented, particularly in relation to the most common site of radiographic analysis, the knee, and possible extensions of this technology to the ankle joint are discussed, along with future challenges.

Sheehan et al. (Chapter 33) report on the use of fast-phase contrast (fast-PC) MRI for *in vivo* assessment of ankle dynamics. Understanding of the *in vivo* kinematics of the talocrural and subtalar joints is of critical importance, clinically, to reduce the impact of impairments on rearfoot function, prevent injury, and improve diagnostic accuracy. Previous work has proven that fast-PC MRI is an effective, accurate technique for the quantification of skeletal dynamics, with results comparable to that of dynamic radiography. The study presents work in which MRI is applied to the assessment of talocrural and subtalar 3D joint kinematics during volitional activities. Results showed that the talocrural and subtalar joints move independently of one another, but were contrary to established anatomical studies.

Talocrural motion accounted for the vast majority of calcaneal-tibial motion in all three directions of rotation. During plantarflexion, inversion and internal rotation were evidenced at the talocrural joint, but were not evident at the subtalar joint.

In Chapter 34, Bruce MacWilliams reports on kinetic assessment of the foot. Despite the recent advances in multisegment kinematic modeling of the foot, no solutions have been presented for determination of the kinetics within the various foot joints. MacWilliams discusses the barriers to kinetic analysis of the foot and presents possibilities whereby current and/or future technologies may help overcome them. Distributed force measures, shear force measurement, data synchronization, pressure sensing, inertial forces, and inverse dynamics are covered. The author cites the integration of pedobarograph data as a special challenge, because these data cannot be channeled through standard analog to digital (A/D) units as EMG or force plate data are. The work presented here illustrates that kinetic foot measurement is possible with current technologies, but extensive processing time and lack of commercial support remain barriers to clinical utility.

As a natural progression from the previous chapter, Miller et al. (Chapter 35) report on the development and testing of a novel triaxial plantar force sensor. This sensor was designed to report plantar foot pressures in the vertical, anterior–posterior (A–P), and medial–lateral (M–L) directions. While force plates can report this information in aggregate terms, the sensor presented here is capable of resolving these forces in the individual segments of the foot. The capability to accurately measure shear forces discretely across the plantar surface has great importance to the potential development of kinetic foot models. Plantar pressure assessment is also important clinically in the diagnosis of foot pathology, assessment of the effect of footwear on gait, and the prevention of plantar ulceration. Calibration and subject testing of the sensor are covered, and future work is proposed to refine the sensor. This work has exciting possibilities, both clinically and in the development of kinetic foot models.

Hansen et al. (Chapter 36) discuss measurement of ankle quasistiffness — the slope of the ankle moment versus dorsiflexion curve — in relation to prosthetic design. Muscles surrounding the ankle–foot complex include passive and active elements relevant during gait. The net effect of these elements could be approximated by a purely passive elastic prosthetic component. The study reports on an investigation into ankle quasistiffness with varying walking speeds. A prosthetic component that is faithful to the physiological response would be able to dynamically adapt to the gait of the user. Data were obtained from 24 able-bodied subjects with an eight-camera motion analysis system. Results showed that the ankle has passive properties during slow gait and active properties during rapid gait.

In Chapter 37, Moreno White at SPARTA, Inc. reports on the development of an advanced biofidelic lower extremity (able) prosthesis. This ongoing research aims to develop a prosthetic ankle capable of mimicking a natural, nonamputee gait. Research involved the creation of complex, dynamic, nonlinear FEMs to approximate the human ankle function, on the basis of clinical data from both able-bodied and amputee subjects. The output of these analyses was used to design prototype ankle components and full-scale ankle assemblies. Testing of these prototype ankles through both mechanical and clinical testing is outlined.

James Otis (Chapter 38) covers the role of robotics in gait simulation and foot mechanics. This chapter covers methods used for characterizing the mechanical properties of joints, as well as the implementation of cadaver models and sophisticated gait simulators to understand the intrinsic kinematics and kinetics of the foot during gait. Robotic technology has previously been applied to quantify mechanical properties of the knee joint, glenohumeral joint, and intervertebral joints of the spine. This technology has the potential to quantify mechanical properties and simulate external loading conditions of the foot during functional activities. The application presented centers on PTTD, which has particularly benefited from the use of cadaver models and gait simulators. The construction of a cadaver model consistent with the physiologic deformity is reported, and the engineering basis and procedure behind the use of robotic technology are outlined.

1.2.2.3 Section E

The text concludes with a discussion by Quatrano and Khan from the National Institutes of Health (NIH) regarding research support applicable to this text. Brief introductions to the NIH and National Center for Medical Rehabilitation Research (NCMRR) are presented to familiarize the reader with the scope and mission of these organizations. To give readers an inclination of the government funding available for research, the 2004 NIH budget was 28 billion dollars, with 82% of this supporting research grants, training, and research and development contracts. The chapter includes an outline for the submission of grant proposals, as well as guidance in beginning research pursuits in medicine and rehabilitation.

REFERENCES

1. Basmajian JV. *Therapeutic Exercise.* 3rd ed. Williams and Wilkins: Baltimore, MD, 1978:1,3,5.
2. Steindler A. *Kinesiology of the Human Body.* Charles C Thomas: Springfield, IL, 1970: 631–632.
3. Muybridge E. *The Human Figure in Motion.* Dover: New York (Reprinted in 1955 from original volume published in 1887).

Part 1

Clinical Applications and Opportunities

Section A

Pediatric Foot and Ankle

2 Clinical Applications of Foot and Ankle Motion Analysis in Children

Peter A. Smith, Sahar Hassani, Adam N. Graf, and Gerald F. Harris

CONTENTS

2.1 INTRODUCTION

Pediatric orthopedists treat a wide variety of children with foot symptoms. Some children present with normal variations such as flexible flat feet. Others have more complicated foot deformities, often in association with muscle imbalance caused by an underlying neuromuscular disorder. Accurate description of these deformities presents a significant challenge. There exists significant variability in the interpretation due to the complexity of foot motion terminology and description.

This chapter outlines several examples of pediatric foot deformities, which are suitable for study with three-dimensional (3D) foot and ankle motion analysis. It demonstrates how motion analysis of the foot can be applied to improve patient care, while highlighting future challenges for a broader range of pediatric applications.

2.2 GAIT ANALYSIS

The function of the foot during gait has been studied for hundreds of years, with important discoveries about periodicity of events, magnitude of forces, and timing of motor unit function.[1–5] In whole-body gait analysis, the foot is modeled as a single rigid segment articulating with the lower extremity.[6] With the evolution of camera and computer technologies, motion analysis has expanded significantly to include detailed descriptions of segmental foot and ankle motion. Multiple markers can be placed in a relatively small area to track subtle motions of small segments. Segmental foot and ankle motion requires a specialized system to track the hallux, forefoot, hindfoot, tibia, and other segments of interest. Adult foot and ankle motion has been shown to produce consistent, accurate quantitative data that can be assessed and statistically analyzed.[7] These data have been useful in analyzing the efficacy of different treatments and evaluating the biomechanical consequences of surgery. It has recently become possible to accurately study the pediatric foot as well.[8–10] A system that accurately measures motion, plantar pressures, and ground reaction forces expands our ability of better describing pathologic gait patterns. While video played in slow motion can reveal significant helpful information on segmental motion patterns, more quantitative, 3D analysis provides improved accuracy of assessment, understanding, and care. Systematic analysis of segmental foot motion and plantar pressures provides a detailed record of gait events, allowing for meaningful dialog among clinicians.

Gait analysis has proven useful in pediatric orthopedics to evaluate children's walking abnormalities at multiple joints for presurgical assessment, postsurgical follow-up, and treatment evaluation.[5,6] It provides a means to differentiate primary problems from secondary compensations. The data include joint angles, angular velocities, angular accelerations, electromyographic (EMG) activities, and plantar foot pressures.[11] Evaluation of segmental foot motion has followed the technical evolution of improved data and collection instruments. The implementation of the four-segment foot model provides greater accuracy for clinical decision making. Children present with a broad range of abnormalities in foot position and motion, ranging from idiopathic, congenital, or neuromuscular causes. It is reasonable to assume that advanced applications of segmental foot motion analysis techniques in

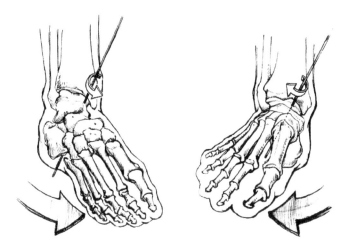

FIGURE 2.1 Left — linked motions of supination, adduction and inversion. Right — pronation, abduction, and eversion.

children will ultimately result in improved treatment.[9,10] To date, little research has been done characterizing foot and ankle motion in children. The current challenge requires establishing and understanding normal pediatric foot patterns and using the data as a comparison for the evaluation of foot pathology.

2.3 FOOT MOTION

The foot and ankle is a complex structure designed to absorb the forces of a step and to support and propel the body forward, while adapting to uneven surfaces or other perturbations. There are 28 bones and 26 joints in each foot and ankle, allowing complex motion in the sagittal, coronal, and transverse planes. Major joints of the foot and ankle are the talocrural (true ankle joint), talocalcaneal (subtalar), transverse tarsal (midtarsal), and metatarsophalangeal. The ankle and subtalar joint together comprise a mechanism of two joints, which are linked in motion.[12,13] The subtalar and multiple other joints participate in the clinically significant combined motions of supination, inversion, and adduction and the corresponding opposite motion of pronation, eversion, and abduction (Figure 2.1). The axes of rotation and range of motion of the ankle, subtalar, and midfoot joints have been studied in cadavers, and elegant models of foot function have been described.[14–20] An understanding of joint motion is helpful in understanding the presentation of foot and ankle motion data, which is presented in three dimensions for each of the four segments: tibia, hindfoot, forefoot, and hallux.

2.4 BIOMECHANICAL MODELS

Several biomechanical models of the foot and ankle have been proposed using cadaver specimens.[1,2,17,18,21] More recently, *in vivo* biomechanical models of the adult foot and ankle using multiple segments have been developed.[22–27] Most models

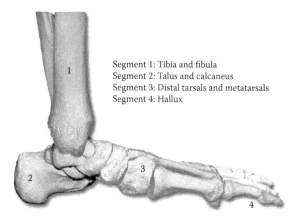

Segment 1: Tibia and fibula
Segment 2: Talus and calcaneus
Segment 3: Distal tarsals and metatarsals
Segment 4: Hallux

FIGURE 2.2 Four segment foot model of the tibia, hindfoot, forefoot/midfoot, and hallux.

represent motion of the tibia in relation to the laboratory and 3D motion of the foot in three additional segments. The motion of each foot segment is referenced to its own more proximal segment. For the pediatric population, there are limited biomechanical models to assess foot and ankle motion. Challenges reported in developing the pediatric foot model include small foot sizes, close marker spacing, and skin motion artifacts.[9,24,28] Many studies do not elaborate on validation procedures, including reliability and accuracy testing. Recently, Myers et al. validated a biomechanical model (The Milwaukee Foot Model) with pediatric applications, which demonstrated accuracy and reliability using a four-segment model.[8] The model segments consist of (1) tibia/fibula, (2) hindfoot (calcaneus, talus, navicular), (3) midfoot/forefoot (cuneiforms, cuboid, metatarsals), and (4) hallux (Figure 2.2).

In the Milwaukee foot and ankle motion analysis system, in order to properly align the marker-based coordinate systems with the underlying bony anatomy, a rotation matrix is determined with the use of radiographic data. The radiographic views are anterior–posterior (A–P), lateral (LAT), hindfoot (HA), and the "Milwaukee view" to determine coronal alignment of the hindfoot (Figure 2.3).[29] This system can be used for both the adult and pediatric population.

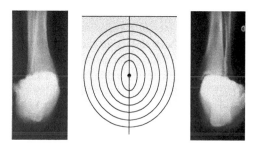

FIGURE 2.3 Radiographic Milwaukee view. The radiograph is taken with the subject standing in a defined alignment referenced to the static gait lab stance position. An ellipse is superimposed on the calcaneal outline to determine the coronal alignment of the hindfoot.

2.5 NORMAL FOOT AND ANKLE MOTION

Patterns of motion of the foot and ankle during normal gait in children appear similar among patients, although a larger sample size and rigorous evaluation of the variability of data has yet to be completed (Figure 2.4). However, the data generated from our laboratory for ten children closely follow previously published data from Johnson and Harris for adults.[7] In addition, motion plots obtained for the tibia, hindfoot, and forefoot are similar to those predicted from biomechanical studies of cadavers and reproduced in textbooks about foot biomechanics.[16,17,30–33]

In foot and ankle motion analysis, the tibia motion is referenced to the laboratory. The motion of the hindfoot, forefoot, and hallux are referenced to their respective proximal segments. Therefore, ankle and subtalar motion is best represented as the motion of the hindfoot relative to the tibia. The midfoot and forefoot segment measures motion of the cuniforms, cuboid, and metatarsals relative to the hindfoot. Most of this motion occurs through the midtarsal joints.

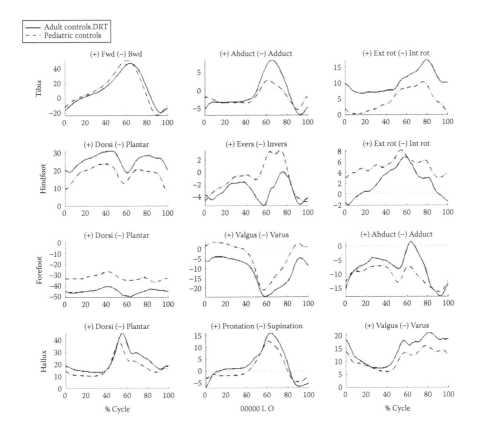

FIGURE 2.4 Three-dimensional foot and ankle motion analysis plots. Pediatric normals ($n = 10$) vs. adult normals ($n = 40$).

2.5.1 Normal Tibial Motion

Tibial motion is measured by markers placed on the lateral and medial malleolus and the medial flat surface of the tibia. There is little variability in sagittal plane tibial motion during normal gait among adults and children, making the tibia a useful reference point for foot motion. The range of motion in the sagittal plane of the tibia is substantial, from approximately 18° of posterior angulation in relation to the laboratory at initial contact to 45° of anterior angulation at foot off. The fact that the range of motion is substantially larger than that measured at the ankle in whole-body gait is because the foot is not always plantigrade during contact. Adduction and abduction of the tibia are related to the foot progression angle during push-off, when the tibia consistently abducts. There is measurable internal rotation of the tibia with load acceptance, which is consistent with theories about the mechanism of action of the ankle and subtalar joint function as a torque converter to convert perpendicular loading to inward rotation.[1,2,21,34]

2.5.2 Normal Hindfoot Motion

The hindfoot segment is referenced to the tibia and demonstrates three rockers in the sagittal plane, which have been described in whole-body gait.[4,6] With heel contact, there is brief plantarflexion during the first 5% of the gait cycle, which corresponds to the first ankle rocker. The second rocker is a period of gradual dorsiflexion of the hindfoot relative to the tibia. The third ankle rocker comprises the last 15% of stance phase. The hindfoot rapidly plantarflexes, which corresponds to push-off from gastrocsoleus activity.

During swing phase, the hindfoot rapidly dorsiflexes to recover to the plantigrade position. In the coronal plane, during the majority of stance, the hindfoot everts and externally rotates. This is consistent with motion through the subtalar joint to accept loading. The measured range of eversion is about 4° on average. Inversion occurs in late stance and proceeds through push-off. There is a single cycle of eversion and inversion, which occurs during swing phase as the ankle recovers dorsiflexion and prepares for heel strike.

2.5.3 Normal Forefoot Motion

The forefoot remains remarkably stationary with respect to the hindfoot in the sagittal plane throughout the gait cycle but supinates in the coronal plane during the last part of stance, just preceding and during push-off. The forefoot pronates and abducts during the early and midswing phases.

2.5.4 Normal Hallux Motion

Hallux motion is consistent among normal subjects. In the sagittal plane, there is 35° of dorsiflexion during the late stance. In the coronal plane, the hallux supinates at initial contact, with 10° of pronation during push-off. For the transverse plane, the hallux exhibits 10 to 15° of valgus throughout the gait cycle.

While these patterns of motion are consistently measured in three dimensions during normal gait, there is variability between subjects. A better understanding of variability will allow more accurate interpretation of pathologic gait patterns.

2.6 CLINICAL CHALLENGES

There exists a wide spectrum of children's foot deformities, which range from congenital to neuromuscular. We have selected common pediatric orthropedic conditions where motion analysis can be applied. Undoubtedly, new applications will arise as the technology advances.

2.7 CEREBRAL PALSY

The most common neuromuscular disorder, cerebral palsy, is a nonprogressive disorder of the brain, which causes abnormal gait or posture. Children with cerebral palsy frequently develop foot and ankle deformities, which interfere with their gait.

2.8 EQUINUS FOOT DEFORMITIES

Ankle equinus is the most common deformity in children with cerebral palsy (Figure 2.5). Ankle equinus is the result of muscle imbalance between overactive plantar flexors (gastrocsoleus) and normal or weakened dorsiflexors. Plantarflexor spasticity is often noted on physical exam. Equinus is often dynamic and associated with an extended posture of the lower extremities, with no fixed muscle contractures. As the child develops a mature gait, fixed equinus contractures can develop, predominately of the gastrocnemius.[35] Contractures of the gastrocsoleus complex are most common in hemiplegia.

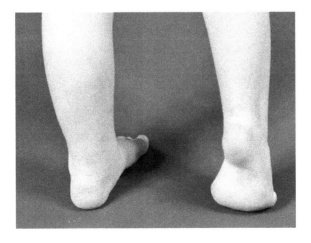

FIGURE 2.5 Right foot equinus in a child with hemiplegic cerebral palsy.

Ankle motion is displayed in whole-body gait analysis, though in this model, the foot is assumed to move as a single unit. Therefore, some important information is not provided. The most common sources of under- or overestimation of ankle equinus are in situations where the foot is excessively abducted and pronated and there is midfoot dorsiflexion, in which case the ankle's dorsiflexion is overestimated. Conversely, when the forefoot is in equinus and cavus, there is overestimation of ankle equinus. Currently, the best way to interpret foot motion measured by whole-body gait analysis is by close analysis of slow motion video. While video analysis will always remain important, the description of accurate foot motion will provide more insight into complex foot deformity dynamics and provide the ability to attribute sagittal plane deformities to different segments of the foot.

2.8.1 VARUS AND VALGUS

Children with cerebral palsy frequently have abnormal coronal plane foot motion with varus and valgus (Figure 2.6).[6,36] These rarely occur in isolation and are commonly associated with hindfoot equinus or, rarely, calcaneus. Significant contracture of the ankle plantar flexors causes all the weight to be placed on the toes or the forefoot, resulting in a decrease in power absorption and a large stress on the mid- and hindfoot.[6,36] As children approach adolescence and gain weight, the foot exhibits permanent structural changes. Whole-body gait analysis, EMG studies, and physical examination have helped the clinician diagnose and treat equinus, but the determination of varus and valgus deformities has relied on observation, EMG, and foot pressure.[35] Measuring significant contributions of midfoot motion in the sagittal and

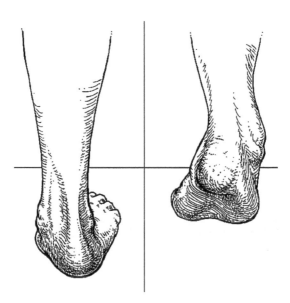

FIGURE 2.6 Foot deformities in cerebral palsy. Left —illustration of planovalgus foot. Right — illustration of equinovarus foot.

coronal, and transverse planes, and separating this from ankle motion would help clinicians direct treatment to the affected joints and understand the exact pathology of abnormal foot positions in cerebral palsy, as well as the effects of intervention.

2.9 PLANOVALGUS FOOT DEFORMITIES

Planovalgus is the most common foot deformity in children with diplegia and quadriplegia (Figure 2.7).[37] Valgus deformity can develop from muscle imbalance, abnormal forces, bony misalignment, and ligamentous laxity. Some children with gastrocsoleus spasticity develop planovalgus due to the increase in force across the hindfoot and midfoot with toe walking. Planovalgus is also associated with external tibial torsion. Spastic and overactive peroneal muscles have been shown to contribute to valgus position. Also contributing to the deformity can be underactivity of the posterior tibialis muscles. The deformity can worsen over time and requires long-term care.

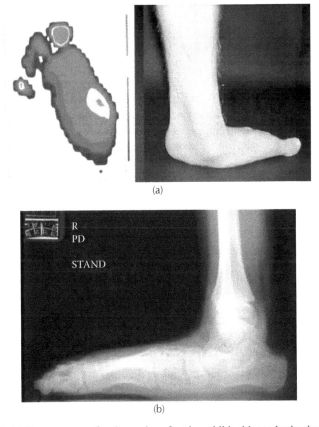

(a)

(b)

FIGURE 2.7 (a) Foot pressure of a planovalgus foot in a child with cerebral palsy. (b) Lateral radiograph of a planovalgus foot in a child with cerebral palsy.

There are a variety of accepted methods for treating planovalgus.[38,39] Bracing is effective in improving gait in young children. Subtalar arthrodesis, calcaneal osteotomies, posterior tibialis advancement, and subtalar fusion have all been proposed as definitive surgical treatments in severe cases in older children. Often, clinical exam and radiographic assessment of planovalgus yields general information, with broad variability and poor specificity. Foot pressure measurements are particularly helpful in documenting the deformity and examining the improvements after surgery (Figure 2.7). Several studies have documented changes in foot pressures after surgery for planovalgus. The usefulness of foot pressure measurements will increase with our understanding of normal and pathological patterns.[40-45] With more experience, preoperative assessment may become routine. Application of foot and ankle motion analysis techniques to the study of the planovalgus foot will improve understanding and treatment.[45]

2.9.1 CASE 1: PLANOVALGUS

A.B. is a 6-yr-old male with a history of diplegic cerebral palsy. He has a moderate planovalgus deformity of the left foot. The patient is a community ambulator and wears an ankle–foot orthosis (AFO). His planovalgus is apparent in the photos (Figure 2.8). On viewing the hindfoot and forefoot plots in the sagittal plane, both the patient's hindfoot and forefoot are deviated toward the neutral (0) point throughout gait. Compared to the normal foot pattern, he has hindfoot plantarflexion and forefoot dorsiflexion, indicating a fixed flat foot throughout the gait cycle. Hindfoot eversion is seen from initial contact through stance with greater transverse plane internal rotation seen through the entire gait cycle. His forefoot exhibits greater valgus during swing phase, but fairly normal alignment with respect to the hindfoot during stance.

Using foot pressures, dynamic foot deformities are best measured by examining the center of pressure (COP) line. At early stance, he lands on his forefoot and later brings the heel down. In the normal foot, the COP line traces the path of the COP from the heel, at initial contact, to toe off, passing through midpoint of the foot. In this child, the COP during the later part of stance is shifted medially from a normal pattern, which is indicative of valgus.

2.9.2 CASE 2: PLANOVALGUS

A.E. is an 8-yr-old male with diplegic cerebral palsy, who presents with severe bilateral flat foot deformity. He was diagnosed with cerebral palsy at 1 yr of age and did not begin to stand or walk until 4 yr of age. His gait has become increasingly worse and he is now ambulating on the medial aspect of both feet at the midfoot region.

His COP line is shifted medially from a normal pattern, indicative of valgus (Figure 2.9). The foot pressure measurement shows an abnormal foot shape, with increased midfoot loading. The foot and ankle plots demonstrate hindfoot plantarflexion shift and forefoot dorsiflexion in the sagittal plane, which correlates with a flattened longitudinal arch. A.E. exhibits bilateral hindfoot valgus during stance. The forefoot is in valgus during swing phase. His forefoot remains abducted throughout stance and swing.

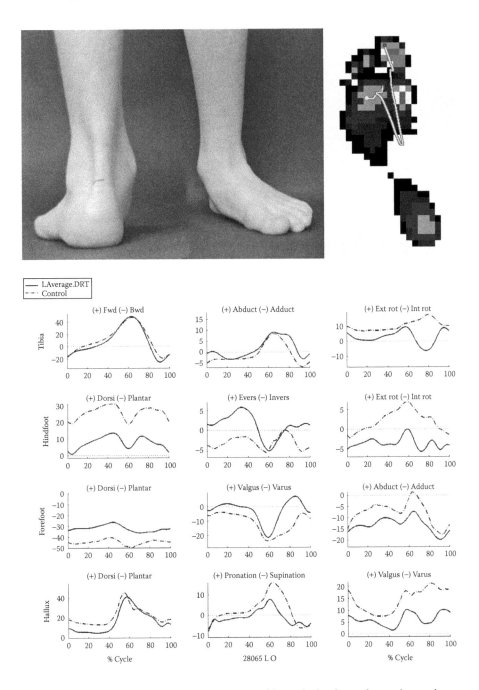

FIGURE 2.8 Case No. 1: A.B. is a 6-yr-old boy with cerebral palsy and a moderate plano-valgus foot deformity of the left foot. Foot pressures and foot and ankle data were acquired for presurgical assessment.

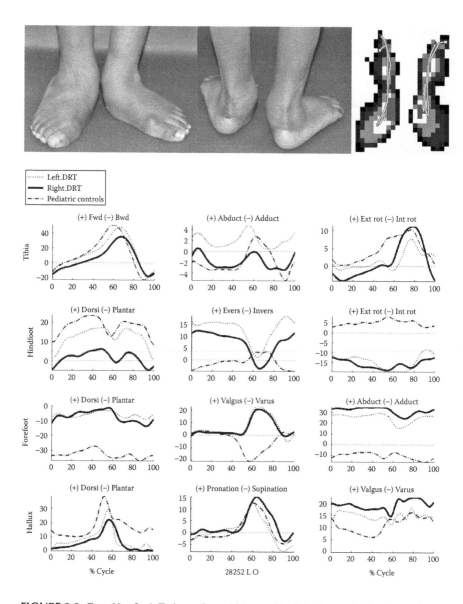

FIGURE 2.9 Case No. 2: A.E. is an 8-yr-old boy with diplegic cerebral palsy and severe bilateral planovalgus foot deformity.

2.10 VARUS FOOT DEFORMITIES

Varus foot deformities are common in young children with cerebral palsy and are associated with equinus (Figure 2.10).[6,36] In toddlers, varus often resolves with observation or bracing. Particularly in diplegia, it can even progress toward the opposite deformity of valgus as children mature. However, in children with hemiplegic cerebral palsy, where one side of the body is more affected, equinovarus

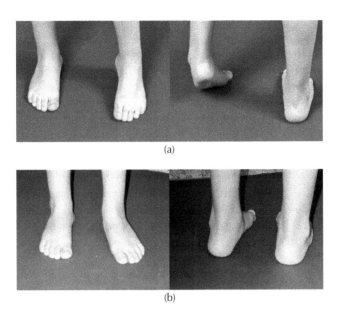

(a)

(b)

FIGURE 2.10 (a) Equinovarus deformity of the left foot in cerebral palsy — preoperative. (b) Correction of equinovarus deformity of the left foot after a split posterior tibial tendon transfer surgery.

commonly persists or worsens. The major cause of the varus hindfoot is overactivity of the posterior tibialis relative to the peroneal evertor muscles. Overactivity of the anterior tibialis must also be evaluated and is commonly present in children with a drop foot or significant varus during the swing phase of gait. The gastrocsoleus, toe flexors, and flexor hallucis are secondary invertors of the foot and can contribute to deformity.[46]

Treatment options for equinovarus vary with the deformity's level of severity and the patient's functional ability and symptoms. Orthotics are commonly prescribed for younger children to provide stability. Injections of BOTOX into the muscle groups such as the posterior tibialis can be helpful for short-term treatment and diagnostic purposes. Despite conservative treatment, with time, a varus deformity may become more severe and symptomatic. Tendon transfer or lengthening surgery can be useful in achieving a plantigrade, brace-free foot in children over 7 yr of age.

Fine wire EMGs can be beneficial for the evaluation and treatment of varus foot deformities, when they are correlated to the phases of the gait cycle. Slow motion video and fine wire EMGs using foot switches to time stance phases have been used to make educated decisions about tendon transfer or lengthening surgery of the varus foot.[47–49] A further refinement can be obtained with foot and ankle motion analysis, which quantifies the motion seen on the video. It is hoped that foot and ankle analysis will improve surgical decision making and evaluation of results. For example, knowledge of the phase and location of gait abnormalities would improve decision making about when to do hindfoot or forefoot tendon transfers or lengthenings. If the varus is most significant during swing phase and the tibialis anterior is active during this period, a split transfer of the tibialis anterior is indicated. If both the tibialis posterior and tibialis anterior are constantly active and the foot postures in equinovarus through all phases of gait, the posterior tibialis can be lengthened and the lateral arm of the anterior tibialis can be transferred to the cuboid. Isolated stance phase varus associated with forefoot abduction or pronation is best treated with a split transfer of the tibialis posterior to the peroneus brevis.[50] If the patient exhibits fixed hindfoot varus, surgical correction by a calcaneal osteotomy may be needed. With experience, an analysis of a patient's foot and ankle data should improve selection of the best surgical options for equinovarus foot deformities.

2.10.1 CASE 3: EQUINOVARUS

L.B. is a 5-yr-old girl with mild left hemiplegic cerebral palsy. L.B. is ambulatory with the aid of a left-sided articulated AFO. She was evaluated for tripping, toe-walking, and intoeing on the left side. She was assessed in the motion analysis laboratory where she exhibited 20° of internal foot progression on the left side. On analysis of slow motion video, the left foot was in varus during stance and in early swing. She recovered foot position to neutral during swing, but she landed with the left foot in slight equinus and varus, with increasing varus during stance phase.

It was felt that her posterior tibialis was the major cause of varus. Based on her clinical examination, x-rays, foot videos, and pressures, L.B. underwent a split posterior tibial tendon transfer. She is now brace free and exhibits a plantigrade foot when she walks without any residual varus, as noted in her foot pressures (Figure 2.11).

2.10.2 CASE 4: CAVOVARUS

K.M. is a 16-yr-old female with bilateral cavovarus feet, with developmental delay, epilepsy, and a diagnosis of diplegic cerebral palsy. She has a progressive cavovarus foot deformity worsening in adolescence. She has had foot pain for the last 3 to 4 yr and has undergone serial casting 2 yr ago, without improvement. She bears weight on the lateral aspect of both her feet. The patient has significant hindfoot varus, which is fixed on her right side (Figure 2.12).

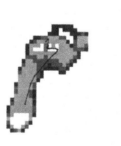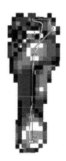

FIGURE 2.11 Case No. 3: L.B. is a 5-yr-old girl with left hemiplegic cerebral palsy and equinovarus foot deformity. Left — preoperative foot pressure. Right — postoperative foot pressure following a left split posterior tibial tendon transfer.

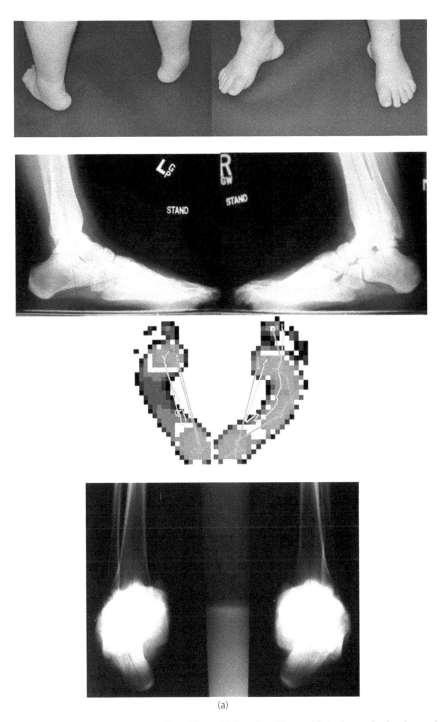

(a)

FIGURE 2.12 Case No. 4: K.M. is a 16-yr-old female with quadriplegic cerebral palsy and bilateral cavovarus feet. These studies were performed for presurgical assessment.

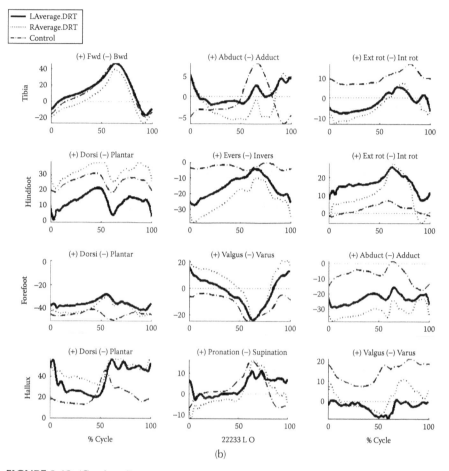

FIGURE 2.12 (Continued).

At the significantly abnormal right foot, her foot and ankle motion analysis shows increased plantar pressure on the lateral part of the foot. The COP line demonstrates a toe-walking pattern, with progression lateral to the central axis of the foot. The left foot shows a more normal loading pattern, and the COP is not abnormally denoted.

Three-dimensional foot and ankle motion analysis shows slightly diminished tibial excursion with increased internal tibial torsion. The hindfoot motion is significantly altered from normal. There is increased hindfoot dorsiflexion, corresponding to an increased calcaneal pitch associated with cavus. In the coronal plane, the hindfoot is in significant varus, which corrects only partially during stance phase. The hindfoot returns to significant varus during swing phase. The forefoot shows increased plantarflexion in relation to the hindfoot (cavus), as well as significant pronation. The analysis demonstrates a significant fixed cavovarus deformity with forefoot pronation. The dynamic motion demonstrates movement occurring through the major joints of the foot, which might predict good long-term function after realignment surgery. Based on these findings, the patient underwent a right split anterior tibial tendon transfer, plantar fascia release, right dorsiflexion first metatarsal osteotomy, and a lateral sliding calcaneal osteotomy. The surgery was designed to address both dynamic and fixed deformities.

2.11 CONGENITAL DEFORMITIES — CLUBFOOT

One of the most common congenital deformities is idiopathic clubfoot, a congenital birth defect characterized by equinus, supination, and inversion of the foot (Figure 2.13). Treatment starts soon after birth and includes serial casting and, rarely, surgery. Although clubfoot is detected and often treated during the first few months of life, there is residual weakness, loss of motion, and deformity, which may cause impairment later in life. Children are followed through their growing years and frequently require secondary procedures. Long-term follow-up is crucial for evaluating different treatments such as surgery vs. casting.[51] In clubfoot, an analysis of both motion and pressure will be useful to evaluate treatment results and predict potential problems in adulthood.[52]

2.11.1 CASE 5: RESIDUAL CLUBFOOT

D.R. is a 17-yr-old female with bilateral clubfoot; she had comprehensive soft tissue release as an infant. She has had several reoperations for recurrent deformity and presented for correction of residual deformity (Figure 2.14). The clinical photographs and videograph demonstrate a plantigrade foot with hindfoot valgus and a dorsal bunion. The foot pressures indicate increased hindfoot pressure with little loading of the metatarsal heads. The COP line passes through the central portion of the foot. This patient shows limited stance phase foot motion in the coronal plane. However, there is significant dynamic forefoot supination in the coronal plane during push-off, and hindfoot plantarflexion is also significant during push-off. This shows that the patient has excessive forefoot motion compensation for limited subtalar motion. Observation of foot pressures shows abnormally high hindfoot loading consistent with weak plantar flexors. Intervention was limited to correction of the first metatarsophalangeal joint.

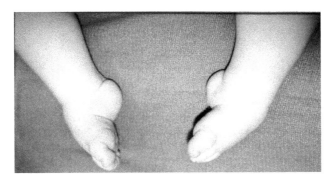

FIGURE 2.13 Congenital clubfoot, uncorrected, in an infant.

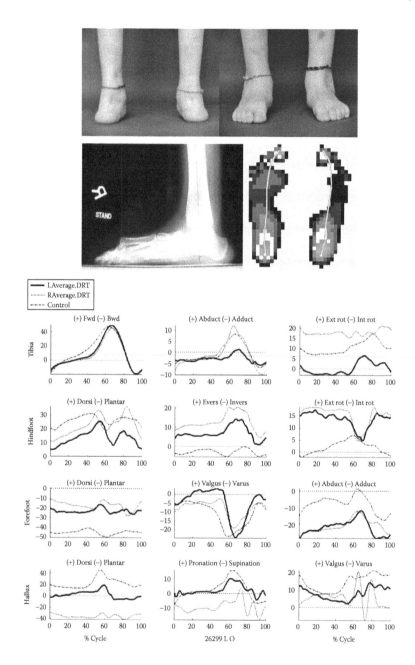

FIGURE 2.14 Case No 5: D.R. is a 17-yr-old female with a history of bilateral clubfeet, who had multiple surgeries as an infant. Foot and ankle data along with foot pressures were used to evaluate her long-term follow-up, and prior to surgery, to correct residual deformities of hindfoot valgus and dorsal bunion.

2.12 OTHER NEUROMUSCULAR DISORDERS

Neuropathic and paralytic disorders such as polio, myelomeningocele, spinal cord injury, Charcot–Marie–Tooth Syndrome, or other neuropathies frequently result in complex foot deformities. All share a common muscle imbalance at the foot, which causes dynamic and, later, static deformity. Children with myelomenigocele typically exhibit increased stance phase knee flexion and increased ankle dorsiflexion associated with gastrocnemius weakness.[53] Orthotics are commonly prescribed. Charcot–Marie–Tooth disease is an inherited condition involving peripheral motor neurons, resulting in progressive muscular weakness of the feet and legs.[16] Patients exhibit foot drop, pes cavus, intrinsic muscle weakness, hammer toes, muscle atrophy of the legs, and peroneal weakness. This condition requires careful evaluation and improves with tendon transfers, stabilizing osteotomies, or fusions. Applications of foot and ankle analysis will improve understanding for surgical decision making and evaluation of results.

2.13 SEVERE FLATFOOT DEFORMITY

Pes valgus, or flatfoot, is a common deformity of the foot and ankle. Flatfeet can be due to genetics, obesity, ligamentous laxity, trauma, or musculoskeletal disorders. Flatfoot deformities maybe flexible or rigid. Flexible flatfeet is a heritable condition in children and adults, occurring in 7 to 22% of the population. The condition is rarely symptomatic but may cause pain with prolonged walking. Symptomatic flexible flatfeet are often associated with tight heel cords. Conservative treatment is usually warranted. Shoe modification, orthotics, and/or therapy are common interventions. Rarely, children present with a severe deformity that requires surgery.

2.13.1 CASE 6: SEVERE FLATFOOT DEFORMITY

A.K. is a 9-yr-old male. He is an independent ambulator with a heel-to-toe reciprocal gait pattern and flatfoot deformity. When standing foot flat, the patient exhibits hindfoot valgus, which partially corrects while doing a toe stand, and the arch also notably reconstitutes. The patient can dorsiflex with knees extended to 20° and plantarflex to 50°. He has a supple forefoot and subtalar joints while the forefoot is easily deformed into a valgus position. This patient has generalized ligamentous laxity. Parents noted that his gait appears to be getting worse as he gets larger. A.K. underwent a gait analysis and foot pressure study showing increased medial forefoot and midfoot weight bearing. The line of progression proceeds medially along the foot during stance. This boy had a particularly severe deformity that was progressive and was felt to benefit from surgery. He underwent a bilateral column lengthening to correct the deformity. In the procedure, a bone graft from the pelvis was inserted into the calcaneous neck to adduct the midfoot and improve calcaneal alignment. During his 1-yr follow-up exam, his foot pressures improved to a more normalized pattern. The heel remains in valgus, but motion of the hindfoot is retained (Figure 2.15).

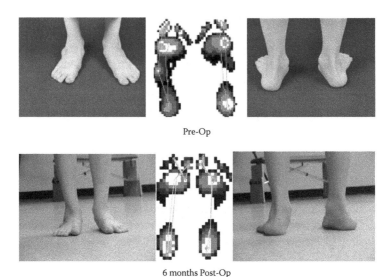

Pre-Op

6 months Post-Op

FIGURE 2.15 Case No. 6: A.K. is a 9-yr-old male with severe flatfoot deformity, idiopathic in nature. He underwent bilateral column lengthening to correct the deformity.

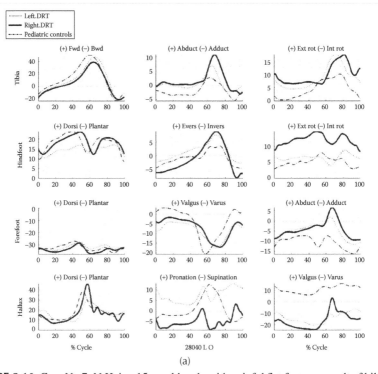

FIGURE 2.16 Case No.7: N.H. is a 15-yr-old male with painful flat feet as a result of bilateral middle talocalcaneal tarsal coalition. The course of treatment for this patient is bilateral talocalcaneal coalition resection.

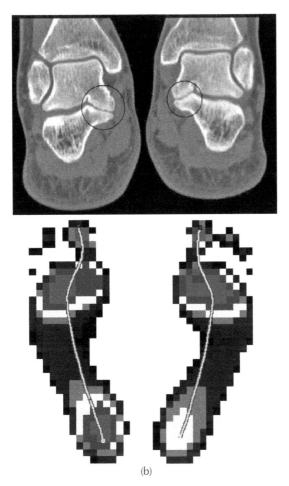

(b)

FIGURE 2.16 (Continued).

2.14 TARSAL COALITION

Tarsal coalition is the union of two or more tarsal bones, caused by fibrous, cartilaginous, or osseous union. The etiology is unknown. Tarsal coalition restricts the
motion of the subtalar joint and when symptomatic, results in a painful flatfoot.

2.14.1 CASE 7: TARSAL COALITION

This is a 15-yr-old male who presented with foot pain interfering with his work,
which involves walking all day (Figure 2.16). He has flat feet, with marked restriction
of subtalar motion. He has pain with attempted passive inversion of his subtalar
joints bilaterally. He has dorsiflexion and plantarflexion of his ankles with no limitation, but he does not reconstitute the medial longitudinal arch when he rises up
on his toes. X-ray findings demonstrate talar breaking as well as poorly defined

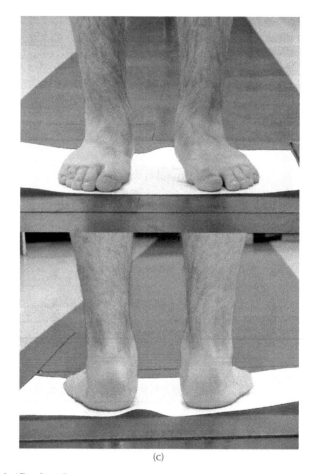

(c)

FIGURE 2.16 (Continued).

middle facet, with blunting of the lateral process of the talus. Computed tomography (CT) scan was performed at an outside institution, which demonstrated middle facet talocalcaneal coalition bilaterally. Three-dimensional foot and ankle motion analysis data show normal tibial motion patterns. In addition, the hindfoot sagittal plane shows all three normal rockers. However, there is no normal ankle inversion motion during stance phase push-off on the hindfoot coronal plane. Rather, the hindfoot gradually everts throughout stance and does not recover until swing phase. The course of treatment for this patient is a bilateral talocalcaneal coalition resection.

2.15 CONCLUSION

Recent technology in pediatric foot and ankle motion analysis and foot pressure assessment will help refine our understanding of gait events at the foot. Pathology of the foot can be better defined and treated using these systems. For example, stance phase stability problems will be quantified with motion, forces, and pressure measurements. Swing phase problems will be characterized with motion analysis. For children with foot disorders, gait analysis and foot pressures have become important tools in pretreatment assessment, surgical decision making, and postoperative follow-up. Clinicians look forward to improved care with advances in technology to measure foot and ankle motion.

REFERENCES

1. Inman, V.T., Ralston, H.J., Todd, F., *Human Walking*, Williams and Wilkins: Baltimore, 1981.
2. Inman, V.T., *Joints of the Ankle*, 2nd ed., Williams and Wilkins: Baltimore, 1991.
3. Marey, M., De la locomotion terrestre, chez les bibier et les quadrupedes, *J l'Anatomie Physiol*, 9, 42, 1973.
4. Perry, J., *Gait Analysis: Normal and Pathological Function*, Slack: Thorofare, NJ, 413–441, 1992.
5. Sutherland, D.H., Olshen, R.A., Biden, E.N., Wyatt, M.P., *The Development of Mature Walking*, Mac Keith Press: London, 1988.
6. Gage, J.R., *The Treatment of Gait Problems in Cerebral Palsy*, Mac Keith Press: London, 2004.
7. Johnson, J., Harris, G., Pathomechanics of posterior tibial tendon insufficiency, *J Biomech*, 2(2), 227–239, 1997.
8. Myers, K., Wang, M., Marks, R., Harris, G., Validation of a multisegment foot and ankle kinematic model for pediatric gait, *IEEE Trans Neural Syst Rehabil Eng*, 12(1), 122–130, 2004.
9. Smith, P., Humm, J., Hassani, S., Harris G.F., Three dimensional motion analysis of the pediatric ankle, In: *Pediatric Gait*, IEEE Press: Piscataway, NJ, 2000, 183–188.
10. Lyon, R., Liu, X., Schwab, J., Harris, G., Kinematic and kinetic evaluation of the ankle joint before and after tendo achilles lengthening in patients with spastic diplegia, *J Pediatr Orthop*, 25(4), 479–483, 2005.
11. Winters, D.A., *The Biomechanics and Motor Control of Human Gait: Normal, Elderly, and Pathological*, 2nd ed., University of Waterloo Press: Waterloo, Ontario, 1991.
12. Close, J.R., Inman, V.T., Poor, P.M., Todd, F.N., The function of the subtalar joint, *Clin Orthop Relat Res*, 50, 159–179, 1967.
13. Wong, Y., Kim, W., Ying, N., Passive motion characteristics of the talocrural and the subtalar joint by dual Eular angles, *J Pediatric Orthop*, 38(12), 2480–2485, 2005.
14. Chen, J., Siegler, S., Schneck, C.D., The three dimensional kinematics and flexibility characteristics of the human ankle and subtalar joint—Part II: Flexibility characteristics, *J Biomech Eng*, 110(4), 374–385, 1988.
15. Gellman, H., Lenihan, M., Halikis, N., Botte, M.J., Giordani, M., Perry, J., Selective tarsal arthrodesis: an in vitro analysis of the effect on foot motion, *Foot Ankle*, 8(3), 127–133, 1987.
16. Mann, R.A., Coughlin, M.J., *Surgery of the Foot and Ankle*, Vol. 1, Mosby: St. Louis, MO, 1992.
17. Mann, R.A., Coughlin, M.J., *Surgery of the Foot and Ankle*, Vol. 2, Mosby: St. Louis, MO, 1992.
18. Ouzounanian, T.J., Shereff, M.J., In vitro determination of midfoot motion, *Foot Ankle*, 10(3), 140–146, 1989.

19. Scott, S.H., Winter, D.A., Talocrural and talocalcaneal joint kinematics and kinetics during the stance phase of walking, *J Biomech*, 24(8), 743–752, 1991.
20. Siegler, S., Chen, J., Schneck. C.D., The three-dimensional kinematics and flexibility characteristics of the human ankle and subtalar joints—Part 1: Kinematics, *J Biomech Eng*, 110(4), 364–373, 1988.
21. Morris, J.M., Biomechanics of the foot and Ankle, *Clin Orthop*, 122, 10–17, 1977.
22. Carson, M., Harrington, M., Thompson, Theologis, T., A four segment in vivo foot model for clinical gait analysis, *Gait Posture*, 8, 73, 1998.
23. Cornell, M.W., McPoil, T.G., Three-dimensional movement of the foot during the stance phase of walking, *J Am Podiatr Med Assoc*, 89(2), 56-66, 1999.
24. Henley, J., Wesdock, Masiello, G., Nogi, J., A new three-segment foot model for gait analysis in children and adults, in Gait and Clinical Movement Analysis Society. Abstract, 6th Annual Meeting, Sacramento, CA, 2001.
25. Kidder, S.M., Abuzzahab, F.S. Jr., Harris, G.F., Johnson, JE., A system for the analysis of foot and ankle kinematics during gait, *IEEE Trans Rehabil Eng*, 4(1), 25–32, 1996.
26. Ortloff, S., Harris, G.F., Wyanarsky, G., Smith, J., Shereff, M., Noninvasive biomechanical analysis of joint motion, *Proc IEEE Eng Med Bio Soc*, 1991, 1962–1963.
27. Udupa, J.K., Hirsch, B.E., Hillstrom, Bauer, G.R., Kneeland, J.B., Analysis of in vivo 3-D internal kinematics of the joints of the foot, *IEEE Trans Biomed Eng*, 45, 1387–1396, 1998.
28. Theologis, T., Harrington, M., Thompson, N., Benson, M., Dynamic foot movement in children treated for congenital talipes equinovarus, *J Bone Joint Surg Br*, 85(4), 572–577, 2003.
29. Johnson, J., Lamdan, R., Granberry, W., Harris, G., Hindfoot coronal alignment: a modified radiographic method, *Foot Ankle Int*, 20(12), 818–825, 1999.
30. Lundberg, A., Kinematics of the ankle and foot: in vivo roentgen stereophotogrammetry, *Acta Orthop Scand Suppl*, 233, 1–24, 1989.
31. Mann, J.T., DuVries' *Surgery of the Foot, Biomechanics of the Foot and Ankle*, Mosby: St. Louis, MD, 1978.
32. Sammarco, G.L., Burstein, A.H., Frankel, V.H., Biomechanics of the ankle: a kinematics study, *Orthop Clin North Am*, 4, 75–96, 1973.
33. Serrafian, S.K., *Anatomy of the Foot and Ankle*, Lippincot: Philadelphia, 1993, 1983.
34. Dontaelli, R., Wolf, S.L., *The Biomechanics of the Foot and Ankle*, Davis: Philadelphia, 1990.
35. Lyon, R., Liu, X., Schwab, J., Harris, G., Kinematic and kinetic evaluation of the ankle joint before and after tendo achilles lengthening in patients with spastic diplegia, *J Pediatr Orthop*, 25(4), 479–483, 2005.
36. Miller, F., *Cerebral Palsy*, Springer Science and Business Media: New York, 2005.
37. Bleck, E.E., *Orthopaedic Management in Cerebral Palsy*, Mac Keith Press: Oxford, 1987.
38. Olson, C.L., Kuo, K.N., Smith, P.A., Long-term results of triple arthrodesis: clinical, radiographic, gait and power analysis, *Orthop Transac*, 17(2), 414, 1994.
39. Smith, P.A., Millar, E.A., Sullivan, R.C., Sta-peg arthrodesis for treatment of the planovalgus feet in cerebral palsy, In: *Clinics in Podiatric Medicine and Surgery: Advances in the Treatment of Pediatric Flatfoot*, IEEE Press: Piscataway, NJ, 17(3), 459–469, 2000.
40. Liu, X., Thometz, J., Tassone, C., Dynamic plantar pressure measurement for the normal subject. Free-mapping model for the analysis of pediatric foot deformities, *J Pediatr Orthop*, 25(1), 103–106, 2005.

41. Noritake, K., Yoshihashi, Y., Miyata, T., Calcaneal lengthening for planovalgus foot deformity in children with spastic cerebral palsy, *J Pediatr Orthop B*, 14(4), 274–279, 2005.

42. Smith, P.A., Harris, G.F., Abu-Faraj, Z., *Human Motion Analysis*, 1st ed., IEEE Press: Piscataway, NJ, 370–386, 1996.

43. Abu-Faraj, Z., Harris, G.F., Abler, J.H., Wertsch, J.J., Smith, P.A., A holter-type microprocessor-based rehabilitation instrument for acquisition and storage of plantar pressure data in children with cerebral palsy, *IEEE Trans Rehabil Eng*, 4(1), 33–38, 1996.

44. Davitt, J., MacWilliams, B., Armstrong, P., Plantar pressure and radiographic changes after distal calcaneal lengthening in children and adolescents. *J Pediatr Orthop*, 21, 70–75, 2001.

45. Abu-Faraj, Z., Harris, G., Smith, P.A., Surgical rehabilitation of the planovalgus foot in cerebral palsy, *IEEE Trans Neural Syst Rehabil Eng*, 9(2), 202–214, 2001.

46. Sutherland, D.H., Varus foot in cerebral palsy: an overview, *Instr Course Lect*, 539, 1993.

47. Chang, C.H., Miller, F., Schuyler, J., Dynamic pedobarograph in evaluation of varus and valgus foot deformities, *J Pediatr Orthop*, 22(6), 813–818, 2002.

48. Chang, C.H., Albarracin, J.P., Lipton, G.E., Miller, F., Long-term follow-up of surgery for equinovarus foot deformity in children with cerebral palsy, *J Pediatr Orthop*, 22(6), 792–799, 2002.

49. Hoffer, M.M., Reiswig, J.A., Garret, A.M., Perry, J., The split anterior tibial tendon transfer in the treatment of spastic varus hindfoot of childhood, *Orthop Clin North Am*, 5, 31–38, 1974.

50. Kling, T.F., Kaufer, H., Hensinger, R.N., Split posterior tibial tendon transfers in children with cerebral spastic paralysis and equinovarus deformity, *J Bone Joint Surg Am*, 67, 186–194, 1985.

51. Ippolito, E., Manacini, F., Di Mario, M., Farsetti, P., A comparison of resultant subtalar joint pathology with functional results in two groups of clubfoot patients treated with two different protocols, *J Pediatr Orthop B*, 14(5), 358–361, 2005.

52. Roche, C., Mattingly, B., Tylkowski, C., Stevens, D.B., Hardy, P.A., Pienkowski, D., Three-dimensional hindfoot motion in adolescents with surgically treated unilateral clubfoot, *J Pediatr Orthop*, 25(5), 630–634, 2005.

53. Abel, M.F., Damiano, D.L., Dias, L., Blanco, J.S., Conaway, M., Miller, F., Dabney, K., Sutherland, D., Chambers, H., Sarwark, J., Killian, J., Doyle, S., Root, L., LaPlaza, J., Widmann, R., Snyder, B., Relationships among musculoskeletal impairments and functional health status in ambulatory cerebral palsy, *J Pediatr Orthop*, 23(4), 535–541, 2003.

3 Functional Gait Analysis in Children Following Clubfoot Releases

Michael Khazzam, J.Y. Roh, Jason T. Long, Peter A. Smith, Sahar Hassani, Gerald F. Harris, Adam N. Graf, and Ken N. Kuo

CONTENTS

3.1 INTRODUCTION

Idiopathic congenital talipes equinovarus (clubfoot) is a common, congenital deformity treated by the pediatric orthopaedic surgeons. Clubfoot is a complex, congenital, contractural malalignment of the bones and joints of the foot and ankle.[19] The goal in the correction of congenital clubfoot is to obtain a painless, straight, plantigrade, mobile foot with reestablishment of anatomic bony relationships, normal radiographic appearance, and which allows the development of a normal gait pattern.[1–6] Following treatment, patients are often reevaluated for potential problems such as overcorrection, residual, and/or recurrent foot deformity which may require further treatment intervention. In attempts to quantify foot function, several authors have used gait analysis[7–17] for an objective assessment in addition to clinical, functional, and radiographic evaluations.

This chapter reviews the pathology and treatment of congenital clubfoot deformity. In addition, results from detailed gait analysis of patients evaluated at long-term follow-ups of corrective clubfoot surgery will be described utilizing both standard gait analysis modeling techniques as well as the most recent advances in motion analysis of the foot and ankle (the multisegmental foot model).

3.2 CONGENITAL CLUBFOOT PATHOANATOMY

Idiopathic congenital clubfoot (Figure 3.1) is characterized by four basic deformities: (1) cavus (plantar flexion of the forefoot or the hindfoot), (2) adductus (forefoot or the midfoot), (3) varus (subtalar joint complex), and (4) equinus (hindfoot). These deformities are not always passively correctable. The primary bony anatomy of the foot involved in this deformity consists of the talus, calcaneus, cuboid, and navicular and their corresponding articulations. The talar neck is medially rotated, shortened, and plantar flexed. Over time, growth of the anterior aspect of the talus is stunted and medial neck deviation continues to grow resulting in a progressive deformity. The calcaneus is shortened and widened, with medial bowing. Malposition of the calcaneus in adduction and inversion under the talus results in hindfoot deformity. The navicular is medially displaced, often abutting the medial malleolus, resulting in forefoot deformity and adduction of the midfoot. The cuboid is medially displaced and inverted on the calcaneus. Cavus (or high arch) deformity develops as a result of forefoot pronation relative to the hindfoot with the entire foot supinated. Varus and adduction deformity of the hindfoot and midfoot result in supination of the forefoot. Additionally, many of the posteromedial structures

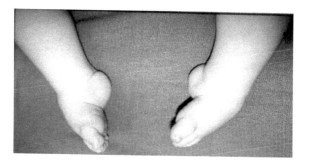

FIGURE 3.1 A congenital deformity of the foot seen in 1 per 1000 births. Cause is unknown.

of the foot and ankle are shortened or contracted including the posterior ankle capsule, gastrocnemius-soleus complex (Achilles tendon), posterior tibialis muscle, long toe flexors, and posterior and medial ligaments of the ankle and tarsal joints.[2,5,18]

3.3 ETIOLOGY

The incidence of clubfoot varies widely with respect to gender, race, and geography. All populations demonstrate a 2.5:1 male-to-female ratio[2,4,19,20] with bilateral disease occurring in approximately 50% of cases.[2,19] There is up to a 30-fold increased risk of clubfoot deformity if the individual has an affected sibling.[4] In untreated clubfoot, at skeletal maturity, the patient often walks on the dorsolateral aspect of the affected foot with limited motion of the subtalar and midtarsal joints.

Although there have been several speculations,[2,4,19] the cause of congenital clubfoot is unknown. Possible causes include intrauterine compression, environmental factors, genetic factors, neurotrophic factors, denervation, abnormal muscle development, vascular anomalies (hypoplasia or absent anterior tibial artery), early amniocentesis, chromosomal abnormalities, or viral infection.

3.4 CLINICAL ASSESSMENT

Physical examination and clinical criteria are the primary diagnostic tools used in the assessment of clubfoot. Patients found to have evidence of congenital clubfoot should have a complete physical examination since there is a higher incidence of associated disorders. Examinations should include detailed neurologic and spine examinations, degree of fixed deformity, joint range of motion, active muscle function, leg length evaluation, thigh and calf circumference, and skin creases. Absence of heel skin crease often exists in severe deformity of the clubfoot.

3.5 RADIOGRAPHIC EXAMINATION

Anteroposterior and lateral views of the foot, which simulate weight bearing, are the standard for preoperative evaluation of clubfoot (Figure 3.2). Measurement of the talocalcaneal angle, tibiotalar angle, calcaneometatarsal V angle, talometatarsal angle, angle of calcaneal dorsiflexion, and talocalcaneal index (summation of the anterior-posterior (AP) and lateral talocalcaneal angles) are all commonly used, but with little data as their prognostic value. Additionally, postoperative radiographic measurements have been reported to have an inconsistent relationship to functional outcome.[21] Overall, radiographic examination of this population has several inconsistencies because of difficulty in correctly positioning the foot. Immature ossific nuclei do not represent the true shape of the tarsal bones; the talus, calcaneus, and metatarsals may be the only ossified bones in the first year of life. Failure to hold the ankle and foot in proper position while taking an x-ray makes flat top talus appear worse radiographically.[2,4,19]

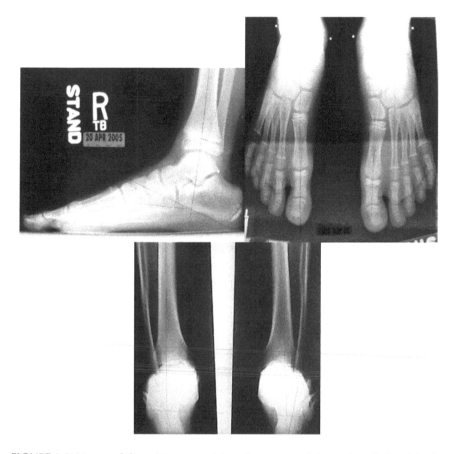

FIGURE 3.2 X-rays of foot. Intersegmental angles measured to create offset matrix for alignment of foot model to bony anatomy. Lateral view and modified coronal plane view to measure tibiacalcaneus angle. Foot positioned perpendicular to plane of x-ray for near orthogonal measurement. (From Johnson JE, Lamdan R, Granberry WF, Harris GF, Carrera GF. *Foot Ankle Int,* 1999; 20(12):818–825. With permission.)

3.6   TREATMENT OPTIONS

The treatment of congenital clubfoot consists of conservative (nonoperative) and operative strategies with the goal being a functional, pain-free, straight, plantigrade foot with good mobility and normal radiographic appearance. It is a common agreement among the pediatric orthopedic community that initial management should be nonsurgical starting during early infancy.[2,4,5,19,21]

3.6.1   NONOPERATIVE TREATMENT

Conservative treatment modalities include serial manipulation and casting, taping, and strapping (Figure 3.3), and functional treatment ("French technique," physical therapy, continuous passive motion, and splinting).[2,4,5,19,21] Manipulation and casting

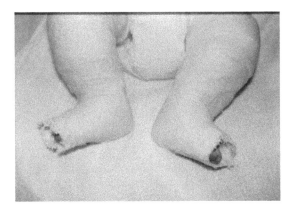

FIGURE 3.3 Casting and bracing are nonsurgical treatment options.

as described by Ponseti et al.[1,2,4,19,21–23] has been the most frequently used technique in the U.S. as the gold standard.

The Ponseti approach of serial gentle manipulation starts with correction of cavus deformity by elevating the first metatarsal or supinating the forefoot relative to the hindfoot. Next, the forefoot is abducted and the hindfoot is everted with the foot in equinus (to allow the calcaneus to freely abduct under the talus and evert into a neutral position) through the subtalar complex. Finally, the equinus deformity is corrected by progressively dorsiflexing the foot, often aided by percutaneous Achilles tenotomy. A toe to groin cast is applied after each manipulation. Attempts to correct equinus before hindfoot varus deformity is corrected result in inappropriate dorsiflexion through the midfoot (rocker bottom deformity).[1,2,4,19,21–23] After the foot is corrected, a brace is applied to keep the foot in an abducted and externally rotated position beyond the walking age.

3.6.2 SURGICAL TREATMENT

Surgical correction may be required for those feet which have failed to respond to conservative manipulative correction, or where one cannot hold the corrected position due to noncompliance of brace wearing. Surgical soft-tissue release must address all of the pathoanatomic structures affected to optimize successful correction (Figure 3.4). There are four regions that may require soft-tissue release: (1) posterior release that includes Achilles tendon lengthening, posterior tibiotalar joint capsulotomy, posterior subtalar joint capsulotomy, posterior talo-fibular and calcaneo-fibular ligaments release, and posterior deltoid ligament release; (2) lateral calcaneocuboid (realigns cuboid with long axis of calcaneus, straightening the lateral border of the foot); (3) plantar fascia (corrects forefoot cavus and realigns the first metatarsal with the talus; and (4) medial release may include posterior tibial tendon lengthening, talonavicular, subtalar and calcaneocuboid capsulotomy, superficial deltoid, spring ligaments, and the knot of Henry (realigns navicular on the talus, moves it away from the medial malleolus, and provides midfoot mobility).[2]

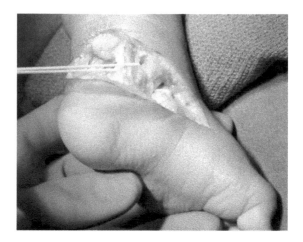

FIGURE 3.4 Surgical treatment: comprehensive clubfoot release performed through a Cincinnati incision.

Posteromedial release as described by Turco et al.[1,2,4,19,21,24] is the first described one-stage clubfoot release. The procedure was further revised and modified by subsequent authors including McKay, Simmons, and Carroll. Bensahel proposed an a la carte procedure instead of universal complete release. Comprehensive clubfoot release often results in a plantigrade foot, which will fit well in a regular shoe. However, a common problem of the surgically released foot is stiffness of the foot at long-term follow-up.

3.7 GAIT ANALYSIS FOR ASSESSMENT OF OUTCOME FOLLOWING CLUBFOOT CORRECTION

3.7.1 PREVIOUS INVESTIGATIONS

There have been several studies[7-17] which have examined the gait of children following treatment for clubfoot deformity. Early studies[8-17] examined gait using a simple model of the ankle–joint complex, which provides only a single axis of kinematic information for the motion of the foot and ankle. The ankle–joint complex method of gait analysis treats the foot and ankle as a rigid structure with the majority of information obtained relative to sagittal plane motion (dorsiflexion/plantarflexion). While this traditional method of lower body gait analysis provides useful information related to the motion of the hips, knees, and ankles, it is unable to provide kinematic insight as to what is occurring at the other joints of the foot during ambulation. As a result, critical information about the hindfoot, forefoot, and hallux are missed since clubfoot affects all of these foot and ankle segments.

More recently, with the development of advanced multisegmental foot modeling, a more accurate assessment of foot and ankle motion during ambulation has been explored. Theologis et al.[7] examined the gait of 20 children following treatment for correction of clubfoot deformity using a three-segment foot model (tibia, hindfoot, and forefoot) in addition to traditional lower body gait analysis.

The authors reported that even though this patient population had good clinical results at follow-up, gait analysis showed residual in-toeing, foot drop, increased midfoot dorsiflexion, and external hip rotation.

3.7.2 CURRENT INVESTIGATION

We performed a retrospective study consisting of 17 patients who all had undergone posteromedial surgical soft-tissue release to correct congenital clubfoot deformity. There were 15 males and 2 females. All patients were evaluated and treated by one surgeon between July 1985 and June 1987 and were available for clinical evaluation and gait analysis at the time of this study. Standard lower extremity gait analysis techniques using the Hayes et al. marker set were employed for collection of kinematic and kinetic data. Additionally, multisegmental foot and ankle temporal–spatial and kinematic data were collected using the Milwaukee Foot Model.[25–28]

3.8 RESULTS OF LOWER BODY GAIT ANALYSIS

3.8.1 TEMPORAL PARAMETERS

Comparison of temporal–spatial parameters between postoperative clubfoot subjects and a database of normal adults demonstrated several significant differences (Table 3.1). Stride length was shortened from 1.28 to 1.19 m ($p < .01$), cadence was reduced from 104.41 to 100.97 steps/min ($p < .0001$), and walking speed was reduced from 1.12 to 1.0 m/sec ($p < .0001$). Walking speed was found to be 89.29% of the normal walking speed. Stance duration of the clubfoot group was prolonged from 61.78% to 63.63% ($p < .05$).

3.8.1.1 Kinematic Results

Several kinematic variables at the ankle, knee, and hip were found to be significantly different in the clubfoot population compared to normal.

3.8.1.1.1 Ankle (Figure 3.5)

Sagittal motion at the ankle of the clubfoot group was significantly decreased ($p < .001$) compared to normal. Specifically, the ankle demonstrated decreased

TABLE 3.1
Temporal–Spatial Parameters

	Temporal–Spatial Data		
	Clubfoot	**Normal**	***p*-Value**
% Stance	63.63 ± 2.39	61.78 ± 2.86	0.04
% Swing	36.37 ± 2.39	38.22 ± 2.86	0.04
Stride length	1.19 ± 0.1	1.28 ± 0.11	0.005
Cadence	100.97 ± 7.92	104.41 ± 7.38	<0.0001
Walking speed	1 ± 0.14	1.12 ± 0.1	<0.0001

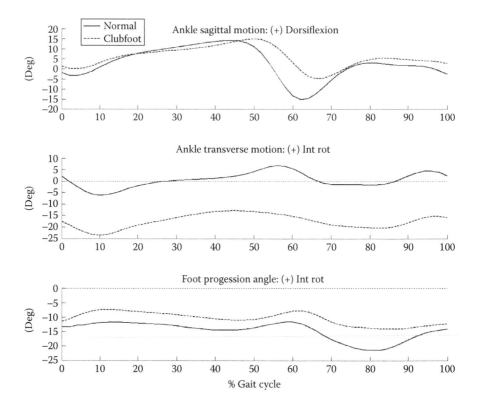

FIGURE 3.5 Ankle kinematics and foot progression angle.

overall range of motion and decreased plantar flexion throughout the gait cycle. Although the first and second ankle rockers appeared to be unaffected by these changes in sagittal ankle motion, the third rocker did appear to be delayed. Transverse ankle motion of the clubfoot group also demonstrated significant kinematic alterations ($p <$ .001) compared to normal. The ankle was more externally rotated and underwent less internal rotation throughout the gait cycle. Although the average foot progression angle of the clubfoot group trended toward more internal rotation, this was found not to be significantly different than normal.

3.8.1.1.2 Knee (Figure 3.6)

Most of the kinematic data about the knee in the clubfoot group were within normal limits. Noteworthy was that the knee of the clubfoot group demonstrated significantly less valgus than normal ($p <$ .001).

3.8.1.1.3 Hip (Figure 3.7)

Hip sagittal motion in the clubfoot group demonstrated significant reductions in both range of motion ($p =$ .008) and flexion ($p =$ .0015) throughout the gait cycle.

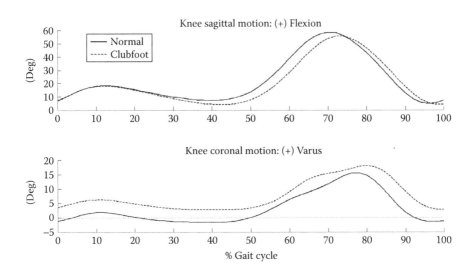

FIGURE 3.6 Knee kinematics.

3.8.1.1.4 Kinetics (Figure3.8)

Ankle plantar flexion moment demand was not significantly different ($p > .05$) than normal. Both average range and maximum ankle internal rotation moment demand were significantly larger ($p < .001$) than normal. Average maximum ankle power generated by the clubfoot group was significantly decreased ($p = 0.0011$) as compared to normal.

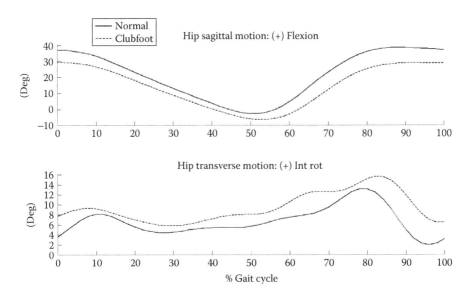

FIGURE 3.7 Hip kinematics.

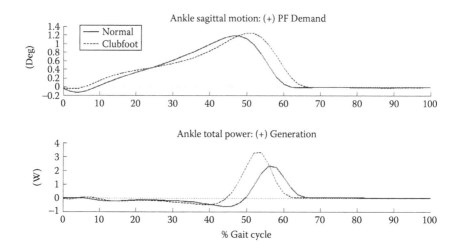

FIGURE 3.8 Ankle kinetics.

3.8.1.2 Case Example

M.F. is a 17-yr-old male with a prior history of surgical correction of right clubfoot deformity. This patient was diagnosed at birth as having a right clubfoot. Treatment began at 2 wk of age with stretching and the application of a cast. This continued serially for about 2 to 3 months, at which time casting treatment was discontinued for financial reasons. Although the foot did show some response to conservative treatment, the child developed recurrent clubfoot deformity within a few months. The patient was seen again at 8 months of age and assessed for surgical clubfoot correction. The patient's father also had a history of right clubfoot deformity, which required three surgical procedures for correction. Physical examination at this time revealed normal range of motion and motor strength of the hips and knees bilaterally. The patient was not yet ambulatory and stood on the lateral border of the right foot. The right foot was held in the equinovarus position, and could only be dorsiflexed up to 15° shy of neutral. The ankle was very tight and in a fixed varus position with the forefoot fixed in adduction. Additionally, no peroneal function could be elicited. The left foot demonstrated normal motor strength and range of motion. The left foot was in normal alignment. On radiograph, the left foot was normal. The right foot exhibited typical clubfoot findings, with marked parallelism between the talus and calcaneus, on both the AP and lateral views, which were not corrected in the forced views. The patient was placed back in a stretching cast until the time of surgery. This long leg cast was placed with the hindfoot in equinus. The cast was changed roughly 1 wk following placement. At 9 months of age, the patient underwent right posteromedial soft-tissue release for correction of the clubfoot deformity and was placed in a long leg cast. At approximately 3 wk following surgery the cast was changed. At this time it was noted that the foot was well corrected and was able to externally rotate 15° and dorsiflex up to 10° past neutral. The patient was placed back in a long leg cast for an additional 4 wk. Six weeks following surgery the cast was removed and the patient was placed in a Moore clubfoot brace for 6 months. At this point, the foot was able obtain 30° of dorsiflexion above neutral with knees extended and had active peroneal function. Following 6 months of bracing the patient was able to actively dorsiflex the foot 15° and plantarflex 15°. The heel was in neutral position, foot supple, and forefoot straight. At this time, the patient walked with a normal heel toe gait and had no limping or tripping.

Approximately 16 yr following surgery, the patient underwent postoperative gait analysis. At this time, the patient had no complaints related to his right foot. The hindfoot demonstrated a small amount of valgus, and the midfoot and forefoot were well aligned. The patient was able to actively dorsiflex past neutral with knees extended. He demonstrated 5/5 motor strength plantar flexion and dorsiflexion, was able to walk on his toes, and had 4/5 eversion strength.

3.8.2 TEMPORAL–SPATIAL RESULTS

The average walking speed for this patient was 1.18 m/sec, the average cadence was 109.28 steps/min, the average stride length was 1.29 m, and the average stance duration of clubfoot was 65.55% of the gait cycle.

3.8.2.1 Kinematic Results (Figure 3.9)

3.8.2.1.1 Tibia

The tibia in this patient was in a position of increased dorsiflexion during load response, which then decreased from midstance through the initial swing phase as compared to normal. The tibia also demonstrated a decreased range of motion in the coronal (abduction/adduction) and transverse (external/internal rotation) planes throughout the gait cycle as compared to normal.

3.8.2.1.2 Hindfoot

The hindfoot of this patient demonstrated decreased dorsiflexion from load response through preswing. Of note was the preservation of the first and third rockers, with alterations observed in the second rocker. Range of motion of the hindfoot was decreased throughout the gait cycle in the transverse plane (external/internal rotation) and the hindfoot was also internally rotated throughout the gait cycle.

3.8.2.1.3 Forefoot

Range of motion of the forefoot was decreased throughout the gait cycle in the sagittal (dorsiflexion/plantarflexion), coronal (valgus/varus), and transverse (abduction/adduction) planes. Additionally, the forefoot maintained a less plantarflexed and abducted position for the majority of the gait cycle.

3.8.2.1.4 Hallux

Range of motion of the hallux was decreased in the sagittal (dorsiflexion/plantarflexion) plane throughout the gait cycle. The hallux also maintained a more plantarflexed and supinated position than normal.

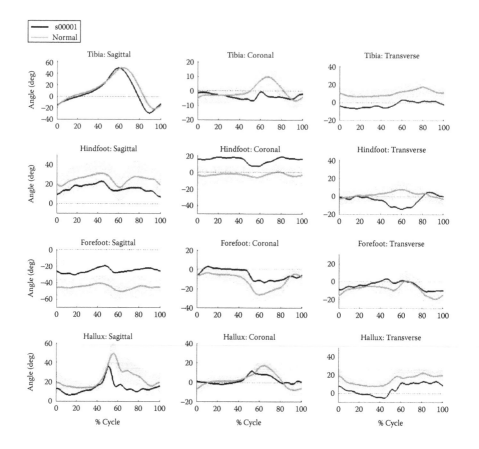

FIGURE 3.9 Case example: foot kinematics.

3.9 DISCUSSION

Although there have been numerous studies examining whole-body gait of patients following surgical correction of clubfoot deformity, this methodology does not allow for assessment of motion beyond the ankle, thereby neglecting the primary area of pathology. To date there has been relatively little published information[7] that quantitatively assesses multisegment foot and ankle motion in the postoperative clubfoot population.

In our examination of 17 subjects following posteromedial soft-tissue release utilizing standard whole-body gait analysis methods we found several temporal–spatial, kinematic, and kinetic alterations compared to normal. Temporal–spatial changes included decreased walking speed, cadence, and stride length, as well as increased stance duration. Kinematic alterations demonstrated by whole-body gait analysis included decreased sagittal ankle range of motion, with preservation of the first and second ankle rockers and a delayed third rocker. The ankle also appeared to be more externally rotated as compared to normal. Kinematic changes at the hip included decreased overall sagittal range of motion as well as decreased flexion/increased extension especially during terminal stance and initial swing as compared to normal. Ankle power was significantly less than normal. These alterations in gait parameters provide evidence that there exist significant changes in ambulation of residual and/or recurrent clubfoot deformity compared with a normal population of adolescents. We also believe that any alterations in kinematics found proximal to the ankle are a result of compensation for changes occurring at the foot and ankle. The details of foot motion abnormalities can only be examined utilizing an advanced multisegment foot and ankle model.

To provide some insight into what is occurring at the foot and ankle (i.e., tibia, hindfoot, forefoot, and hallux) we analyzed a patient following surgical correction of unilateral clubfoot deformity using the Milwaukee Foot Model. This analysis demonstrated several kinematic alterations including decreased tibial range of motion in both the coronal and transverse planes; decreased dorsiflexion and transverse plane range of motion of the hindfoot, with increased internal rotation of the hindfoot; and decreased range of motion of the forefoot (sagittal, coronal, and transverse planes) and hallux (sagittal). Unlike what was demonstrated by whole-body gait, there was preservation of the first and third ankle rockers and an abnormal second rocker. Additionally, the sagittal position of the hindfoot indicates flattening of the plantar arch.

In conclusion, this study indicates that over time there are several gait abnormalities that develop in patients following surgical clubfoot correction and may indicate residual and or recurrent foot and ankle deformity. This pathology cannot be fully examined using traditional whole-body gait analysis methods and requires more advanced foot and ankle gait analysis, which is able to provide information regarding motion of multiple segments of the foot. Although what we have presented here is preliminary data, it does provide evidence that using the Milwaukee Foot Model provides insight into some of this missing data. Further study of multisegmental foot and ankle kinematics in this population may prove useful in assessing treatment outcome as well as provide information as to the appropriate timing for additional treatment interventions.

REFERENCES

1. Laaveg SJ, Ponseti IV. Long-term results of treatment of congenital clubfoot. *J Bone Joint Surg Am,* 1980;62A:23–31.
2. Roye DP, Roye BD. Idiopathic congenital talipes equinovarus. *J Am Acad Orthop Surg,* 2002;10(4):239–248.
3. Ippolito E, Farsetti P, Caterini R, Tudisco C. Long-term comparative results in patients with congenital clubfoot treated with two different protocols. *J Bone Joint Surg Am,* 2003;85A(7):1286–1294.
4. Cummings RJ, Davidson RS, Armstrong PF, Lehman WB. Congenital clubfoot. *J Bone Joint Surg Am,* 2002;84A(2):290–308.
5. Noonan KJ, Richards BS. Nonsurgical management of idiopathic clubfoot. *J Am Acad Orthop Surg,* 2003;11(6):392–402.
6. Dobbs MB, Rudzki JR, Purcell DB, Walton T, Porter KR, Gurnett CA. Factors predictive of outcome after use of the ponseti method for the treatment of idiopathic clubfoot. *J Bone Joint Surg Am,* 2004;86A(1):22–27.

7. Theologis TN, Harrington ME, Thompson N, Benson MKD. Dynamic foot movement in children treated for congenital talipes equinovarus. *J Bone Joint Surg Am,* 2003;85B(4):572–577.

8. Sawatzky BJ, Sanderson DJ, Beauchamp RD, Outerbridge AR. Ground reaction forces in gait in children with clubfeet: a preliminary study. *Gait Posture,* 1994;2: 123–127.

9. Karol LA, Concha MC, Johnston CE. Gait analysis and muscle strength in children with surgically treated clubfeet. *J Pediatr Orthop,* 1997;17(6):790–795.

10. Alkjaer T, Pedersen ENG, Simonsen EB. Evaluation of the walking pattern in clubfoot patients who received early intensive treatment. *J Pediatr Orthop,* 2000;20(5): 642–647.

11. Davies TC, Kiefer G, Zernicke RF. Kinematics and kinetics of hip, knee and ankle of children with clubfoot after posteromedial release. *J Pediatr Orthop,* 2001;21(3): 366–371.

12. Tareco J, Sala DA, Scher DM, Lehman WB, Feldmen DS. Percutaneous fixation in clubfoot surgery: a radiographic and gait study. *J Pediatr Orthop,* 2002;11(2): 139–142.

13. Muratli HH, Dagli C, Yavuzer G, Celebi L, Bicimoglu A. Gait characteristics of patients with bilateral clubfeet following posteromedial release procedure. *J Pediatr Orthop,* 2005;14(3):206–211.

14. O'Brien SE, Karol LA, Johnston CE. Calcaneus gait following treatment for clubfoot: preliminary results of surgical correction. *J Pediatr Orthop,* 2004;13(1):43–47.

15. Asperheim MS, Moore C, Carroll NC, Dias L. Evaluation of residual clubfoot deformities using gait analysis. *J Pediatr Orthop,* 1995;4B(1):49–54.

16. Otis JC, Bohne WHO. Gait analysis in surgically treated clubfoot. *J Pediatr Orthop,* 1986;6(2):162–164.

17. Karol LA, O'Brein SE, Wilson H, Johnson CE, Richards BS. Gait analysis in children with severe clubfeet: early results of physiotherapy versus surgical release. *J Pediatr Orthop,* 2005;25(2):236–240.

18. Irani RN, Sherman MS. The pathological anatomy of idiopathic clubfoot. *Clin Orthop Relat Res,* 1972;84:14–20.

19. Mosca VS. The foot. In: *Lovell and Winter's Pediatric Orthopaedics.* 5th ed. Philadelphia: Lippincot-Raven, 1996:1153–1161.

20. Lochmiller C, Johnson D, Scott A, Risman M, Hecht JT. Genetic epidemiology study of idiopathic talipes equinovarus. *Am J Med Genet,* 1998;79:90–96.

21. Herring JA, ed. *Tachdjian's Pediatric Orthopaedics.* 3rd ed. Philadelphia: WB Saunders Company, 2002:922–959.

22. Ponseti IV, Campos J. Observations on pathogenesis and treatment of congenital clubfoot. *Clin Orthop Relat Res,* 1972;84:50–59.

23. Ponseti IV, Smoley EN. Congenital clubfoot: the results of treatment. *J Bone Joint Surg Am,* 1963;45A:261–275.

24. Turco VJ. Surgical Correction of the clubfoot: one-stage postereomedial release with internal fixation: a preliminary report. *J Bone Joint Surg Am,* 1971;53A:477–497.

25. Johnson JE, Kidder SM, Abuzzahab FS. Three-dimensional motion analysis of the adult foot and ankle. In: Harris GF, Smith P, Eds. *Human Motion Analysis.* New York: IEEE Press, 1996:351–369.

26. Johnson JE, Lamdan R, Granberry WF, Harris GF, Carrera GF. Hindfoot coronal alignment: a modified radiographic method. *Foot Ankle Int,* 1999;20(12):818–825.

27. Kidder SM, Abuzzahab FS, Harris GF. A system for the analysis of the foot and ankle kinematics during gait. *IEEE Trans Rehabil Eng,* 1996;4(1):25–32.

28. Abuzzahab FS, Harris GF, Kidder SM. Foot and ankle motion analysis system instrumentation, calibration and validation. In: Harris GF, Smith P, Eds. *Human Motion Analysis.* New York: IEEE Press, 1996:152–166.

29. Kadaba MP, Ramakrishnan HK, Wootten ME. Measurement of lower extremity kinematics during level walking. *J Orthop Res,* 1990;8(3):383–392.
30. Kadaba MP, Ramakrishnan HK, Wootten ME, Gainey J, Gorton G, Cochran GV. Repeatability of kinematic, kinetic, and electromyographic data in normal adult gait. *J Orthop Res,* 1989;7(6):849–860.

4 Dynamic Plantar Pressure Characteristics and Clinical Applications in Patients with Residual Clubfoot

Xue-Cheng Liu and John Thometz

CONTENTS

4.1 INTRODUCTION

Nearly 20 yr ago, Simons[15] established the standard radiographic measures used to assess clubfoot. Six commonly measured radiographic parameters were reported. However, those angle measurements were specifically designed for children before walking and also required complex techniques for foot positioning, which is particularly difficult between the ages of 2 months and 2 yr. Movement of the foot in those patients often resulted in inaccuracy of the radiographic measurements.[8] In spite of these clinical controversies when using standard radiographic measurements, clinicians continue to apply these measurements to assess children who are able to walk.

Radiographs provide a method to evaluate the structure of the foot during weight bearing. However, these static measurements more accurately represent the anatomical alignment rather than the function of the foot during gait. In previous studies by Cavanagh et al.,[6] it was reported that the arch height expressed by the first metatarsal inclination (lateral view) was one of the dominant factors in predicting peak pressures under the heel and the first metatarsal head during walking. Our data on the residual clubfoot did not support this correlation between the lateral talus-first metatarsal angle and peak pressures. This study was done by comparing radiographs and EMED plantar pressure results of 61 idiopathic clubfeet in 39 children at an average of 8 yr-status post complete subtalar release.[17] Radiographic measures were obtained using the standard method outlined by Simons and pressure data were collected for eight regions of the foot. Pearson correlation analysis was performed, and the most significant correlation was found between the calcaneal-first metatarsal angle in the lateral radiographic view ($r = .72$) and the midfoot contact area. In the antero-posterior (AP) view, there was only mild correlation between the talus-first metatarsal angle and both the peak pressure and plantar contact area. The results of this study indicate that radiographs are insufficient to assess foot function in clubfoot.

The clubfoot is a complex deformity involving the ankle, subtalar and midtarsal joints, and forefoot in which motion or deformity at one joint can have unknown effects on the others. Residual deformities after conservative or surgical correction of clubfoot are not uncommon and occur in a variety of forms.[18] These residual deformities may be seen as a dynamic supination deformity of the forefoot, which would never be detected by standard x-rays. Although the Dimeglio classification of clubfoot was established based upon clinical examination in the sagittal, coronal, and transverse planes (including soft–soft feet, soft > stiff feet, stiff > soft feet, and stiff–stiff feet),[10] it was primarily used to assess feet in the early stage of pathology. There have been few classifications of the residual clubfoot deformity based upon functional assessment. With the advent of more advanced methods of assessing plantar pressure such as the EMED pressure system,[1,5,9] we can better determine foot function that may correlate with dynamic plantar pressure distribution. Since the 1990s, dynamic foot pressure analysis has been applied clinically with a variety of foot deformities, and a series of studies using this technology was introduced for the assessment of clubfeet. The greatest differences in peak pressure between club-feet and normal feet occurred in the region of the midfoot.[9] However, indications of the correct surgical procedures as determined by the plantar pressure patterns have not been developed.

The goal of this chapter is (1) to characterize the dynamic plantar pressure patterns in the resistant or relapsed clubfoot; (2) to correlate treatment options with pressure patterns, showing a case study of plantar pressure change following surgical procedures; and (3) to investigate the influence of shoe wear on the distribution of pressure under clubfoot.

4.2 MATERIAL AND METHODS

Twenty-six idiopathic clubfeet in 17 children, treated by complete subtalar release, were examined by radiography, physical examination, and the EMED foot pressure system (Novel Electronics, St. Paul, MN). The EMED plantar pressure system is a platform to measure pressure under the bare foot. Mean length of follow-up for clubfoot patients was 7 yr and 5 months, ranging from 4 yr and 3 months to 14 yr and 1 month. A total of 68 normal children (6 to 16 yr) were tested as a control group. Five of 26 clubfeet were assessed by both the EMED foot pressure system

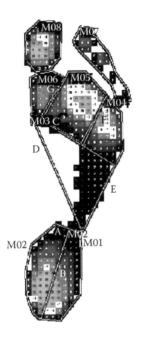

FIGURE 4.1 Eight regions of free-mapping model.

and Pedar insole pressure system (PEDAR mobile system, NOVEL, Germany). Subjects were asked to step on the EMED pressure system (4 sensors/cm^2, 50 Hz) three times with each foot during normal walking. The in-shoe plantar pressure system is designed to measure pressure distribution and contact area between the foot and shoe. This system consists of a PEDAR data collective box, 12 V power supply, software, video, PCMCIA card, four pairs of different sizes of sensor matrices, synchronization device, and the calibration device. The PEDAR mobile system scans with a speed of 10,000 sensors per second and takes samples at 50 Hz.

The plantar pressure of each foot was divided into eight regions using a free-mapping method.[13] The first two masks are delineated by circumscribing the heel to the point where the arch narrowing begins (Figure 4.1). Here a line along the anterior area of the heel is drawn (line A). A line bisecting this heel region (line B) separates the first two masks with the lateral mask being designated as mask 1 (M01) and the medial as mask 2 (M02). The midfoot regions are created by first drawing a diagonal line connecting the medial and lateral points where the arch flares and reaches its greatest width (line C). Lines are drawn from the medial and lateral ends of this line to connect to the outermost points of the anterior margin of masks 1 and 2 (lines D and E). This sets the boundaries of the midfoot (M03). The remaining anterior, medial, and lateral borders are the natural shape of the foot, excluding the toes. Two additional lines are drawn at right angles to the diagonal line (line C), which separates the forefoot from the midfoot (lines F and G). These two lines separate the fifth metatarsal (M04) from the fourth, third, and second metatarsals (M05), thus isolating the first metatarsal (M06). The seventh mask is made by circumscribing the phalanges from digits 2 to 5 (M07). The eighth mask is made by circumscribing the hallux (M08). The free-mapping method is able to locate eight plantar anatomical landmarks, including the lateral and medial heel; midfoot; first, third, and fifth metatarsal heads; lateral toes (second to fourth toe together); and hallux.

According to Simon's radiographic index,[15] we measured seven parameters on the AP and lateral radiographs. On the AP, the measurements included the talocalcaneal angle (AP-TC), calcaneal-fifth metatarsal angle (AP-CM5), and talus-first metatarsal angle (AP-TM1). On the lateral radiograph the measurements included the talocalcaneal angle (lateral-TC), talus-first metatarsal angle (lateral-TM1), calcaneal-first metatarsal angle (lateral-CM1), and first to fifth metatarsal angle (lateral-M1-5). Using these masks the following variables were analyzed: (1) peak pressure (N/cm^2), (2) maximal mean pressure (N/cm^2), (3) contact area (cm^2), (4) contact time as a function of stance phase, (5) pressure time integral, (6) force time integral, (7) instant of peak pressure as a function of stance phase, and (8) instant of maximum force as a function of stance phase. We then calculated the mean and standard deviation for all variables and compared their means between the normals and patients with clubfeet using the Student's t-test. Different pressure patterns will be classified in terms of their plantar contact area, peak pressure, and trajectory of center of pressure (COP); then the percentage of clubfeet with similar classified pressure patterns will also be computed.

4.3 RESULTS

There were significant differences in specific regions of the foot ($p < .05$). The mid-MT region of clubfoot patients had an increased plantar contact area as compared to the normals (19.6 vs. 17.8), and the first metatarsal (MT) and hallux had a lesser contact area (4.3 vs. 5.9, 6 vs. 7.4, respectively). The greatest difference in peak pressure and loading between clubfeet and normal feet was in the regions of the midfoot and hallux. The midfoot had an increased peak pressure and loading (9.8 vs. 6.7, 2.9 vs. 1.8, respectively), and the hallux had a decreased peak pressure and loading (15.5 vs. 26.9, 3.6 vs. 5.8, respectively). A delayed roller time of the hallux was seen (86.8% vs. 82.1%).

Based upon the differences between clubfoot and normal foot, five different pressure patterns were classified as following:

Pattern A: A lateral shift of the COP on the forefoot and increased peak pressure on the lateral region of the forefoot (Figure 4.2A), which occur in 27% of clubfeet.

Pattern B: An absence of COP on the heel (Figure 4.2B), which is found in 5% of clubfeet.

Pattern C: A decreased contact area on the first metatarsal head (Figure 4.2C), which is seen in 27% of clubfeet.

Pattern D: An increased midfoot contact area (Figure 4.2D), which is displayed in 21% of clubfeet.

Pattern E: An increased peak pressure on the midfoot (Figure 4.2E), which is shown in 16% of clubfeet.

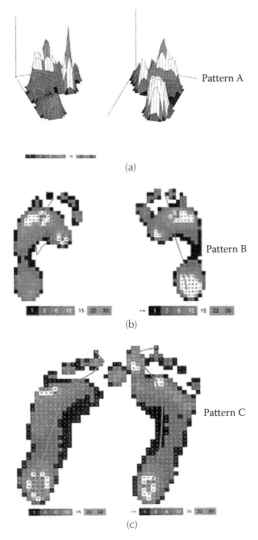

FIGURE 4.2 (a) A lateral shift of the COP and increased peak pressure on the forefoot. (b) An absence of COP on the heel. (c) A decreased contact area on the first metatarsal head. (d) An increased midfoot contact area. (e) An increased peak pressure on the midfoot.

A persistent COP medial deviation on the heel at initial contact was seen in 121 of 134 normal feet (75.4%) (Figure 4.3). This was coupled with a short interruption of the rise of the first peak pressure curve (a notch) and higher peak pressure on the medial heel than the lateral heel following heel strike. These three graphic signs indicate the mechanism of shock absorption caused by pronation movement at the subtalar joint. In patients with clubfeet, there was the absence of shock absorption by deceleration of the foot at initial contact or pronation movement of the subtalar joint following the heel-strike in 92% of cases.

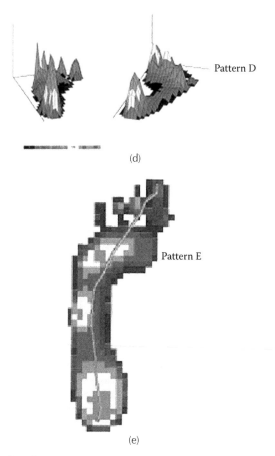

FIGURE 4.2 (Continued).

Indications for surgical procedures were considered based upon pressure distribution patterns in combination with radiographic measurements and physical examination of the foot. Most likely, tendon Achilles lengthening, usually Z-lengthening, would be adopted if pattern B (an absence of COP or advancement of COP at the heel) was identified. Pattern B indicates that there is contracture of the tendon Achilles and results in the absence of heel-strike or midfoot cavus deformity. After the complete subtalar release, we had 8% of clubfoot patients remaining in dynamic hindfoot varus deformity, confirmed by absence of medial deviation of the COP on the heel. In the case of pattern B and the absence of the medial deviation of COP, a shortening of the lateral column of the foot — the Dwyer procedure, would be suggested. The Dwyer procedure consists of a closing wedge osteotomy of the calcaneus for persistent hindfoot varus.

Pattern A (a lateral shift of the COP and increased peak pressure on the lateral region of the forefoot) or pattern C (a decreased contact area on the first metatarsal head)

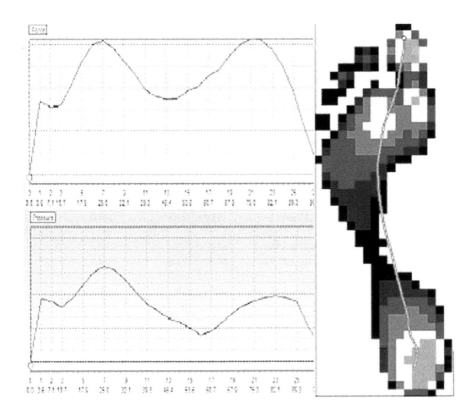

FIGURE 4.3 Pressure–time, force–time, and plantar pressure in a normal foot.

may represent a supination deformity of the forefoot, sometimes coupled with forefoot adduction. Indications for surgical procedures include closing wedge cuboid osteotomy, opening wedge cuneiform osteotomy, and split anterior tibial tendon transfer to the cuboid.

Pattern D, with increased midfoot contact area, usually demonstrates a breaking down of the midfoot, which stems from the malalignment of the medial column of the foot, consisting of the talus, navicular, medial cuneiform, and first ray. If this deformity was seen alone, a medial arch support orthosis was usually prescribed.

Pattern E, with increased peak pressure on the lateral midfoot, was noted as either midfoot breaking down or midfoot supination. Surgical options would include the methods mentioned above (the combination of transcuneiform osteotomy with closing cuboid and opening cuneiform osteotomy).

Considerable effects were noted with the use of shoe wear in patients with clubfoot. Table 4.1 shows significant changes of peak pressure and force, as well as plantar contact area. There were extensive increases of the plantar contact area of the forefoot and remarkable reduction of the maximal forces and peak pressure on the middle forefoot. Likewise, reduced pressure–time and force–time occurred in the middle forefoot.

TABLE 4.1

Significant Changes of Pressure Metrics with or without Shoe Wear in Clubfoot ($p < .05$)

Metrics	Pedar (Mean ± sd)	EMED (Mean ± sd)	p-Value
Contact area			
m04	7.99 ± 1.6	4.33 ± 1.52	0.04
m06	7.45 ± 1.6	3.02 ± 1.51	0.04
Max. force			
m05	19.01 ± 13.52	53.31 ± 9.95	0.04
Peak pressure			
m05	10.47 ± 4.22	25.2 ± 14.75	0.04
Contact time%			
m01	84.9 ± 13.01	61.02 ± 8.08	0.04
m08	34.41 ± 11.43	66.17 ± 17.46	0.04
Pressure–time			
m05	2.01 ± 1.18	5.04 ± 2.88	0.04
Force-time			
m03	4.85 ± 3.95	10.07 ± 2.53	0.04
m05	3.22 ± 2.77	13.24 ± 4.3	0.04

4.4 CASE REPORT

AP is a white male and was born with severe bilateral idiopathic clubfoot. There were no complications surrounding the pregnancy or delivery. No family history of clubfoot was reported. Treatment was initiated at 2 wk of life in a series of manipulations and long leg casting. He received bilateral complete subtalar releases at the age of 6 months. Following the first surgery, both his feet were nicely plantigrade. However, bilateral forefoot adductus has been observed since then. After a relapse of his clubfoot deformity, he had a second surgery at 5 yr of age. He was evaluated with a series of AP and lateral x-rays on the foot, followed by plantar pressure analysis before and after foot surgery. Table 4.2 shows that all of his angles in the AP and lateral view x-rays were improved after the first surgery, complete subtalar release at 6 months of age, as compared to those at the age of 4 months. However, 4 yrs later, his lateral calcaneus-first metatarsal angle increased to an abnormal level. Following second foot surgery, his talocalcaneal index remained more than 40°, but the osseous alignment with the first metatarsal in both the lateral and AP views (AP-talo-first metatarsal, lateral talo-first metatarsal, lateral calcaneus-first metatarsal) were not improved (Figure 4.4a and Figure 4.4b).

Table 4.3A and Table 4.3B indicate that pressure metrics of his left clubfoot improved significantly following the second foot surgery. After the second surgery, his plantar contact area on the first metatarsal head and hallux increased to normal range. Reduced peak pressures on the heel and hallux and increased peak pressure on the midfoot were corrected — so did loading on those anatomical areas (Table 4.3A and Table 4.3B, Figure 4.5). Based upon pedometric data

TABLE 4.2
Evaluation of the Left Clubfoot over 5 yrs (Degrees)

X-Rays	Normal	4 Months	6 Months (First Surgery)	4 Yrs	5 Yrs (Second Surgery)
AP-talocalcaneal	20°–40°	10°	22°	30°	19°
AP-talus-first met	0–15°	−32°	−18°	−15°	21°
Lateral-talocalcaneal	25–50°	12°	45°	30°	24°
Lateral-talus-first met	−1°–10°	15°	11°	14°	28°
Lateral-calcaneus-first met	0–40°	17°	57°	40°	50°
Lateral-first-fifth met	11°–21°	8°	12°	26°	24°
T-C index	>40°	22°	67°	60°	43°

(Figure 4.5), defined by 24 zones under the foot, his COP was remarkably shifted medially in the zones of 22, 19, 15, 11, 7, and 2, especially in the forefoot region; this showed that the COP moved from zone 3 (before surgery) to zone 2 (after surgery) following bony osteotomy and tendon transfer. Additionally, medial deviation of the COP in the zones of 22 to 18 at heel strike was noted, which is indicative of normal heel valgus and subtalar motion following surgery as opposed to pre-surgery. His hallux internal rotational angle was reduced from 27° to 21°, and his

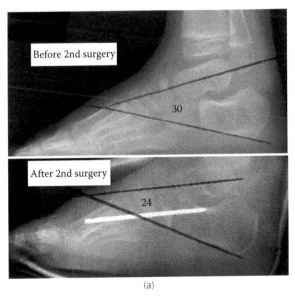

(a)

FIGURE 4.4 (a) Comparison of talocalcaneal angle in the lateral view before and after the second surgery. (b) Comparison of talo-first metatarsal angle in the AP view before and after the second surgery.

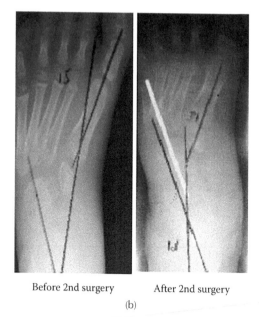

Before 2nd surgery After 2nd surgery

(b)

FIGURE 4.4 (Continued).

foot progression angle was also improved from 8.2° to 1.3° of internal rotation with respect to walking direction.

His second surgery included closing wedge cuboid osteotomy, opening wedge medial cuneiform osteotomy, and split anterior tibial tendon transfer. A medial

TABLE 4.3A
Comparison of Peak Pressure on the Left Clubfoot before and after Second Surgery

Mask Parameter	Area (cm²)			Peak Pressure (N/cm²)		
	Normal	Pre-OP	Post-OP	Normal	Pre-OP	Post-OP
M01 (lateral-heel)	13.2 ± 3.5	11.3	18.3	25.1 ± 10.4	02.5	40.3
M02 (medial-heel)	12.9 ± 3.6	11.4	16.0	27.2 ± 11.9	06.0	35.5
M03 (midfoot)	17.2 ± 8.4	13.8	23.8	6.7 ± 3.5	13.0	10.2
M04 (fifth metatarsal head)	6.3 ± 2.6	3.6	8.8	14.4 ± 11.2	17.8	20.7
M05 (third metatarsal head)	17.8 ± 3.8	19.0	12.6	22.6 ± 11.3	29.8	22.3
M06 (first metatarsal head)	5.9 ± 1.9	0.8	4.0	16.1 ± 9.5	08.0	16.3
M07 (two to fifth toes)	6.7 ± 2.2	2.8	8.6	14.2 ± 7.9	08.7	13.7
M08 (hallux)	7.4 ± 1.8	4.5	7.1	26.9 ± 15.1	9.5	25.0

TABLE 4.3B
Comparison of Peak Pressure on the Left Clubfoot before and after Second Surgery

Mask Parameter	Pressure–Time Integrals [(N/cm²)–s]			Instant of Peak Pressure [%ROP]		
	Normal	Pre-OP	Post-OP	Normal	Pre-OP	Post-OP
M01 (lateral-heel)	4.9 ± 2.5	0.2	6.6	13.3 ± 8.0	25.9	04.5
M02 (medial-heel)	5.3 ± 2.8	0.5	6.6	14.5 ± 7.9	25.9	04.5
M03 (midfoot)	1.8 ± 1.1	3.4	2.9	46.2 ± 15.9	70.4	71.9
M04 (fifth metatarsal head)	3.8 ± 2.8	3.7	4.3	64.9 ± 14.2	77.8	76.6
M05 (third metatarsal head)	6.5 ± 3.4	5.1	4.7	79 ± 8.3	85.2	84.3
M06 (first metatarsal head)	4.5 ± 2.6	0.4	3.0	69.3 ± 13.8	82.6	85.5
M07 (two to fifth toes)	2.8 ± 2.6	0.4	3.0	83.9 ± 8.4	82.6	82.0
M08 (hallux)	5.8 ± 4.3	0.7	4.2	82.1 ± 7.1	96.2	88.8

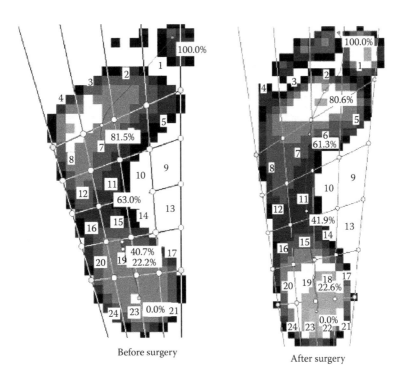

Before surgery   After surgery

FIGURE 4.5 Changes of plantar contact area and peak pressures before and after second surgery.

incision was made over the proximal first metatarsal, medial cuneiform, and navicular. The insertion of the anterior tibial tendon on the base of the first metatarsal was identified and was freed up. The most medial portion of the tendon was dissected off and split to the most proximal portion of the incision. The tendon was grabbed with the tendon passer and then turned to the cuboid. A 3 cm incision was made over the cuboid and a large osteotome was then used under fluoroscopic guidance to perform a closing wedge osteotomy of the cuboid. The wedge of bone was removed. A straight transverse osteotomy on the medial cuneiform was made and a bone graft from the cuboid was inserted into the interval of the cuneiform.

4.5 DISCUSSION

Dynamic plantar pressure analysis has been applied clinically for clubfeet since the 1990s. The technique has already improved our understanding of the foot and its function. The objective documentation of foot function before and after treatment has been greatly enhanced. The study with a dynamic pedobargraph in the evaluation of varus and valgus foot deformities found that a coronal index of the pedobargraph, determined by comparing the pressure–time integral under the medial column with that under the lateral column of the foot, is highly correlated with clinical assessment and provides better information than radiographic measurement in differentiating the clinical categories ($r = .90$).[7] Chang et al. agreed that the clinical assessment is still the primary tool to determine general features, but it is difficult to apply an objective measurement and the pedobargraph should be a primary tool to measure the severity of deformities of the foot. The 30-yr follow-up of the treatment of idiopathic clubfoot[9] performed pedobarographic and electrogoniometric analyses in addition to the clinical outcomes and radiographic studies. They showed that the clinical outcome could not be predicted from the radiographic result, and the clinical result should be considered from the standpoint of pain and limitation of function. Our experience has shown that the dynamic plantar pressure has become a routine tool in the follow-up of the treated clubfoot and to effectively evaluate the residual clubfoot deformity.

Gait analysis has been utilized in the assessment of the clubfoot deformity. It has defined walking patterns in terms of their ankle joint movement and torque.[2,4] Pressure patterns have not been completely characterized for residual clubfoot deformities. Three-dimensional gait analysis showed reduced range of motion of the ankle joint for patients with clubfeet. These gait patterns only indicate weaker plantar flexor and talar flattening.[4] Our study divided plantar pressures into five patterns that represent different foot deformities. These five pressure patterns derived from the residual clubfoot deformities during walking included forefoot adduction and supination, midfoot cavus or supination, and hindfoot varus. Cooper et al. also recognized decreased peak pressure in the heel region coupled with the increased pressures in the mid-part of the clubfoot.[9] This pattern is similar to our type B, having an absence of COP on the heel. In their patient population, they also discovered a mild lateral transfer of weight-bearing as compared to normal feet, and this pattern is the same as our type A.

We attempted to find a relationship between treatment recommendation and pressure patterns. Our experience taught us that the dynamic plantar pressure analysis is able to assist in decision-making for treatment. A common residual deformity that may be seen following the management of clubfoot is a dynamic supination deformity of the forefoot, which can be easily detected by dynamic plantar pressure analysis. Static clinical examination may present with normal alignment of the forefoot, but the dynamic plantar pressure shows both pattern A and pattern C (lateral shift COP and reduced contact area in the region of the first metatarsal head). The presence of a strong anterior tibialis with weak peroneals is often the cause for this deformity.[18] The anterior tibial tendon transfer to the dorsum of the foot is a procedure that has been devised to correct persistent dynamic supination deformity.[18] In a study of 27 clubfeet that underwent the anterior tibialis tendon transfer, this procedure was found to improve muscle balance and correct the dynamic supination deformity and progression of recurrence of clubfoot deformity.[11]

The fixed forefoot supination deformity, demonstrated by both clinical examination and abnormal pressure distribution (patterns A and C), was often a result of an incomplete release of the calcaneocuboid joint[16] or improper position of the navicular with respect to the talus.[3] A number of procedures have been previously described for correction of angular and rotational deformities, but many do not address the full deformity.[14] Hoffman et al. used the opening wedge medial cuneiform osteotomy to reliably correct forefoot adductus, however, it failed to correct supination. Evans' procedure involved distal calcaneocuboid joint wedge osteotomy and fusion, but it did not resolve adduction deformity distal to the midfoot.[14] A combination of opening wedge medial cuneiform osteotomy, closing wedge cuboid osteotomy, and truncated wedge middle and lateral cuneiform osteotomy is an effective method to correct both the angular and rotational deformities.[18]

Based on the results, we found that a medial shift curve of the COP on the heel at the heel strike occurred in 75.4% of 134 normal feet as compared to 8% of 26 clubfeet. Huber et al.[12] agreed that an interruption in the rise of the pressure–time curve and a short medial deviation of the COP path immediately after heel strike are reliable and objective characteristics of pronation movement of the subtalar joint. They found that 79% of 24 clubfeet had a demonstrable pronation movement with 87 points on the Orthopaedic Foot and Ankle Society Score (OFAS), and 21% did not have pronation movement of the subtalar joint with 57 points on OFAS. They concluded that an idiopathic clubfoot with preserved hindfoot pronation has a better long-term prognosis.

Shoe wear reduced the peak pressure and ground reaction force over the forefoot and did not fundamentally change the COP trajectory. This indicates that regular shoe wear does not alter residual clubfoot alignment.

Our case report is an example of analyzing dynamic plantar pressure patterns and using them to indicate the surgical procedures. Following the closing wedge cuboid osteotomy, opening wedge medial cuneiform osteotomy, and split anterior tibial tendon transfer, improved clinical results (normal foot progression angle, reduced hallux internal rotation angle, and normal hindfoot valgus) were observed. This work indicates that these combined surgical procedures are an effective method for successful treatment of the residual clubfoot deformity.

4.6 CONCLUSION

Five dynamic plantar pressure patterns were seen in patients with residual clubfeet. They represent a variety of foot deformities that have followed surgical intervention. These dynamic pressure features provide valuable functional analysis of the clubfoot deformity and assist clinical decision-making in tandem with clinical examination and radiography.

REFERENCES

1. Alexander, I.J, Chao, E., Johnson, K.A., The assessment of dynamic foot-to-ground contact forces and plantar pressure distribution: a review of the evolution of current techniques and clinical applications. *Foot Ankle.* 11(3), 152, 1990.
2. Alkjer, T., Pedersen, E.G., Simonsen, E.B., Evaluation of the walking pattern in clubfoot patients who received early intensive treatment. *J Pediatr Orthop.* 20, 642, 2000.
3. Atar, D., Lehman, W., Tarsal navicular position after complete soft-tissue clubfoot release. *Clin Orthop Relat Res.* 295, 252, 1999.
4. Bach, C.M., Wachter, R., Stockl, B., Gobel, G., Nogler, M., Frischhut, B., Significance of talar distortion for ankle mobility in idiopathic clubfoot. *Clin Orthop Relat Res.* 398, 196, 2002.
5. Bowen, T.R., Miller, F., Castagno, P., Richards, J., Lipton, G., A method of dynamic foot-pressure measurement for the evaluation of pediatric orthopaedic foot deformities. *J Pediatr Orthop.* 18(6), 789, 1998.
6. Cavanagh, P.R., Morag, E., Boulton, A.J., Young, M.J., Deffner, K.T., Pammer, S.E., The relationship of static foot structure to dynamic foot function. *J Biomech.* 30(3), 243, 1997.
7. Chang, C.H., Miller, F., Schuyler, J., Dynamic pedobargraph in evaluation of varus and valgus foot deformities. *J Pediatr Orthop.* 22, 813, 2003.
8. Cook, D.A., Breed, A.L., Cook, T., DeSmet, A.D., Muehle, C.M., Observer variability in the radiographic measurement and classification of metatarsus adductus. *J Pediatr Orthop.* 12, 86, 1992.
9. Cooper, D.M., Dietz, F.R., Treatment of idiopathic clubfoot — a thirty-year follow-up note. *J Bone Joint Surg Am.* 77A, 1477, 1995.
10. Dimeglio, A., Bensahel, H., Souchet, P., Bonnet, F., Classification of clubfoot. *J Pediatr Orthop B.* 4, 129, 1995.
11. Ezra, E., Hayek, S., Gilai, A., Khermosh, O., Wientroub, S., Tibialis anterior tendon transfer for residual dynamic supination deformity in the treated clubfoot. *J Pediatr Orthop.* 9, 207, 2000.
12. Huber, H., Dutoit, M., Dynamic foot-pressure measurement in the assessment of operatively treated clubfeet. *J Bone Joint Surg Am.* 86, 1203, 2004.
13. Liu, X.C., Thometz, J., Tassone, C., Lyon, R., Brady, M., Dynamic plantar pressure distribution in normal subjects: free-mapping model for the analysis of pediatric foot deformities. *J Pediatr Orthop.* 25(1), 103, 2005.
14. Pohl, M., Nicole, R., Transcuneiform and opening wedge medial cuneiform osteotomy with closing wedge cuboid osteotomy in relapsed clubfoot. *J Pediatr Orthop.* 23, 70, 2003.

15. Simons, G.W., A standardized method for the radiographic evaluation of clubfeet. *Clin Orthop Relat Res.* 135, 107, 1978.
16. Taraf, Y., Carrol, C., Analysis of the components of the residual deformity in clubfeet presenting for reoperation. *J Pediatr Orthop.* 12, 207, 1992.
17. Thometz, J., Liu, X.C., Tassone, C., Klein, S., Predictors of dynamic foot function in post-surgical clubfoot by foot radiographs. *J Pediatr Orthop.* 25(2), 249, 2005.
18. Thometz, J., Pediatric foot and ankle. *Curr Opin Orthop.* 11, 438, 2000.

5 Three-Dimensional Magnetic Resonance Imaging Modeling of Normal and Surgically Treated Clubfeet

Chester Tylkowski, Vishwas Talwalkar,
David Pienkowski, Christopher Roche,
and Brian Mattingly

CONTENTS

5.1 INTRODUCTION

Clubfoot is a common congenital deformity that can be seen in children with obvious neurologic injury as in myelomeningocele, or with other syndromic associations, such as arthrogryposis. Most commonly, the deformity is an isolated one without a clear etiology and is referred to as idiopathic. The condition is characterized by severe soft tissue contractures and malformation of the osteocartilaginous structures of the immature foot. The pathologic anatomy may also include aberrant muscles, nerves, and blood vessels.[1–5] Treatment for this disorder has included manipulation, casting, physical therapy, continuous passive motion, taping, limited surgical release, extensive surgical release, tendon transfers, osteotomy, and arthrodesis, or some combination of these modalities. The goal of all treatment methods is to obtain a painless plantigrade foot while preserving as much strength and mobility as possible. Optimal therapy remains controversial, and outcomes have been unpredictable. Gross range of motion of the joints of the foot is commonly used as an outcome measure but lacks reproducibility and precision. Documentation of clubfoot deformity continues to be by radiographic angular measurements despite the fact that such measurements have several limitations in their accuracy and precision.[6–9] Data published demonstrate a large range of acceptable values in the normal foot.[8-15] The precision of radiographic measurements is least in the most immature, primarily cartilaginous foot.[15] Clinical outcomes do not correlate well to radiographic measurements. These limitations diminish the utility of radiographic measurements to accurately quantify the anatomic deformity. The most fundamental limitation of two-dimensional (2D) radiographic imaging is the inability to accurately represent the complex three-dimensional (3D) structure of the foot. Three-dimensional imaging by computed tomography (CT) has been used extensively for assessment of clubfoot, following treatment.[16–21] This modality allows for excellent imaging of bony structures, but requires significantly more radiation exposure than plane radiography. CT is a very useful tool for 3D evaluation of morphology in adults, but is unable to accurately image cartilage, making it less useful in the skeletally immature. Magnetic resonance imaging (MRI) and computer-based image analysis have recently been used to create 3D virtual models of bone, cartilage, soft tissues, and joints.[22–31] The ability to image bony and cartilaginous structures without ionizing radiation is particularly well suited to pediatric orthopedic conditions, including clubfoot. Three-dimensional modeling of articular surfaces allows for quantitative evaluation of joint surfaces and joint congruity.

5.2 MATERIALS AND METHODS

5.2.1 RESEARCH SUBJECTS

Seven subjects (mean age: 13.0 ± 2.8 yr) with idiopathic unilateral clubfoot previously treated between ages 1 and 2 yr by serial casting followed by posterior–medial surgical release were recruited into this Institutional Review Board–approved study. Clinical examination by a pediatric orthopedist confirmed that the surgical treatment of each clubfoot resulted in a plantigrade weight-bearing foot. None of the subjects had any secondary bony procedures. Each contralateral foot was also determined to be clinically normal.

5.2.2 IMAGING TECHNIQUE

There were four distinct stages used to assess the 3D hindfoot tarsal morphology (Figure 5.1): (1) quasistatic MRI of each subject's hindfoot, (2) 3D computer reconstruction of the resulting images, (3) geometric modeling of the computer-reconstructed anatomy (this included an assessment of bone volume, bone area, and the fitting of geometric models to each hindfoot bone and articular surface), and (4) assessment of the quality of fit for each geometric model.

In the first stage, each subject's lower limbs were separately secured at neutral position in a commercially available, MRI-compatible ankle-positioning device

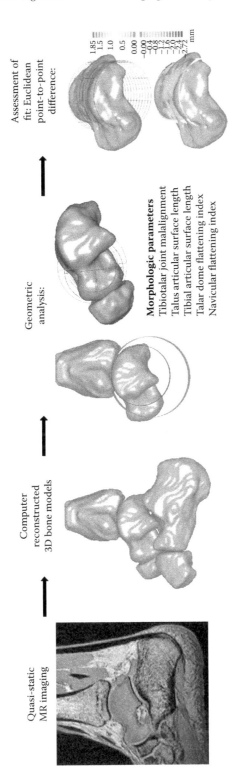

FIGURE 5.1 Illustrated summary of the methodology used.

(CHAMCO™, Miami, FL) as they reclined supine in the bore of a Siemens 1.5 T MRI. The MRI used a 3D FISP (fast imaging in the steady state MRI protocol) to produce 64 high-resolution T_1/T_2-weighted images of each subject's lower limbs.[24]

5.2.3 IMAGE RECONSTRUCTION ANALYSIS

In the second stage, the MR images of each subject were imported as raw data (data type = short 1, header size = 6144 bytes, endianess = big endian, and a voxel size = 0.9375 mm × 0.9375 mm × 1.5 mm or 1.0 mm, depending upon slice thickness) into the image reconstruction software Amira (TGS, Inc.). Once imported, the distal tibia, talus, calcaneus, navicular, and cuboid bones were manually segmented, inter-polated, and smoothed to assemble 3D models of each bone. After each bone model was created, it was saved and imported into the surface-modeling software I-DEAS Freeform (EDS, Inc.).[24,33]

5.2.3.1 Geometric Modeling

In the third stage, the size of each bone (surface area and volume) was computed. The articular surfaces of each joint were then geometrically modeled by using cylinders, spheres, or planes of varying dimensions and creating a best-fit geometric model. The articular surfaces of the tibiotalar, anterior and middle (continuous) subtalar, posterior subtalar, and calcaneocuboid joints were modeled with cylinders of varying radii and placed in male–female configurations, relative to models. The articular surfaces of the talonavicular joint were modeled with either one male–female sphere or two male–female spheres of varying radii, where the radius of each sphere corresponded to the greater and lesser curvatures of the modeled articular surfaces. Each of the geometric models closely approximated the ideal articular surface shapes described by Sarrafian (Figure 5.2).[34] In the fourth stage, the quality of fit was quantified by the average Euclidean point-to-point perpendic-ular difference between the articular surface and the geometric model (Figure 5.3).

5.2.3.2 Tarsal Morphological Parameters

The reliability of the morphological parameter used was determined by quantifying the accuracy and precision of the geometric modeling technique. This was accom-plished by modeling ping-pong balls and polyvinylchloride pipes of known radii, as determined by a coordinate measuring machine and comparing these known radii values to the experimentally determined radii values. The usefulness of each mor-phological parameter was defined by its ability to quantitatively distinguish the primary deformities associated with the clubfoot pathological anatomy. The primary osseous deformities associated with the clubfoot included: a flattened talar dome[1,2,35]; a deformed talar head[15,36]; a wedge-shaped navicular with a deformed articular surface; a single, deformed subtalar joint; and a deformed calcaneocuboid articular surface.[37]

The specific morphological parameters measured were tarsal volume, tarsal surface area, articular surface area, articular surface length, difference in articular surface length, joint malalignment, the degree of talar flattening, and the degree of

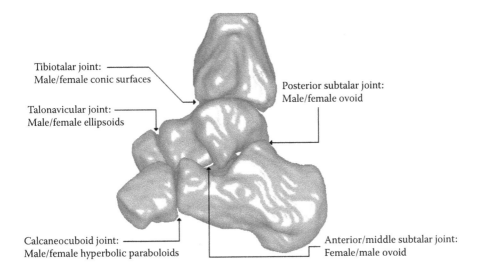

Tibiotalar joint:
Male/female conic surfaces

Posterior subtalar joint:
Male/female ovoid

Talonavicular joint:
Male/female ellipsoids

Calcaneocuboid joint:
Male/female hyperbolic paraboloids

Anterior/middle subtalar joint:
Female/male ovoid

FIGURE 5.2 Summary of tarsal articular surfaces studied.

navicular flattening. The first four parameters are routine and self-explanatory. Differences in articular surface lengths were measured for the tibiotalar joint by calculating the difference in arc length of the cylinders that represented these two joint surfaces. This was accomplished by computing the distance between the articular surface extremes — the chord. The articular surface length was approximated by the arc length (Equation 5.1):

$$Arc\ Length = D * \left(\arcsin\left(\frac{C}{D}\right) \right) \tag{5.1}$$

where D denotes the diameter of the cylinder used to model the articular surface and C denotes the chord of the articular surface. The difference in articular surface length was determined by subtracting the distal tibia articular surface length from the talar dome articular surface length. Articular surface length and the difference in articular surface length were both used to quantify joint size. Theoretically, the functional relevance of this parameter is that an increase in the difference of articular surface length should predict an increase in talus sagittal rotation.

Joint malalignment was measured in the tibiotalar and posterior subtalar joints by calculating the angle of deviation between the cylinders describing the joint surface. The angle of deviation (Equation 5.2) was quantified by the ratio of the vector dot product of the cylinder position vectors and the product of the magnitudes of the cylinder position vectors:

$$Angle\ of\ Deviation = \arccos \frac{\vec{A} \cdot \vec{B}}{|A| * |B|} \tag{5.2}$$

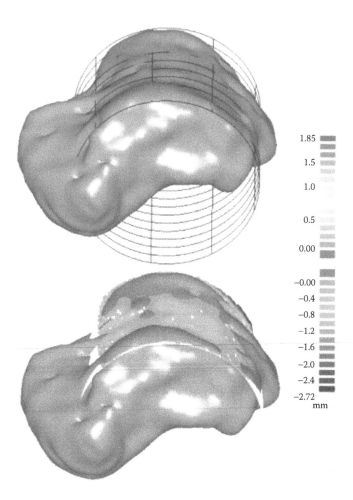

FIGURE 5.3 Representative Euclidian perpendicular difference between the geometric model (top figure) and the articular surface (bottom figure)

where $\vec{A}$ and $\vec{B}$ are the position vectors that describe the talus and tibia or calcaneus cylinders, respectively; and $|A|$ and $|B|$ are the magnitudes of the position vectors that describe the talus and tibia or calcaneus cylinders, respectively. Theoretically, the functional relevance of this parameter is that an increase in the angle of deviation should predict a decrease of in-plane motion and an increase of out-of-plane motion.

The degree of talar flattening was quantified by the talar flattening index (Equation 5.3) — a parameter adopted from one similarly developed by Hjelmstedt and Sahlstedt.[35]

$$Talar\ Flattening\ Index = \frac{Trochlea\ Curvature}{Talar\ Length} \qquad (5.3)$$

The talar flattening index has been shown to be functionally relevant because it correlates with dynamic joint motion, however, not static motion. [38] Finally, the degree of navicular flattening was quantified by the navicular flattening index:

$$Navicular\ Flattening\ Index = \frac{Greater\ Navicular\ Curvature}{Navicular\ Length} \quad (5.4)$$

5.2.4 DATA ANALYSIS

Two-tailed paired t-tests were used to compare the mean values of tarsal volume, tarsal surface area, and articular surface area between the unilateral surgically treated clubfoot and the contralateral normal foot. If the corresponding differences were significant, it was concluded that surgical treatment did not restore "normal" tarsal size or joint size in the unilateral clubfoot. Second, a two-tailed unpaired t-test was used to compare the mean values of the remaining morphological parameters between the same groups. If the corresponding differences were significant, a similar conclusion was drawn. p-Values less than .05 were considered indicative of significant differences.

5.3 RESULTS

The geometric modeling technique quantified spherical surface curvature with an accuracy of 96%, cylindrical surface curvature with an accuracy of 97%, and measured surface area and volume with accuracies of 92 and 89%, respectively. The technique used was able to assemble the MR images into 3D volumes with a coefficient of variation (COV), a measurement of precision of 0.19%, geometrically model the 3D volumes with a COV of 0.14%, calculate the surface areas with a COV of 0.30%, and compute bone volumes with a COV of 0.40%.[27]

The talus, calcaneus, navicular, and cuboid in the surgically treated clubfeet were smaller in volume (20–36% less, $p < .001$) and had less total surface area (16–28%, $p < .002$) than the corresponding bones in the contralateral normal feet (Table 5.1 and Table 5.2). The areas of the articulating surfaces of the distal tibia, talus, and navicular in the surgically treated clubfeet were also smaller (25–40% less, $p < .05$) than those in the contralateral normal feet (Table 5.3). Mean articulating surface areas in the surgically treated feet of the calcanei at the posterior subtalar joints and the cuboids at the calcaneocuboid joints trended slightly less (Table 5.3) than the corresponding values in the controls. No difference was observed at the calcaneocuboid joint (Table 5.3).

Radii of the cylinders and spheres, which were used to model the curvature of each articular surface, were the basis from which other morphological parameters were derived and subsequent comparisons made (Table 5.4). Mean values for the articulating surface areas of the talus and tibia in the tibiotalar joints of the surgically treated feet and contralateral normal feet are shown in Table 5.5. Treated clubfoot-related differences in articulating surface length on an absolute and differential

TABLE 5.1

Comparison of the Average Tarsal Volumes in the Contralateral Normal and the Unilateral Surgically Treated Adolescent Clubfoot

Bone	Volume (mm³)		Percent Difference	p-Value
	Clinically Normal	Surgically Treated		
Talus	37,822 ± 8,057	24,299 ± 6,228	35.8	.001
Calcaneus	60,364 ± 18,240	46,301 ± 13,102	23.3	.001
Navicular	9374 ± 2829	7426 ± 2683	20.8	<.001
Cuboid	12,591 ± 3,060	10,017 ± 2,257	20.4	.001

TABLE 5.2

Comparison of the Average Tarsal Surface Area in the Contralateral Normal and the Unilateral Surgically Treated Adolescent Clubfoot

Tarsal Surface Area (mm²)	Clinically Normal	Surgically Treated	Percent Difference	p-value
Talus	6812 ± 1170	4889 ± 959	28.2	<.001
Calcaneus	9807 ± 2383	7932 ± 1743	19.1	.002
Navicular	2676 ± 647	2231 ± 641	16.7	.002
Cuboid	3018 ± 609	2540 ± 481	15.8	.001

TABLE 5.3

Comparison of the Average Tarsal Articular Surface Area in the Contralateral Normal and the Unilateral Surgically Treated Adolescent Clubfoot

Articular Surface Area (mm²)	Clinically Normal	Surgically Treated	Percent Difference	p-Value
Talus, tibiotalar joint	1107 ± 328	666 ± 245	39.9	.043
Tibia, tibiotalar joint	661 ± 173	484 ± 127	26.9	.005
Talus, talonavicular joint	783 ± 115	587 ± 148	25.0	.009
Navicular, talonavicular joint	487 ± 136	354 ± 139	27.3	.004
Talus, posterior subtalar joint	487 ± 114	335 ± 116	31.2	.027
Calcaneus, posterior subtalar joint	512 ± 120	459 ± 149	10.4	NS
Calcaneus, calcaneocuboid joint	536 ± 120	532 ± 145	0.8	NS
Cuboid, calcaneocuboid joint	537 ± 141	502 ± 114	6.5	NS

Note: NS, not specified.

TABLE 5.4
Comparison of Articular Surface Curvature in the Contralateral Normal and Unilateral Surgically Treated Adolescent Clubfoot

Articular Surface	Curvature (mm)		Percent Difference	p-Value
	Clinically Normal	Surgically Treated		
Talus, tibiotalar	22.3 ± 1.5	20.5 ± 1.7	8.1	.068
Tibia, tibiotalar	28.8 ± 3.8	27.8 ± 11.0	3.6	NS
Talus, talonavicular	17.2 ± 2.7	22.2 ± 7.4	29.2	NS
Navicular, talonavicular	21.0 ± 1.9	30.7 ± 12.8	46.3	.070
Talus, talonavicular greater curvature	18.2 ± 3.1	22.9 ± 8.9	26.0	NS
Navicular, talonavicular greater curvature	20.2 ± 2.3	36.7 ± 17.1	82.2	NS
Talus, talonavicular lesser curvature	15.2 ± 1.7	22.8 ± 12.1	49.6	NS
Navicular, talonavicular lesser curvature	19.4 ± 2.6	40.7 ± 37.6	109.8	NS
Talus, posterior subtalar	24.3 ± 8.3	36.1 ± 14.1	48.5	NS
Calcaneus, posterior subtalar	21.4 ± 6.2	23.9 ± 6.6	11.5	NS
Talus, anterior/middle subtalar	13.6 ± 3.1	14.0 ± 3.8	2.6	NS.
Calcaneus, anterior/middle subtalar	25.3 ± 4.0	21.7 ± 4.9	14.3	NS
Calcaneus, calcaneocuboid vertical	17.2 ± 5.2	25.5 ± 4.3	48.3	.059
Cuboid, calcaneocuboid vertical	19.8 ± 5.3	20.3 ± 6.8	2.8	NS
Calcaneus, calcaneocuboid transverse	18.6 ± 7.1	18.9 ± 7.2	1.2	NS
Cuboid, calcaneocuboid. transverse	18.8 ± 3.2	26.0	NA	NA

Note: NS, not specified; NA, not applicable

(78.4%) basis are clearly attributable to shape alterations in the talus, but not in the tibia (Table 5.5). The navicular in the clubfeet were also flatter than those in the contralateral normal feet. The mean navicular flattening index in the surgically treated clubfeet was 85.7% larger ($p = .029$) than those of the contralateral normal feet (Table 5.5). In the surgically treated foot, the talus was flatter, as quantified by the talar flattening index, which trended ($p = .062$) 15.4% larger than the value for the contralateral normal foot. One of the subjects in this study displayed a talus with a true "flat top" (Figure 5.4).

TABLE 5.5

Comparison of the Morphologic Parameters in the Contralateral Normal and Unilateral Surgically Treated Adolescent Clubfoot

Morphological Parameter	Clinically Normal	Surgically Treated	Percent Difference	*p*-Value
Tibiotalar joint misalignment	4.76° ± 3.47°	7.64° ± 4.01°	60.6	NS
Posterior subtalar joint misalignment	11.96° ± 8.63°	16.77° ± 13.99°	40.2	NS
Talus articular surface length, tibiotalar joint	38.70 ± 8.32 mm	28.72 ± 5.35 mm	25.8	.029
Tibia articular surface length, tibiotalar joint	29.34 ± 3.65 mm	26.70 ± 3.78 mm	9.0	NS
Difference in tibiotalar articular surface length	9.36 ± 5.14 mm	2.02 ± 2.94 mm	78.4	.011
Talar dome flattening index	0.377 ± 0.035	0.435 ± 0.064	15.4	.062
Navicular flattening index	0.748 ± 0.154	1.389 ± 0.665	85.7	.029

Note: NS, not specified.

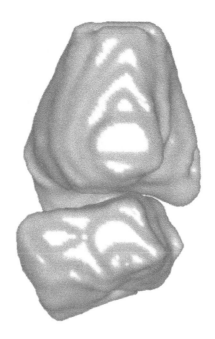

FIGURE 5.4 Three-dimensional computer reconstruction of a "flattened talus" from a subject's surgically treated clubfoot.

5.4 DISCUSSION

Although it has been established that clubfeet are smaller than contralateral normal feet, the results of this study provide new 3D quantitative information regarding the shape and size of the hindfoot complex. The talus, calcaneus, navicular, and cuboid in the unilateral surgically treated clubfoot were significantly smaller in surface area (20–36%) and volume (16–24%) than the corresponding tarsals in the contralateral normal foot. Also, the articular surfaces of the distal tibia, talus, and navicular in the clubfoot were smaller (27–40%) and flatter (up to 86%). This documented discrepancy in shape and size is part of the pathology of clubfeet. The long-term effect of treatment on morphology is not well described. The present quantitative morphological data, obtained from adolescents, complements the morphological and architectural data Itohara et al. obtained from 5-month-old infants[22] and the CT-based 3D architectural and qualitative shape data presented by Ippolito et al.[19]

The morphological data presented are consistent with the findings of prior anatomic studies. Stindel et al.[39] used MR reconstruction to calculate tarsal volumes in ten normal adult feet. They noted that the mean (± SD) volume of the talus, calcaneus, navicular, and cuboid were 36,380 mm³ ± 7,773 mm³, 66,719 mm³ ± 15,653 mm³, 10,787 mm³ ± 2,675 mm³, and 12,208 mm³ ± 2,260 mm³, respectively. Considering normal variability and the expected size difference between the adult and adolescent tarsals, their results are in excellent agreement (4–15% difference) with the values presented here.

Two different studies by Cahuzac et al.[28,31] used MR reconstruction to compare the size of the tarsal ossific nuclei in the contralateral normal and unilateral infant clubfoot. They noted that the mean volume of the talar, calcaneal, and navicular ossification centers in the infant clubfeet were 40, 20, and 15% smaller, respectively, than those of the contralateral normal foot. The magnitude of these differences (35.8, 23.3, and 20.8%, respectively), although they measure only the ossific nuclei, is consistent with the differences obtained from the present study. A similar study by Itohara et al.[22,40] also reported similar findings.

Sarrafian[34] determined that the mean curvature of the trochlea in the adult talus was 20 mm and this is consistent with the results (22.3 mm ± 1.5 mm) presently reported from the normal foot. Laidlaw[41] reported that the average curvature of the posterior facet in the adult calcaneus was 30 mm (range: 12–40 mm); this is also in line with the present results (21.4 ± 6.2 mm). Despite the large differences in means, no statistically significant differences were detected in articular surface curvatures between the tarsals from the contralateral normal and surgically treated clubfeet. This was likely due to the small sample sizes and large variability of this measurement as note by the size of the standard deviations.

Hjelmstedt and Sahlstedt[35,42] reported a value for the talar flattening index in the normal foot (0.365 ± 0.045) and this value is within 3.3% of the value (0.377 ± 0.035) presently determined for the contralateral normal foot. Bach et al.[38] measured the mean talar flattening index of nine treated clubfeet (0.597, range = 0.31–1.33) and, given the small sample sizes of both studies and the intrinsic variability of club foot morphology, this value is consistent with that presently reported (0.435 ± 0.064). Two independent studies[43,44] found talar flattening in only 1.5% of clubfeet, whereas other reports[45,46] noted talar flattening in 68 and 74% of subjects, respectively. This discrepancy may be due to differences in measurement technique, parallax errors of radiographic visualization and interpretation, or small sample size fluctuations. Although the present study made no attempt to estimate the incidence of talar flattening, it presents a methodology that will obviate the errors inherent in 2D radiographs.

A minor limitation to the accuracy of the present technique is its dependence upon the resolution of the MR images and the technician's ability to discern and outline the images from which the software assembles and geometrically models the bone volumes. A slightly more important limitation concerns the actual geometric models used. Spheres, cylinders, and planes are merely first approximations to the complex articular surface anatomy. More complex shapes (conic sections, parabolas, etc.) may fit better, but also introduce complexities of description and comparison that were considered unfavorable trade-offs, and thus were not considered further. It is important to note that only the subchondral bone surface was modeled, rather than the actual articulating cartilage surface. This is not a major concern as long as subchondral bone shape reflects cartilage shape. Subsequent research efforts should pursue a 3D reconstruction of articular cartilage morphology with comparable shape modeling and quantification.

In conclusion, described here is a technique to use MR images to construct 3D models of nonosseous structures. This allows for 3D modeling of the developing foot of the infant, child, adolescent, and adult as the proportion of cartilage and bone changes with growth. The 3D parameters developed allow for the accurate documentation of morphologic changes and alterations in articular surface shape. The method provides a tool to quantify changes in the growing foot, as influenced by pathology and/or treatment.

REFERENCES

1. Settle, G., The anatomy of congenital talipes equinovarus: sixteen dissected specimens. *J Bone Joint Surg,* 1963; 45A:1341–1354.
2. Irani, R.N., Sherman M.S., The pathological anatomy of idiopathic clubfoot. *Clin Orthop Relat Res,* 1972; 84:14–20.
3. Carroll, N.C., McMurtry, R., Leete, S.F., The pathoanatomy of congenital clubfoot. *Orthop Clin North Am,* 1978; 9(1):225–232.
4. Shapiro, F., Glimcher, M.J., Gross and histological abnormalities of the talus in congenital clubfoot. *J Bone Joint Surg [Am],* 1979; 61(4):522–530.
5. Hootnick, D.R., et al., Confirmation of arterial deficiencies in a limb with necrosis following clubfoot surgery. *J Pediatr Orthop B,* 1999; 8(3):187–193.
6. Katz, M.A., et al., Plain radiographic evaluation of the pediatric foot and its deformities. *Univ Pa Orthop J,* 1997; 10:30–39.
7. Roye, B.D., et al., Patient-based outcomes after clubfoot surgery. *J Pediatr Orthop,* 2001; 21(1):42–49.
8. Beatson, T.R., Pearson J.R., A method of assessing correction in club feet. *J Bone Joint Surg Br,* 1966; 48(1):40–50.
9. Simons, G.W., Analytical radiography of club feet. *J Bone Joint Surg Br,* 1977; 59B(4):485–489.

10. Aronson, J., Puskarich C.L., Deformity and disability from treated clubfoot. *J Pediatr Orthop,* 1990; 10(1):109–119.
11. Herbsthofer, B., et al., Significance of radiographic angle measurements in evaluation of congenital clubfoot. *Arch Orthop Trauma Surg,* 1998; 117(6–7):324–329.
12. Heywood, A.W.B., The mechanics of the hindfoot in clubfoot as demonstrated radiographically. *J Bone Joint Surg,* 1964; 46B:102–107.
13. Price, C.T., Congenital clubfoot. *J Fla Med Assoc,* 1979; 66(1):104–107.
14. Templeton, A.W., McAlister, W.H., Zim, I.D., Standardization of terminology and evaluation of osseous relationships in congenitally abnormal feet. *Am J Roentgenol Radium Ther Nucl Med,* 1965; 93:374–381.
15. Vanderwilde, R., et al., Measurements on radiographs of the foot in normal infants and children. *J Bone Joint Surg Am,* 1988; 70(3):407–415.
16. Johnston, C.E., II, et al., Three-dimensional analysis of clubfoot deformity by computed tomography. *J Pediatr Orthop B,* 1995; 4(1):39–48.
17. Huppert, B.J., et al., Single-shot fast spin-echo MR imaging of the fetus: a pictorial essay. *Radiographics,* 1999; 19:S215–S227.
18. Ippolito, E., et al., A comparison of resultant subtalar joint pathology with functional results in two groups of clubfoot patients treated with two different protocols. *J Pediatr Orthop B,* 2005;14(5):358–361.
19. Ippolito, E., et al., The influence of treatment on the pathology of club foot. CT study at maturity. *J Bone Joint Surg Br,* 2004; 86(4):574–580.
20. Ippolito, E., et al., A radiographic comparative study of two series of skeletally mature clubfeet treated by two different protocols. *Skeletal Radiol,* 2003; 32(8):446–453.
21. Ippolito, E., et al., Long-term comparative results in patients with congenital clubfoot treated with two different protocols. *J Bone Joint Surg Am,* 2003; 85A(7):1286–1294.
22. Itohara, T., et al., Assessment of talus deformity by three-dimensional MRI in congenital clubfoot. *Eur J Radiol,* 2005; 53(1):78–83.
23. Itohara, T., et al., Assessment of the three-dimensional relationship of the ossific nuclei and cartilaginous anlagen in congenital clubfoot by 3-D MRI. *J Orthop Res,* 2005; 23(5):1160–1164.
24. Roche, C., et al., Three-dimensional hindfoot motion in adolescents with surgically treated unilateral clubfoot. *J Pediatr Orthop,* 2005; 25(5):630–634.
25. Ippolito, E., et al., Validity of the anteroposterior talocalcaneal angle to assess congenital clubfoot correction. *AJR Am J Roentgenol,* 2004; 182(5):1279–1282.
26. Saito, S., et al., Evaluation of calcaneal malposition by magnetic resonance imaging in the infantile clubfoot. *J Pediatr Orthop B,* 2004; 13(2):99–102.
27. Talwalkar, V., et al. Quantifying 3D Motion of the Pediatric Hindfoot in Treated Clubfoot by Magnetic Resonance Imaging, Pediatric Orthopaedic Society of North America. 2002. Salt Lake City, Utah.
28. Cahuzac, J.P., et al., Assessment of the position of the navicular by three-dimensional magnetic resonance imaging in infant foot deformities. *J Pediatr Orthop B,* 2002; 11(2):134–138.
29. Pekindil, G., et al., Magnetic resonance imaging in follow-up of treated clubfoot during childhood. *Eur J Radiol,* 2001; 37(2):123–129.
30. Sullivan, R.J., Davidson, R.S., When does the flat-top talus lesion occur in idiopathic clubfoot? Evaluation with magnetic resonance imaging at three months of age. *Foot Ankle Int,* 2001; 22(5):422–425.
31. Cahuzac, J.P., et al., Assessment of hindfoot deformity by three-dimensional MRI in infant club foot. *J Bone Joint Surg Br,* 1999; 81(1):97–101.

32. Mattingly, B., et al., Three-dimensional in vivo motion of adult hind foot bones. *J Biomech,* 2005. Published on-line (16 February 2005).

33. Sarrafian, S., *Anatomy of the Foot and Ankle*. Philadelphia: J.B. Lippincott, 1993.

34. Hjelmstedt, A., Sahlstedt, B., Talar deformity in congenital clubfeet. An anatomical and functional study with special reference to the ankle joint mobility. *Acta Orthop Scand,* 1974; 45(4):628–640.

35. Carroll, N.C., Congenital clubfoot: pathoanatomy and treatment. *Instr Course Lect,* 1987; 36:117–121.

36. Pirani, S., Zeznik, L., Hodges, D., Magnetic resonance imaging study of the congenital clubfoot treated with the Ponseti method. *J Pediatr Orthop,* 2001; 21(6):719–726.

37. Bach, C.M., et al., Significance of talar distortion for ankle mobility in idiopathic clubfoot. *Clin Orthop Relat Res,* 2002; (398):196–202.

38. Stindel, E., et al., 3D MR image analysis of the morphology of the rear foot: application to classification of bones. *Comput Med Imaging Graph,* 1999; 23(2):75–83.

39. Itohara, T., et al., Assessment of the three dimensional relationship of the ossific nuclei and cartilaginous anlages in congenital clubfoot by 3-D MRI. 51st Annual Meeting of the Orthopaedic Research Society, Washington, D.C., 2005.

40. Laidlaw, P.P., The varieties of the os calcis. *J Anat Physiol,* 1904; 38:133.

41. Hjelmstedt, E.A.,Sahlstedt, B., Arthrography as a guide in the treatment of congenital clubfoot. Findings and treatment results in a consecutive series. *Acta Orthop Scand,* 1980; 51(2):321–334.

42. Dunn, H.K., Samuelson, K.M., Flat-top talus. A long-term report of twenty club feet. *J Bone Joint Surg Am,* 1974; 56(1):57–62.

43. Keim, H.A., Ritchie, G.W., "Nutcracker" treatment of clubfoot. JAMA, 1964; 189: 613–615.

44. Cooper, D.M., Dietz, F.R., Treatment of idiopathic clubfoot. A thirty-year follow-up note. *J Bone Joint Surg Am,* 1995; 77(10):1477–1489.

45. Hutchins, P.M., et al., Long-term results of early surgical release in club feet. *J Bone Joint Surg Br,* 1985; 67(5):791–799.

6 Dynamic Foot Pressure in the Early Evolution of Foot Deformities in Children with Spastic Cerebral Palsy

Chris Church, Nancy Lennon, Scott Coleman, John Henley, Mary Nagai, and Freeman Miller

CONTENTS

6.1 INTRODUCTION

Children with spastic cerebral palsy (CP) are at risk for developing a mixture of foot deformities as they mature. Although CP is caused by a static encephalopathy, the associated musculoskeletal pathology is dynamic and influenced by a number of factors. Factors that may contribute to the deformities of the feet and ankles include spasticity, muscle imbalance, contracture, bony torsion, joint instability, and disordered biomechanics during weight-bearing and ambulation.[1] Although there is a general consensus regarding the principles of management of the foot and ankle in children with CP, there is little agreement on the specifics of orthopaedic intervention.

The majority of flexible foot and ankle deformities can be conservatively treated with appropriate shoe selection or bracing. However, orthopedic surgeons have many different opinions with regards to the optimal brace choice for a given foot and ankle deformity.[2–7]

Many children with CP ultimately develop stiff, painful, and unbraceable foot and ankle deformities. Foot and ankle surgeries account for approximately 25 to 30% of all surgical procedures performed on ambulatory children with CP to improve their gait function.[8] As with the conservative management of these foot and ankle deformities, little consensus exists regarding the optimal surgical procedures to correct the various foot and ankle deformities observed in these patients. Numerous soft-tissue releases and tendon transfers have been described in the literature to correct both flexible and stiff foot and ankle deformities seen in children with CP.[9–11] The correction of stiff foot and ankle deformities frequently requires a combination of soft-tissue proce-dure(s), an osteotomy, and a joint fusion. Furthermore, the optimal timing for the surgical treatment of these severe foot and ankle deformities is unknown.[8,12–16]

The lack of agreement in the literature regarding the nonsurgical and surgical treatment of foot and ankle deformities in children with CP reflects the current lack of knowledge of the natural history of these foot and ankle deformities in this population. Presently, the impact of nonsurgical and surgical treatment on the natural history of the dynamic foot and ankle deformities in these children is unknown. The purpose of this prospective study is to document the natural history of dynamic foot and ankle deformities seen in young children with CP, using the technology in the gait analysis lab.

6.2 MATERIAL AND METHODS

6.2.1 SUBJECTS

Subjects included 10 typically developing 2-yr-olds and 51 children with CP between 21 and 42 months (average age, 32 ± 6 months). Thirty-five subjects with CP com-pleted a 6-month follow-up (38 ± 6 months old), and 19 completed a 1-yr follow-up (44 ± 6 months old). Subjects had a wide variety of baseline function. Children were included with spastic hemiplegia ($n = 12$), diplegia ($n = 34$), and quadriplegia ($n = 5$), who were able to ambulate with or without an assistive device. Gross Motor Function Classification System scores varied from I to IV (I, $n = 27$; II, $n = 14$; III, $n = 8$; IV, $n = 2$).[17] Subjects' involved feet were considered individually with $n = 90$ for initial visit, $n = 61$ for the 6-month follow-up, $n = 33$ for the 1-yr follow-up, and $n = 20$ for typically developing 2-yr-olds. Testing protocol involved videotaping gait, dynamic foot pressure recordings, physical exam, parent questionnaire, and Gross Motor Function Measure section D. This chapter focuses on the dynamic foot pressure results.

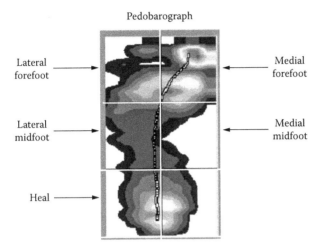

FIGURE 6.1 Foot pressure data divided into the five areas for analysis.

6.2.2 Foot Pressure

Dynamic foot pressure during walking was collected for three right and three left gait cycles on each subject using the Tekscan HR Mat measurement system (Boston, MA) and was analyzed using laboratory-specific software. A coronal plane pressure index (CPPI) was utilized to identify dynamic foot valgus or varus pressure patterns during walking. This measurement technique and its validation have been previously described in the *Journal of Pediatric Orthopedics*.[13]

To calculate the CPPI, the foot pressure data are rotated using the software to align the long axis of the foot with the line of forward progression. The model next separates the foot into three equal length segments (hindfoot, midfoot, and forefoot). There is another split into medial and lateral halves (Figure 6.1).

The summated pressure over stance phase for each segment is monitored as well as the time–pressure integral or impulse of each segment. From these data, the CPPI is calculated from the impulses recorded from the lateral forefoot (LF), medial forefoot (MF), lateral midfoot (LM), and medial midfoot (MM) as follows:

$$CPPI = \frac{(MM + MF) - (LM + LF)}{MM + MF + LM + LF} \times 100$$

6.2.3 Statistics

Statistical analysis was completed by grouping subjects and by analyzing subjects individually due to the subjects' wide spectrum of initial walking status and high degree of variability in foot pressure patterns. Subjects (both typically developing 2-yr-olds, and subjects with CP) were compared to a normal database established from 50 typically developing children (age range 4 to 18 yr). Z-tests were used to compare groups as a whole to the normal population. Individual children were considered to have made significant change, or a significant abnormality was considered to be present, if a z-score change of greater than 0.8 was seen. Feet were considered valgus if the CPPI z-score was 0.8 or higher, and varus if the CPPI z-score was -0.8 or lower. Trend analyses were also completed using repeated-measures ANOVAs.

6.3 RESULTS

6.3.1 CHILDREN WITH NORMAL DEVELOPMENT

Significant differences in dynamic pressure patterns during walking were observed between typically developing 2-yr-olds and normal reference values for older children (age 4 to 18 yr). The 2-yr-old children have a greater tendency for valgus foot pressure patterns with a higher CPPI ($p = .002$, average z-score 0.76), higher pressure in the MM segment ($p = .003$), lower pressure in the LF segment ($p = .001$), lower pressure in the LM ($p = .006$), and decreased pressure in the MF ($p = .027$). Typically developing 2-yr-olds demonstrate limited progression of weight onto the forefoot as a whole compared to normal children age 4 to 18 yr (Figure 6.2).

Additionally, the average pressure impulse in the heel segment is normal, but the 2-yr-olds have a higher degree of variability in the timing to heel rise, ranging from initiation of heel rise at 20 to 90% of stance phase.

6.3.2 CHILDREN WITH CP

6.3.2.1 Initial Visit for Subjects with CP

The dynamic foot pressure patterns of the subjects with CP at initial evaluation reveal a strong tendency toward valgus distribution, similar to that found in the group of typically developing 2-yr-olds, compared to a normal population of children age 4 to 18 yr.

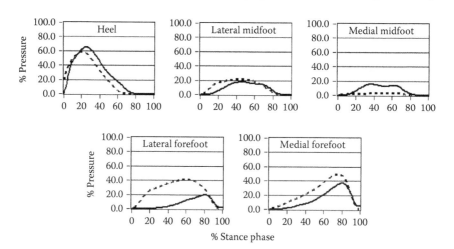

FIGURE 6.2 Two-year-old typically developing children demonstrate valgus foot pressure patterns compared to 4- to 18-yr-old children (Solid line indicates 2-yr-old norms; dashed line indicates 4- to 18-yr-old norms). Pressure on the Y-axis is normalized to the maximum pressure recorded from the foot pressure data.

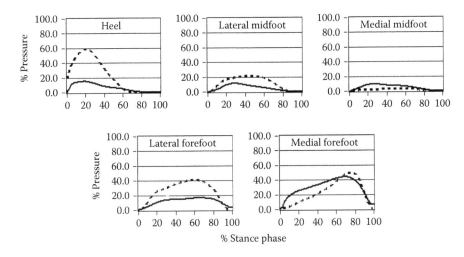

FIGURE 6.3 Children with CP age 2 to 3 yr show a strong tendency toward valgus foot pressure (Solid line indicates subjects with CP at their initial evaluation; dashed line indicates 4- to 18-yr-old norms).

The mean CPPI value for our subjects' (with CP) feet was two standard deviations above the normal mean ($p = .001$). Figure 6.3 demonstrates the average pressure distribution for subjects with CP at their initial evaluation. Significantly high MM and MF pressure, and low LM and forefoot pressure were present ($p = .001$ for all values).

Of the 51 subjects with CP that completed the initial visit, 80% had valgus foot position during walking, 2% had varus position, and 18% had neither varus nor valgus disposition. Similar effects were seen regardless of diagnosis (Figure 6.4).

A significantly high prevalence of "toe-walking" was also noted with 86% of feet analyzed demonstrating reduced heel contact ($p = .001$).

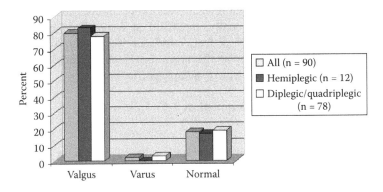

FIGURE 6.4 Valgus tendency is present regardless of initial diagnosis in subjects with CP.

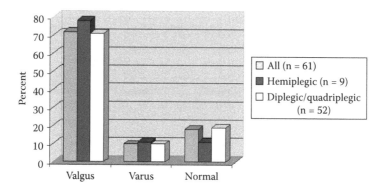

FIGURE 6.5 Valgus tendency continues regardless of initial diagnosis at 6-month follow-up in subjects with CP.

6.3.2.2 Dynamic Foot Development at 6-Month Follow-Up for Subjects with CP

The valgus foot pressure distribution continues in the subjects at the 6-month follow-up evaluation regardless of initial diagnosis (Figure 6.5). CPPI continues to be significantly more valgus than in the normal population ($p = .001$). MM pressure continues to be significantly increased, and LM and forefoot pressures continue to be significantly decreased compared to normal ($p = .001$ for all values). MF pressure continues to be elevated, but significance is questionable ($p = .039$).

Repeated-measures ANOVA testing shows that CPPI tends to move in the varus direction ($p = .033$), with increasing pressure on the lateral side of the foot and decreasing pressure on the medial side, regardless of initial foot position, similar to the trend found in children with normal development. Trends were found when analyzing changes in impulses in the specific sections of the foot, but none of these were found to be significant. MM ($p = 0.41$) and forefoot ($p = 0.11$) pressures tended to decrease from the initial evaluation to the 6-month follow-up. LM ($p = .094$) and forefoot ($p = .086$) pressures tended to increase at the 6-month reevaluation compared to pressures recorded at the initial evaluation. Significance was likely limited by the wide variety of our patient population, small number of subjects, and small effect size.

Looking at patients individually, the CPPI at 6-month follow-up showed increased lateral pressure in 31% of feet considered, increased medial pressure in 10%, and no change in 54%. Similar effects are seen if feet are divided up by initial classification (hemiplegic or diplegic/quadraplegic; Table 6.1).

6.3.2.3 Dynamic Foot Development at 1-Yr Follow-Up in Subjects with CP

The valgus foot pressure distribution continues in the subjects at the 1-yr follow-up evaluation regardless of initial diagnosis (Figure 6.6). CPPI continues to be significantly more valgus than the normal population ($p = .001$). MM pressure continues to be significantly increased ($p = .12$), and LM and forefoot pressures continue to

TABLE 6.1
CPPI Tends to Demonstrate Increased Lateral Pressure at 6-Month Follow-Up, Compared to Initial Evaluation in Subjects with CP

	All ($n = 61$)	Hemipleic ($n = 9$)	Di/Quadriplegic ($n = 52$)
Increased lateral pressure	19/61 = 31%	2/9 = 22%	17/52 = 33%
Increased medial pressure	7/61 = 11%	0/9 = 0%	7/52 = 13%
No change	35/61 = 57%	7/9 = 78%	28/52 = 54%

be significantly decreased compared to normal ($p = .001$). MF pressure continues to be elevated, but no longer to a significant level ($p = .091$).

When looking at individual foot segments, repeated-measures ANOVA analysis shows a significant trend with increasing pressure in the LF ($p = .004$) over the course of the year. Other trends in the variables considered were found to be insignificant, though there was a trend showing decreasing MM pressure over the year ($p = .16$).

When looking at the foot as a whole, at the 6-month visit, the CPPI showed some tendency toward more lateral pressure, but at the 1-yr follow-up there seemed to be no pattern evident though the majority of the subjects with CP continue to have valgus pressure distribution (Table 6.2).

6.3.2.4 Variability

Variability was determined by averaging the standard deviations of the subjects CPPI values for three recorded foot pressure measurements. These values were analyzed using the data from the children who completed all three evaluations (initial, 6 months, and 1-yr follow-up). Mean variability in subjects' CPPI, who have CP, at

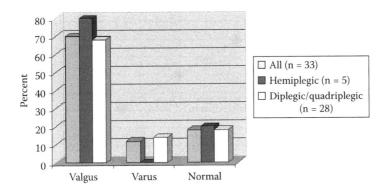

FIGURE 6.6 Valgus tendency is present regardless of initial diagnosis at 1-yr follow-up in subjects with CP.

TABLE 6.2

Changes in CPPI at 1-Yr Follow-Up Compared to 6-Month Follow-Up in Subjects with CP

	All ($n = 33$)	Hemipleic ($n = 5$)	Di/Quadriplegic ($n = 28$)
Increased lateral pressure	6/33 = 18%	1/5 = 20%	5/28 = 18%
Increased medial pressure	11/33 = 33%	1/5 = 20%	10/28 = 36%
No change	16/33 = 8%	3/5 = 60%	13/28 = 46%

initial visit is 17.1 ± 11.6. Mean variability in normal 2-yr-olds is 18.3 ± 11.9. Mean variability in the normal 4- to 18-yr-old population is 14.8 ± 6.0. Variability tends to decrease over the course of time from initial evaluation (17.1 ± 11.6) to 6 months (16.3 ± 9.4) and 1-yr follow-up (14.1 ± 9.7; Figure 6.7). Upon the initial evaluation, children with the most severely involved feet ($n = 27$; children with valgus feet greater than three standard deviations from normal values) showed less variability (13.5 ± 8.5; Figure 6.8).

Variability in foot pressure distribution seems to decrease with age and is decreased in feet with greater deformity.

6.3.2.5 Botox and Surgical Intervention

A small number of subjects underwent Botox injections ($n = 2$, four involved feet), or surgical intervention ($n = 3$, six involved feet) during the study. In the subjects receiving Botox in their gastrocnemius muscles, 50% showed increases in valgus foot positioning by greater than one standard deviation.

In the children undergoing surgical intervention (one bilateral Achilles tendon lengthenings, two bilateral hip adductor and hamstring lengthenings), 83% of feet

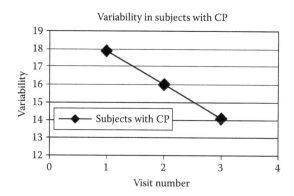

FIGURE 6.7 Variability seems to decrease with age in children with CP. Visit 1 = initial evaluation, visit 2 = 6-month follow-up, visit 3 = 1-year follow-up.

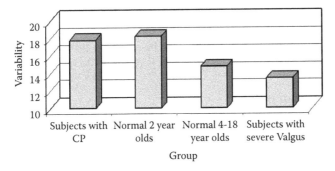

FIGURE 6.8 Variability of dynamic foot pressure appears to be dependent on age and severity of foot deformity.

showed an increase in valgus pressure distribution. While the number of subjects was very small, it suggests the need for further research to determine the effects of Botox and surgical intervention on foot pressure distribution.

6.4 DISCUSSION

Findings from this longitudinal study demonstrate that dynamic foot pressure patterns are still evolving in typically developing 2-yr-old children as demonstrated by the differences in this group compared to a group with mature walking patterns. This finding is consistent with the work of Sutherland and colleagues[18], who identified the changes in temporal–spatial and kinematic patterns before age four and described their relationship to maturational processes. It appears that these processes also influence the normal development of dynamic foot pressure distribution during walking. A similar phenomenon also appears to be present in young children with CP during the early development of walking. Findings from this study also reveal that a large percentage of children with CP demonstrate a trend towards improvement in early pes valgus.

The natural history of foot position in both children with normal development and children with CP changes rapidly in early childhood, which has implications in the development of plan of care. The presence of valgus foot position is quite prevalent in both typically developing new walkers and young children with CP. A large percentage of children with CP demonstrate improvement in the degree of weight-bearing foot valgus during the early maturation of walking. At the 1-yr follow-up, the average subject with CP continued to have moderate planovalgus, so perhaps this trend for planovalgus resolution is delayed or interrupted in children with CP. One-year follow-up seems to show some children with CP continue to have improvements in their dynamic foot position (i.e., decreasing valgus), but some children show no improvement, and some also show progressive deformity. Further research is required to determine what factors determine which progression, and eventually what interventions, would be beneficial. Further analysis is indicated to correlate motor function, spasticity, range of motion, and other factors with the dynamic foot development.

Further study is also required to determine at what point children with hemiplegia develop more typical equinovarus presentation. Use of Botox in the ankle plantarflexors and surgical intervention in the LE seem to be related to increasing valgus based on preliminary data presented. Further research is necessary to quantify this effect.

6.5 CONCLUSION

The current treatment of foot deformities in children with CP is inconsistent and informed decisions to develop plan of care are difficult to make without the knowledge of the natural history of the population. Foot position changes in early childhood in both children with normal development and children with CP. The trend in early development in both children with normal development and children with CP is to have some resolution of planovalgus foot position. Further research is indicated to describe factors that influence change in dynamic foot pressure.

REFERENCES

1. Muir D, Angliss, RD, Nattrass, GR, Graham HK. Tibiotalocalcaneal arthrodesis for severe calcaneovalgus deformity in cerebral palsy, *J Pediatr Orthop*, 25(5), 651–656, 2005.
2. Radtka SA, Skinner SR, Johanson ME. A comparison of gait with solid and hinged ankle-foot orthoses in children with spastic diplegic cerebral palsy, *Gait Posture*, 21(3), 303–310, 2005.
3. Buckon CE, Thomas SS, Jakobson-Huston S, Moor M, Sussman M, Aiona M. Comparison of three ankle-foot orthosis configurations for children with spastic diplegia, *Dev Med Child Neurol*, 46(9), 590–598, 2004.
4. Smiley SJ, Jacobsen FS, Mielke C, Johnston R, Park C, Ovaska GJ. A comparison of the effects of solid, articulated, and posterior leaf-spring ankle-foot orthoses and shoes alone on gait and energy expenditure in children with spastic diplegic cerebral palsy, *Orthopaedics*, 25(4), 411–415, 2002.
5. Radtka SA, Skinner SR, Dixon DM, Johanson ME. A comparison of gait with solid, dynamic, and no ankle-foot orthoses in children with spastic cerebral palsy, *Phys Ther*, 77(4), 395–409, 1997.
6. Crenshaw S, Herzog R, Castagno P, Richards J, Miller F, Michaloski G, Moran E. The efficacy of tone-reducing features in orthotics on the gait of children with spastic diplegic cerebral palsy, *J Pediatr Orthop*, 20(2), 210–216, 2000.
7. Carlson WE, Vaughan CL, Damiano DL, Abel MF. Orthotic management of gait in spastic diplegia, *Am J Phys Med Rehabil*, 76(3), 219–225, 1997.
8. Andreacchio A, Orellana CA, Miller F, Bowen TR. Lateral column lengthening as treatment for planovalgus foot deformity in ambulatory children with spastic cerebral palsy, *J Pediatr Orthop*, 20(4), 501–515, 2000.
9. Lyon R, Liu X, Schwab J, Harris G. Kinematic and kinetic evaluation of the ankle joint before and after tendo achilles lengthening in patients with spastic diplegia, *J. Pediatr Orthop*, 25(4), 479–482, 2005.
10. Moran MF, Sanders JO, Sharkey NA, Piazza SJ. Effect of attachment site and routing variations in split tendon transfer of tibialis posterior, *J Pediatr Orthop*, 24(3), 298–303, 2004.

11. Liggio FJ, Kruse R. Split tibialis posterior tendon transfer with concomitant distal tibial derotational osteotomy in children with cerebral palsy, *J Pediatr Orthop,* 21(1), 95–101, 2001.

12. Noritake K, Yoshihashi Y, Miyata T. Calcaneal lengthening for planovalgus foot deformity in children with spastic cerebral palsy, *J Pediatr Orthop B,* 14(4), 274–279, 2005.

13. Chang CH, Miller F, Schuyler J. Dynamic pedobarograph in evaluation of varus and valgus foot deformities, *J Pediatr Orthop,* 22(6), 813–818, 2002.

14. Chang CH, Albarracin JP, Lipton GE, Miller F. Long-term follow-up of surgery for equinovarus foot deformity in children with cerebral palsy, *J Pediatr Orthop,* 22(6), 792–799, 2002.

15. Davids JR, Mason TA, Danko A, Banks D, Blackhurst D. Surgical management of hallux valgus deformity in children with cerebral palsy, *J Pediatr Orthop,* 21(1), 89–94, 2001.

16. Miller F. *Cerebral Palsy.* 1st edition. Springer Science+Business Media, Inc, New York, 2005.

17. Palisano et al. Gross motor function classification system for cerebral palsy, *Dev Med Child Neurol,* 39, 214–223,1997.

18. Sutherland D, Olshen R, Bichen E, Wyatt M. *The Development of Mature Walking.* Cambridge University Press (1991).

7 Plantar Pressure-Based Quantitative Assessment of Subtalar Arthrodesis in the Rehabilitation of the Planovalgus Foot Deformity

Ziad O. Abu-Faraj, Gerald F. Harris, and Peter A. Smith

CONTENTS

7.1   INTRODUCTION

The human foot is a versatile biomechanical structure comprising 26 bones, 29 joints, 42 muscles, and a number of tendons and ligaments. In the lifetime of a normal individual, the foot travels anywhere between 100,000 and 160,000 km and is susceptible to varying forces/pressures with each footstep.[1] During the stance phase of walking, this extraordinary structure provides weight-bearing support, propulsive forces for locomotion, and shock absorption for distribution of impact forces during foot-to-ground contact.[2] Being the final segment in the lower extremity linkage system, the foot must transmit the forces of locomotion to the adjacent environment. To be effective, this transmission must be adapted to diversities in terrain while preserving both stability and load distribution.[3] Menkveld et al. described four functional tasks that are accomplished by the foot during stance: (i) acceptance of impact load at heel strike, (ii) terrain acclimation during weight acceptance, (iii) stability and load distribution during foot flat, and (iv) propulsion for forward progression during push-off.[4] To endure the consequences resulting from these difficult tasks, the foot and ankle complex must be structurally robust, yet reliable and stable.

A pathological foot is inevitably challenged in the performance of the above functional tasks with a resultant change in plantar load distribution. Consequently, there may develop focal areas of high pressure, which can affect stability and serve as sources of discomfort and pain. Such anomalies could be manifested in the following nonexclusive enumerative list of foot pathologies: pes planovalgus, pes cavus, talipes equinovarus (club foot), talipes calcaneovalgus, plantar fasciitis, metatarsus adductus, hallux valgus, hammer toe, claw toes, osteochondritis (Köhler's disease), and plantar interdigital neuroma (Morton's neuroma).

To better understand the biomechanics of the foot and the effectiveness of therapeutic and surgical interventions in the correction and treatment of foot disorders, it is essential to identify objective measures of foot dynamics. Ground reaction forces and plantar pressure measurements, whose characteristics have long been of interest to many investigators,[5–45] are fundamental to the study of foot dynamics, in both health and pathology. This chapter addresses the event-related alterations in plantar pressure distribution resulting from subtalar arthrodesis (fusion), which is a corrective and rehabilitative treatment of the planovalgus foot deformity secondary to cerebral palsy.[46–50]

7.2 PLANTAR PRESSURES: A CLINICAL BACKGROUND

Foot pathologies usually affect foot function and gait adversely. Hutton and Stokes reported that by studying the mechanical consequences of these pathologies, a better understanding of the progress of the disorders and a more refined evaluation of the effectiveness of therapeutic intervention was possible.[3] To date, several measurement techniques have been utilized in the study of the normal and pathological foot. The focus of these studies includes the anesthetic foot resulting from diabetes mellitus and Hansen's disease,[51–53] evaluation of therapeutic footwear for the insensitive foot,[54,55] distance running,[56] and orthopaedic walkers.[57] Plantar foot ulcers have been reported to be the primary cause of impairment in individuals with diabetes mellitus and leprosy.[52] In 1982, Brand stated that leprosy was the primary cause of loss of sensation in the foot in at least parts of the world such as Asia and Africa.[58] In 1993, Reiber reported that as many as 14 million individuals in the U.S. with diabetes will undergo pathological alterations in their lower extremities.[59] Also in 1993, Levin et al. reported an estimated 60,000 major amputations associated with diabetes in the U.S. each year.[60] In 1959, Kosiak carried out a series of experiments on 16 mongrel dogs in which he applied high pressures for short time intervals and low pressures repeated over longer periods.[61] Kosiak demonstrated that for ischemic ulceration, there is an inverse relationship between pressure and time, and that this relationship is hyperbolic. Brand reported that necrosis could result from small pressure if that pressure is maintained all day.[53] Brand also stated that the vast majority of all wounds and ulcers on insensitive feet are not generated by coincidental injury or by ischemia from continuous pressure, but from repetitive moderate stresses on the same part of the foot.[53,62] These occurrences are observed in patients with diabetes mellitus, leprosy, syringomyelia, spina bifida, and other sensory neuropathies.[62,63] Hence, by repeated measurements of plantar pressure distributed while ambulating in a natural setting for extended periods of time, one should be able to gain objective insight regarding plantar weight-bearing patterns indicative of the biomechanical transfer of load through the structure of the foot. Such measurements would allow one to identify areas of repetitive stress on the plantar surface of the normal and abnormal foot in an objective manner.

7.3 CEREBRAL PALSY AND THE PLANOVALGUS FOOT

In 1862, physician William John Little described the condition recognized at present as cerebral palsy.[64] Cerebral palsy is defined as a static encephalopathy representing a group of nonprogressive neuromuscular conditions caused by injury to the immature central nervous system during its early stages of development: fetal, perinatal, and infantile.[65] It is physically manifested by altered motor and sensory functions affecting posture and movement. Ever since Little's description, the intricate rehabilitative challenges that fall under this universal diagnosis have been addressed by patients as well as their families, medical practitioners, and healthcare professionals. These comprise, but are unquestionably not limited to, neurologists, orthopedists, developmental pediatricians, physical therapists, psychologists and psychiatrists, occupational and speech therapists, kinesiologists, and biomedical engineers.

The prevalence of cerebral palsy has not changed appreciably over the past two decades. This has been to the surprise of numerous investigators who have felt that the incidence should be decreasing. Although the incidence of cerebral palsy varies among different published reports, the most often quoted is 1.5 to 2.5 per 1000 live births.[66–68] The occurrence is higher in regions where there is insufficient prenatal care and accompanying prematurity. Several factors have been reported to contribute to the etiology of cerebral palsy. These include infections during pregnancy, head trauma at birth, head injury in childhood, anoxic brain damage, vascular accidents following treatment of brain tumor, involvement of the central nervous system from encephalitis, and other viral diseases.[69]

The anatomic location and severity of central nervous system injury determines the type and degree of involvement.[70] Hemiplegic involvement characterizes a child with one side affected, the arm more so than the leg. A diplegic child has equal involvement of the right and left sides with relative sparing of the upper extremities in comparison to the lower limbs. Quadriplegia or total body involvement refers to a child with all four limbs involved to a significant degree. Patients with diplegic and quadriplegic distribution frequently go on to develop planovalgus foot deformity, which is progressive and can be debilitating.[71–74]

Planovalgus foot deformity is characterized by valgus of the hindfoot and a pronated posture of the midfoot with a flattened longitudinal arch (Figure 7.1).

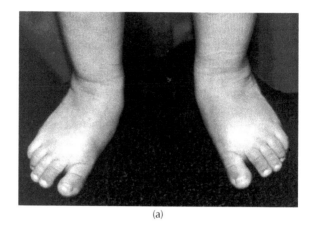

(a)

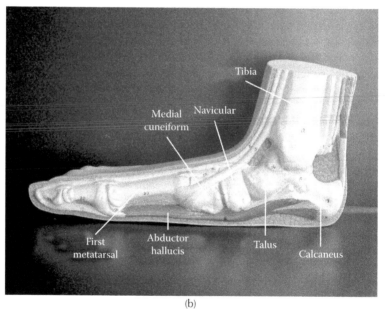

(b)

FIGURE 7.1 (a) Planovalgus foot deformity in a child with spastic cerebral palsy. The medial longitudinal arch is absent and the forefoot is pronated and deviates laterally. The medial midfoot is prominent. (b) A cast model (3B Scientific GmbH, Hamburg, Germany) revealing the medial section of the planovalgus foot.

Hindfoot valgus reflects a divergence of the longitudinal axis of the talus and the calcaneus in both the sagittal and transverse planes. The distal talus lies medial to the substance of the calcaneus. In the midfoot, the navicular slides laterally with respect to the talar head, with a corresponding shift of the calcaneal–cuboid joint. The talar head becomes prominent, both medially and plantarly, because the talus plantarflexes after losing the support of the plantar ligaments. The prominence normally causes discomfort during shoe wearing and calluses might develop.

Difficulties occurring comprise poor stance phase stability, shoe-wear problems, and impaired push-off power during ambulation.[71] The deformity is also commonly accompanied with hallux valgus at the metatarsophalangeal joint.[75]

Planovalgus foot deformity is thought to result from an imbalance in the evertors and invertors of the foot as a consequence of poor selective motor control. Surgical treatment focuses on subtalar joint stabilization to prevent excessive hindfoot valgus.[73,74,76] This could be achieved by limiting joint motion with a staple,[77] use of a polyethylene insert,[78] or fusion of the subtalar joint.[79–83] Osteotomies of the planovalgus foot are also performed, such as medial osteotomy of the calcaneus[84] or lateral column lengthening osteotomy of the calcaneus.[85,86] Rehabilitation after surgery is intended to provide better stance phase stability, swing phase foot clearance, and a more efficient walking pattern.

In most available studies, outcomes of subtalar arthrodesis are based upon subjective criteria with results ranging from 60 to 90% signifying *good* to *excellent*.[79–83,85,87] These studies depend only on reports of physical examination supplemented by radiographic analyses. The accuracy of these studies is limited by clinical assessment and relies on such vague criteria as *regular shoe wear* and *plantigrade foot*. There is no definition of what constitutes a *satisfactory* foot, and indisputably, there are no quantitative indices that can be used to describe results in a clinical series.

This study was designed to investigate the multistep dynamic plantar pressure distribution in hemiplegic and diplegic children and adolescents with cerebral palsy.[46–50] A group of children with planovalgus foot deformity secondary to spastic cerebral palsy was evaluated preoperatively and following subtalar arthrodesis for rehabilitation of the foot deformity. The key hypothesis behind this study was that an objective description of plantar foot dynamics would yield a better understanding of the biomechanics of the planovalgus foot, as well as providing a quantitative measure of the effectiveness of surgical intervention in the correction and rehabilitative treatment of this disorder.

7.4 MATERIALS AND METHODS

7.4.1 PLANTAR PRESSURE SYSTEM

A Holter-type, portable, microprocessor-based, in-shoe, plantar pressure data acquisition system was utilized to record the dynamic plantar pressure history in the pediatric population that participated in this study. The system has extended the recording and processing capacity necessary to monitor the long-term biomechanical characteristics addressed earlier. Moreover, these measurements provide the means for determining the effectiveness of corrections for the planovalgus deformity, both surgical and rehabilitative. System instrumentation has been described in previous works.[46–50,88–93]

The Holter-type system consists of 12 discrete conductive polymer pressure sensors. The unit is mounted in a $21 \times 12 \times 3$ cm^3 case, weighs less than 350 g, and is fully portable; children carry it in a belt-pack during free unrestricted ambulation. The system allows real-time recording of both pressure and temporal distance gait parameters for up to 2 hr during normal daily activities. The microprocessor employs custom software, written in C, which controls data acquisition and sensor calibration. Recorded plantar pressure and calibration data are uploaded into a personal computer (PC) for further processing, analysis, and display. This computer is used to initialize the portable unit and upload the recorded plantar pressure data and sensor calibration data. Additional PC software converts raw voltage data into pressure metrics, determines various gait parameters, conducts statistical analyses, and displays results.[90,92]

Plantar pressure data are sampled at a rate of 40 Hz (samples per second). The sampling rate was based on published and experimental studies.[94-96] Antonsson and Mann reported that 99% of the spectral power from barefoot walking across a Kistler force platform (Kistler Instrument Corp., Amherst, NY) was below 15 Hz, 98% below 10 Hz, and over 90% below 5 Hz. The authors stated that in order to preserve 99% of the signal power in gait, positional fidelity must be maintained up to 15 Hz, which for a sampled system requires a *minimum* sampling rate of 30 Hz.[94] In 1989, Acharya et al. reported similar findings for in-shoe plantar pressures.[95] In 1991, Zhu et al. conducted time–domain analyses to establish an adequate sampling rate for in-shoe plantar pressure measurements. The authors investigated a series of sampling frequencies ranging from 5 to 200 Hz. The authors reported that signals sampled at 20 Hz were not significantly different from signals sampled at 200 Hz.[96] Thus, the selected sampling rate of 40 Hz was considered adequate for the current study.

Force Sensing Resistors[TM] (FSR, Interlink Electronics, Camarillo, CA), generally termed as conductive polymer force (pressure) sensors, were chosen to measure the discrete in-shoe plantar pressures. Our group has investigated several of the existing transducers utilized both commercially and for research.[97-100] These comprise capacitive sensors, piezoelectric sensors, strain gage transducers, and FSRs. The FSR was found to offer numerous advantages, such as flexibility, durability, reliability, overload tolerance, electronic simplicity, and low cost. In the absence of pressure, the FSR maintains an open circuit. Pressure results in increased shunting of the conductive layer causing the FSR resistance to drop. At no load, the sensor provides a stand-off resistance greater than 10 MΩ. With increasing pressure, the sensor resistance drops following a power law. The sensor used in this study was the Interlink rectangular FSR with the following dimensions: 29 mm length × 15 mm width, and 11 mm active sensing diameter. The sensor overall thickness is 0.5 mm. A photograph of this sensor is presented in Figure 7.2. Pressure computations were determined by dividing the measured vertical forces over the active sensing area (380 mm²). In 1988, Maalej et al. explored the static and dynamic characteristics of the conductive polymer force (pressure) sensors.[98] The authors reported that the hysteresis was between 5 and 10% of full pressure scale of 0 to 1.2 MPa. The maximal pressure nonrepeatability for increasing pressure at any data point was between 5 and 8% of full scale. Additionally, the authors reported that the rise-time of the sensor was determined by measuring the time between 10 and 90% of maximal output response to an impulse created by a hammer strike, and was about 0.26 ms during the rising and falling edges of the impulse response.[98] The sensor exhibits greater sensitivity at low pressures. The nonlinearity of the sensor was compensated for by using the calibration lookup tables. The maximum temperature-related drift was -0.8%/°C. Since the sensor is sealed, it is insensitive to humidity.[30] These cumulative empirical outcomes supported the selection of the FSR for the measurement of plantar pressures.

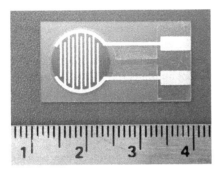

FIGURE 7.2 The 11 mm diameter rectangular FSR used in this study.

Sensors were positioned within predetermined anatomic areas beneath the calcaneus (CAL), medial midfoot (MMF), lateral midfoot (LMF), medial metatarsal head (MMH), lateral metatarsal head (LMH), and hallux (HAL). These six discrete anatomic areas were recognized as fundamental in analyzing the pediatric foot during ambulation.[46–50] These sites have also been shown to present pressure gradients closely associated with biomechanical variations and foot pathology in other studies.[28,30,96] Individual pathology and surgical intervention were also considered in this study. The six discrete sensor locations are illustrated in Figure 7.3. To support a symmetrical gait pattern

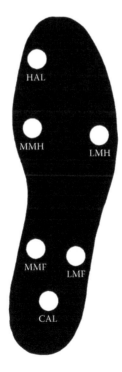

FIGURE 7.3 The six discrete sensor locations: CAL, MMF, LMF, MMH, LMH, and HAL. The illustration represents the operated foot, whether it is the right foot, the left foot, or both.

during subject testing, the insoles were instrumented bilaterally for all study patients, although the analysis focused only on measurements obtained from the operated feet.

Sensor sites within the defined plantar anatomic areas were determined through a combination of clinical examination and a qualitative footprint impression recording technique using an APEX foot imprinter (APEX, S. Hackensack, NJ).[30] The aim behind this procedure was to determine the precise coordinates of the highest load center within each anatomic area. Accordingly, each subject walked barefoot on the APEX mat, which had been evenly inked and covered with an APEX orthotic paper. The operator then aligned the APEX paper on the insole to lay out the primary sensor locations. Due to pathological asymmetries, the same protocol was followed to determine sensor locations on the contralateral foot. The test was repeated three times; subsequently, for each test, the location of the highest load area center within each of the six plantar anatomic areas was determined. Areas of high pressures were correlated with the darkest areas on the APEX orthotic paper. The three obtained centers for every anatomic area were then averaged to determine the sensor location within that area. Sample foot impressions, obtained with the APEX foot imprinter, for a child with planovalgus foot deformity and a normal child with no impairment are depicted in Figure 7.4.

To decrease excessive hysteresis due to bending, a small (15 mm diameter, 0.55 mm thick) stainless steel disc was mounted to the back of each sensor to keep it flat throughout the gait cycle. Sensors were embedded within the insole material. The upper insole layer was carefully carved to accept the sensors and thin metal backings, which were flush mounted with the insole surface. Subjects could not perceive the presence of the sensors and metal backings in the insole while ambulating. The instrumented insoles were fitted into a pair of standard canvas tennis shoes (Converse Chuck Taylor All Star®, Converse Inc., North Andover, MA). These shoes were selected in order to minimize support provided by the shoe structure, while offering a suitable platform for the instrumented insole. The existing structure of the shoes was not altered. Each test individual received a customized pair of instrumented insoles and a separate pair of shoes.

To better characterize sensor output during the stance phase of walking, a dynamic force application unit, consisting of a compression lever, a precalibrated 440 N strain gage load cell, and preamplifier, was used to calibrate the FSRs. Dynamic loads with durations similar to those of stance-phase foot contact (≤620 ms) were applied to each sensor during calibration. Resulting calibration data from each sensor and the load cell were then automatically transferred to the PC unit, where a piecewise linear calibration table was located for converting voltage data into pressure values. To compensate for temperature sensitivity, a Plexiglas™ oven (Rohm and Haas Corp., Philadelphia, PA), surrounding the calibration apparatus and the instrumented insole, was used to calibrate the sensors at 36°C.[30] This temperature simulated the in-shoe temperature environment. The overall system error, during actual usage and interface mechanics, has been reported in previous works.[33,93]

7.4.2 Patient Testing

This study comprised 12 children and adolescents (eight males and four females) with planovalgus foot deformity secondary to spastic cerebral palsy. The study was

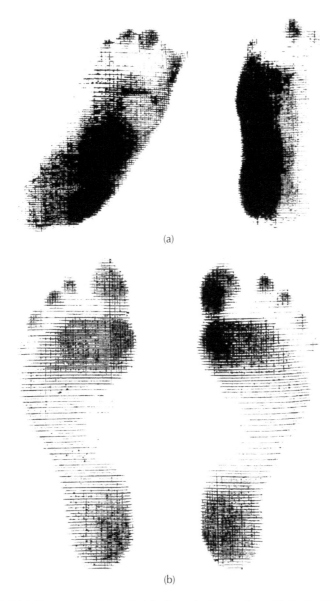

(a)

(b)

FIGURE 7.4 (a) Preoperative left and right footprint impressions obtained with the APEX foot imprinter from a child with planovalgus foot deformity secondary to spastic cerebral palsy. The medial foot areas exhibit higher pressure loading, as indicated by the darkness of the ink, resulting from the planovalgus deformity. (b) Left and right APEX foot impressions obtained from a nonimpaired child. This picture is provided for comparison purposes.

conducted at the Chicago Unit of Shriners Hospitals for Children. Preoperatively, patients ranged in age from 9.0 to 17.2 yr (mean $\pm$ SD = 13.1 $\pm$ 2.6 yr), and had a mean height of 146.0 $\pm$ 18.4 cm, and mean body mass of 47.8 $\pm$ 19.6 kg. These patients were examined just before surgery, and at 6 and 12 months following

TABLE 7.1
Preoperative Demographic Data for the Pediatric Population
That Participated in This Study

Patient Initials	Operated Limb	Gender	Age (yr)	Height (cm)	Body Mass (kg)
CB	R	M	11.6	111.8	20.0
EP	L	M	9.0	124.0	26.2
JK	B	F	11.6	135.9	25.0
JL	B	M	11.2	144.8	42.2
JM	R	M	17.2	175.3	80.8
KB	L	F	11.1	146.1	31.8
KC	R	M	14.9	167.6	51.1
MA	B	M	16.0	154.9	61.3
NO	B	F	14.2	153.7	74.9
RD	L	M	12.9	134.1	52.4
RR	B	M	11.0	140.2	47.9
SR	R	F	16.3	163.8	60.4

Note: R, right; L, left; B, bilateral; M, male; F, female.

subtalar arthrodesis for correction of the foot deformity. A single patient was incapable of participating in the 12 months plantar pressure analysis follow-up evaluation due to personal reasons, but was capable of completing a gait analysis follow-up. Subtalar arthrodesis was performed on 17 feet following the methods of Dennyson and Fulford.[79] Five patients received bilateral subtalar arthrodesis, while seven patients underwent unilateral subtalar fusion, four on the right foot and three on the left foot. Preoperative demographic data for the study population are presented in Table 7.1.

During the acquisition of plantar pressures, the instrumented subjects walked continuously at their respective freely selected natural cadences on a smooth 21 m concrete walkway in the mall area of the hospital. Acclimation to the examination shoes and establishment of a constant-temperature shoe environment was provided during a 30 min pretest stabilization period.[24,27,30] Several data-gathering sessions were conducted for each subject with a 10 min rest period in between. Steps around the ends of the walkway were excluded to eliminate any altered gait patterns during the turn maneuver. During all trials, a log was maintained to document the timing of any unusual gait activities. To avoid the possibility of discomfort and fatigue, tests were limited to less than 400 steps (200 strides) per trial. None of the subjects experienced blisters or pain during the test trials. Following data acquisition, and to verify the integrity of the acquired raw pressure data, the different trials for each subject were then analyzed graphically for evident errors. Accordingly, the best multistep trial was selected for the data analysis. Nevertheless, the first trial for each subject was excluded from the data analysis because of possible variations in initial gait.

7.4.3 DATA ANALYSIS

From the collected raw pressure–time data of each trial, the following metrics were processed at each of the six discrete sensor locations: peak pressures (kPa), sensor contact durations (ms), and pressure–time integrals (kPa.s). These metrics have demonstrated their usefulness in previous clinical studies.[5,24,31,33,101–107] Peak pressure was defined as the maximum vertical pressure experienced throughout a single step cycle. Contact duration was defined as the elapsed time between initial foot–sensor–ground contact (signal excursion above no-load base line of 5% or more) and return to no-load base line (within 5%). The no-load threshold was identified for each sensor during calibration. The pressure–time integral was defined as the area under the pressure–time curve during a single step cycle. Subsequently, the mean (M), standard deviation (SD), and coefficient of variation (CV) values were calculated for each of the pressure metrics, per subject, by sensor location, and over the entire selected trial. These resulting values were then used in the evaluation of the study outcome. The CV (equal to $SD \times M^{-1} \times 100\%$) offers a measure of consistency.[108,109]

Temporal-distance gait parameters were also derived from each of the recorded pressure–time multistep trials. These included: number of strides (1 stride = 2 steps), stride time (s), stride length (cm), cadence (steps/min), walking speed (cm/s), and foot-off (% gait cycle). Values obtained from the selected trial for each patient were then used in the evaluation of the study outcome.

Even though follow-up measurements were acquired at 6 months postsurgery, these measurements were not considered in this study. At 6 months postsurgery, patients may still be recovering from the surgical procedure. These patients could experience pain and endure discomfort and fatigue during gait. Adequate time for a surgical recovery results in a better stance phase stability, swing phase foot clearance, and a more normal walking pattern. Accordingly, in this study the overall assessment of surgery addresses the pre- and 12-month postoperative outcomes.

Pre- and postoperative alterations in the study results were evaluated by implementing a Wilcoxon Signed Rank Test using Sigma Stat® statistical software (Jandel Scientific Software, San Rafael, CA) with 95% confidence interval. The Signed Rank Test method was chosen for this study because it is a nonparametric procedure, which does not necessitate the assumption of normality or equal variance. This method is best suitable when it is required to determine whether the effect of a single treatment on the same individuals is significant and when the treatment effects are not normally distributed with the same variances. These requirements correlate well with the settings presented in this study, namely that subtalar arthrodesis is performed on a heterogeneous group of patients with planovalgus foot deformity secondary to cerebral palsy. Subsequently, the Wilcoxon Signed Rank Test was conducted in this study with the null hypothesis that subtalar fusion treatment had no effect on the subject. Comparisons of pre- vs. 12-month postoperative results were performed by executing a series of paired-difference tests on all investigated study parameters with $n = 17$, the number of operated limbs. Accordingly, for any investigated metric, if the computed p-value for the data from two test comparisons was less than or equal to 0.05, the variations in measurements were considered statistically significant.

TABLE 7.2

Preoperative Plantar Pressure Distribution by Sensor Location for the Study Population

Sensor Location	Peak Pressure (kPa)			Contact Duration (ms)			Pressure–Time Integral (kPa·s)		
	Mean	SD	CV (%)	Mean	SD	CV (%)	Mean	SD	CV (%)
CAL	127.5	149.4	117.2	371.1	372.2	100.3	27.6	30.2	109.4
MMF	197.1	112.4	57.0	647.6	193.2	29.8	75.5	48.6	64.4
LMF	53.4	65.7	123.0	345.1	323.1	93.6	16.9	25.2	149.1
MMH	248.5	192.0	77.3	747.6	178.1	23.8	86.3	67.0	77.6
LMH	53.2	63.8	119.9	424.9	341.4	80.3	17.5	16.2	92.6
HAL	303.0	412.8	136.2	627.6	233.4	37.2	77.4	66.9	86.4

7.5 RESULTS

7.5.1 PLANTAR PRESSURE OUTCOMES

Plantar pressure distribution outcomes for the preoperative and 1-yr postoperative metrics are presented in Table 7.2 and Table 7.3, respectively. The overall means, intersubject standard deviations, and coefficients of variation are presented in each table by sensor location and for every investigated plantar pressure parameter.

Preoperatively, the smallest metric values were consistently observed at the LMF, LMH, and CAL sensors. The peak values for all three metrics were prominent at the remaining plantar locations, specifically at the MMF, MMH, and HAL sensors. Postoperatively, the smallest values were seen at the CAL region for peak pressures and contact durations, and at the LMH for pressure–time integrals. Metric values were uniformly distributed amongst the remaining sensor locations. Generally, mean peak pressures prevailed on the medial aspect of the foot preoperatively, while postoperatively the mean peak pressures were more uniformly redistributed laterally.

TABLE 7.3

1-Yr Postoperative Plantar Pressure Distribution by Sensor Location for the Study Population

Sensor Location	Peak Pressure (kPa)			Contact Duration (ms)			Pressure–Time Integral (kPa·s)		
	Mean	SD	CV (%)	Mean	SD	CV (%)	Mean	SD	CV (%)
CAL	82.3	66.8	81.2	445.6	478.6	107.4	65.7	152.5	232.1
MMF	168.4	91.4	54.3	826.0	543.5	65.8	77.4	76.7	99.1
LMF	136.3	78.3	57.4	882.3	529.4	60.0	66.2	54.1	81.7
MMH	154.2	144.6	93.8	850.6	315.8	37.1	69.9	65.1	93.1
LMH	114.1	143.4	125.7	601.8	416.1	69.1	44.6	39.9	89.5
HAL	225.2	303.0	134.5	650.2	489.8	75.3	77.6	67.4	86.9

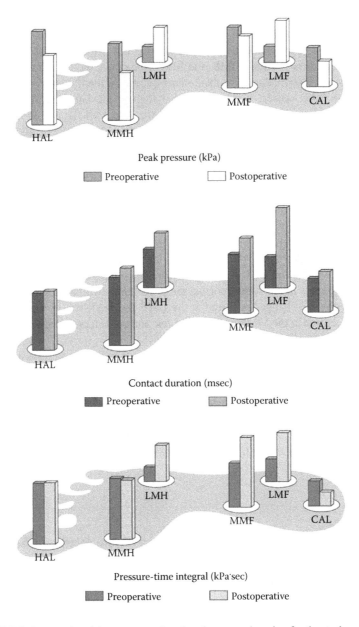

FIGURE 7.5 Bar graphs of the mean metric values by sensor location for the study population during the pre- and postoperative tests: peak pressures (top); contact durations (middle); and pressure–time integrals (bottom).

The same tendency was demonstrated for contact durations and pressure–time integrals. Pattern distributions of the overall mean plantar pressure metric values from the pre- and postoperative assessments are depicted in Figure 7.5 by sensor location.

Recalling that the CV is a measure of consistency, it could provide an indicator about the intersubject variability in the collected data. Preoperatively, the CV exceeded the 100% range for the peak pressures at the CAL, LMF, LMH, and HAL sensors, while at the medial, MMF, and MMH locations, the CV remained moderately below the 100% values. For the contact durations, the CV exceeded the 100% range at the CAL sensor; it was somewhat high at the lateral, LMF, and LMH sensors; and it was relatively low medially at the HAL, MMH, and MMF sensors. For the pressure–time integral, the CV exceeded the 100% range at the CAL and LMF locations; it was slightly below the 100% range for the remaining sensor locations, namely under the MMF, MMH, LMH, and HAL sensors.

Postoperatively, the CV remained in excess of the 100% range for the peak pressures at the LMH and HAL sensors with negligible changes; it was notably reduced at the CAL and LMF sensors; and it remained almost unchanged at the MMF and MMH sensor locations. For the contact durations, the CV remained invariably above the 100% range at the CAL location, whereas slight reductions were seen at the LMF and LMH sensor locations, and moderate increases occurred at the MMF, MMH, and HAL sites. Finally, for the pressure–time integrals, the CV remained in excess of the 100% range at the CAL sensor with a substantial increase, whereas negligible changes occurred at the LMF and HAL sensor locations, slight increases occurred at the MMF and MMH sites, and considerable reduction occurred at the LMF sensor location.

The pre- vs. 12-month postoperative alterations in mean plantar pressure metrics for the study population are presented in Table 7.4 by sensor location. Alterations in plantar pressures following foot surgery showed statistically significant ($p \leq .05$) increases in all three pressure metrics at the LMF and LMH sensor locations. Statistically significant alterations in metric values were not observed at the remaining plantar locations, although subtalar fusion resulted in noticeable decreases in mean peak pressures at the CAL, MMF, MMH, and HAL sensors. Mean contact

TABLE 7.4
Postoperative Alterations in Mean Plantar Pressure Metrics by Sensor Location for the Study Population

Sensor	Peak Pressure		Contact Duration		Pressure–Time Integral	
Location	Change (%)	p-Value	Change (%)	p-Value	Change (%)	p-Value
CAL	−35.5	0.358	+20.1	0.119	+138.0	0.855
MMF	−14.6	0.561	+27.5	0.489	+2.4	0.847
LMF	+155.2[a]	0.002[a]	+155.6[a]	<0.001[a]	+291.0[a]	<0.001[a]
MMH	−37.9	0.074	+13.8	0.274	−19.0	0.464
LMH	+114.4[a]	0.007[a]	+41.6[a]	0.025[a]	+154.8[a]	0.002[a]
HAL	−25.7	0.151	+3.6	0.847	−8.9	0.421

[a]Significant changes, within a 95% confidence-limit interval.

Peak Pressure

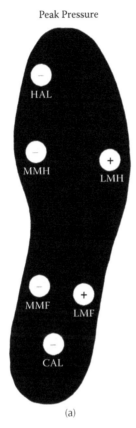

(a)

FIGURE 7.6 Postoperative redistribution in mean plantar pressure metrics by sensor location for the pediatric population evaluated in this study: (a) peak pressure, (b) contact duration, and (c) pressure–time integral. Statistically significant changes, within a 95% confidence-limit interval, are shown in boldface. (Alterations in metric values are represented by a + for increase and a - for decrease.)

durations also increased at the remaining plantar locations; noticeable increases in contact durations occurred at the CAL, MMF, and MMH, while only a mild increase in this metric was observed at the HAL. Mean pressure–time integrals increased markedly at the CAL and mildly at the MMF, while slight decreases in this metric were noticeable at the MMH and HAL. Figure 7.6 demonstrates a qualitative redistribution in the postoperative mean plantar pressure metrics for the study group by sensor location.

7.5.2 TEMPORAL-DISTANCE OUTCOMES

The pre- and postoperative temporal-distance parameter values for the study group are shown in Table 7.5. This table presents the overall means and intersubject standard deviations for every examined temporal-distance parameter. The table also

Contact Duration

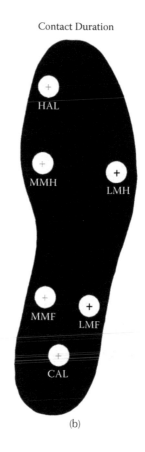

(b)

FIGURE 7.6 (Continued).

provides the pre- vs. 12-month postoperative variations in these metrics for the study population. Alterations in temporal-distance parameters exhibited the following outcomes: the mean stride time increased slightly from 1.40 to 1.49 s (p = .644), the mean stride length decreased significantly from 61.79 to 53.28 cm (p =.040), the mean cadence decreased from 93.62 to 86.81 steps/min (p = .459), the mean walking speed decreased from 49.54 to 40.05 cm/s (p = .064), and the mean foot-off value increased from 74.14 to 77.42% of gait cycle (p = .132).

The temporal and stride characteristics revealed that preoperatively the study group was significantly below normal gait values with a mean walking speed of only 0.49 m/s. In normal gait, the mean walking speed is approximately 1.0 m/s. Besides the stride length, there were no statistically significant alterations in walking speed or other stride characteristics following foot surgery in the pediatric population involved in this study.

Pressure-time Integral

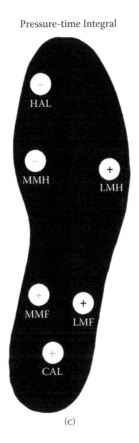

(c)

FIGURE 7.6 (Continued).

TABLE 7.5
**Pre- and Postoperative Temporal-Distance Parameter Values
for the Study Population**

Temporal Distance Parameter	Preoperative Mean	SD	Postoperative Mean	SD	Pre- vs. Postsurgical Comparisons Change (%)	p-Value
Strides	136.4	28.4	119.8	31.5	—	—
Stride time (s)	1.4	0.4	1.5	0.4	+6.4	0.644
Stride length (cm)	61.8	21.6	53.3	19.9	−13.8	0.040
Cadence (steps/min)	93.6	25.6	86.8	20.4	−7.3	0.459
Walking speed (cm/s)	49.5	24.1	40.0	20.5	−19.2	0.064
Foot-off (% gait cycle)	74.1	8.7	77.4	7.4	+4.4	0.132

7.6 DISCUSSION

In this study, the dynamic plantar pressure distribution in hemiplegic and diplegic children with planovalgus foot deformity has been determined. The participating cerebral palsied children were evaluated just prior to surgery and at 12 months subsequent to subtalar arthrodesis for the correction of the foot deformity. The assessment of this study group revealed a heterogeneous population with unilateral and bilateral pathology. This heterogeneity was evidenced by the excessively high values in the CV.

The clinical outcomes of this study were graded as *good* and *excellent* in all the 17 feet operated on for planovalgus foot deformity. This appraisal was based on standard clinical measurements, which include standing anteroposterior (AP) and lateral radiographs of the foot, clinical examination of the foot, and analysis of shoe wear. It is vital to point out here that there is a likelihood to overcorrect a subtalar arthrodesis and produce an abnormal varus or valgus deformity, opposite of the original. In such a possibility, the result of the procedure would be graded as *poor.* In fact, none of the patients in the current study were overcorrected into a varus position. This assertion is based on the clinical examinations and radiographs. Standing AP and lateral radiographs were obtained on all patients, and in all patients they showed a solid subtalar fusion in an anatomic position. There were no nonunions or screw failures. Figure 7.7 shows a lateral radiograph of subtalar arthrodesis.

Although clinical methods for grading the foot are frequently used, they remain subjective and vulnerable to interobserver variability. This study intended first to show the feasibility of quantitative techniques in the clinical assessment of the foot, and second that they are capable of showing quantifiable differences before and after surgery, which might be expected from the type of surgical procedure performed in the study. Subsequently, the study objective was to demonstrate that these techniques may well be utilized to enhance the standard clinical measures.

The Holter-type, portable, in-shoe, plantar pressure data acquisition system utilized in this study was able to demonstrate concrete alterations in dynamic foot pressures following surgery. The redistribution in peak pressures obtained

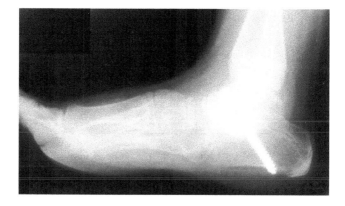

FIGURE 7.7 Lateral radiograph of subtalar arthrodesis. A screw transfixes the talus to the calcaneus in a neutral position, and a bone graft is positioned to fuse the subtalar joint.

postoperatively, mostly at the midfoot and metatarsal head regions, correlates well with the effect of subtalar arthrodesis, which stabilizes the midfoot and provides alignment between the talus and navicular, preventing excessive pronation of the forefoot. The lateral increase in contact durations suggests that it is the result of the formation of new plantar weight-bearing areas reflective of the biomechanical transfer of load through the structure of the foot following subtalar fusion. Moreover, the lowest values in the CV occurring preoperatively at the medial foot, mainly at the MMF and MMH sensors, suggest a common pattern of foot loading in all test subjects. This highly correlates with the biomechanical characteristics of the planovalgus foot.

It should be mentioned that contemporary portable plantar pressure data acquisition systems, whether those developed for research or commercially available ones, are capable of measuring only the vertical or normal component of the forces (pressures) exerted on the plantar aspect of the foot. It has been reported that shear stress is much more critical to the foot and is not easy to measure.[62] Even though shear stress has been implicated in the etiology of ulcers on the plantar surface of the diabetic foot, little research has been conducted to isolate or describe these effects.[110] Currently, there is no commercial sensor designed to determine the discrete AP and mediolateral (ML) shear forces beneath the sole of the foot. In addition, only a few investigators have reported on the development of shear sensors, however, with varying results.[110–114]

The development of a multiaxis force (pressure) sensor, capable of measuring vertical pressures as well as AP and ML shear pressures, would be a considerable progress in this field, and would aid in the identification of patients with a high risk of tissue breakdown.

The clinical benefits of subtalar arthrodesis have been better stance phase stability, reduced callus formation, and improved shoe wear. This study was designed to better understand, in a quantitative manner, the event-related changes in the planovalgus foot resulting from subtalar joint stabilization as a corrective and rehabilitative treatment of this deformity. On the basis of the outcomes obtained in this study, it is hoped that prospectively procedures with different approaches could be compared. Furthermore, the technology is at hand to objectively describe the biomechanics of the normal and pathologic foot and ankle, and the effectiveness of surgical and rehabilitative interventions.

REFERENCES

1. Levin ME. Pathogenesis and management of diabetic foot lesions. In: Levin ME, O'Neal LW, Bowker JH; Editors. *The Diabetic Foot*, 5th Edition. St. Louis: Mosby-Year Book, Inc., Chapter 2, pp. 17–60, 1993.
2. Klenerman L. Functional anatomy. In: Klenerman L; Editor. *The Foot and Its Disorders*, 3rd Edition. Oxford: Blackwell Scientific Publications, Chapter 1, pp. 1–9, 1991.
3. Hutton WC and Stokes IAF. The mechanics of the foot. In: Klenerman L; Editor. *The Foot and Its Disorders*, 3rd Edition. Oxford: Blackwell Scientific Publications, Chapter 2, pp. 11–25, 1991.
4. Menkveld SR, Knipstein EA, Quinn JR. Analysis of gait patterns in normal school-aged children. *J Pediatr Orthoped*, Vol. 8, No. 3, pp. 263–267, 1988.

5. Bauman JH and Brand PW. Measurement of pressure between the foot and shoe. *Lancet*, March, pp. 629–632, 1963.

6. Lereim P and Serek-Hanssen F. A method of recording pressure distribution under the sole of the foot. *Bull Prosthet Res*, Vol. 20, pp. 118–125, 1973.

7. Hennacy RA and Gunther R. A piezoelectric crystal method for measuring static and dynamic pressure distributions in the feet. *J Am Podiatr Assoc*, Vol. 65, No. 5, pp. 444–449, 1975.

8. Spolek GA, Day EE, Lippert FG, Kirkpatrick GS. Ambulatory-force measurement using an instrumented-shoe system. *Exp Mech*, Vol. 15, pp. 271–274, 1975.

9. Miyazaki S and Iwakura H. Foot-force measuring device for clinical assessment of pathological gait. *Med Biol Eng Comput*, Vol. 16, pp. 429–436, 1978.

10. Frost RB and Cass CA. A load cell and sole assembly for dynamic pointwise vertical force measurement in walking. *Eng Med*, Vol. 10, pp. 45–50, 1981.

11. Henning EM, Cavanagh PR, Albert HT, Macmillan NH. A piezoelectric method of measuring the vertical contact stress beneath the human foot. *J Biomed Eng*, Vol. 4, pp. 213–222, July 1982.

12. Soames RW, Blake CD, Scott JRR, Goodbody A, Brewerton DA. Measurement of pressure under the foot during function. *Med Biol Eng Comput*, Vol. 20, pp. 489–495, 1982.

13. Boulton AJM, Hardisty CA, Betts RP, Franks CI, Worth RC, Ward JD, Duckworth T. Dynamic foot pressure and other studies as diagnostic and management aids in diabetic neuropathy. *Diabetic Care*, Vol. 6, No. 1, pp. 26–33, 1983.

14. Chao EY, Laughman RK, Schneider E, Stauffer RN. Normative data of the knee joint motion and ground reaction forces in adult level walking. *J Biomech*, Vol. 16, No. 3, pp. 219–233, 1983.

15. Polchaninoff M. Gait analysis using a portable, microprocessor based segmental foot force measuring system. In: *Proceedings of the IEEE 7th Annual Symposium on Computer Applications in Medical Care*, Silver Spring, MD, 1983. New York: Institute of Electrical and Electronic Engineers, Inc., pp. 897–899.

16. Boulton AJM, Franks CI, Betts BP, Duckworth T, Ward JD. Reduction of abnormal foot pressures in diabetic neuropathy using a new polymer insole material. *Diabetic Care*, Vol. 7, No. 1, pp. 42–46, 1984.

17. Miyazaki S and Ishida A. Capacitive transducer for continuous measurement of vertical foot force. *Med Biol Eng Comput*, Vol. 22, pp. 309–316, 1984.

18. Maffei P and Power-Barnes MR. Computerized gait analysis: a quantitative diagnostic tool. *Diagnosis*, II, pp. 23–27, 1984.

19. Cavanagh PR, Henning EM, Rodgers MM, Sanderson DJ. The measurement of pressure distribution on the plantar surface of diabetic feet. In: Whittle M and Harris D; Editors. *Biomechanical Measurement in Orthopaedic Practice*. Oxford: Clarendon Press, Chapter 20, pp. 159–166, 1985.

20. Chizeck HJ, Selwan PM, Merat FL. A foot pressure sensor for use in lower extremity neuroprosthetic development. In: Brubaker C, Editor: *RESNA '85 Proceedings of the 8th Annual Conference, Memphis, TN, June 1985*. Washington, DC: RESNA Press, pp. 379–381, 1985.

21. Hermens HJ, de Waal CA, Buurke J, Zilvold G. A new gait analysis system for clinical use in a rehabilitation center. *Orthopedics*, Vol. 9, pp. 1669–1675, 1986.

22. Boulton AJM, Betts RP, Franks CI, Newrick PG, Ward JD, Duckworth T. Abnormalities of foot pressure in early diabetic neuropathy. *Diabetic Med*, Vol. 4, No. 3, pp. 225–228, 1987.

23. Boulton AJM, Betts RP, Franks CI, Ward JD, Duckworth T. The natural history of foot pressure abnormalities in neuropathic diabetic subjects. *Diabetic Res*, Vol. 5, pp. 73–77, 1987.

24. Gross TS and Bunch RP. Measurement of discrete vertical in-shoe stress with piezo-electric transducers. *J Biomed Eng*, Vol. 10, pp. 261–265, 1988.

25. Harris GF, Riedel SA, Weber RC. Validation and preliminary study of the AAMRL/BBD portable force dosimeter. In: *Proceedings of the 34th International Instrumentation Symposium (ISA), Albuquerque, NM, May 1988*. Triangle Park, NC: Instrument Society of America, pp. 391–396.

26. Brodsky JW, Kourosh S, Mooney V. Objective evaluation and review of commercial gait analysis systems. In: *Proceedings of the American Orthopedic Foot and Ankle Society, Las Vegas, NV, February 1989*. Park Ridge, IL: American Orthopedic Foot and Ankle Society, p. 24, 1989.

27. Gross TS and Bunch RP. Discrete normal plantar stress variations with running speed. *J Biomech*, Vol. 22, No. 6/7, pp. 699–703, 1989.

28. Zhu H, Maalej N, Webster JG, Tompkins WJ, Bach-y-Rita P, Wertsch JJ. An umbilical data-acquisition system for measuring pressures between the foot and shoe. *IEEE Trans Biomed Eng*, Vol. 37, No. 9, pp. 908–911, 1990.

29. Snow RE, Williams KR, Holmes GB. The effects of wearing high heeled shows on pedal pressure in women. *Foot Ankle*, Vol. 13, No. 2, pp. 85–92, 1992.

30. Wertsch JJ, Webster JG, Tompkins WJ. A portable insole plantar pressure measurement system. *J Rehab Res Dev*, Vol. 29, No. 1, pp. 13–18, 1992.

31. Chang AH, Abu-Faraj ZU, Harris GF, Shereff MJ, Nery J. Multistep measurement of plantar pressure alterations with the use of metatarsal pads. *Foot Ankle Int*, Vol. 15, No. 12, pp. 654–660, 1994.

32. Phillipson A, Dhar S, Linge K, McCabe C, Klenerman L. Forefoot arthroplasty and changes in plantar foot pressures. *Foot Ankle Int*, Vol. 15, No. 11, pp. 595–598, 1994.

33. Abu-Faraj ZO, Harris GF, Chang AH, Shereff MJ. Evaluation of a rehabilitative pedorthic: plantar pressure alterations with scaphoid pad application. *IEEE Trans Rehab Eng*, Vol. 4, No. 4, pp. 328–336, 1996.

34. Abu-Faraj ZU, Harris GF, Chang AH, Shereff MJ, Nery J. Quantitative evaluation of plantar pressure alterations with metatarsal and scaphoid pads. In: Harris GF and Smith PA; Editors. *Human Motion Analysis: Current Applications and Emerging Horizons*. Piscataway, NJ: IEEE Press, pp. 387–406, 1996.

35. Rozema A, Ulbrecht JA, Pammer SE, Cavanagh PR. In-shoe plantar pressures during activities of daily living: implications for therapeutic footwear design. *Foot Ankle Int*, Vol. 17, No. 6, pp. 352–359, 1996.

36. Wu G and Chiang JH. The effect of surface compliance on foot pressure in stance. *Gait Posture*, Vol. 4, pp. 122–129, 1996.

37. Novacheck TF. The biomechanics of running. *Gait Posture*, Vol. 7, pp. 77–95, 1998.

38. Femery V, Moretto P, Hespel JM, Lensel G. Plantar pressure biofeedback device for foot loading. In: Henning E and Stacoff A, Editors. *Proceedings of the 5th Symposium on Footwear Biomechanics, Zurich, Switzerland*, pp. 36–37, 2001.

39. Kirtley C. An instrumented insole for kinematic and kinetic gait measurements. In: Henning E and Stacoff A, Editors. *Proceedings of the 5th Symposium on Footwear Biomechanics, Zurich, Switzerland*, pp. 52–53, 2001.

40. Chang CH, Miller F, Schuyler J. Dynamic pedobarograph in evaluation of varus and valgus foot deformities. *J Pediatr Orthopaed*, Vol. 22, pp. 813–818, 2002.

41. Femery V, Moretto P, Renaut H, Lensel G, Thevenon A. Analyse des asymétries baropodométriques lors de la marche chez le sujet valide: application à l'étude des asymmetries chez l'enfant infirme moteur cerebral. *Ann Réadaptation Méd Phys*, Vol. 45, pp. 114–122, 2002.

42. Perttunen J. Foot loading in normal and pathological walking. Academic Dissertation, Faculty of Sport and Health Sciences, University of Jyväskylä, Finland, 2002.

43. Smith BT, Coiro DJ, Finson R, Betz RR, McCarthy J. Evaluation of force-sensing resistors for gait event detection to trigger electrical stimulation to improve walking in the child with cerebral palsy. *IEEE Trans Neural Syst Rehab Eng*, Vol. 10, No. 1, pp. 22–29, 2002.

44. Weijers RE, Walenkamp GHIM, van Mameren H, Kessels AGH. The relationship of the position of the metatarsal heads and peak plantar pressure. *Foot Ankle Int*, Vol. 24, No. 4, pp. 349–353, 2003.

45. Wu G and Hitt J. Ground contact characteristics of Tai Chi gait. *Gait Posture*, Vol. 22, No. 1, pp. 32–39, 2005.

46. Harris GF, Smith PA, Abler J, Abu-Faraj Z, Millar EA. Biomechanical evaluation of the planovalgus foot in cerebral palsy: a microprocessor-based insole system. In: *Proceedings of the 8th Annual East Coast Clinical Gait Laboratory Conference, May 5–8, 1993, Mayo Clinic, Rochester, MN*, pp. 125–126.

47. Abu-Faraj ZO, Harris GF, Abler JH, Smith PA, Wertsch JJ. A Holter-type microprocessor-based rehabilitation instrument for acquisition and storage of plantar pressure data in children with cerebral palsy. *IEEE Trans Rehab Eng*, Vol. 4, No. 1, pp. 33–38, 1996.

48. Smith PA, Harris GF, Abu-Faraj ZU. Biomechanical evaluation of the planovalgus foot in cerebral palsy. In: Harris GF and Smith PA; Editors. *Human Motion Analysis: Current Applications and Emerging Horizons*. Piscataway, NJ: IEEE Press, pp. 370–386, 1996.

49. Smith PA, Abu-Faraj ZO, Wertsch JJ, Abler JH, Harris GF. System and study of planovalgus foot deformity in children with cerebral palsy. Abstract: *Proceedings of the 2nd Medical Engineering Week of the World, May 26–30, 1996, Taipei, Taiwan, People R.O.C.*, p. 152.

50. Abu-Faraj ZO, Harris GF, Smith PA. Surgical rehabilitation of the planovalgus foot in cerebral palsy. *IEEE Trans Neural Syst Rehab Eng*, Vol. 9, No. 2, pp. 202–214, 2001.

51. Levin ME. Saving the diabetic foot. *Med Times*, Vol. 108, No. 5, pp. 56–62, 1980.

52. Birke JA and Sims DS. Plantar sensory threshold in the ulcerative foot. *Lepr Rev*, Vol. 57, pp. 261–267, 1986.

53. Brand PW. Repetitive stress in the development of diabetic foot ulcers. In: Levin ME, O'Neal LW; Editors. *The Diabetic Foot*, 4th Edition. St. Louis: C.V. Mosby Co., Chapter 5, pp. 83–90, 1988.

54. Bauman JH, Ling JPG, Brand PW. Plantar pressures and trophic ulceration: an evaluation of footwear. *J Bone Joint Surg*, Vol. 45B, No. 4, pp. 652–673, 1963.

55. Schaff PS and Cavanagh PR. Shoes for the insensitive foot: the effect of a "rocker bottom" shoe modification on plantar pressure distribution. *Foot Ankle*, Vol. 11, No. 3, pp. 129–140, 1990.

56. Cavanagh PR and Lafortune MA. Ground reaction forces in distance running. *J Biomech*, Vol. 13, No. 5, pp. 397–406, 1980.

57. Birke JA and Nawoczenski DA. Orthopedic walkers: effect on plantar pressures. *Clin Prosthet Orthot*, Vol. 12, No. 2, pp. 74–80, 1988.

58. Brand PW. The insensitive foot (including leprosy). In: Jahss MH; Editor. *Disorders of the Foot*, Vol. 2. Philadelphia: WB Saunders Co., Chapter 46, pp. 1266–1286, 1982.

59. Reiber GE. Epidemiology of the diabetic foot. In: Levin ME, O'Neal LW, Bowker JH; Editors. *The Diabetic Foot*, 5th Edition. St. Louis: Mosby-Year Book, Inc., Chapter 1, pp. 1–15, 1993.

60. Levin ME, O'Neal LW, Bowker JH. Preface. In: Levin ME, O'Neal LW, Bowker JH; Editors. *The Diabetic Foot*, 5th Edition. St. Louis: Mosby-Year Book, Inc., pp. xvii–xxii, 1993.

61. Kosiak M. Etiology and pathology of ischemic ulcers. *Arch Phys Med Rehab*, February, pp. 62–69, 1959.

62. Brand PW. Repetitive stress on insensitive feet: the pathology and management of plantar ulceration in neuropathic feet. Department of Health, Education, and Welfare, Carville, LA, 1975.

63. Hall OC and Brand PW. The etiology of the neuropathic plantar ulcer: a review of the literature and a presentation of current concepts. *J Am Podiatr Assocn*, Vol. 69, No. 3, pp. 173–177, 1979.

64. Little WJ. On the influence of parturition, difficult labours, premature birth, and asphyxia neonatorum on the mental and physical condition of the child, especially in relation to deformities. *Trans Obstet Soc Lond*, Vol. 3, p. 253, 1862.

65. Bax MCO. Terminology and classification of cerebral palsy. *Develop Med Child Neurol*, Vol. 6, p. 295, 1964.

66. Blair E and Stanley JJ. An epidemiological study of cerebral palsy in Western Australia, III: postnatal etiology. *Develop Med Child Neurol*, Vol. 24, pp. 575–585, 1982.

67. Hensleight PA, Fainstate T, Spencer R. Perinatal events and cerebral palsy. *Am J Obstetr Gynecol*, Vol. 154, pp. 978–981, 1986.

68. Nelson KB and Ellenberg JH. Antecedents of cerebral palsy: multivariate analysis of risk. *N Engl J Med*, Vol. 315, No. 2, pp. 81–86, 1986.

69. Schwartz SI, Shires GT, Spencer FC. Orthopaedics. In: *Principles of Surgery*, 5th Edition. New York: McGraw-Hill, pp. 1879–2020, 1989.

70. Aiona MD. Human motion analysis: a method of outcome assessment in selective dorsal rhizotomy. In: Harris GF and Smith PA; Editors. *Human Motion Analysis: Current Applications and Emerging Horizons*. Piscataway, NJ: IEEE Press, pp. 303–317, 1996.

71. Gage JR. Gait analysis in cerebral palsy. In: *Clinics in Developmental Medicine*, No. 121, London: Mac Keith Press, 1991.

72. Bonnett G, Rang M, Jones D. Varus and valgus deformities of the foot in cerebral palsy. *Develop Med Child Neurol*, Vol. 24, pp. 499–503, 1982.

73. Bleck EE. *Orthopaedic Management in Cerebral Palsy*. Oxford: Mac Keith Press, p. 282, 1987.

74. Fulford GE. Surgical management of ankle and foot deformities in cerebral palsy. *Clin Orthopaed*, pp. 253–255, 1990.

75. Renshaw TS, Sivke KB, Drennan JC. The management of hallux valgus in cerebral palsy. *Develop Med Child Neurol*, Vol. 21, pp. 202–208, 1970.

76. Green WT and Grice DS. The surgical correction of the paralytic foot. *Instructional Course Lecture at the American Academy of Orthopaedic Surgeons*, Vol. 10, p. 343, 1953.

77. Crawford AH, Kucharzyk D, Roy DR, Bilbo J. Subtalar stabilization of the planovalgus foot by staple arthrodesis in young children who have neuromuscular problems. *J Bone Joint Surg*, Vol. 72A, p. 840, 1990.

78. Smith SD and Millar EA. Arthroriesis by means of a subtalar polyethylene peg implant for correction of hindfoot pronation in children. *Clin Orthopaed*, Vol. 181, pp. 15–23, 1983.

79. Dennyson WG and Fulford R. Subtalar arthrodesis by cancellous grafts and metallic fixation. *J Bone Joint Surg*, Vol. 58B, p. 507, 1976.

80. Grice DS. An extraarticular arthrodesis of the subastragular joint for correction of paralytic feet in children. *J Bone Joint Surg*, Vol. 34A, p. 927, 1952.

81. Grice DS. Further experience with extraarticular arthrodesis of the subtalar joint. *J Bone Joint Surg*, Vol. 37A, p. 246, 1955.

82. Seymour N and Evans DK. A modification of the Grice subtalar arthrodesis. *J Bone Joint Surg*, Vol. 50B, No. 2, p. 372, 1968.

83. Smith JB and Westin GW. Subtalar extraarticular arthrodesis. *J Bone Joint Surg*, Vol. 50A, p. 1027, 1968.

84. Koutsogiannis E. Treatment of mobile flat foot by displacement osteotomy of the calcaneus. *J Bone Joint Surg*, Vol. 53B, No. 1, pp. 96–100, 1971.

85. Armstrong G. Evans elongation of lateral column of the foot for valgus deformity. *J Bone Joint Surg*, Vol. 57B, p. 530, 1975.

86. Mosca VS. Calcaneal lengthening for valgus deformity of the hindfoot: results in children who had severe, symptomatic flatfoot and skewfoot. *J Bone Joint Surg*, Vol. 77A, No. 4, pp. 500–512, 1995.

87. Barrasso JA, Wile PB, Gage JR. Extraarticular subtalar arthrodesis with internal fixation. *J Pediatr Orthopaed*, Vol. 4, p. 555, 1984.

88. Abu-Faraj ZU, Harris GF, Wertsch JJ, Abler JH, Vengsarkar AS. Holter system development for recording plantar pressures: design and instrumentation. *Proceedings of the IEEE Engineering in Medicine & Biology Society, November 3–6, 1994, Baltimore, MD*, Vol. 16, pp. 934–935.

89. Harris GF, Abu-Faraj ZU, Wertsch JJ, Abler JH, Vengsarkar AS. A Holter type system for study of plantar foot pressures. Abstract: *Proceedings of the 1st Medical Engineering Week of the World, September 25–29, 1994, Taipei, Taiwan, People R.O.C.*, p. 252.

90. Vengsarkar AS, Abler JH, Abu-Faraj ZU, Harris GF, Wertsch JJ. Holter system development for recording plantar pressures: software development. *Proceedings of the IEEE Engineering in Medicine & Biology Society, November 3–6, 1994, Baltimore, MD*, Vol. 16, pp. 936–937.

91. Harris GF, Abu-Faraj ZU, Wertsch JJ, Abler JH, Vengsarkar AS. A Holter type system for study of plantar foot pressures. *J Biomed Eng*, Vol. 1, pp. 233–239, 1994; Also in *Biomed Eng Appl, Basis Commun*, Vol. 7, No. 4, pp. 409–415, 1995.

92. Wervey RA, Abler JH, Abu-Faraj ZU, Harris GF, Wertsch JJ. Data preview software for interactive review of Holter type plantar pressure data. *Proceedings of the IEEE Engineering in Medicine & Biology Society, September 20–23, 1995, Montréal, Canada*, Vol. 17, 2 pp.

93. Abu-Faraj ZO, Harris GF, Abler JH, Wertsch JJ. A Holter-type, microprocessor-based, rehabilitation instrument for acquisition and storage of plantar pressure data. *J Rehab Res Dev*, Vol. 34, No. 2, pp. 187–194, 1997.

94. Antonsson EK, Mann RW. The frequency content of gait. *J Biomech*, Vol. 18, pp. 39-47, 1985.

95. Acharya KR, Harris GF, Riedel SA, Kazarian L. Foot magnitude and spectral frequency content of heel strike during gait. *Proc IEEE Eng Med Biol Soc*, Vol. 11, pp. 826-827, 1989.

96. Zhu H, Harris GF, Wertsch JJ, Tompkins WJ, Webster JG. A microprocessor-based data-acquisition system for measuring plantar pressures from ambulatory subjects. *IEEE Trans Biomed Eng*, Vol. 38, No. 7, pp. 710–714, 1991.

97. Kothari M, Webster JG, Tompkins WJ, Wertsch JJ, Bach-y-Rita P. Capacitive sensors for measuring the pressure between the foot and shoe. *Proc IEEE Eng Med Biol Soc*, Vol. 10, pp. 805–806, 1988.

98. Maalej N, Bhat S, Zhu H, Webster JG, Tompkins WJ, Wertsch JJ, Bach-y-Rita P. A conductive polymer pressure sensor. *Proc IEEE Eng Med Biol Soc*, Vol. 10, pp. 770–771, 1988.

99. Bhat S, Webster JG, Tompkins WJ, Wertsch JJ. Piezoelectric sensor for foot pressure measurements. *Proc IEEE Eng Med Biol Soc*, Vol. 11, pp. 1435–1436, 1989.

100. Patel A, Kothari M, Webster JG, Tompkins WJ, Wertsch JJ. A capacitance pressure sensor using a phase-locked loop. *J Rehab Res Dev*, Vol. 26, No. 2, pp. 55–62, 1989.

101. Wertsch JJ, Loftsgaarden JD, Harris GF, Zhu H, Harris JL. Plantar pressures with contralateral versus ipsilateral cane usage. *Arch Phys Med Rehab*, Vol. 71, p. 772, 1990.

102. Zhu H, Wertsch JJ, Harris GF. Asymmetry of plantar pressure during normal walking. *Arch Phys Med Rehabn*, Vol. 71, p. 808, 1990.

103. Zhu H. Acquisition and analysis of plantar pressure data. Ph.D. Dissertation, Marquette University, Milwaukee, Wisconsin, 100 pp., 1991.

104. Zhu H, Harris GF, Alba HM, Wertsch JJ. Effect of walking cadence on plantar pressures. *Arch Phys Med Rehab*, Vol. 72, p. 834, 1991.

105. Zhu H, Wertsch JJ, Harris GF, Loftsgaarden JD, Price MB. Foot pressure distribution during walking and shuffling. *Arch Phys Med Rehab*, Vol. 72, pp. 390–397, 1991.

106. Zhu H, Wertsch JJ, Harris GF, Alba HM, Price MB. Sensate and insensate in-shoe plantar pressures. *Arch Phys Med Rehab*, Vol. 74, pp. 1362–1368, 1993.

107. Wertsch JJ, Frank LW, Zhu H, Price MB, Harris GF, Alba HM. Plantar pressures with total contact casting. *J Rehab Res Dev*, Vol. 32, No. 3, pp. 205–209, 1995.

108. Bendat JS and Piersol AG. *Random Data: Analysis and Measurement Procedures*, 2nd Edition. New York: Wiley Interscience, p. 254, 1986.

109. Ott L. *An Introduction to Statistical Methods and Data Analysis*, 3rd Edition. Boston, MA: PWS-Kent Publishing, p. 419, 1988.

110. Lebar AM, Harris GF, Wertsch JJ, Zhu H. An optoelectric plantar "shear" sensing transducer: design, validation, and preliminary subject tests. *IEEE Trans Rehab Eng*, Vol. 4, No. 4, pp. 310–319, 1996.

111. Tappin JW, Pollard J, Beckett EA. Method for measuring 'shearing' forces on the foot. *Clin Phys Physiol Meas*, Vol. 1, No. 1, pp. 83–85, 1980.

112. Pollard JP, LeQuesne LP, Tappin JW. Forces under the foot. *J Biomed Eng*, Vol. 5, pp. 37–40, 1983.

113. Laing P, Deogan H, Cogley D, Crerand S, Hammond P, Klenerman L. The development of the low profile Liverpool shear transducer. *Clin Phys Physiol Meas*, Vol. 13, No. 2, pp. 115–124, 1992.

114. Lord M, Hosein R, Williams RB. Method for in-shoe shear stress measurement. *J Biomed Eng*, Vol. 4, No. 3, pp. 181–186, 1992.

8 Chemodenervation and Motion Assessment

Susan Sienko Thomas and Jeffrey D. Ackman

CONTENTS

8.1 BOTULINUM TOXIN TYPE A

Botulinum toxin is one of the most potent bacterial toxins known to man, and has been used both as a chemical weapon and as a therapeutic tool. To date, seven serologically distinct serotypes of botulinum toxin have been recognized and are designated as types A to G, with A being the most potent.[1] These serotypes possess similar molecular weights and a common subunit structure. Human intoxication occurs with labeled types A, B, C, E, and sometimes F.[1] Botulinum toxin A was first utilized in the treatment of strabismus in nonhuman primates in 1973, and Scott reported on its use in humans as an alternative to strabismus surgery in 1981.[2] Since 1989, the U.S. Food and Drug Administration (FDA) has approved botulinum toxin A for the treatment of strabismus, blepharospasm, hemifacial spasm, cervical dystonia, and, more recently, wrinkles. Utilization of botulinum toxin A for the management of spasticity in children with cerebral palsy began in the late 1980s and continues today, though it remains off-label for this use in the U.S.[3]

Botulinum toxin type A, produced by *Clostridium botulinum*, is a single-chain polypeptide that binds with a high affinity and specificity to the receptor on the cell surface of presynaptic membranes of cholinergic motor neurons (Figure 8.1).[4] The inhibitory action of botulinum toxin A occurs by rapid binding of the toxin to the presynaptic nerve ending. The toxin then becomes intracellular and prevents acetylcholine release from presynaptic vesicles by enzymatic cleavage of essential polypeptides. This chemodenervation by chemical blockade produces a reversible,

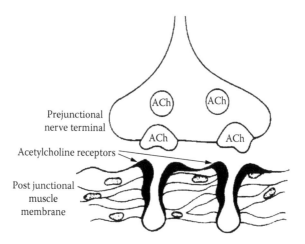

FIGURE 8.1 Representation of a normal motor neuron.

dose- and distribution-dependent flaccid paralysis usually lasting 12 to 16 weeks.[5,6] Recovery occurs by sprouting of new nerve terminals, accompanied by regeneration of the old terminals. Intramuscular injection of botulinum toxin type A reduces spasticity within 12 to 72 hrs, with a clinical effect lasting 3 to 6 months. Injections can be repeated every 16 weeks, but no more frequently than every 8 weeks. Because of its high-binding affinity, little if any type A toxin reaches the systemic circulation, and no cases of the clinical syndrome of botulism have been reported following administration of commercially available and regulated preparations.[7]

8.2 MOUSE MODELS OF SPASTICITY

Beginning in the 1980s, spastic mouse models were introduced to aid in the understanding of the pathophysiology of spasticity seen in children with cerebral palsy and to determine the subsequent impact of therapeutic interventions offered to these children.[8–10] Ziv et al. found that in comparison to normal, muscle growth in the spastic mouse was slower and markedly reduced in relation to bone growth, thus leading to the development of muscle contractures. In 1994, Cosgrove and Graham evaluated the use of botulinum toxin A in the hereditary spastic mouse to determine whether the paralysis imposed by the use of botulinum toxin A facilitated the growth of muscle, thus reducing the development of muscle contracture.[10] They found that an injection of botulinum toxin A to the spastic muscles of mice permitted longitudinal growth of the musculotendinous unit, specifically in the muscular portion of the unit.[10]

8.3 CHILDREN WITH CEREBRAL PALSY

In children with cerebral palsy, contractures are purported to arise from muscle fibers that are shorter (i.e., have fewer sarcomeres in series) than normal.[11] Most children with cerebral palsy have hypertonicity, which is manifested by spasticity, a velocity-dependent increase in the tonic stretch reflexes with exaggerated tendon jerks, resulting from hyperexcitability of the stretch reflex.[12] Lieber and Friden found that the flexor carpi ulnaris muscle in children with cerebral palsy had normal fiber lengths yet extremely long sarcomere lengths, even though the spastic muscle was shorter than normal.[13] In this group of children, the longer sarcomere lengths enabled the shorter muscles (less fibers in a series) to span from origin to insertion,[14,15] leading to excessive passive tension in the muscle to achieve normal muscle length.[11] In addition, spastic muscle has also been shown to have a decreased resting sarcomere length with nearly double the elastic modulus compared with normal muscle cells.[14]

Equinus (toe walking), one of the most common deformities in children with cerebral palsy, may be dynamic, resulting from overactivity of the gastrocnemius–soleus complex or static, secondary to a fixed contracture.[16] It was postulated that botulinum toxin type A injections into select spastic muscles of children with cerebral palsy would weaken the muscles and allow them to be stretched, thus creating an environment conducive to longitudinal muscle growth, or at least prevent or delay progressive muscle shortening. However, there is no evidence to date that utilization of botulinum toxin A facilitates longitudinal muscle growth in children with or without cerebral palsy.

8.4 ASSESSMENT OF THE EFFICACY OF BOTULINUM TOXIN TYPE A

A combination of static and dynamic measures has been employed in both the clinical and the research settings to assess the efficacy of botulinum toxin A at reducing equinus. Static components of equinus are routinely measured with passive range of motion of the ankle with the knee either flexed or extended in order to give an indication of muscle length of both the gastrocnemius and the soleus. Dynamic components are measured with the modified Tardieu scale, which consists of two measures: the first is the point of resistance to a rapid velocity stretch (R1),[17] and the second is the greatest magnitude of dorsiflexion achieved with slow stretch (R2). "R1" or the "catch" is the result of an overactive stretch reflex, whereas "R2" represents the fixed component or contracture. The difference between "R1" and "R2" represents the dynamic component, with a larger difference representing the reflexive component of the gastrocnemius muscle (spasticity), while a smaller difference indicates limitation from muscle contracture rather than spasticity.[18] Although the reliability of clinical measures is often questioned, standardization of testing procedures, consideration of the positioning of proximal and distal segments, and the utilization of the same experienced examiner improve the accuracy and reliability of these measures.[19]

Due to the difficulty in differentiating between static and dynamic deformity, it may be beneficial to assess the contractures functionally during gait.[20] This can be accomplished through a three-dimensional computerized assessment of gait. Kinematics (description of the joint motion without regard to the forces that cause the motion) and kinetics (the forces and torques that cause the motion of the body)[21] provide a dynamic assessment of motion and forces about all of the joints during the dynamic activity of walking. Although ankle motion during the entire gait cycle is important, specific kinematic variables such as peak dorsiflexion at initial stance, mid-stance, and mid-swing are often utilized as key indicators of successful outcome following various treatment interventions aimed at improving ankle motion. While sagittal plane ankle kinematics determine whether the motion of the ankle normalizes following treatment intervention, kinetic parameters such as ankle moment quotient [(AMQ), description of the double bump ankle moment often attributed to ankle clonus], peak power generation, and ankle power quotient [(APQ), description of the triphasic power curve], provide insight into the dynamic strength and spasticity changes following therapeutic interventions.[4,22]

Initial randomized studies evaluating the efficacy of botulinum toxin A in the gastrocnemius reported a lack of significant improvement in passive range of motion at the ankle (fixed muscle length); however, dynamic ankle motion, as measured by the confusion test, physician rating scale (PRS), and computerized gait analysis, demonstrated significant improvements following the injection of botulinum toxin A.[23,25] These initial findings support the premise that the inhibition of acetylcholine release facilitates muscle relaxation and subsequently impacts the dynamic component of gastrocnemius function more than the static. While the use of botulinum toxin A has gained widespread acceptance in the clinical management of focal muscle spasticity in children with cerebral palsy, the impact of botulinum toxin A on muscle length and function remains unclear. Some authors have reported a lack of improvement in passive ankle motion following botulinum toxin A,[23,26,27] while others have demonstrated significant gains in range of motion.[28–31] These conflicting reports on the passive range of motion may be explained by the findings of Cosgrove et al., who reported an inverse relationship between the therapeutic response and the patient's age, with younger children demonstrating a greater increase in passive ankle motion than older children.[32] In addition, it has been reported that the effectiveness of botulinum toxin A decreases with age, consistent with the increasing development of fixed contractures.

Kinematic and kinetic evaluations of children with cerebral palsy following botulinum toxin A injection have also demonstrated contradictory findings. While some authors report significant improvements in ankle dorsiflexion at initial contact, midstance and mid-swing,[23,27,29,31] others have found only slight improvements in dynamic ankle motion, which are not significant.[26,33] Kinetic variables such as peak power generation show no change following an injection of botulinum toxin A,[26,29,34] and AMQ and APQ demonstrate inconsistent findings with reports of either improvements[34] or no change.[29] Although gait analysis provides a quantitative method of assessing dynamic motion and forces, the findings are inconclusive with respect to the efficacy of botulinum toxin A at improving walking patterns in all children.

Boyd et al. stratified the response level to botulinum toxin A in children with cerebral palsy utilizing a combination of clinical measures and gait analysis and found that not all children have a universally favorable response. Only 5% of children were considered to be "golden responders," as they achieved and maintained functional goals for more than 12 months, 75% were clinical responders in whom some of their goals were met and a functional gain was maintained between 6 and 23 months, and 20% were minimal or nonresponders.[35] The question is how do we separate out preinjection those that would respond and those that would not? More specifically, how do we gain greater insight into the dynamic vs. the fixed component of muscle shortening? Musculoskeletal models have been developed and utilized to enhance our understanding of movement abnormalities and to provide a theoretical basis for assessing and planning treatment.[36] These models provide information about biomechanical parameters that are not easily measured, such as muscle lengths, moment arms of muscles, and force and moment-generating capacities.[36] Musculoskeletal models are combined with the computerized gait analysis data to determine dynamic muscle length during gait. Although the musculoskeletal geometry and locations of various origins and insertions vary between the models, some of the musculoskeletal models utilize the musculoskeletal geometry of normal adult males,[37] while others have utilized magnetic resonance imaging (MRI) data from both able-bodied children and children with cerebral palsy.[39,40] Musculoskeletal models have been found to provide a basis for identifying patients who will likely benefit from surgical intervention and those who may not,[36] in addition to bestowing insight into our understanding of the changes in functional outcome following alterations to biomechanical alignment.

8.5 MUSCULOSKELETAL MODELING

Musculoskeletal length models are beginning to be utilized to assess the muscle length in children with either dynamic or fixed equines and subsequently determine the impact of muscle length on the efficacy of surgical and pharmacological interventions at the ankle. Wren et al. evaluated two groups of children with either dynamic or fixed equinus during gait. While abnormally short muscle lengths were found in the dynamic group and the fixed group preoperatively, the fixed group also demonstrated shorter static muscle lengths and higher dynamic-to-static ratios of muscle length, which did not change significantly after surgical intervention to the gastrocnemius muscle. The differentiation between these two groups of children as a function of their muscle length may facilitate treatment planning and subsequently determine the outcome of different treatment options.

Utilizing data from three-dimensional gait analysis, anthropometric measurements of the children taken from MRI scans, and a simple model of muscle length, Eames et al. were able to determine the dynamic and fixed components of muscle shortening to overall muscle length in 39 children treated with botulinum toxin A.[41] They found that there was a mean increase in muscle length during gait of 1.5% and that there was a strong correlation between the dynamic component measured before the injection and the maximum response measured as a change in gastrocnemius length during gait. Therefore, children with a greater dynamic component to their gait had a greater response to an injection of botulinum toxin A as demonstrated by the increase in muscle length postinjection. These authors felt that gait analysis had a role in determining which patients are likely to benefit from botulinum toxin A injection in the gastrocnemius muscle.

Bang et al. evaluated the muscle lengths of children with cerebral palsy before and after botulinum toxin A injection and found that although the gastrocnemius length improved by 0.44 cm on average for the entire group, nine of the limbs in eight patients demonstrated a paradoxical decrease in the gastrocnemius muscle lengths following an injection of botulinum toxin A.[39] Closer evaluation of this group of patients revealed the presence of genu recurvatum prior to treatment. They found that although the tibia and ankle portion of the gastrocnemius length increased postinjection, the decrease in the knee portion of the muscle length minimized the absolute gains postinjection, and thus they suggested that utilization of the dynamic length of the soleus is of greater use than the gastrocnemius in children with dynamic equinus and genu recurvatum.

Evaluating the effect of botulinum toxin A on the hamstrings of patients with crouch gait, Thompson et al.[42] found that several of the hamstring muscles that were to be injected had adequate muscle length prior to injection. Following injection, only the muscles that were short preinjection showed a significant improvement in excursion, whereas muscles with adequate muscle length did not. They attributed their findings to the fact that botulinum toxin A acts on the dynamic component of the spasticity in the short muscle, which is not present to the same extent in a muscle that has adequate length. Despite the lack of increase in muscle length as measured with musculoskeletal modeling, Thompson et al. also found that for the group as a whole, the knee kinematics improved significantly. Thus botulinum toxin A can impact the dynamic element of the contracture as measured with kinematic data; however, it may produce relatively small changes in absolute muscle length.[42]

In our multicenter study comparing the efficacy of botulinum toxin A alone, casting alone, or the combination of botulinum toxin A and casting at reducing the dynamic equinus during gait in children with spastic cerebral palsy, it was found that botulinum toxin A alone provided no improvement in ankle kinematics, velocity, and stride length, while casting alone and botulinum toxin A casting were effective in the short- and long-term management of dynamic equinus.[26] Ankle kinematics and kinetics, passive ankle range of motion, and Tardieu were utilized to determine the efficacy of each treatment. These findings are in conflict with many of the clinical reports and randomized studies reported.[35,24,43] Perhaps the utilization of musculoskeletal modeling may provide additional insight into the discrepancy between our findings and those of other authors. Below are two examples of children treated with botulinum toxin A only. Initial clinical and ankle kinematic measurements were similar between the two children; however, muscle length modeling demonstrates different findings before and after treatment.

8.6 CASE STUDIES

Case 1 is an 8-yr-old male with a diagnosis of spastic left hemiplegia who walked with dynamic equinus on the left. He was evaluated preinjection and 3 months postinjection with both passive range of motion, Ashworth and Taridieu scales and quantitative gait analysis. His preinjection range of motion at the ankle was 15° dorsiflexion, with the knee flexed and 5° with the knee extended. Gastrocnemius spasticity, as measured with the Ashworth scale, demonstrated a score of 2, while the Tardieu scale was −10°. Postinjection, the range of motion at the ankle was 15° dorsiflexion with the knee flexed and 10° with the knee extended. The Ashworth scale demonstrated a score of 2, while the Tardieu scale was 5°. Ankle kinematic graphs demonstrate a double bump ankle pattern usually indicative of ankle spasticity preinjection, which was eliminated postinjection (Figure 8.2). An improvement in

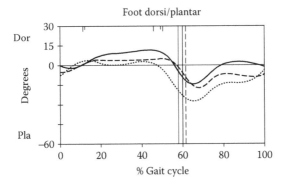

FIGURE 8.2 Case 1: Representation of ankle kinematics pre– and post–botulinum toxin A injection. Solid black line with standard deviation bar — normal database; dotted line — pre-botulinom toxin A; dashed line — post-botulinum toxin A.

dorsiflexion during mid- to late-stance and throughout swing was found, in addition to the elimination of his double bump ankle pattern. Assessment of the gastrocnemius (Figure 8.3) and soleus (Figure 8.4) muscle lengths demonstrates shorter than normal muscle lengths preinjection, which improve in muscle length 3 months after botulinum toxin A, especially during mid- to late-stance.

Case 2 is an 8-yr-old female with a diagnosis of spastic hemiplegia, who presented with dynamic equinus of the left. She was evaluated preinjection and 3 months postinjection, with both passive range of motion, Ashworth and Tardieu scales and quantitative gait analysis. Her preinjection range of motion at the ankle was 25° dorsiflexion with the knee flexed and 15° with the knee extended. The Ashworth scale demonstrated a score of 2, while the Tardieu scale was –10°. Postinjection, the

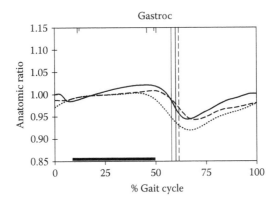

FIGURE 8.3 Case 1: Representation of gastrocnemius muscle length pre– and post–botulinum toxin A injection. Solid black line with standard deviation bar — normal database; dotted line — pre-botulinom toxin A; dashed line — post-botulinum toxin A.

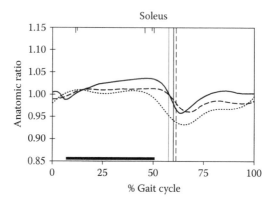

FIGURE 8.4 Case 1: Representation of soleus muscle length pre– and post–botulinum toxin A injection. Solid black line with standard deviation bar — normal database; dotted line — pre-botulinom toxin A; dashed line — post-botulinum toxin A.

range of motion at the ankle was 25° dorsiflexion with the knee flexed and 25° with the knee extended. The Ashworth scale demonstrated a score of 2, while the Tardieu scale was 0° or neutral. Ankle kinematic graphs demonstrate a double bump ankle pattern usually indicative of dynamic ankle spasticity preinjection, which remained postinjection, although a slight increase in maximum dorsiflexion was noted (Figure 8.5). Prior to the injection, gastrocnemius length (Figure 8.6) during stance was only slightly reduced from normal, while swing phase length was short during mid- to late-swing. The soleus muscle (Figure 8.7) was shorter than normal throughout most of the cycle. Following the injection of botulinum toxin A, there were only slight improvements in muscle length of either the gastrocnemius or the soleus.

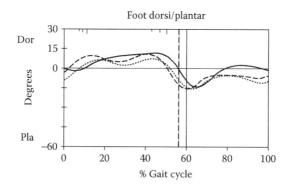

FIGURE 8.5 Case 2: Representation of ankle kinematics pre– and post–botulinum toxin A injection. Solid black line with standard deviation bar — normal database, dotted line — pre-botulinum toxin A; dashed line — post-botulinum toxin A.

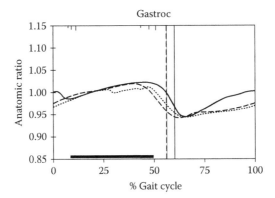

FIGURE 8.6 Case 2: Representation of gastrocnemius muscle length pre– and post–botulinum toxin A injection. Solid black line with standard deviation bar — normal database; dotted line — pre-botulinum toxin A; dashed line —post-botulinum toxin A.

8.7 SUMMARY AND CONCLUSIONS

Muscle length models provide further insight into the changes following botulinum toxin A injections; however, limitations to the musculoskeletal models must be reduced and the accuracy with which the models represent the individuals with musculoskeletal impairments needs to be enhanced before models, and subsequently simulations, can be used clinically to guide treatment decisions.[36] In order to gain further insight into the potential difference in the architecture of the medial gastrocnemius, Shortland et al. evaluated normal adults and children in addition to children with spastic diplegia using ultrasound images.[44] They found that the architectural

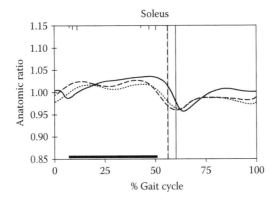

FIGURE 8.7 Case 2: Representation of soleus muscle length pre– and post–botulinum toxin A injection. Solid black line with standard deviation bar — normal database; dotted line — pre-botulinum toxin A; dashed line — post-botulinum toxin A.

variables of the muscle were similar for normally developing adults and children. In addition, they also found that the architecture of the medial gastrocnemius did not differ greatly between normally developing children and children with cerebral palsy; however, deep fascicle angles were consistently smaller at any ankle joint angle in children with spastic diplegia.[44] Further to this study, Fry et al. utilized three-dimensional ultrasound to determine the differences in the muscle architecture and morphology of normally developing children and children with cerebral palsy and found that children with cerebral palsy have a shorter medial gastrocnemius muscle belly than their peers.[45] These findings suggest that the muscle bellies of children with spastic diplegia do not grow as rapidly as the long bone, and thus their tendons adapt to a greater length under conditions of increased tension.[45] The combination of the morphological measurements that are made possible by the ultrasound technique can produce patient-specific mechanical characteristics of the actuators. These may then be incorporated into the current models providing a mechanism with which one can relate individual muscle impairment to function and determine the impact of treatment interventions on the individual.

Clinical measures of dynamic and static lengths of the gastrocnemius (passive range of motion), dynamic ankle range of motion during gait (kinematics), and muscle length (modeling) measurements have demonstrated that children with cerebral palsy have varying degrees of dynamic and fixed equinus; however, further investigation is required to determine the continuum on which treatments such as casting, bracing, physical therapy, botulinum toxin A, and orthopedic surgery should be offered. While some treatments such as botulinum toxin A appear to impact the dynamic component of muscle length rather than fixed, the combination of botulinum toxin A and casting may address both the fixed and the dynamic components of equinus gait, leading to greater improvement in both clinical and dynamic outcome measures.

Fifty-two percent of children have been reported to undergo tendoachilles lengthenings following a minimum of three injections of botulinum toxin A,[46] therefore improvements in ankle dorsiflexion and increases in muscle length are transient for a percentage of children and a problem that requires surgical intervention. While the utilization of botulinum toxin A may delay the need for orthopedic surgery to a time where the outcomes are more predictable in some children, the data available to date would appear to dispute the premise that relaxing the muscle via botulinum toxin A allows or promotes longitudinal muscle growth. The question that remains is whether the use of botulinum toxin A altered the course of the other 48% of children and what distinguishing features can be recognized between the two groups, which will facilitate the identification of which children would benefit from botulinum toxin A injection.

ACKNOWLEDGMENTS

The authors would like to acknowledge and thank Bruce MacWilliams, PhD, and Robin Dorociak, BS, for their technical assistance in the development of the ankle motion and muscle length graphs and Cathleen Buckon, MS, for her editorial assistance.

REFERENCES

1. Jankovic, J., Brin, M., "Botulinum toxin: historical perspective and potential new indications," In: Mayer, N.H., Simpson D.M., eds. *Spasticity: Etiology, Evaluation, Management and the Role of Botulinum Toxin*, New York: We Move, 2002, 100.
2. Scott, A., "Botulinum toxin injection of eye muscles to correct strabisumus," *Trans Am Opthalmol Soc*, 79:734, 1981.
3. Koman, L.A., Mooney, J.F., Smith, B., et al., "Managament of cerebral palsy with botulinum-a toxin: preliminary investigation," *J Pediatr Orthop*, 13:489, 1993.
4. Graham, H.K., Aoki, K.R., Autti-Ramo, I., et al., "Recommendations for the use of botulinum toxin type A in the management of cerebral palsy," *Gait Posture*, 11:67, 2000.
5. Bakheit, A.M.O., Severa, S., Cosgrove, A., et al., "Safety profile and efficacy of botulinum toxin A (Dysport) in children with muscle spasticity," *Dev Med Child Neurol*, 43:234, 2001.
6. Koman, L.A., Mooney, J.F., Smith, B.P., et al., "Management of spasticity in cerebral palsy with botulinum-a toxin: report of a preliminary, randomized, double-blind trial," *J Pediatr Orthop*, 14:299, 1994.
7. Koman, L.A., Mooney, J.F., Smith, B.P., "Neuromuscular blockade in the management of cerebral palsy," *J Child Neurol*, 11(suppl 1):23, 1996.
8. Ziv, I., Blackburn, N., Rang, M., et al., "Muscle growth in normal and spastic mice," *Dev Med Child Neurol*, 26:94, 1984.
9. Wright, J., Rang, M., "The spastic mouse and the search for an animal model of spasticity in human beings," *Clin Orthop Relat Res*, 253:12, 1990.
10. Cosgrove, A.P., Graham, H.K., "Botulinum toxin A prevents the development of contractures in the hereditary spastic mouse," *Dev Med Child Neurol*, 36:379, 1994.
11. Delp, S., "What causes increased muscle stiffness in cerebral palsy," *Muscle Nerve*, 27:131, 2003.
12. Lance, J., "Spasticity: disorders of motor control " In: Feldman, R., Young, R., and Koella, W., eds. *Symposium Synopsis*, Chicago: Year Book Publishers, 1980:185.
13. Lieber, R., Friden, J., "Spasticity causes a fundamental rearrangement of muscle-joint interaction," *Muscle Nerve*, 25:265, 2002.
14. Friden, J., Lieber, R., "Spastic muscle cells are shorter and stiffer than normal cells," *Muscle Nerve*, 27:157, 2003.
15. Lieber, R., Steinman, S., Barash, I., et al., "Structural and functional changes in spastic skeletal muscle," *Muscle Nerve*, 29:615, 2004.
16. Rosenthal, R., Simon, S., "The vulpius gastocnemius-soleus lengthening," In: Sussman, M., ed. *The Diplegic Child*, Rosemont, IL: American Academy of Orthopaedic Surgeons, 1992:355.
17. Boyd, R., Graham, H., "Objective measurement of clinical findings in the use of botulinum toxin type A for the management of children with cerebral palsy," *Eur J Neurol*, 6(suppl 4):23, 1999.
18. Boyd, R., "A physiotherapy perspective on assessment and outcome measurement of children with cerebral palsy," In: Scrutton, D., Damiano, D., Mayston, M., eds. *Management of the Motor Disorders of Children with Cerebral Palsy*, London: MacKeith Press, 2004:52.
19. Stuberg, W., Fuchs, R., Meaner, J., "Reliability of goniometric measurements of children with cerebral palsy," *Dev Med Child Neurol*, 30:657, 1988.
20. Perry, J., Giovn, P., Harris, L., et al., "The determinants of muscle action in the hemiparetic lower extremity and their effect on the examination procedure," *Clin Orthop Relat Res*, 131:71, 1978.

21. Schwartz, M., "Kinematics of normal gait," In: Gage, J., ed. *The Treatment of Gait Problems in Cerebral Palsy*, London: MacKeith Press, 2004:99.

22. Boyd, R.N., Pliatsios, V., Starr, R., et al., "Biomechanical transformation of the gastroc-soleus muscle with botulinum toxin A in children with cerebral palsy," *Dev Med Child Neurol*, 42:32, 2000.

23. Sutherland, D.H., Kaufman, K.R., Wyatt, M.P., et al., "Injection of botulinum A toxin into the gastrocnemius muscle of patients with cerebral palsy: a 3-dimensional motion analysis study," *Gait Posture*, 4:269, 1996.

24. Sutherland, D.H., Kaufman, K.R., Wyatt, M.P., et al., "Double-blind study of botulinum A toxin injections into the gastrocnemius muscle in patients with cerebral palsy," *Gait Posture*, 10:1, 1999.

25. Koman, L.A., Mooney, J.F., Smith, B.P., et al., "Botulinum toxin type a neuromuscular blockade in the treatment of lower extremity spasticity in cerebral palsy: a randomized, double-blind, placebo-controlled trial," *J Pediatr Orthop*, 20:108, 2000.

26. Ackman, J., Russman, B., Thomas, S., et al., "Comparing botulinum toxin A with casting for treatment of dynamic equinus in children with cerebral palsy," *Dev Med Child Neurol*, 47:620, 2005.

27. Corry, I.S., Cosgrove, A.P., Duffy, C.M., et al., "Botulinum toxin A compared with stretching cast in the treatment of spastic equinus: a randomised prospective trial," *J Pediatr Orthop*, 19:304, 1998.

28. Flett, P.J., Stern, L.M., Waddy, H., et al., "Botulinum toxin A versus fixed cast stretching for dynamic calf tightness in cerebral palsy," *J Paediatr Child Health*, 35:71, 1999.

29. Metaxiotis, D., Siebel, A., and Doederlein, L., "Repeated botulinum toxin a injections in the treatment of spastic equinus foot," *Clin Orthop Relat Res*, 394:177, 2002.

30. Ubhi, T., Bhakta, B.B., Ives, H.L., et al., "Randomised double blind placebo controlled trial of the effect of botulinum toxin on walking in cerebral palsy," *Arch Dis Child*, 83:481, 2000.

31. Wissel, J., Muller, J., Baldauf, A., et al., "Gait analysis to assess the effects of botulinum toxin type A treatment in cerebral palsy: an open-label study in 10 children with equinus gait pattern," *Eur J Neurol*, 6:S63, 1999.

32. Cosgrove, A.P., Corry, I.S., and Graham, H.K., "Botulinum toxin in the management of the lower limb in cerebral palsy," *Dev Med Child Neurol*, 36:386, 1994.

33. Bottos, M., Benedetti, M., Salucci, P., et al., "Botulinum toxin with and without casting in ambulant children with spastic diplegia: a clinical and functional assessment," *Dev Med Child Neurol*, 45:758, 2003.

34. Zurcher, A.W., Molenaers, G., Desloovere, K., et al., "Kinematics and kinetic evaluation of the ankle after intramuscular injection of botulinum toxin a in children with cerebral palsy," *Acta Orthop Belg*, 67:475, 2001.

35. Boyd, R., Graham, J., Nattrass, G., et al., "Medium-term response characterization and risk factor analysis of botulinum toxin type A in the management of spasticity in children with cerebral palsy," *Eur J Neurol*, 6(suppl 4):S37, 1999.

36. Arnold, A., Delp, S., "The role of musculoskeletal models in patient assessment and treatment," In: Gage, J., ed. *The Treatment of Gait Problems in Cerebral Palsy*, London: MacKeith Press, 2004:165.

37. Delp, S., Loan, J., Hoy, M., et al., "An interactive graphics-based model of the lower extremity to study orthopaedic procedures," *IEEE Trans Biomed Eng*, 37:757, 1990.

38. Wren, T.A., Do, K.P., and Kay, R.M., Gastrocnemius and soleus lengths in cerebral palsy equinus gait — difference between children with and without static contracture and effects of gastrocnemeius recession. *J. Biomech*, Scp, 37(9): 1321–7, 2004.

39. Bang, M., Chung, S., Kim, S., et al., "Change of dynamic gastrocnemius and soleus muscle length after block of spastic calf muscle in cerebral palsy," *Am J Phys Med Rehabil*, 81:760, 2002.
40. Eames, N., Baker, R., Cosgrove, A., "Defining gastrocnemius length in ambulant children," *Gait Posture*, vol. 6. 9, 1997.
41. Eames, N.W.A., Baker, R., Hill, N., et al., "The effect of botulinum toxin A on gastrocnemius length: magnitude and duration of response," *Dev Med Child Neurol*, 41:226, 1999.
42. Thompson, N., Baker, R., Cosgrove, A., et al., "Musculoskeletal modelling in determining the effect of botulinum toxin on the hamstrings of patients with crouch gait," *Dev Med Child Neurol*, 40:622, 1998.
43. Desloovere, K., Molenaers, G., Jonkers, I., et al., "A randomized study of combined botulinum toxin type A and casting in the ambulant child with cerebral palsy using objective outcome measures," *Eur J Neurol*, 8(suppl 5):75, 2001.
44. Shortland, A., Harris, C., Gough, M., et al., "Architecture of the medial gastrocnemius in children with spastic diplegia," *Dev Med Child Neurol*, 44:158, 2002.
45. Fry, N., Gough, M., Shortland, A., "Three-dimensional realisation of muscle morpology and architecture using ultrasound," *Gait Posture*, 20:177, 2004.
46. Koman, L.A., Smith, B.P., Tingley, C.T., et al., "The effect of botulinum toxin type A injections on the natural history of equinus foot deformity in paediatric cerebral palsy patients," *Eur J Neurol*, 6(suppl 4):19, 1999.

9 Equinovarus Foot: Electromyography Analysis and Clinical Outcome

Michael Aiona, Robin Dorociak, Molly Nichols, and Rosemary Pierce

CONTENTS

9.1   INTRODUCTION

Neuromuscular deficits in patients with cerebral palsy cause a variety of bone and joint deformities. One common deformity is the equinovarus foot. This multiplane deformity consists of equinus at the ankle and inversion at the subtalar joint. An imbalance of forces across these two joints is responsible for this deformity.

9.2   NORMAL ANATOMY/KINESIOLOGY OF FOOT AND ANKLE

Foot position during gait is controlled by muscle-generated forces and by body weight (the ground reaction force). In the equinovarus foot, the muscles of interest are those affecting subtalar joint movements. The axis of rotation of this complex joint is oriented in the sagittal plane approximately 45° from posterior plantar to dorsal anterior. In the transverse plane, it is directed 23° medially.[1]

The muscular invertors of the foot consist of the posterior tibialis, soleus, and the anterior tibialis. Though the peroneal muscles are evertors of the foot, body weight provides the greatest eversion force during stance phase. The anterior tibialis functions to dorsiflex the foot in swing phase, assisting in foot clearance as well as controlling ankle plantar flexion at initial foot contact. The posterior tibialis, active in stance phase, controls foot position around the subtalar joint as the ground reaction force moves laterally across the foot.

9.3 EQUINOVARUS FOOT PATHOMECHANICS

In patients with cerebral palsy, the resultant abnormal mechanical alignment along with weak, spastic muscles can produce an abnormal gait pattern. Obtaining a plantigrade foot is an essential part of the treatment of these complex multilevel gait deformities. The goal of correction of any significant foot deformity should be improved pressure distribution along the sole of the foot, allowing brace tolerance and shoe fitting. As such, the plantigrade foot is an essential part of the treatment goals in these complex multilevel gait deformities. The foot functions biomechanically much like a lever at the ankle joint, modulating the influence of the ground reaction force on proximal joints during gait. As the point of application of this force vector moves along the plantar surface of the foot during stance phase, structural foot deformities may alter its normal direction of progression during weight bearing.

Various combinations of overactivity and weakness of the anterior tibialis and posterior tibialis muscles produce varus in the foot. While each muscle performs different functions during gait, each has been implicated as causing foot deformity.

Though equinovarus is predominantly a stance phase issue, swing phase abnormalities can cause this deformity. The anterior tibialis inserts on the medial cuneiform and the first metatarsal close to the subtalar axis of rotation. With slight inversion of the foot, it becomes a stronger invertor of the foot by being in a more mechanically advantageous position, tipping the balance of power across the subtalar joint toward inversion. Recent studies have supported the significant influence of foot position on the moment arms of the anterior tibialis and posterior tibialis about the subtalar joint axis.[2] Out-of-phase posterior tibialis activity in swing phase may cause the foot to land in an inverted position at initial foot contact, causing the direction of the ground reaction force to remain medial to the axis of rotation of the subtalar joint and diminishing the everting effect of body weight. Stance phase activity of the anterior tibialis may add to the deformity if the foot is already prepositioned in inversion.

9.4 CLINICAL IMPLICATIONS OF THE EQUINOVARUS FOOT

The clinical impact of the equinovarus foot is the abnormal plantar pressure distribution with resultant pain and callus formation. Specifically, pressure on the base of the fifth metatarsal is a sign of the persistent varus position of the foot with the head of the metatarsal involved with significant equinus (Figure 9.1a, b). Significant

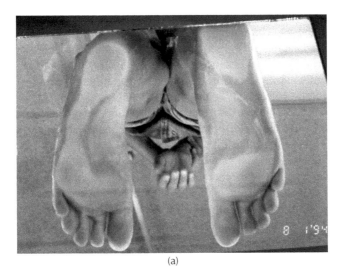

(a)

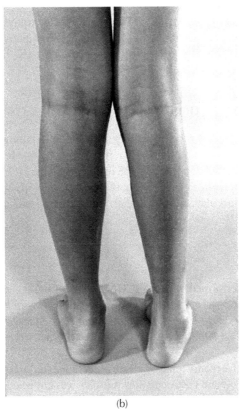

(b)

FIGURE 9.1 (a) Plantar Pressure on the sole of the foot demonstrating excessive lateral weighing typical of an inverted varus foot; (b) view of the inverted heel position in the weight-bearing position.

deformity may make it difficult to tolerate brace wear. Patients are more prone to ankle sprains, and some have metatarsal stress fractures from the persistent abnormal loading. The indications for surgery would include an unbraceable foot, pain, progressive deformity, and, on occasion, the hope of making the foot brace free.

As two potential muscles are implicated as the etiology of the deformity, the surgical procedure performed would require defining the major deforming force. Described procedures include the isolated posterior tibialis lengthening, split anterior tibialis transfer, split posterior tibialis transfer, or a combination of the above.[3–15] The clinician presently evaluates the strength of the anterior tibialis, the position of the foot during observational gait, the tightness and spasticity of each muscle, and the passive correctability of the foot to determine the choice of the procedure. Though results have been generally good, failures have been noted. Some authors have proposed that more in-depth evaluation of muscle activity would enhance the percentage of good results, as nonphasic muscle activity could be identified.[16–18]

9.5   EMG ASSESSMENT OF EQUINOVARUS FOOT STUDY

We reviewed our treatment experience to determine if electromyogram (EMG) firing patterns influence the outcome of the surgically managed equinovarus foot in patients with cerebral palsy. This study design was approved by the Institutional Review Board (IRB).

9.6   STUDY POPULATION

Inclusion criteria included surgical management of an equinovarus foot, pre- and post-op 3D gait analysis with preoperative fine wire assessment of posterior tibialis activity. Twenty-six ambulatory patients (28 limbs, mean age 11.2 ± 3.3) with cerebral palsy (16 with hemiplegia, 7 with spastic diplegia, 1 with spastic quadriplegia, and 2 unknown neuromuscular disorders) met these criteria and constitute the study population.

9.7   METHODS

Gait analysis was performed with a VICON 6-camera motion analysis system collected at 50 Hz. The markers were placed in accordance with the VICON Clinical Manager (VCM) model to generate the kinematic data. Surface and fine wire electrodes were placed to simultaneously record muscle activity with a Motion Lab Systems MA-300.

The activity of the rectus femoris, vastus medialis, vastus lateralis, medial hamstring, tibialis anterior, and gastrocnemius muscles was collected with surface EMG. Posterior tibialis muscle activity for the affected limb was collected using fine wire EMG. Placement of the fine wire electrode in the posterior tibialis muscle was confirmed by electrical stimulation. Data collection rate for fine wire and surface EMG was 800 Hz with 20 Hz high pass and 300 Hz low pass. For this study, EMG data for gastrocnemius, anterior tibialis, and posterior tibialis were analyzed.

Kinematics and kinetics were processed with VCM. EMG data were linear enveloped also using VCM. Three representative trials were chosen for analysis (for a few subjects, only two representative trials were available). Anterior tibialis and gastrocnemius surface EMG data were collected simultaneously during walking trials. Posterior tibialis fine wire EMG data were collected during subsequent walking trials. An Excel® spreadsheet was used to extract the EMG data into 2% increments of the gait cycle. EMG data were normalized to maximum signal activity during the entire gait cycle for each trial. An ensemble average of the three trials was created. To categorize on/off activity, a 20% threshold was applied to account for potential baseline signal noise. Less than 20% of normalized maximum signal activity was "off," with greater than 20% classified as "on."

The mean percent gait cycle for foot off, opposite foot off, and opposite foot contact was calculated for the three representative trials for each subject. The gait cycle was divided into phases:

- Loading: 0 to 8%
- Stance: 16 to 50%
- Preswing: 8% of gait cycle preceding foot off
- Initial swing: 8% of gait cycle following foot off
- Terminal swing: 92 to 100%

Muscle activity was considered to be "on" for a phase if the majority (>80%) of the phase points were "on." EMG activity profiles for each of the three muscles were created.

Clinical outcomes were categorized using a modification of the Kling criteria.[9] Excellent (E) was a plantigrade foot in valgus. Satisfactory (S) was a foot with improved lateral pressure, though with some residual increase. A poor (P) result was an uncorrected foot. The use of a brace was not a discriminating criterion as the ability of patients to voluntarily dorsiflex the foot was variable, and the goal of the surgery is to achieve a plantigrade, braceable foot.

9.8   RESULTS

Fifty percent (14/28) of feet had an excellent result though one patient required one further operation to achieve the final result. Eighteen percent (5/28) had a satisfactory result with some mild residual deformity not requiring further intervention. Two of these patients had an initial excellent correction but had a recurrent though mild deformity. Therefore, almost 70% of patients had significant improvement at final follow-up. Despite having more than one surgical attempt at correction, 9 feet were still classified as a poor result with unimproved persistent significant lateral weight-bearing pressure. Interestingly, these residual deformities did not appear to prevent successful ambulation (Table 9.1).

The literature appears to distinguish two main categories of abnormal muscle activity that would suggest specific recommended interventions, stance phase anterior tibialis activity, and swing phase posterior tibialis activity. These specific patients were separately analyzed.

TABLE 9.1
Overall Results of Surgical Treatment

Procedure	Result		
	E	S	P
Split anterior tibialis transfer + posterior tibialis lengthening	3	3	6
Isolated posterior tibialis lengthening	9	0	1
Split posterior tibialis transfer	2	2	2

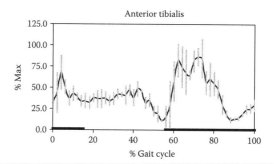

FIGURE 9.2 Stance phase anterior tibialis activity (non-phasic). Black bar represents normal expected timing.

TABLE 9.2
Results in Feet with Stance Phase Anterior Tibialis Activity

Procedure	Result		
	E	S	P
Anterior tibialis procedure	2	2	5
No anterior tibialis procedure	6	1	0

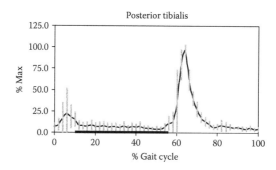

FIGURE 9.3 Swing phase posterior tibialis activity (non-phasic). Black bar represents normal expected timing.

Significant anterior tibialis activity in stance would indicate the need for anterior tibialis transfer (Figure 9.2). Sixteen feet had anterior tibialis activity in stance phase. Nine had a split anterior tibialis transfer with only four feet achieving satisfactory or excellent results and five having poor results. Of the five poor results, two had technical surgical problems requiring retensioning of the transferred arm. Interestingly, 86% of the feet that did not have any anterior tibialis intervention despite stance phase activity did well with acceptable clinical outcomes. This would suggest that the mere presence of anterior tibialis activity in stance phase does not mean a procedure addressing that specific muscle is necessary to obtain a good result (Table 9.2).

The second category of nonphasic muscle activity involves the posterior tibialis muscle (Figure 9.3). If swing phase activity was present, then some posterior tibialis procedure was recommended. All patients underwent some sort of intervention on the posterior tibialis muscle. An intramuscular lengthening was performed in the majority of the cases, with six cases undergoing split posterior tibialis transfer (Table 9.3).

A majority of feet with isolated lengthening appear to have had an excellent result and never went on to have further surgical intervention. Three feet had initially excellent results, but had recurrence with time and required further procedures including repeat lengthening. Of the four poor results, further surgery was performed including tendon transfer to achieve a better foot position. This would imply that swing phase posterior tibialis activity might be prognostic for a good result with stance phase anterior tibialis activity potentially more difficult to treat.

Though all patients met the prerequisite of a passively correctable deformity, it is clear that age at surgery influenced outcome. Though clinically it was felt that the deformity was correctable, the older patient may have a more "rigid" deformity not as amenable to tendon transfer alone. In fact, of all of the poor results, only one patient was under the age of ten at the time of surgery. Interestingly, the majority of older patients underwent anterior tibialis surgery, perhaps skewing the analysis of this particular surgery toward poorer results (Table 9.4).

In analyzing the poor results, it is difficult to evaluate the adequacy of the surgical technique. Though some patients underwent further surgery to retension the transferred tendon, it is difficult to know if some of the less than satisfactory results were due to the difficulty in setting the correct tension on the transferred or lengthened muscle.[19–21] It is assumed that any obvious technical failures would have been addressed with further surgery, though acceptance of a less than optimal result may have been the choice of some patients and families as the amount of improvement

TABLE 9.3
Results in Feet with Swing Phase Posterior Tibialis Activity

Procedure	Result		
	E	S	P
Intramuscular (IM) lengthening	10	1	4
Split posterior tibialis transfer (SPPT)	2	2	2

TABLE 9.4
Results Based on Age at Initial Surgical
Treatment

	Result		
Age at Surgery	E	S	P
Less than 10-yr-old	9	3	1
Greater than 10-yr-old	5	2	8

was sufficient. Indeed, the majority of patients were clinically and functionally improved despite residual deformity.

9.9 COMPARISONS WITH CURRENT LITERATURE AND INDICATIONS FOR SURGERY

As this study included three different surgical procedures, comparison to the literature can be done only if the procedures are analyzed separately. Barnes and Herring reported the outcomes of a split anterior tibialis transfer with posterior tibialis lengthening in the management of an equinovarus foot in patients with cerebral palsy.[5] The criteria for the procedure was a flexible foot with adequate anterior tibialis strength. Assessment of the patient did not include gait analysis or EMG data. Twenty-four of the twenty-eight feet had good results with only four failures. Two failures were because the anterior tibialis was not of adequate strength and two had more rigid deformities, which were unlikely to respond to tendon transfer alone. The findings of our study would support those two conclusions. Patients with good functional anterior tibialis strength defined as adequate dorsiflexion in swing phase measured by computerized gait analysis had excellent results with anterior tibialis transfer. Age played a role in our poor results, implying a greater degree of rigidity in patients over 10 yr, accounting for the higher failure rate.

Green et al. reported good results in 16/16 patients with split posterior tibialis transfer, though two required calcaneal osteotomies to correct fixed varus.[10] If equinus was present, then a split posterior tibialis procedure was performed. In their experience, the anterior tibialis is weak in many of these patients. They noted significant posterior tibialis EMG activity with all showing swing phase activity with continuous activity in some patients. O'Byrne et al. had similar good results while incorporating the use of gait analysis in the assessment and management of this deformity.[11] They also felt the presence of equinus in swing phase would indicate the anterior tibialis is weak and a split posterior tibialis procedure should be recommended. However, in both studies, the majority of the patients underwent concomitant heelcord lengthening, implying a fixed ankle deformity. Thus the anterior tibialis would not be expected to dorsiflex the foot in the face of a fixed deformity. In addition, there are no data to support whether transfer is better than lengthening alone. Their implication is that if the foot is in equinus in swing phase, a split transfer would be recommended. All patients in our study had the posterior tibialis addressed in some manner, agreeing with Kling that this appears to be the main deforming force.[9] Over two thirds of the feet had good results with a simple intramuscular posterior tibialis lengthening, a much easier procedure than a transfer. However, a selection bias may be present, as the treating physician may have chosen an isolated lengthening for those individuals with a milder deformity. We were unable to define which additional factors would predict which procedure to perform.

9.10 DISCUSSION

Joint deformity in patients with cerebral palsy is the result of an imbalance of the forces that control position. Many soft-tissue procedures on muscles and tendons are meant to balance those forces to correct deformity. The use of EMG activity as promoted in the literature to determine the surgical choice and influence outcome did not routinely achieve excellent results in our study. Stance phase anterior tibialis activity and swing phase posterior tibialis activity are examples of muscles firing out of phase. This would seem to imply the need to address these muscles in the management of the deformity. However, with these criteria, analysis of our data and outcomes did not yield predictable results.

The causes of equinovarus foot deformity can be multiple. It may be a prepositioning issue with the foot held in "enough" inversion to cause the ground reaction force to stay medial to the subtalar joint axis. The ground reaction force would maintain the foot in inversion, causing increased lateral pressure on the foot. Persistent stance phase force imbalance, maintaining the foot in inversion, may also be a causative factor. The challenge is determining how much is too much or too little. The complexity of the subtalar axis and its relationship to the ground reaction force add to this challenging problem.

What areas of further development may improve this predictability? The authors and others[22] believe better definition of the muscle force, a more detailed kinematic model of the foot, and improved analysis and assessment capabilities of dynamic foot pressure would be the key future developments needed to further understanding and treatment of this foot deformity.

9.10.1 COMPONENTS OF FORCE

What are the components of force and what are the barriers to accurate measurement? Factors involved in determining the effects of muscles on the joints of the foot include: the timing of contraction, the muscle force generated, the muscle length and excursion, and the moment arm. Some or all of these elements may be abnormal in the patient with cerebral palsy. Current movement analysis and foot assessment tools are being developed in hopes of improving the accurate measurement of the subtalar joint during gait.

9.10.2 CURRENT ASSESSMENT TOOLS AND LIMITATIONS

Force generation requires the timely, selective electrical activation (i.e., phasic activity) of the muscle by the nervous system. The electrical activity of the muscle can be measured through the use of the electromyogram. Electrodes are placed on the surface in anatomically correct locations to measure the activity of the muscle. Advantages of surface EMG include the noninvasive nature of the technique and the sampling of a broader area of muscle. However, surface EMG signal may be affected by skin resistance, amount of subcutaneous tissue, and the potential for cross talk with adjacent muscles, and is limited to muscles directly under the skin surface. To measure the activity of muscles not accessible through surface techniques, a fine wire electrode may be placed through the insertion of a needle into those muscles. Sampling of fine wire data is specific to the area at the tip of the electrode, unlike the broad area of the surface electrode. Verification of fine wire placement requires stimulation, which may be painful to the subject. Though its use is needed for specific deep muscles, its application for many muscles is of limited or no use in the pediatric population.

Though EMGs demonstrate when a muscle is active and when it is silent, it is uncertain whether there is a correlation between the amplitude of the signal and the strength of the contraction.[23] In this study, a majority of feet with stance phase anterior tibialis activity and no surgery on this muscle did well. It may be that the strength of the muscle could not influence foot position, as it may be too weak to control body weight during stance phase. This is a prime example where strength, not activity, is the more relevant issue. Though the activity can be measured, separating muscle activity that is a primary cause of problems from reactive muscle activity required to maintain upright posture through compensatory mechanisms has been difficult to tease out from the data.

Biologic force is generated by muscle contraction. At the cellular level in patients with cerebral palsy, the biologic elements may be affected. Increased sarcomere length, less muscle excursion, and greater stiffness have all been reported. At the organ level, muscle dysfunction can be caused by inappropriate firing (phasic or nonphasic activity), weakness, diminished length, and excursion.[19,24]

At the clinical assessment level, manual muscle tests can be used to determine the strength of muscles influencing foot position. Isolating the contribution of each muscle is difficult. The resistance applied by the clinician can vary from day to day and from observer to observer. Mechanical devices to measure strength have been used. A hand-held dynamometer is easy to use, is portable, and can provide some quantitative data. Though some report good reliability with this measure, technical aspects including its use and application may make it inaccurate in some hands.[25,26] Specialized mechanical devices have been employed to measure strength. The joint is moved through a range of motions both passively to measure resistance and actively to measure torque generation. These are accurate and reproducible measures of muscle force–generating capacity. However, this *in vitro* measure does not necessarily reflect the power generation during a functional activity such as walking. Only the sagittal plane of the ankle has been evaluated extensively using specialized mechanical devices with none specifically for the complex motions of the foot.

Another area of need is the development of a more sophisticated kinematic model of the foot. Though gait analysis is well established as an accurate measure of kinematics of the lower extremity, the foot presents greater challenges. The foot is a complex entity with small bones, multiple joints, and 3D motions. Markers have to be small and placed on bony landmarks that may be distorted secondary to deformities of the foot. An improved foot model must separate the foot movements into anatomically based, relevant directions that can be clinically applied for defining causes and determining treatments. Motions may need to reflect summations of multiple joints, as the number and size of the bones present great challenges for measurement of each joint. Motions within the foot are small in magnitude, making precision even more critical. Many researchers and clinicians are developing working models describing foot motion,[27–31] some of which are covered in other chapters in this text.

Incorporating kinematic data, ground reaction force measurement, and anatomic measurements can yield kinetic data. One component of kinetic data is moment arm distance, which is not a static value as movement of a joint alters this measurement. Using anthropomorphic data, known anatomical structure, and 3D joint kinematics, the distance can be calculated with the generation of instantaneous moment data.[20,21]

An example of joint motion implying a degree of adequate strength is clearly demonstrated in the three patients with excellent results with the split anterior tibialis transfer, who had adequate "active" dorsiflexion seen in swing phase in the preoperative gait analysis. Unfortunately, a number of patients have an equinus component to their deformity, which prevents normal dorsiflexion motion in swing phase. This lack of motion does not necessarily imply anterior tibialis weakness, as the passive motion is not present to make this assessment accurate. More techniques will have to be developed to quantify muscle force production in hopes of answering questions of causation in the equinovarus foot.

The necessary forces needed to modulate the movement may require eccentric or concentric muscle contractions. Combining EMG activity and muscle length measures can assist in determining whether true power generation or absorption is occurring. One could propose that if a deformity were occurring with progressive muscle shortening, this would be pathologic. If the muscle is not shortening, it may be a modulating factor attempting to maintain or avoid positioning of a pathologic nature. With a more detailed kinematic model of the foot, EMG activity, kinetic, and muscle length data, more accurate, objective assessment would become possible in the foot.

An additional area of further development is foot pressure measurement analysis. Present technology can depict the static cumulative pressure on the sole of the foot. Dynamic foot pressure evaluations depict the pressure in designated areas of the foot over time, graphically representing the pressure pattern from foot contact to foot-off (Figure 9.4). This allows the generation of a central line of pressure to determine if the foot is loaded laterally or medially. In the equinovarus foot, persistent pressure on the lateral border of the foot occurs throughout stance.[32] Defining relevant variables from the data can be a clinical challenge. Photographic overlays, pressure area integration, and the use of nonvertical force measurement are examples of different ways to interpret the data.

Though each of the clinically available measurement devices has a slightly different approach, they should be integrated with the kinematics of the entire lower extremity. For example, proximal joints can influence the initial contact and positioning of the foot during gait. Though the foot pressure measure may show heel contact pressure, exaggerated knee extension and hip flexion can compensate for an

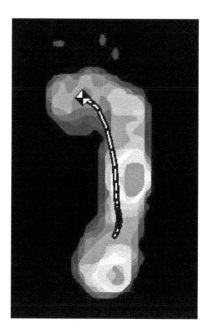

FIGURE 9.4 Pedobarograph demonstrating the excessive lateral pressure with areas of force concentration at the base of the 5th metatarsal

equinus positioning of the foot. It is well known that apparent equinus at the ankle may be secondary to knee flexion deformity, thus the pressure tracing would not be reflective of the actual anatomy of the foot. Though this measure is reliable and accurate in measuring actual foot pressure, it must be incorporated with other measures in order to assist in determining causation of the deformity.

In summary, patients with an equinovarus foot have difficulty with uneven pressure distribution of the foot and can have resulting functional limitations. Though a few surgical approaches are well accepted in treating the equinovarus foot, choosing which one to perform is still a dilemma for some clinicians. We propose that continued refinement of an accurate kinematic foot model, along with improved definition of muscle force, length, and strength will advance the understanding of the equinovarus foot in patients with cerebral palsy and thus lead to improved treatment outcomes.

REFERENCES

1. Close, J.R., et al. The function of the subtalar Joint, *Clin Orthop Relat Res*, 50, 159, 1967.
2. Piazza, S.J., et al. Changes in muscle moment arms following split tendon transfer of tibialis anterior and tibialis posterior, *Gait Posture*, 14, 271, 2001.
3. Ruda, R. and Frost, H.M. Cerebral palsy. Spastic varus and forefoot adductus, treated by intramuscular posterior tibial tendon lengthening, *Clin Orthop Relat Res*, 79, 61, 1971.

4. Johnson, W.L. and Lester, E.L. Transposition of the posterior tibial tendon, *Clin Orthop Relat Res*, 245, 223, 1989.
5. Barnes, M.J. and Herring, J.A. Combined split anterior-tibial tendon transfer and intramuscular lengthening of the posterior tibial tendon. Results in patients who have a varus deformity of the foot due to spastic cerebral palsy, *J Bone Joint Surg Am*, 73, 734, 1991.
6. Vogt, J.C. Split anterior tibial transfer for spastic equinovarus foot deformity: retrospective study of 73 operated feet, *J Foot Ankle Surg*, 37, 2, 1998.
7. Hoffer, M.M., Barakat, G., and Koffman, M. 10-year follow-up of split anterior tibial tendon transfer in cerebral palsied patients with spastic equinovarus deformity, *J Pediatr Orthop*, 5, 432, 1985.
8. Hoffer, M.M., et al. The split anterior tibial tendon transfer in the treatment of spastic varus hindfoot of childhood, *Orthop Clin North Am*, 5, 31, 1974.
9. Kling, T.F., Kaufer, H., and Hensinger, R.N. Split posterior tibial-tendon transfers in children with cerebral spastic paralysis and equinovarus deformity, *J Bone Joint Surg Am*, 67, 186, 1985.
10. Green, N.E., Griffin, P.P., and Shiavi, R. Split posterior tibial-tendon transfer in spastic cerebral palsy, *J Bone Joint Surg Am*, 65, 748, 1983.
11. O'Byrne, J.M., et al. Split tibialis posterior tendon transfer in the treatment of spastic equinovarus foot, *J Pediatr Orthop*, 17, 481, 1997.
12. Kagaya, H., et al. Split posterior tibial tendon transfer for varus deformity of hindfoot, *Clin Orthop*, 323, 254, 1996.
13. Saji, M.J., et al. Split tibialis posterior transfer for equinovarus deformity in cerebral palsy. Long-term results of a new surgical procedure, *J Bone Joint Surg Br*, 75, 498, 1993; Erratum in: *J Bone Joint Surg Br*, 76, 683, 1994.
14. Synder, M., Kumar, S.J., and Stecyk, M.D. Split tibialis posterior tendon transfer and tendo-achillis lengthening for spastic equinovarus feet, *J Pediatr Orthop*, 13, 20, 1993.
15. Chang, C.H., et al. Long-term follow-up of surgery for equinovarus foot deformity in children with cerebral palsy. *J Pediatr Orthop* 22, 792, 2002.
16. Barto, P.S., Supinski, R.S., and Skinner, S.R. Dynamic EMG findings in varus hindfoot deformity and spastic cerebral palsy, *Dev Med Child Neurol*, 26, 88, 1984.
17. Wills, C.A., Hoffer, M.M., and Perry, J. A comparison of foot-switch and emg analysis of varus deformities of the feet of children with cerebral palsy, *Dev Med Child Neurol*, 30, 227, 1988.
18. Perry, J. and Hoffer, M.M. Preoperative and postoperative dynamic electromyography as an aid in planning tendon transfers in children with cerebral palsy, *Arch Phys Med Rehabil*, 85, 77, 2004.
19. Friden, J., Ponten, E., and Lieber, R.L. Effect of muscle tension during tendon transfer on sarcomerogenesis in a rabbit model, *J Hand Surg*, 25, 138, 2000.
20. Piazza, S.J., et al. Effects of tensioning errors in split transfers of tibialis anterior and posterior tendons, *J Bone Joint Surg Am*, 85, 858, 2003.
21. Hui, J.H., Goh, J.C., and Lee, E.H. Biomechanical study of tibialis anterior tendon transfer, *Clin Orthop*, 349, 249, 1998.
22. Fuller, D.A., et al. The impact of instrumented gait analysis on surgical planning: treatment of spastic equinovarus deformity of the foot and ankle, *Foot Ankle Int*, 23, 738, 2002.
23. Perry, J., et al. Predictive value of manual muscle testing and gait analysis in normal ankles by dynamic electromyography, *Foot Ankle*, 6, 254, 1986.
24. Koh, T.J. and Herzog, W. Increasing the moment arm of the tibialis anterior induces structural and functional adaptation: implications for tendon transfer, *J Biomech*, 31, 593, 1998.

25. Taylor, N.F., Dodd, K.J., and Graham, H.K. Test-retest reliability of hand-held dynamometric strength testing in young people with cerebral palsy, *Arch Phys Med Rehabil*, 85, 77, 2004.

26. Boiteau, M., Malouin, F., and Richards, C.L. Use of a hand-held dynamometer and a Kin-Com dynamometer for evaluating spastic hypertonia in children: a reliability study, *Phys Ther*, 75, 796, 1995.

27. Kidder, S.M., et al. A system for the analysis of foot and ankle kinematics during gait, *IEEE Trans Rehabil Eng*, 4, 25, 1996.

28. MacWilliams, B.A., Cowley, M., and Nicholson, D.E. Foot kinematics and kinetics during adolescent gait, *Gait Posture*, 17, 214, 2003.

29. Myers, K.A. et al. Validation of a multisegment foot and ankle kinematic model for pediatric gait, *IEEE Trans Neural Syst Rehabil Eng*, 12, 122, 2004.

30. Leardini, A., et al. An antomically based protocol for the description of foot segment kinematics during gait, *Clin Biomech*, 14, 528, 1999.

31. Carson, M.C., et al. Kinematic analysis of a multi-segment foot model for research and clinical applications: a repeatability analysis, 34, 1299, 2001.

32. Chang, C.H., Miller, F., and Schuyler, J. Dynamic pedobarograph in evaluation of varus and valgus foot deformities, *J Pediatr Orthop*, 22, 813, 2002.

10 Lower Extremity Characterization of Walker-Assisted Gait in Children with Spastic Diplegic Cerebral Palsy

Kelly M. Baker, Lucy Lu, Stephen S. Klos,
Kathy Reiners, Jeffrey D. Ackman, John Klein,
Jeffrey P. Schwab, and Gerald F. Harris

CONTENTS

10.1 INTRODUCTION

Cerebral palsy (CP) is a nonprogressive clinical syndrome, which is a symptom of injury to an immature brain.[1] Studies have concluded that the prevalence of CP is 2.0 to 2.5 per 1000 live births worldwide.[2,3] CP is linked to a variety of events including low birth weight and perinatal ischemia/asphyxia. The prognosis includes delayed developmental head control, sitting, standing, walking, and/or independent ambulation. It is also associated with impaired sensations, cognitive defects, speech problems, and bowel/bladder control problems. Other general symptoms can include postural instability, spasticity, abnormal muscle tone, uncoordinated and restricted voluntary movement, and cocontractions of agonist and antagonist muscle groups. These symptoms can cause ambulation difficulties including decreased walking speed, decreased stride length, abnormal joint static, dynamic joint angles, and increased energy expenditure.

There are three main types of CP: spastic, athetoid, and ataxic. The most prevalent is the spastic type, which includes 60 to 80% of CP patients. This condition causes stiff, irregular, or uncoordinated movement in one or more muscles. In most cases, the lower extremity (LE) muscles are most affected.[4] The spastic group is further classified into hemiplegic (one-side affected) or diplegic (both-sides affected). Spastic diplegic is the most common form of CP. Spastic diplegic CP predominantly affects the lower extremities, but in more severe cases it can affect the upper extremities (UEs) as well.[1]

Many children with CP are prescribed walkers to help maintain stability in ambulation. Little quantitative information is available about how walkers affect a patient's UE and LE motion. Most existing analysis is subjective and mainly qualitative. Because walker effects on the body are vague, there are no quantitative guidelines for walker prescription, which specifically consider individual patient conditions.

With several different types of walkers on the market, it can be difficult to prescribe a particular type of walker to patients. The two most-commonly prescribed walkers are the anterior walker and the posterior walker. These two types of walkers are used differently. As patients ambulate with an anterior walker, which is positioned in front of them, they push the walker forward and then step into it from behind. As the patients ambulate with a posterior walker, which is positioned behind them, they pull the walker behind them after stepping out of it. The two walking patterns create different body positioning and affect the overall gait pattern. There has been some evidence that the different placement positions of the walkers create dissimilar postures, which affect the motion of the body,[5–10] and one of the most well-known theories supporting posterior walker prescription is that posterior walkers force a more upright trunk position.[9] However, the quantitative data to support this theory are based on pelvic tilt or visual assessment.

There is some controversy as to which of the two major types of walkers is more effective and best matched to the user. Many feel that the posterior walker decreases double support time, trunk/hip/knee flexion, and energy expenditure, and increases swing phase, stride length, and overall gait stability.[7,9] However, others have found that there is no significant difference in step length.[8] In general, LE motion analysis of children with CP is part of clinical routine. Studies that have examined walker-assisted gait with this population of children have mainly reported on the gait temporal and spatial data[5,6] or the energy expenditure.[9]

Many LE motion data studies have not involved the use of walkers, and those that have involved walkers have not fully quantified the motion.[7–9] In fact, the authors that involved walkers in their studies only reported on pelvic tilt, hip flexion, and knee flexion at initial contact, mid-stance, preswing, and mid-swing. No graphical display has been given of the overall motion, and the ankle joint has not been considered.

Ounpuu presented patterns of gait pathology in children with CP and explored the general LE characteristics.[11] While detailed, the study did not delineate specific subset characteristics including type, distribution, assistive device usage, or bracing. Stout and Gage also described LE motion of children with CP with a focus on children with hemiplegia.[12] Novacheck also described LE motion of two children with spastic diplegic CP, but his patients did not use assistive devices when tested.[13]

In summary, few studies have analyzed LE motion in children with CP using walkers, and those that have are not complete characterizations. This work presents LE kinematic results from a comparative study of anterior and posterior walkers. Results from 11 children with spastic diplegic CP using anterior and posterior walkers are presented. Gait temporal and stride parameters (GTPs) are also analyzed and differences between the two walker types are highlighted. The analysis and data presented in this study may aid as future research evolves in pediatric walker-assisted motion and walker prescription.

10.2 METHODS

Our study took place at Shriners Hospital for Children (SHC), in Chicago, IL, and at the Medical College of Wisconsin (MCW) Department of Orthopaedic Surgery in Milwaukee, WI. Institutional Review Board (IRB) approvals were obtained from all institutions involved, and thorough training sessions were completed to coordinate the gait lab systems. To ensure consistency, the same personnel traveled between institutions to conduct the visit procedures.

We randomly selected 11 patients with CP (age 12.3 ± 3.8 yr) to participate in the study. The inclusion criteria for participation required patients to have spastic diplegic CP; to be between 5 and 18 yr of age; to be community ambulators who used either an anterior or a posterior walker for a minimum of one month; to have no surgery within one year of starting the study; to have no botulinum toxin type A within six months of starting the study; to have an Ashworth score less than or equal to 2 (meaning slight increase in tone) at the elbow joint; and to be fully willing to comply with the study's requirements. The chosen Ashworth score was to make sure patients were able to use both types of walkers.

A total of three visits were required for this study. During the first visit, our group completed a pre-evaluation screening of each participant to assure eligibility and IRB compliance. It was during this visit that we explained the risks involved in the study (e.g., mechanical malfunction of any measurement system or a potential walkway hazard) to patients and parents/guardians, and informed the patients and parents/guardians that all procedures followed institutional IRB regulations.

During the second visit, patients completed a motion analysis testing period while using the posterior walker. Coincidentally, at the start of the study, all 11 children used posterior walkers. This was not a requirement for participation. Following the second visit, patients were taught how to use the anterior walker and then used this new walker in their everyday environments for a minimum of a one-month period. During this acclimation period, phone calls were placed to parents to monitor patient progress. At the end of this one-month period, patients returned to the lab and were retested under identical conditions using the anterior walker.

For the posterior and anterior walker visits, our protocol consisted of two parts: (1) motion analysis and (2) statistical analysis.

10.2.1 PART 1: MOTION ANALYSIS

A 15-camera Vicon Motion Analysis System (MAS) (Oxford Metrics, Oxford, UK) was used at MCW and a 12-camera Vicon MAS was used at SHC (Figure 10.1).

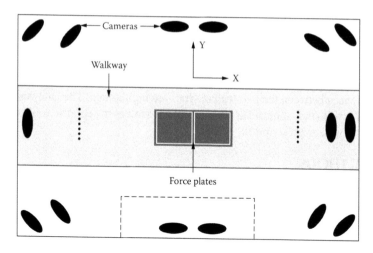

FIGURE 10.1 Motion analysis laboratory schematic.

Our group obtained pediatric anterior walkers (Sunrise Medical, Model 7783, 7781, 7780, Longmont, CO) and posterior walkers (Kaye Products, Inc, Model W2B-W4B, Hillsborough, NC). We used the Helen Hayes marker set to help analyze LE motion and GTPs (Figure 10.2). LE landmarks included the sacrum at the level of the posterior superior iliac spine (PSIS); the anterior superior iliac spines (ASIS); wands, laterally on the thighs; the lateral epicondyle of the knees; lateral wands, mid-shaft of the fibula; the lateral maleolus of the ankles; the calcaneous; and the dorsum of the foot just proximal to the head of the second metatarsals.

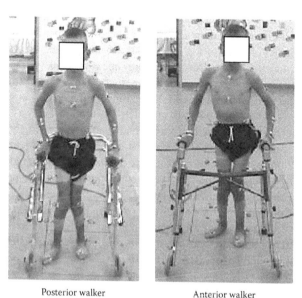

Posterior walker   Anterior walker

FIGURE 10.2 Patient using a posterior walker and an anterior walker.

The walkers were adjusted so that the top of the walker was aligned with the ulnar styloid when the subject stood beside the frame with arms held loosely in a relaxed position. Walkers were fit to the needs of each subject. A static trial with the subject standing still in the center of the capture volume was performed. Subjects then walked through a capture volume for a minimum of five trials. This was to ensure that we obtained at least three valid bilateral gait cycles. An acceptable gait cycle was defined as foot strike to ipsilateral foot strike with no marker dropout.[14]

After collection, data were processed through a Woltring filter and a LE Plug-in-Gait model, which was developed by Vicon MASs. This LE model is the most accepted model in use in the clinical community. The model uses the filtered data to calculate pelvis, hip, knee, and ankle angles, by use of the standard Euler rotation method. All joint angles are determined by comparing the distal segment relative to the proximal. All resulting data were graphed using Polygon, a software tool produced by Vicon Motion Systems. Once each gait cycle was plotted, it was exported to an ASCII file and saved for statistical analysis.

10.2.2 PART 2: STATISTICAL ANALYSIS

The LE kinematic data, including joint angles and corresponding gait cycle intervals, were input into a database. The gait cycle interval data, for each joint of each patient, were analyzed using the Fourier method.[15-18] This technique allowed us to analyze the continuous gait data accurately and it provided a method to describe the entire population. A Fourier regression model was fit to each LE joint (pelvis, hips, knees, and ankles) of each patient. The Fourier regression models were of the form:

$$Y_{ij} = \alpha_0 + \sum_{i=1}^{j} \alpha_i \sin(2\pi_i/100) + \beta_i \cos(22\pi_i/100) + error$$

where Y_{ij} was a specific joint value, i was a percentage of the gait cycle (which ranged from $i = 0, 2...100$, in the raw data, because the Vicon system outputs every 2% for the LE), and j represented each trial (which ranged from $j = 1, 2...t$, where t was the total number of trials for the patient). f was the maximum number of sine and cosine terms used by the model; α_0, α_1, β_1 were regression coefficients; and the error term was random and normally distributed with a mean of zero.

Model selection for each patient involved two steps. First, we determined the maximum number of terms used in each model, f. Due to the amount of data, we needed to simplify our output while maintaining a "good prediction" of joint angles. f was chosen based on curve prediction using a subset of our data. A "good prediction" was determined by evaluating an adjusted R^2 value (R_A^2) for each selected f. $R_A^2 = 1 - (n - 1/n - p - 1)(1 - R^2)$, where n was the number of trials times the number of percentage points in a gait cycle (51 in our case. so $n = 51 * t$), p was the number of terms in the model ($p = 2*f + 1$), and $R^2 = \sum_{i=0}^{100} t\,(\hat{Y}_i - \bar{Y})^2 / \sum_{i=0}^{100} \sum_{j=1}^{t}(Y_{ij} - \bar{Y})^2$. In the R^2 calculation, $\hat{Y}_i$ was the predicted joint value for each percent gait cycle, and $\bar{Y}$ was the mean of each patient's set of trials.

In determining f, we started analyzing the R_A^2 from f equals zero. We gradually increased f until the largest R_A^2 value was found. By definition, the f with the largest R_A^2 value was the best estimator. According to our analysis, the best value for f was determined to be six for all joints and we fixed it at six for the second step of the model selection.

The second part of the model selection process was to make the model more patient specific by determining which sine and cosine terms were significant to the patient's motion. To ascertain this, a stepwise model selection method was used. This procedure involved analyzing the p-values from a partial F-test obtained from the addition of each term. The partial F-statistic (F_P) was $F_P = (R^2 - R_R^2)/(1 - R^2)((51 * t) - p - 1)/q$, where R_R^2 was the coefficient of multiple determination from the reduced model, t was the number of trials, p was the number of terms in the reduced model, and q was the difference between the number of terms in the new model and the reduced model. Once F_P was calculated, a p-value was found by looking at the F-distribution, with q being the first degree of freedom and $((51 * t) - p - 1)$ being the second degree of freedom. If a p-value was less than 0.15, then the corresponding term was included in the model, otherwise it was excluded. This stepwise process started with no sine or cosine terms in the model and gradually included each term until all terms were checked.

Once we determined the patient-specific model at each joint, α_0, α_l, β_l were estimated by using the least square method and were represented as the vector $\hat{\beta}$, where $\hat{\beta} = (X'X)^{-1}X'Y$ and $\hat{\beta} = (\hat{\alpha}_0, \hat{\alpha}_1, \cdots, \hat{\alpha}_f, \hat{\beta}_1, \hat{\beta}_2, \cdots, \hat{\beta}_f)$. X was expressed as

$$
X = \begin{pmatrix}
1 & \sin\left(\dfrac{2\pi * 0 * 1}{100}\right) & \sin\left(\dfrac{2\pi * 0 * 2}{100}\right) & \cdots & \sin\left(\dfrac{2\pi * 0 * f}{100}\right) & \cdots & \cos\left(\dfrac{2\pi * 0 * f}{100}\right) \\
1 & \sin\left(\dfrac{2\pi * 0 * 1}{100}\right) & \sin\left(\dfrac{2\pi * 0 * 2}{100}\right) & \cdots & \sin\left(\dfrac{2\pi * 0 * f}{100}\right) & \cdots & \cos\left(\dfrac{2\pi * 0 * f}{100}\right) \\
\cdots & \cdots & \cdots & \cdots & \cdots & \cdots & \cdots \\
1 & \sin\left(\dfrac{2\pi * 0 * 1}{100}\right) & \sin\left(\dfrac{2\pi * 0 * 2}{100}\right) & \cdots & \sin\left(\dfrac{2\pi * 0 * f}{100}\right) & \cdots & \cos\left(\dfrac{2\pi * 0 * f}{100}\right) \\
1 & \sin\left(\dfrac{2\pi * 2 * 1}{100}\right) & \sin\left(\dfrac{2\pi * 2 * 2}{100}\right) & \cdots & \sin\left(\dfrac{2\pi * 2 * f}{100}\right) & \cdots & \cos\left(\dfrac{2\pi * 2 * f}{100}\right) \\
\cdots & \cdots & \cdots & \cdots & \cdots & \cdots & \cdots \\
1 & \sin\left(\dfrac{2\pi * 100 * 1}{100}\right) & \sin\left(\dfrac{2\pi * 100 * 2}{100}\right) & \cdots & \sin\left(\dfrac{2\pi * 100 * f}{100}\right) & \cdots & \cos\left(\dfrac{2\pi * 100 * f}{100}\right)
\end{pmatrix}
$$

where each row represented a patient's trial with all gait cycle percentages grouped together. Y was a vector of joint angles ($Y = Y_{01}, Y_{02} \ldots Y_{0t}, Y_{21} \ldots Y_{100,t}$). After the coefficient values were determined, a unique predicted expression could be stated for all patients' joints. The predicted expressions took the form $\hat{Y}_i = \hat{\alpha}_0 + \sum_{l=1}^{f} \hat{\alpha}_l \sin(2\pi i l / 100) + \hat{\beta}_l \cos(2\pi i l / 100)$, where $\hat{Y}_i$ were the predicted joint values at each one percentage point for each patient. We still used f for the simplicity of the expression; however, some of the terms equal zero because of the second step in the model selection process.

To develop the average characteristic joint curves of the patients ($n = 11$), the predicted characteristic patient curves were averaged for all patients. $\overline{Y}_i = 1/N$ $\sum_{k=1}^{N} \hat{Y}_i^k$ was the expression used to determine the joint values at the ith percentage points ($\overline{Y}_i$) and $\hat{Y}_i^k$ was the predicted value for the kth patient at the ith percentage point of the gait cycle. The 99% confidence interval (CI) for each percent of the gait cycle was ($\overline{Y}_i - 2.5758 * std.err_i$, $\overline{Y}_i + 2.5758 * std.err_i$), where $std.err_i$ was the standard error determined by the expression

$$std.err_i = \sqrt{\sum_{k=1}^{N} (\hat{Y}_i^k - \overline{Y}_i)^2 / N\ (N-1)} \ .$$

The CI was plotted with the characteristic curve.

Furthermore, statistical analysis of the individual segments and joints of the LE model was compared to find significant differences between the anterior and posterior data (the significant level was set to 0.01). A pointwise comparison (Wilcoxon Signed Rank Test) was used to test data at each tenth percentage point.

10.3 RESULTS

LE sagittal plane characteristic curves are shown in Figure 10.3. These curves are representative of 11 patients with spastic diplegic CP using anterior and posterior walkers. Minimum and maximum values for each joint are listed in Table 10.1. The pelvis motion mimicked a double bump pattern. There was a 20° anterior tilt offset in comparison to normal unassisted gait with both walkers. Patients had a slightly greater amount of anterior tilt using the posterior walker. The minimum and maximum pelvic tilts for the patient when using the anterior walker were 21.9 and 26.3°, respectively. The minimum and maximum pelvic tilts for the patient when using the posterior walker were 23.1 and 26.6°, respectively.

The hip motion on both left and right sides demonstrated a large flexion bias and a right-ward phase shift. On the left side, patients using posterior walkers had a slightly greater amount of hip flexion than when using anterior walkers. On the right side, patients using anterior walkers had a slightly greater amount of hip flexion for the first half of the gait cycle, but had a lesser amount of hip flexion than when using posterior walkers during the second half of the gait cycle. The minimum and maximum angles for the anterior walker user on the right side were 17.3 and 49.6°, respectively, and on the left side were 16.0 and 46.3°, respectively. The minimum and maximum angles for the posterior walker user were 19.0 and 52.3°, respectively, on the right side, and 20.6 and 50.8°, respectively, on the left side.

The knee motion exhibited a large flexion offset on the left and right sides using anterior and posterior walkers. Neither knee demonstrated a large flexion curve during the loading response. In fact, instead, the knees attempted to extend instead of flex. There was persistent knee flexion at mid-stance and a slightly diminished amount of knee flexion during swing. During swing, the amount of knee flexion that occured as the leg moved was rightward shifted (delayed). Patients using the posterior walker tended to be slightly more flexed at the knee joint than when they used

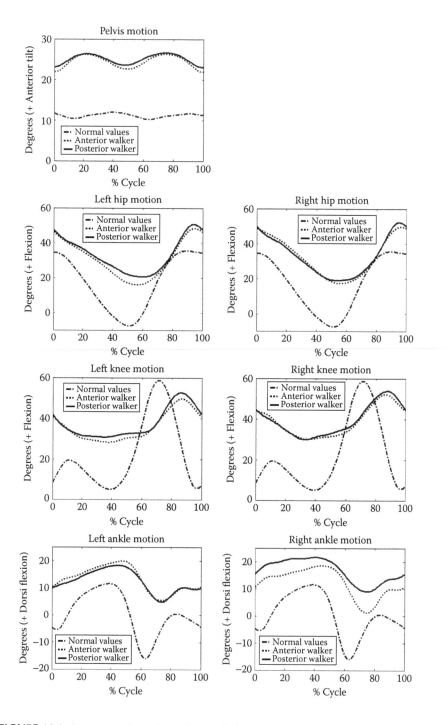

FIGURE 10.3 Average sagittal plane characteristic curves of the pelvis, hips, knees, and ankles (*n* = 11).

TABLE 10.1
Average Minimum and Maximum Values for
Pelvis, Hips, Knees, and Ankles

			Peak Values	
Segment	Walker	Side	Min Angle	Max Angle
Pelvis	Anterior	Right	22.0°	26.5°
		Left	21.6°	26.5°
	Posterior	Right	22.8°	26.5°
		Left	22.6°	26.8°
Hip	Anterior	Right	17.3°	49.6°
		Left	16.0°	46.3°
	Posterior	Right	19.0°	52.3°
		Left	20.6°	50.8°
Knee	Anterior	Right	30.1°	52.1°
		Left	28.2°	49.6°
	Posterior	Right	29.9°	53.9°
		Left	30.7°	52.6°
Ankle	Anterior	Right	1.3°	18.5°
		Left	5.4°	19.9°
	Posterior	Right	9.0°	21.6°
		Left	4.9°	18.2°

the anterior walker. The minimum and maximum knee joint angles that occurred when using the anterior walker were 30.1 and 52.1°, respectively, on the right side, 28.2 and 49.6°, respectively, on the left side. The minimum and maximum knee joint angles found when using the posterior walker were 29.9 and 53.9°, respectively, on the right side, and 30.7 and 52.6°, respectively, on the left side.

At the ankle joint, there was a dorsiflexion offset on both right and left sides, using either type of walker. The dorsiflexion was greater on the right side when using the posterior walker, but tended to be larger on the left side when using the anterior walker. The patients showed a loss of the first rocker regardless of which walker was used. There was diminished dorsiflexion range from the first to second rocker, and diminished plantarflexion range from the second to third rocker with respect to normal. The minimum and maximum joint angles that occurred during ankle motion were 1.3 and 18.5°, respectively, on the right side, and 5.4 and 19.9°, respectively, on the left side, during anterior walker usage. During posterior walker usage, the minimum and maximum joint angles were 9.0 and 21.6° on the right side, and 4.9 and 18.2° on the left side.

When comparing the asymmetry of the joints (e.g., right hip to left hip) at each tenth percentage point, we found that there were no significant differences in hip, knee, or ankle joint motion during either anterior or posterior walker use (Table 10.2). When comparing patients' anterior and posterior walker data at each tenth percentage point, there were no significant differences in joint motion found between the two types of walkers (Table 10.3).

TABLE 10.2

Asymmetrical Analysis of the LE Joints (Left Side–Right Side), p-Values Are Given for Each Tenth Percentage

Percent Gait Cycle	Pelvis		Hip		Knee		Ankle	
	Anterior	Posterior	Anterior	Posterior	Anterior	Posterior	Anterior	Posterior
0	0.6	0.3	0.2	0.2	0.2	0.2	0.9	0.05
10	0.7	1.0	0.1	0.4	0.1	0.2	0.8	0.03
20	0.6	0.8	0.2	0.7	0.3	0.4	1.0	0.05
30	0.7	0.7	0.4	0.8	0.6	0.8	0.8	0.1
40	0.9	0.1	0.5	0.3	0.4	1.0	0.8	0.2
50	0.9	0.2	0.5	0.3	0.7	0.9	0.6	0.5
60	1.0	0.6	0.5	0.6	0.3	0.3	0.8	0.6
70	0.7	0.8	0.9	0.9	0.2	0.3	0.4	0.4
80	0.9	0.9	0	0.5	0.1	0.5	0.4	0.4
90	0.4	0.3	1.0	1.0	0.4	0.2	0.9	0.2
100	0.6	0.3	0.2	0.2	0.2	0.2	0.9	0.05

Table 10.4 presents the GTP results. The average walking speed for an anterior walker user (0.38 m/sec) was slightly faster than it was for a posterior walker user (0.34 m/sec), though not significant. Patients who used the anterior walker also exhibited an increase in cadence (left side: 79.0 steps/min; right side: 77.4 steps/min) in comparison to posterior walker use (left side: 72.5 steps/min; right side: 73.4 steps/min), though again this was not significant. Stride length and step length showed no significant change between walkers.

TABLE 10.3

Walker Comparison Analysis (Anterior Walker–Posterior Walker), p-Values Are Given for Each Tenth Percentage

Percent Gait Cycle	Pelvis	Hip		Knee		Ankle	
		Left	Right	Left	Right	Left	Right
0	0.5	0.6	0.7	0.4	0.8	0.8	0.3
10	0.6	0.7	0.5	0.9	0.5	0.2	0.3
20	0.9	0.5	0.5	0.5	0.9	0.5	0.3
30	0.9	0.5	0.6	0.3	0.8	0.5	0.4
40	1.0	0.2	0.8	0.2	0.7	0.5	0.5
50	0.9	0.1	0.7	0.3	0.4	0.4	0.7
60	0.8	0.1	0.5	0.3	0.4	0.9	0.6
70	0.9	0.4	0.5	1.0	0.5	0.9	0.2
80	0.9	0.6	0.9	0.2	0.6	0.9	0.2
90	0.8	0.4	0.5	0.2	0.5	0.9	0.4
100	0.5	0.6	0.7	0.4	0.8	0.8	0.3

TABLE 10.4
Average GTPs for 11 Patients with CP Using Anterior and Posterior Walkers

GTPs	Side	Anterior Walker	Posterior Walker
Walking speed (m/sec)		0.38	0.34
Cadence (steps/min)	L	79.0	72.5
	R	77.4	73.4
Stride length (m)	L	0.6	0.5
	R	0.6	0.6
Step length (m)	L	0.3	0.3
	R	0.3	0.3

10.4 DISCUSSION

The motivation of this work was to understand how anterior and posterior walkers interface with children who have CP and to determine if there were any significant differences in the effect the two types of walkers have on the children. We accomplished this by analyzing the LE sagittal plane kinematics of the pelvis, hip, knee, and ankle, as well as the GTPs. We examined asymmetries between left and right sides and significant differences between the two walkers. At the pelvis, the motion exhibited a double bump pattern characteristic of unassisted gait in CP. This pattern was observed when using both types of walkers and was commonly associated with hip flexion offset. Increased flexion occurred once during the stance phase and once during the swing phase. It was evident that this pattern was used to advance the limbs forward as the body ambulated and was characteristic of children with a diplegic gait. Posterior walker patients had a greater anterior tilt than anterior walker patients, but there was no statistically significant difference in pelvic tilt between either type of walker. This was contrary to what some other researchers have suggested, although the population size in the current study is greater.[7–9]

At the hip joint, there was a flexion bias throughout the gait cycle and a diminished dynamic range in comparison to a normal unassisted gait. There was a lack of hip extension during mid-stance and a flexion peak toward the end of the swing phase, which was unique to spastic diplegic CP–assisted gait. In general, the extension and flexion peaks were delayed in comparison to normal. No statistically significant differences were found at the hip joints between using the two walkers, and the hips proved to be symmetrically related. However, when using the posterior walker, the hip joint was slightly more flexed on the left side throughout the gait cycle and during the second half of the gait cycle on the right side in comparison to the anterior walker. While reports are limited, some other studies show increased hip extension at initial contact and mid-stance with a posterior walker.[7–9] It was difficult to compare results however as left and right side data were combined in several of these studies.[7,9] The current study does not show any significant differences at initial contact or mid-stance. A larger sample size and consideration of other factors, such as body positioning within the walker and UE kinematics, might yield different results.

Knee kinematics demonstrated a loss of the load response normally seen at the beginning of the gait cycle, with an early extension of the knee joint. The knees were persistently flexed throughout the gait cycle and the range of motion was decreased bilaterally at the knee. As seen with the hip, the flexion peak at the knee was delayed when compared to normal. When patients used the posterior walker, the knees tended to be more flexed than when they used the anterior walker, although these differences were not significant. These results are in agreement with those of Logan.[7] Park et al. reported less knee flexion at initial contact with the posterior walker in a study of ten subjects. Greiner et al. reported mixed results in a small study of five subjects. Statistically there were no differences between patients' knee joint motion, bilaterally or between walkers.

Ankle motion showed reduced plantarflexion during the first rocker and a decreased dynamic range during the second rocker. A lack of plantarflexion was noted during terminal stance (third rocker). The subjects exhibited a bilateral decrease in dynamic plantarflexion at toe-off with increased dorsiflexion when compared to normal in swing phase. In general, these characteristic curves showed a decrease in dynamic range throughout the gait cycle. There were some slight asymmetries at the ankle joint, but they were not significant, and there were no differences in ankle joint motion (pattern or excursion) between using the anterior and posterior walkers. No statistically significant asymmetry was seen in comparing the left and right ankle motion. More flexion was noted on the left with the anterior walker and on the right with the posterior walker. This may be related to the distribution of spasticity.

The population showed slight decreases in cadence, stride length, and walking speed with posterior walker use. These changes were not statistically significant.

10.5 CONCLUSION

This preliminary study gives some insight into the differences between anterior and posterior walker use by children with CP. It provides sagittal plane characteristic curves of the pelvis, hip, knee, and ankle joints of 11 patients. All joints showed a flexion bias with walker usage. The pelvis demonstrated a double bump pattern. Hip motion lacked a dynamic range of extension and included a flexion peak during the latter portion of the gait cycle. Knee motion showed no loading response. Ankle motion displayed diminished dynamic ranges in the first, second, and third rockers. No significant kinematic differences existed in the sagittal plane between anterior and posterior walkers usage. No significant asymmetry existed at the hip, knee, or ankle joints. GTP results did not indicate statistically significant differences between anterior and posterior walker usage. These data lay the groundwork for future investigation into LE kinematics resulting from walker usage. The sample size used in this analysis is small, although it is larger than other studies currently reported. Further work continues to examine the kinematics in a larger population and to include the effects on the UEs resulting from walker usage. Inclusion of recognized and clinically accepted outcomes measures is another objective for future study. The overarching goal is to provide a better understanding of walker dynamics while pursuing more effective means for prescription and evaluation.

ACKNOWLEDGMENT

This study was made possible through a grant from the National Institute of Disability and Rehabilitation Research (NIDRR) #H133G010069.

REFERENCES

1. Plessis, A.J.D., Mechanisms and manifestations of prenatal and perinatal brain injury, In *The Treatment of Gait Problems in Cerebral Palsy*, Gage, J.R., Ed., Mac Keith Press: London, 2004, chap. 2.
2. Reddihough, D. and Collins, K., The epidemiology and causes of cerebral palsy, *Aust J Physiother*, 49, 7–12, 2003.
3. Hagberg, B., et al., Changing panorama of cerebral palsy in Sweden. VIII. Prevalence and origin in the birth year period 1991–94, *Acta Paediatr*, 90, 271–277, 2001.
4. Wren, T.A.L., Rethlefsen, S., and Kay, R.M., Prevalence of specific gait abnormalities in children with cerebral palsy: influence of cerebral palsy subtype, age, and previous surgery, *J. Pediatr Orthop*, 25, 79–83, 2005.
5. Levangie, P.K., et al., The effects of the standard rolling walker and two posterior rolling walkers on gait variables on normal children, *Phys Occup Ther Pediatr*, 9, 19–31, 1989.
6. Levangie, P.K., et al., The effects of posterior rolling walkers vs. the standard rolling walker on gait characteristics of children with spastic cerebral palsy, *Phys Occup Ther Pediatr*, 9, 1–17, 1989.
7. Logan, L., Byers-Hinkley, K., and Ciccone, C.D., Anterior versus posterior walkers: a gait analysis study, *Dev Med Child Neurol*, 32, 1044–1048, 1990.
8. Greiner, B.M., Czerniecki, J.M., and Deitz, J.C., Gait parameters of children with spastic diplegia: a comparison of effects of posterior and anterior walkers, *Arch Phys Med Rehabil*, 74, 381–385, 1993.
9. Park, E.S., Park, C.I., and Kim, J.Y., Comparison of anterior and posterior walkers with respect to gait parameters and energy expenditure of children with spastic diplegic cerebral palsy, *Yonsei Med J*, 42, 180–184, 2001.
10. Bachschmidt, R.A., et al., Quantitative study of walker-assisted gait in children with cerebral palsy: anterior versus posterior walkers, *Arch Phys Med Rehabil*, 2005.
11. Ounpuu, S., Patterns of gait pathology, In *The Treatment of Gait Problems in Cerebral Palsy*, Gage, J.R., Ed., Mac Keith Press: London, 2004, chap. 14.
12. [12]Stout, J. and Gage, J.R., Hemiplegia: pathology and treatment, In *The Treatment of Gait Problems in Cerebral Palsy*, Gage, J.R., Ed., Mac Keith Press: London, 2004, chap. 19.
13. Novacheck, T.F., Diplegia and quadriplegia: pathology and treatment, In *The Treatment of Gait Problems in Cerebral Palsy*, Gage, J.R., Ed., Mac Keith Press: London, 2004.
14. Perry, J., *Gait Analysis: Normal and Pathological Function*, Slack Inc.: New York, 1992.

15. VanBogart, J.J., et al., Effects of the toe-only rocker on gait kinematics and kinetics in able-bodied persons, IEEE TSNRE 12/2005.
16. Wong, M.A., Simon, S., and Olshen R.A., Statistical analysis of gait patterns of persons with cerebral palsy, *Stat Med*, 2, 345–354, 1983.
17. Klein, J., Stastistical issues in randomized clinical trials in motion analysis, In *Proc. IEEE/EMBS*, Chicago, 1997, 2909-13.
18. Fisher, L.D. and Van Bell, G., *Biostatistics: A Methodology for the Health Sciences*, John Wiley and Sons: New York, 1993.

11 Response to Balance Perturbation: A Strategy for Pediatric Assessment

Adam N. Graf, Joseph Krzak, and Gerald F. Harris

CONTENTS

11.1 INTRODUCTION

Postural stability in children is fundamental in achieving independent stance, gait, and higher-level gross motor skills. The foot and ankle contribute significantly to postural control by providing a contact area to the support surface and the primary joints that respond to certain balance perturbations. Children with neuromuscular disorders have deficits in response to perturbations of balance and often require assistive devices or orthoses to accommodate them. This chapter presents a set of quantitative parameters to examine responses to perturbations of standing balance during translations and rotations about the ankle joint. It includes specific examples from children with cerebral palsy (CP), with and without lower extremity bracing.

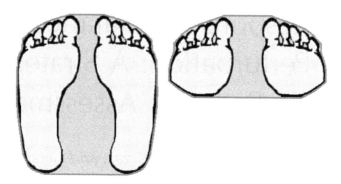

FIGURE 11.1 Base of support (BOS): BOS for a normal subject (left) and a subject up on their toes (right).

The body maintains equilibrium during quiet standing through complex neuromuscular and musculoskeletal systems. If the body is stable, it will have the ability to resist disruption to equilibrium and return to its original state if disturbed. The body segments are capable of changing orientation to maintain mechanical stability. As these segments are moved to assume a certain posture, other segments must adjust in order to maintain stability and equilibrium. The foot and ankle are critical in maintaining balance and controlling equilibrium due to their proximity to the support surface. The reaction forces between the feet and the support surface can be summed over the entire contact area, described as the center of pressure (COP). It is at this point where the ground reaction forces are balanced. The COP is a point found within the base of support (BOS), described by the contact perimeter around the feet and support surface (Figure 11.1). The center of mass (COM) is the average location of the mass of the body. It is the point at which the total mass may be considered to be concentrated, with respect to the pull of gravity. If a line is drawn from the COM vertically downward onto the support surface, it must fall within the boundaries of the BOS and directly onto the COP to be in equilibrium. The human body is inherently unstable due to the fact that the COM is carried above the support surface, roughly located at the level of the pelvis and anterior to the ankle joints when standing in an upright posture (Figure 11.2). In the first postnatal year, the COM is proportionately higher than in older children due to the size of the head and smaller limbs. As a child begins to walk, the distance between the floor and the COM is very small compared to that of an adult.[27] In the child, the COM is at the level of the twelfth thoracic vertebra and descends to the level of the second sacral vertebra with physical maturity (slightly higher in males).[33]

Reaction forces are exerted by the support surface directly onto the feet. This results in a "bottom up" (support surface orientated) linkage on the basis of these reaction forces. The basic system has been described in forms of an inverted pendulum model.[8] The receptors on the soles of the feet and proprioceptive inputs from foot muscles perceive these forces. This sensory information allows for the formation of an internal representation of the support conditions and selection of

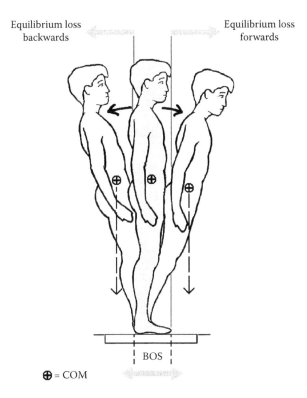

Equilibrium loss
backwards

Equilibrium loss
forwards

BOS

⊕ = COM

FIGURE 11.2 Movement of COM: As the COM moves outside the BOS, balance equilibrium is lost.

the appropriate actuators for optimizing equilibrium maintenance.[6] The combination of muscle responses that allow maintenance of standing stability are termed "sway synergies."

As Nashner and Woollacott[7] have described, balance is controlled by neurally programmed synergies with the coupling of muscles serving to stabilize ankle sway. They worked to prove the theory of Nicholai Bernstein that the nervous system organizes movement in a hierarchical manner, with higher levels of the nervous system activating groups of muscles constrained to act as a unit. These synergies are necessary due to the difficulty the brain would endure if it was forced to independently regulate the vast number of motions of the many mechanical linkages of the body and the activities of the associated muscle groups.[26]

Nashner and Woollacott's results showed that in response to backward platform translations, the body swayed anteriorly, stretching the gastrocnemius muscle. Thus the gastrocnemius was the first muscle activated in a synergy followed sequentially by the hamstrings and paraspinal muscles at 20 msec intervals. Noteworthy is the fact that the gastrocnemius response was slower than a simple stretch reflex response, suggesting that it involves more complex neural pathways. In a forward translation, the tibialis anterior is stretched because of backward sway. Following the activation of the tibialis is the quadriceps, then the abdominal muscles.

By rotating the subject's support surface, the authors isolated motion to the ankle, eliminating motion at the other joints. The rotation of the platform about the ankle joint in both the toes-down and toes-up directions caused the same groups of lower extremity muscles to activate as with forward and backward translations, respectively. This led to the conclusion that movement at the ankle joint from a support surface perturbation was activating a synergistic response in multiple muscles, termed the "ankle strategy."

The ankle strategy is a synergy most commonly used to respond to small perturbations where the support surface is firm. If a perturbation that the ankle strategy could not accommodate were to occur, the intact central nervous system is capable of shifting to other postural movement strategies. The hip or stepping strategies are utilized when perturbations are faster or larger in amplitude, the support surface is compliant or small, or the perturbation forces the COM outside the BOS of the feet.[9–14]

By the age of 7 to 10, children have shown the ability to achieve similar postural responses to those of adults.[5,21–25] Children younger than 7 yr often have less efficient and effective responses characterized by the movement of individual body segments and joint angle changes at the hip, knee, and ankle. Sundermier et al.[37] found that, with maturity, children utilize the muscle synergy associated with the ankle strategy (gastrocnemius followed by hamstrings and paraspinals in the forward sway direction and tibialis quadriceps and abductors in the backward sway direction) in response to postural perturbation and tended to have shorter times to COP stabilization and shorter COP paths during recovery. Children in lower developmental or younger age groups utilized single muscle onset organization, with increased peak muscle torques at the knee.

Some of the more recent research has explained that in the event of an unexpected perturbation to static balance, recovery is reliant upon not only the magnitude of the torque produced about the lower extremity joints but also the latency of onset following the perturbation.[18] It is suggested that there is a correlation between parameters related to the speed of torque generation onset and the magnitude of perturbation from which recovery can be achieved.

Children with neuromuscular disorders such as CP often have poor directional specificity, with antagonists activating before agonists, delayed onset of muscle activity, poor sequencing of muscle synergies, muscle coactivation, and decreased ability to generate sufficient force amplitudes or modulate the force amplitude to react to a perturbation to balance.[17,28,29] They may also have abnormal muscle tone, muscle weakness, loss of selective muscle control, and/or bony deformities. These impairments can cause deficiencies in the typical muscle synergies associated with the ankle, hip, and stepping strategies, as well as loss of range of motion at the foot and ankle. This adversely affects postural stability and responses to perturbations. Impairments associated with toe walking, in-toeing, and other foot deformities common in CP can alter the size and shape of the BOS, thus limiting the distance the COP can move before balance is lost (Figure 11.1).

Treating balance from the neuromuscular standpoint is difficult. Woollacott and Shumway-Cook[30,36] have demonstrated that training children with CP to improve responses to unexpected perturbations is possible but requires multiple repetitions.

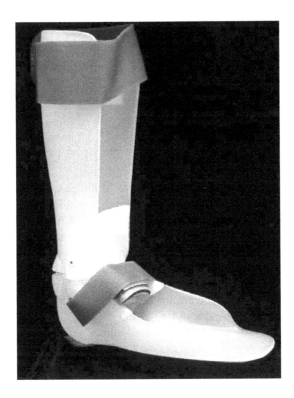

FIGURE 11.3 Articulated (or hinged) ankle foot orthosis.

One way to enhance children's functional abilities is to improve their BOS.[31] This can be done by prescribing an ankle foot orthosis (AFO). AFOs have also been shown to improve ankle kinematics during stance phase, increase step and stride length, decrease cadence, and decrease energy costs in walking, while improving walking/running/jumping skills.[31]

The articulated ankle foot orthosis (AAFO or hinged AFO pictured in Figure 11.3), which allows the ankle to dorsiflex during gait and restricts plantar flexion, is examined in this study, under conditions of postural perturbations. The objective of the study was to use a simple balance assessment protocol to analyze sway energy and other postural metrics in a small group of children with diplegic CP, who used AAFOs. Results include tests from a series of normal children for comparison.

11.2 MATERIALS AND METHODS

This cross-sectional description study examines ten nondisabled children aged 6 to 17 yr (Table 11.1) and compares them to several children with diplegic CP. Only children with no known foot or ankle pathologies and normal foot patterns during gait were included in the control group. Children between the ages of 6 and 12 yr

TABLE 11.1
Demographics

Subject Type	Control	Cerebral Palsy
Number of subjects	10	5
Age (average yr)	12 (range 7–16)	8 (range 6–12)
Sex	7 males, 3 females	2 males, 3 females

were also chosen based on a clinical diagnosis of diplegic CP. Functionally, each of the children were placed into a Gross Motor Function Classification System (GMFCS) as described by Palisano et al. of Level II: ("Children walk indoors and outdoors, and climb stairs holding onto a railing but experience limitations walking on uneven surfaces and inclines, and walking in crowds or confined space. Children have at best only minimal ability to perform gross motor skills such as running and jumping").[39] Each of these children had been previously using an AAFO for greater than 2 yr. For these subjects, the AAFO was prescribed to control dynamic equinus during gait. The design of the AAFO (Figure 11.3) consisted of a tibial shaft length, 3 cm distal to the fibular head, rubber ankle joint allowing for free dorsiflexion with a 0-degree plantar flexion stop, a flexible toe break, and strapping at the tibia and over the talus to maintain enclosure of the hindfoot and forefoot to the footplate.

All participants were fully informed of the study and signed a consent authorization approved by the Institutional Review Board. All of the children were given a brief physical exam of their foot and ankle where their joint range of motion and muscle spasticity was assessed.

11.2.1 NeuroCom EquiTest System

The patient testing was done with the SMART EquiTest® System (Clackamas, OR). This provides objective assessment of balance control and postural stability under dynamic test conditions designed to reflect the challenges of daily life. The system provides assessment capabilities on either a stable or unstable support surface and in a stable or dynamic visual environment. The system utilizes a dynamic 18 in. × 18 in. dual force plate (Figure 11.4) with rotation and translation capabilities. It contains force sensors to measure the vertical and horizontal (shear) forces exerted by the subject's feet.[1] The force sensors outputs data in digitized counts that are normalized to weight where 5.12 counts = 1.0 lb (11.24 counts = 1.0 kg).[2]

Following a physical examination of the ankle and foot, subjects were placed standing in the NeuroCom SMART EquiTest System®, where they were secured with a harness for safety (Figure 11.5).[2] Their feet where aligned in specific positions on the dual force plates in order to maintain a proportional BOS. Taller subjects' feet were spread apart further and shorter subjects' feet were kept closer to produce an equally proportioned BOS as described in the NeuroCom protocol. The lateral

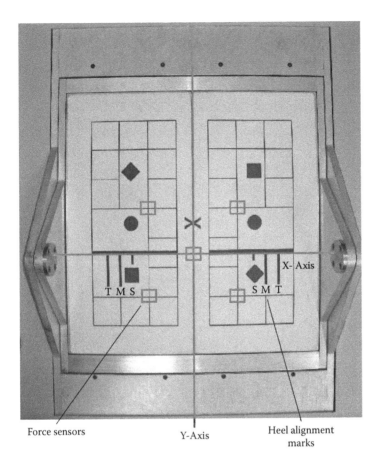

Force sensors   Y-Axis   Heel alignment
      marks

FIGURE 11.4 NeuroCom EquiTest SMART System: NeuroCom EquiTest Dual Forceplate view from above. Allows translation in the +/– *y*-axis or rotation around the *x*-axis. Five force transducers measure shear and vertical forces. The subject's feet are aligned to the markings (T, M, S) according to height.

calcaneus was positioned according to the following height specifications: (S) Short — 30 to 55 in., (M) Medium — 56 to 65 in., and (T) Tall — 66 to 80 in. (the S,M,T designations correspond to the heel alignment markers of Figure 11.4). The scaling was done by entering the subject's height into the EquiTest system, with the foot placements calculated from a demographics database. The axis of the ankle joint was aligned to the rotational axis (*x*-axis) of the force plate.

Prior to testing, the subjects were advised to stand as relaxed and comfortable as possible while maintaining their balance. They were then instructed to keep their feet still, stand upright, and look straight ahead. They were continually reassured that if they should lose their balance, the restraining harness would support them as well as the test operator. They were also videotaped for review.

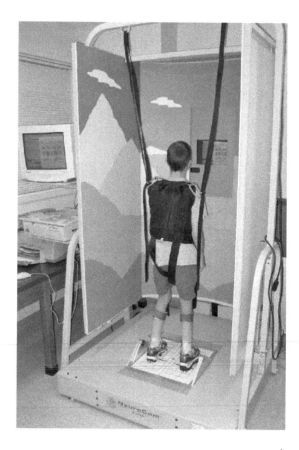

FIGURE 11.5 NeuroCom Dual Forceplate: Subject is secured with a harness and feet are placed according to height.

11.2.1.1 NeuroCom EquiTest Tests

The first test administered was the Motor Control Test (MCT). This assesses the ability of the automatic motor system to quickly recover following an unexpected external disturbance. Sequences of small, medium, or large platform translations in forward and backward directions elicit automatic postural responses. The sizes of the translations are scaled to the child's height to produce proportional sway distur-bances. Small translations are threshold stimulus; large translations produce a max-imal response; and medium translations fall between the two extremes. There are three trials of each size translation in each direction (forward and backward). There is a random delay of 1.5 to 2.5 sec between trials. Random delays prevent the subject from predicting the platform movement and ensure that responses reflect an unantic-ipated response. The translation of the surface is at a constant speed in one horizontal direction, with the movement lasting less than 1 sec. This results in displacement of the subject's center of gravity (COG) away from center in the opposite direction, relative to the BOS (Figure 11.6).[2]

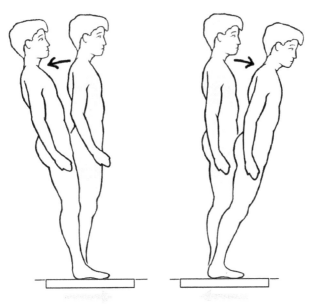

Forward/backward translations

FIGURE 11.6 Motor control test forward/backward translation.

The Adaptation Test (ADT) was the second test performed. This assesses a patient's ability to minimize sway when exposed to surface irregularities and unexpected changes in support surface inclination. The feet are aligned as with the MCT. Sequences of platform rotations in the toes-up or toes-down direction elicit automatic motor responses (Figure 11.7). The axis of movement is at the ankles, with each trial rotation lasting 400 msec and uniform in amplitude (8°) for all trials and subjects. There is a random delay between trials of 300 to 500 msec, with a total of five trials in each rotational direction. For each platform rotation trial, a sway energy score quantifies the magnitude of the force response required to overcome induced postural instability.[3]

11.2.1.1.1 MCT Data and Analysis

The results provide a means for assessment of the child's balance and posture. The MCT data address the subject's weight symmetry, latency, and amplitude scaling. The clinically based parameters used for postural stability assessment are described elsewhere.[17–20] Those selected for inclusion in the current study are listed below.

Weight Symmetry: The symmetry of weight-bearing on the right and left sides of the force plate. A score of 100 implies even weight distribution, >100 favors right, <100 favors left. This measurement is taken prior to the translation.

Latency: This is the time in milliseconds from the plate translation to the subject's active response to the movement. There is also a composite latency

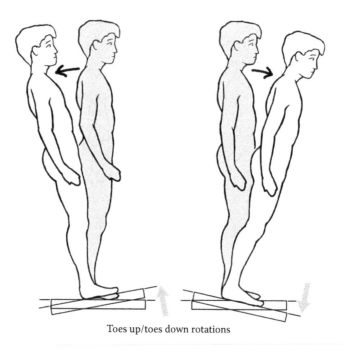

Toes up/toes down rotations

FIGURE 11.7 Adaptation test anterior/posterior rotation.

score that reflects the average latency for right and left legs, in both directions of the translation.

Amplitude Scaling: This shows the force amplitude of the subject's active
response to each translation. For each translation, the system imparts a
known amount of forward or backward angular momentum to the body. To
stop the sway and return the body to its initial position, the active force
response must impart an angular momentum in the opposite direction and
approximately twice as large as that created by the translation. One half of
the response momentum is required to halt the further sway; the other half
moves the body back in the opposite direction.[4]

11.2.1.1.2   ADT Data and Analysis

Movement of the body causes sway or excursion of the COP and/or COG. The ADT
score quantifies how well the patient can minimize AP sway after unexpected support
surface rotations. The ADT data illustrate the magnitude of the force response
required to overcome sway induced by sequences of toes-up and toes-down rotational
disturbances.[3] The four load cells imbedded in the force plate each transmit force
information to the computer at a frequency of 100 Hz. This allows for the calculation
of the location of the COP. The program calculates a nondimensional "sway energy"
function during each of the rotation trials (see below). Falls are scored by a 0 and
excluded from the group statistics. Falls occur at any time the subject moves a foot

from an original position, when the walls or safety straps are used for support, or when the harness is used to maintain posture.

11.2.1.1.2.1   Sway Energy Calculation[15]

1. The program twice differentiates the *y*-axis vertical force position trace, giving *PY'* and *PY''*, and calculates the root mean squares of each, giving *PY'* (*RMS*) and *PY''* (*RMS*).
2. The program then calculates the weighted sum of the RMS velocity *PY'* and acceleration *PY''* using the following formula:

$$Sway\,Energy = C1*PY'(RMS) + C2*PY''(RMS)$$

where *C1* and *C2* are weighted constants used to give dimensionless energy values:

$$C1 = \frac{1}{in/sec}$$

$$C2 = \frac{0.25}{sec^2}$$

11.2.1.2   Statistics

Mean and standard deviation were determined from each of the test's scores. A one-way analysis of variance (ANOVA) was done to compare group means. This returns a *p*-value for the null hypothesis that all samples in the groups are drawn from the same population. Significance was set at $p < .05$.

11.3   RESULTS

11.3.1   MCT RESULTS (TABLE 11.2)

11.3.1.1   Weight Symmetry

The trials with the CP subjects wearing braces had a slightly lower group average value for weight symmetry (91.83) than the CP subjects barefoot (99.37) or the control subjects (98.09). There was not a significant difference between any of the groups. Since no difference was found between sides, the left and right side measurements were averaged together. A score less than 100 implies the subject is supporting more weight on the left side; greater than 100 implies right side.

11.3.1.2   Latency

The control group population exhibited the quickest active response time to the various size translation perturbations. The greatest differences were found between the CP subjects who were barefoot and the control group for the large forward

TABLE 11.2
Motor Control Test Group Averages

	Translation (3 trials each)	Weight Symmetry	Latency (msec)	Amplitude Scaling	Strength Symmetry	Composite Score
Control group barefoot	Small B	95.27	152.79	1.10	98.18	
	Medium B	96.36	140.00	2.53	103.27	
	Large B	97.91	139.64	3.43	99.64	
	Small F	98.73	148.64	1.27	107.44	
	Medium F	99.09	134.64	2.23	104.64	
	Large F	101.18	152.48	3.06	104.27	
	Overall average	98.09(7.08)	144.70(21.97)	2.27(2.12)	102.91(12.15)	133.63(15.36)[a]
CP subjects barefoot	Small B	97.80	177.75[a]	0.30[a]	100.00	
	Medium B	95.00	164.00[a]	1.20	91.50	
	Large B	98.00	154.00	1.70[a]	90.00	
	Small F	103.40	171.00[a]	0.50	88.67	
	Medium F	99.40	151.00	0.90[a]	88.67	
	Large F	102.60	186.00[a]	1.00[a]	91.50	
	Overall average	99.37(12.98)	152.50(36.15)	0.93(0.78)	91.72(13.83)	164.40(10.45)[a]
CP subjects with AAFO	Small B	86.20	174.16[a]	0.40	100.00	
	Medium B	94.20	180.83[a]	0.80[a]	100.00	
	Large B	90.60	177.25[a]	1.40[a]	89.20	
	Small F	88.00	193.33[a]	0.70	80.00	
	Medium F	95.00	211.00[b]	1.30	56.00	
	Large F	97.00	194.75[a]	1.90[a]	85.00	
	Overall average	91.83(14.09)	188.55(36.64)	1.08(1.06)	85.03(22.08)	188.25(13.47)

[a]p-Value < .01 when compared to control group.
[b]p-Value < .01 when compared to control group and CP barefoot group.
Overall average — average over all of the translations sizes with standard deviation in parentheses.

translations (LFT), medium backwards translations (MBT), small backwards translations (SBT), and small forward translations (SFT). The population of CP subjects when braced exhibited the slowest latency scores overall and had significant differences from the control group for all of the translations. When comparing the CP subjects barefoot and braced trials, the average latency for the barefoot group was less. The only significant difference was found in the MBT trials, with the CP barefoot population responding at an average of 164 msec and the CP braced group responding 180.8 msec after the perturbation.

11.3.1.3 Amplitude Scaling

The average amplitude scaling, or the measurement of the strength of the subject's active response, was found to be the highest in the control group and lowest in the CP subjects' barefoot trials. Significant differences were exhibited between the control group and CP subjects barefoot for the large translations in both the forward and backward directions. There were also significantly weaker responses from the LBT, LFT, MFT, and SBT from the CP subjects barefoot. The CP subjects braced population had significantly weaker responses than the control group from LBT, LFT, and MBT, but no significant differences were found between CP populations.

11.3.1.4 Composite Score

The average overall MCT score, or composite score, was lowest for the control group and highest for the CP subjects when braced. There were significant differences between the controls and both CP groups with a *p*-value of .019 between the CP populations.

11.3.2 ADT RESULTS (TABLE 11.3)

11.3.2.1 Toes-Up

The ADT measures sway energy for toes-up and toes-down rotational perturbations to the standing platform. The control subjects recorded an average sway energy score of 73.33 for all five trials. The CP subjects were unable to maintain a standing posture for all of the trials when not wearing their prescribed AAFOs, recording a fall each time. The CP subjects faired only slightly better with the braces on, with only 8 out of 25 trials recorded as nonfalls, with an average sway energy score of 103.4.

11.3.2.2 Toes-Down

The control subjects minimized their AP sway in the toes-down trials compared to the toes-up trials, with an average sway energy score for the controls of 56.4, 110.8 for the CP subjects barefoot, and 129.0 for the CP subjects with AAFOs. There were significant differences in this test between the controls and the CP barefoot population ($p < .01$), and the controls and the CP braced population ($p < .01$).

11.4 DISCUSSION

Impairments associated with CP, such as spasticity, muscle weakness, immature/disorganized muscle synergies, and coactivation of proximal–distal and agonist–antagonist musculature, have several effects on balance. These include decreasing the BOS, impairing medial-arch reactions, placing mechanical restrictions on joint range of motion, and not providing an effective lever arm in the ankle and foot. The use of lower extremity bracing has been shown to be an effective intervention for the impairments of children with CP during gait, but controversial in addressing the resulting balance deficits.[31,34,35] There have been mixed findings on bracing's functional gains. The pediatric assessment strategy used in this pilot study of children with CP, using AFOs, can help identify possible benefits.

We examined five subjects with CP barefoot and braced, as well as ten control subjects in various tests of balance. We used an assessment strategy implemented by the NeuroCom Smart EquiTest System, which has been shown to be a useful tool in the assessment of balance dysfunction.[2,15] The use of specific protocols such as the MCT and ADT adequately replicate real-life situations including recovery

TABLE 11.3
Adaptation Test Group Average Sway Energy Score

		Trial 1	Trial 2	Trial 3	Trial 4	Trial 5	Overall Average[a]	p-Value
Toes-up	Control group barefoot	89.60	77.64	69.36	65.05	65.00	73.33(25.27)	
	CP subjects barefoot	fall	fall	fall	fall	fall	fall	
	CP subjects with AAFO[b]	94.00	128.00	111.00	97.00	87.00	103.40(22.21)	
	Controls vs. CP subjects barefoot							.00
	Controls vs. CP subjects braced							.002
	CP subjects braced vs. barefoot							.00
Toes-down	Control group barefoot	66.36	52.00	54.55	53.91	55.18	56.40(21.08)	
	CP subjects barefoot	120.00	111.50	115.50	100.00	107.00	110.80(20.56)	
	CP subjects with AAFO	126.00	135.75	130.80	131.00	121.80	129.07(37.14)	
	Controls vs. CP subjects barefoot							<.000
	Controls vs. CP subjects braced							<.000
	CP subjects braced vs. barefoot							.4827

[a]Standard deviations in parentheses.
[b]Only 8 out of 25 trials were not falls.

from an unexpected slip, surface irregularities, and changes in inclination.[16] The subject testing was performed quickly and easily, taking no more than 15 to 20 min per subject. The time efficiency would support the use of these tests during a clinic visit or gait analysis. The output data were clear and understandable, providing an index of the subject's functionality. There are default reports provided by NeuroCom, but the data can also be exported in raw form. The raw form is in digital counts, which allows for additional analysis.

Figure 11.8 and Figure 11.9 display raw subject data. Figure 11.8 includes two plots tracking the COP during the MCT. The x–y axis represents the dual force plate support surface. The x-axis aligns with the axis of rotation of the ankle joint. The top plot shows the COP motion during a forward translation for a normal subject. The trial begins with collecting data during static standing until the perturbation occurs at 0.50 sec. The COP is tracked during the static standing and as the subject responds to the perturbation, until the trial ends at 2.50 sec. This type of plot can also be seen for a backward translation in the bottom plot. Examination of the forward translation plot shows that the COP initially moves posteriorly, but also to the right; then once the translation stops, the COP moves forward and to the left. Notice that the COP does not end at its starting location. Rather, it ends in a more posterior location, possibly in anticipation of another translation. The bottom plot of the backward translation tracks the COP as it moves forward and to the right in response to the translation, then back and to the left, ending slightly posterior to the original location.

Figure 11.9 is an example of another plot that displays MCT data. It shows the force measured by each of the five force sensors on the force plates during a single trial. There are left–right side and front–rear sensors, as well as a centrally located shear sensor. The first 0.50 sec is static standing, at which point the perturbation occurs. A baseline measurement is taken from each sensor during the static standing part of the trial. This static measurement is then subtracted from the force measured after the perturbation; so the plot represents the change in force due to the translation. The first parts of the curves are flat since the subject is quietly standing. After the forward translation, the subject's weight shifts rearward, then to the front, and then oscillates to the rear again. The top plot in this figure is an average of the normal subjects during the forward translation, the middle plot is a CP subject barefoot, and the bottom plot is the same subject braced. Comparison of these plots illustrates that the barefoot trial has the weakest force response. The magnitude of the response in the braced trial is closer to normal, and the normal subjects have the strongest response.

Examination of Table 11.2 shows that the control group had the quickest responses to the translational perturbations, while the CP subjects wearing their braces were the slowest, on average. This implies that AFO and shoe wear had some type of dampening effect on the perception of the perturbation. However, the braced subjects presented with higher amplitude in strength of response than the unbraced CP subjects (Figure 11.8). This suggests that once the braced subjects did sense the translation, they were able to exert more force to return their COP back to within a position of stability within their BOS. The increase in force amplitude could be attributed to several reasons. The AAFO provides extrinsic support to the ankle and

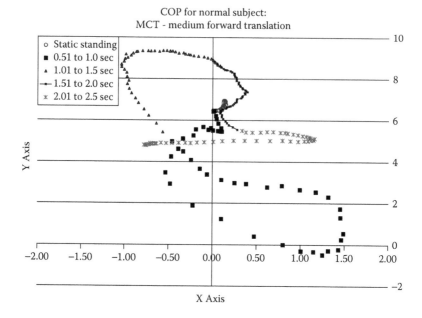

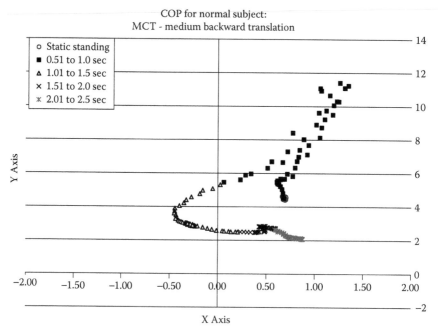

FIGURE 11.8 Example data: These plots trace the COP during a forward translation (top) and backward translation (bottom). The static standing portion of the trial is represented by the circles. The perturbation occurs after 0.50 sec. Data are sampled at 100 Hz.

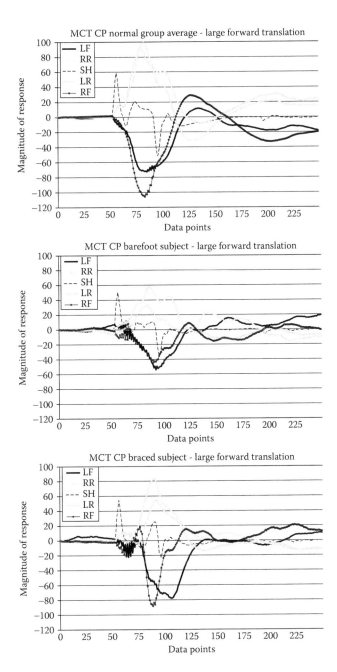

FIGURE 11.9 Example data: These plots display the magnitude of the force response for the group of normal subjects (top), and a CP subject barefoot (middle) and braced (bottom). The normal subjects have the highest magnitude, with the CP subjects having a stronger response with their braces on. LF, left front force sensor on force plate; RF, right front; LR, left rear; RR, right rear; and SH, shear sensor.

foot, which the musculature in a child with CP cannot. Much of the available research on the effect of orthoses on children with CP focuses on impairment level measures that encompass changes to anatomical structure and physiologic function. It is questionable that these corrections have led to functional gains.[31] The goal of bracing is to place the foot and ankle in appropriate alignment, thus improving the BOS and providing a rigid support lever. As a result, balance reactions may be enhanced.

The subjects with CP also responded slower, on average, to the forward translations, with their braces on, than to the backward translations. This could be due to the mechanical restrictions of the AAFO, which do not allow for plantar flexion. There were no significant differences between the groups when looking at the weight or strength symmetry. This would be an expected result in diplegic subjects, with bilateral bracing.

The ADT, which measures sway by rotating the support surface in the toes-up or toes-down direction about the ankle joint, showed significant differences between the control group and the CP group, with and without braces. In the toes-up direction, none of the CP subjects were able to remain standing after the perturbation without braces. According to Bleck (1987),[39] even children with spastic diplegia, who walk without aids, generally have poor equilibrium reactions and so may fall backward with very little provocation. This holds true with our subjects who all fell during the ADT toes-up trials even though the AAFO allows for foot dorsiflexion. Falls were most likely due to the hyperactive stretch reflex in the gastrocsoleus muscle and/or mechanical limitations in the ankle joints. The gastrocsoleus was not able to stretch in response to the change in surface inclination, and the children simply tipped over backwards, falling into the harness, or were forced to take a step. Performance on the ADT requires adequate ankle range of motion and muscle strength, as well as effective motor adaptation. During the first (unexpected) trials, the initial disruptive responses were corrected by secondary responses in the opposing muscles. With each subsequent trial in normal subjects, initial reactions were attenuated and secondary responses strengthened to reduce overall sway.[2]

When braced, the subjects were able to resist the disturbance and regain equilibrium during 8 out of 25 trials (32%). Potential explanations for why some were able to resist falls are:

- The mechanical strength of the brace and shoe were able to support the body.
- The COP of children with CP is shifted more anteriorly than that of normal children. The use of footwear and AFOs that resist plantar flexion enabled the children to shift their COP more posteriorly to allow for a more balanced starting point.[32]
- By wearing shoes and braces the BOS is increased, allowing for the COP to move a greater distance without traveling outside the BOS.
- By providing an extrinsic support and a rigid lever to work from, an AFO allows the muscles crossing the ankle and foot to have more effective levers to generate force, aiding in the treatment of lever arm dysfunction (LAD). Gage (2004) explains that bones constitute the levers upon which muscles act, and lever arm dysfunction describes the bony distortions and positional deformities that alter the leverage relationships between bone and muscle.[19]

- LAD is present in the feet of children with CP, thus affecting the amount of torque that can be generated in response to a perturbation to standing balance.

In the ADT toes-down trials, there were also significant differences between the control group and the CP subjects, but not between the braced and unbraced trials. The fact that none of the subjects fell during these trials was somewhat surprising, because the AAFO does not allow for plantar flexion. The toes-down rotation of the platform creates a flexion moment at the knee since that is the next joint available with free motion, allowing the subjects to adequately respond to the platform rotation. Although there were no significant differences between the braced and unbraced trials, the braced trials had a higher sway energy score on average. The higher score implies that a greater magnitude of force is required to overcome the induced postural instability. This could be necessary due to the greater latency in response, which occurs when wearing the brace.

The ankle and hip strategy respond to sagittal plane balance perturbations. They are defined by their motion in that plane, though, as seen in Figure 11.8, the COP moves laterally as well as anteriorly/posteriorly even though the support surface motion was restricted to sagittal motion. This nonsagittal motion could be further measured with the use of a three-dimensional motion capture system. Kinematics along with electromyography (EMG) data would also be useful to observe muscle strategies and supplement the balance testing done with the NeuroCom system. These additions would add time to testing, but would provide useful data on full body responses to balance disruptions.

11.5 CONCLUSION

Previous research has shown the effectiveness of lower extremity bracing on improving the level of impairment in children with CP. However, it is questionable whether these improvements translate into functional gains with regard to balance. The initial findings of this study show that children with CP are deficient in reacting to unexpected perturbations to standing balance and that bracing of the ankle and foot may help accommodate the loss of balance under certain circumstances. As found in this study, an efficient assessment of balance could be a helpful aid in determining the functionality of assistive devices during balance perturbations.

Potential research in this area will include testing a larger sample size with the same protocol. This could be used to study children with hemiplegia, quadriplegia, lower motor neuron disorders, as well the effects of other types of assistive devices. The inclusion of three-dimensional motion data as well as EMG would further supplement a balance assessment.

REFERENCES

1. Jacobson, G.P., Newman, C.W., Kartush, J.M. *Handbook of Balance Function Testing*. St Louis: Mosby Year Book, 1993.
2. NeuroCom International, Inc. *EquiTest Manual, EquiTest System Operators Manual Version 7.04*, MCT-8, 2000.

3. Bronstein, A.M., Brandt, T., Woollacott, M. *Clinical Disorders of Balance Posture and Gait*. New York: Arnold, 1996:1.

4. Nashner, L.M. Fixed patterns or rapid postural responses among leg muscles during stance. *Exp Brain Res* 1977; 30: 13–24.

5. Shumway-Cook, A., Woollacott, M. *Motor Control: Theory and Practical Applications*. Baltimore, M.D: Williams & Wilkins, 1995.

6. Horak, F.B., Nashner, L.M. Central programming of postural movements: adaptation to altered support surface configurations. *J Neurophysiol* 1986; 55: 1369–1381.

7. Nashner, L.M., Woollacott, M., The organization of rapid postural adjustments of standing humans: an experimental-conceptual model. In: Talbott, R.E., Humphrey, D.R., eds. *Posture and Movement*. New York: Raven Press, 1979: 243–257.

8. Nashner, L.M., McCollum, G. The organization of human postural movements: a formal basis and experimental synthesis. *Behav Brain Sci* 1985; 8: 135–172.

9. Macpherson, J.M. How flexible are muscle synergies. In: Humphrey, D.R., Freund H-J, eds. *Motor Control: Concepts and Issues*. Chichester: John Wiley, 1991: 33–47.

10. Moore, S.P., Rushmer, D.S., Windus, S.L., Nashner, L.M. Human automatic postural responses: responses to horizontal perturbations of stance in multiple directions. *Exp Brain Res* 1988; 73: 648–658.

11. Woollacott, M., Roseblad, B., Hofsten, von C. Relation between muscle response onset and body segmental movements during postural perturbations in humans. *Exp Brain Res* 1988; 72: 593–604.

12. Bouisset, S., Zattara, M. Segmental movement as a perturbation to balance? Facts and concepts. In: Winters, J.M., Woo S.L.Y., eds *Multiple Muscle Systems: Biomechanics and Movement Organization*. New York: Springer, 1990: 498–506.

13. Crenna, P., Frigo, C. A motor program for the initiation of forward-orientated movements in man. *J Physiol* 1991; 437: 635–653.

14. Winter, D.A. *Biomechanics and Motor Control of Human Movement*. New York: John Wiley, 1990: 80–84.

15. NeuroCom International, Inc. NeuroCom Products: EquiTest. Oct. 10, 2005. http://www.onbalance.com/neurocom/products/EquiTest.aspx.http://www.onbalance.com/neurocom/protocols/motorImpairment/mct.aspx.http://www.onbalance.com/neurocom/protocols/motorImpairment/adt.aspx.

16. Lockhart, T.E. Relationship between postural control and slip response among different age groups. *Gait Posture* 2002; 16: S125–S126.

17. Burtner, P.A., Qualls, C., and Woolacott, M.H. Muscle activation characteristics of stance balance control in children with spastic cerebral palsy. *Gait Posture* 1998; 8: 163–174.

18. Robinovitch, S.N., Heller, B., Lui, A., and Cortez, J. Effect of strength and speed of torque development on balance recovery with the ankle strategy. *J Neurophysiol* 2002; 88: 613–620.

19. Gage, J.R. *The Treatment of Gait Problems in Cerebral Palsy*. London: Mac Keith Press, 2004: 3.

20. Bax, M., Goldstein, M., Rosenbaum, P., Leviton, A., and Paneth, N. Proposed definition and classification of cerebral palsy. *Dev Med Child Neurol* 2005; 47: 571–576.

21. Bhattacharya, A., Shukla, R., Dietrich, K., Bornshein, R., and Berger, O. Effect of early lead exposure on childrens postural balance. *Dev Med Child Neurol* 1995; 37: 861–878.

22. Di Fabio, R.P., Foudriat, B.A. Responsiveness and reliability of a pediatric strategy score for balance. *Physiother Res Int* 1996; 1(3): 180–194.

23. Shimizu, K., Asai, M., Takata, S., and Watanabe, Y. The development of equilibrium function in childhood. In: Taguchi, K., Igarashi, M., Mori, S., eds. *Vestibular and Neural Front*. New York: Elsevier Science BV, 1994: 183–186.

24. Horak, F.B., Shumway-Cook, A., Crowe, T.K., and Black, F.O. Vestibular function and motor proficiency of children with impaired hearing, or with learning disability and motor impairment. *Dev Med Child Neurol* 1988; 30: 64–79.

25. Shumway-Cook, A., Woollacott, M.H. *Motor Control Theory and Practical Applications*. Baltimore: Williams & Wilkins, 1995:3–6.

26. Berstein, N. *Co-Ordination and Regulation of Movements*. New York: Pergamon Press, 1967.

27. Forssberg, H., Nashner, L.M. Ontogenetic development of postural control in man: adaptation to altered support and visual conditions in stance. *J Neurosci* 1982; 2: 545–552.

28. Nashner, L.M., Shumway-Cook, A., and Marin, O. Stance postural control in select groups of children with cerebral palsy: deficits in sensory organization and muscular coordination. *Exp Brain Res* 1983; 49: 393–409.

29. Brogren, E., Hadders-Algra, M., and Forssberg, H., Postural adjustments in sitting children with spastic diplegia. *Dev Med Child Neurol* 1996; 33: 379–388.

30. Woollacott, M., Shumway-Cook, A., Hutchinson, S., Ciol, M., Price, R., and Kartin, D. Effect of balance training on muscle activity used in recovery of stability in children with cerebral palsy: a pilot study. *Dev Med Child Neurol* 2005; 47: 455–461.

31. Kott, K.M., Held, S.L. Effects of orthoses on upright functional skills of children and adolescents with cerebral palsy. *Pediatr Phys Ther* 2002; 14: 199–207.

32. Morris, C., Orthotic management of children with cerebral palsy. *J Prosth Orth* 2002; 14: 150–158.

33. Magee, D.J. *Orthopedic Physical Assessment*. 3rd ed. Philadelphia: W.B. Saunders Company, 1997.

34. Harris, S.R., Riffle, K. Effects of inhibitive ankle-foot orthoses on standing balance in a child with cerebral palsy. *Phys Ther* 1986; 66: 663–667.

35. Taylor, C.L., Harris, S.R. Effects of ankle-foot orthoses on functional motor performance in a child with spastic diplegia. *Am J Occup Ther* 1986; 40: 492–494.

36. Shumway-Cook, A., Hutchinson, S., Kartin, D., Price, R., and Woollacott, M. Effect of balance training on recovery of stability in children with cerebral palsy. *Dev Med Child Neurol* 2003; 45: 591–602.

37. Sundermier, L., Woollacott, M., Roncesvalles, N., and Jensen, J. The development of balance control in children: comparisons of EMG and kinetic variables and chronological and developmental groupings. *Exp Brain Res* 2001; 136: 340–350.

38. Palisano, R., Rosenbaum, P., Walter, S., Russell, D., Wood, E., and Galuppi, B. Gross motor function classification system for cerebral palsy. *Dev Med Child Neurol* 1997; 39: 214–233.

39. Bleck, Egene *Orthopaedic Management in Cerebral Palsy*. Mac Keith Press: Oxford: Blackwell Scientific Publications Ltd. 1987.

Section B

Adult Foot and Ankle

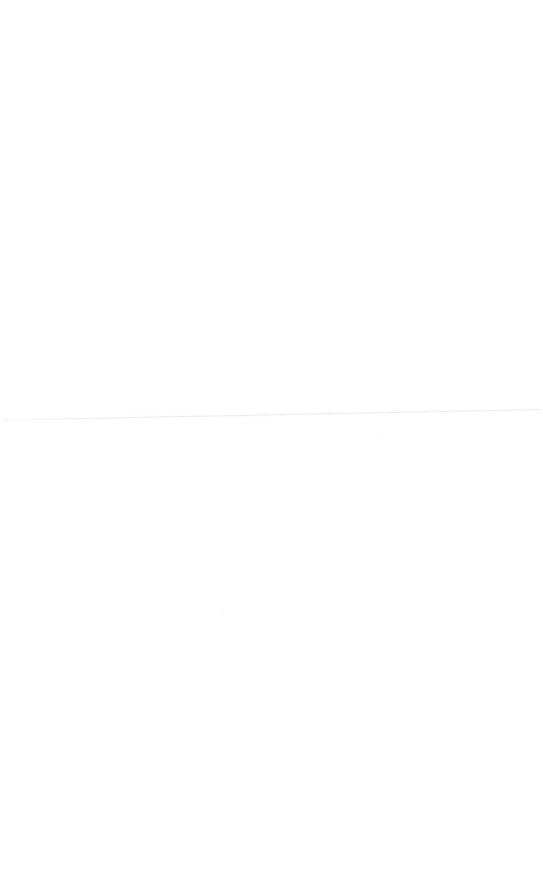

Section B

Adult Foot and Ankle

12 Gait Analysis in Posterior Tibial Tendon Dysfunction: Pre- and Postoperative Analysis Compared to a Normal Population

Richard M. Marks, Jason T. Long,
and Gerald F. Harris

CONTENTS

12.1 INTRODUCTION

Dysfunction of the posterior tibial tendon may result in a pathologic flatfoot deformity, and if not appropriately addressed through conservative measures (rest, rehabilitation, and/or bracing), surgical intervention is necessary to correct the resulting deformity and restore function of the limb.

Presently, there are several operative choices commonly utilized by orthopedic surgeons to address posterior tibial tendon dysfunction (PTTD).[1–9] While surgeons have evaluated the radiographic and clinical results of various surgical procedures,[2,7,9–12] the temporal and kinematic effects of surgical intervention have not been evaluated. The development of quantitative gait analysis has added to the evaluation of musculoskeletal and neurological impairments of the lower extremities, and has been particularly helpful in the evaluation of numerous pediatric abnormalities.

Traditional techniques for gait analysis measure joint kinematics in three dimensions at the hip, knee, and ankle, modeling each limb segment (pelvis, thigh, tibia, foot) as a single rigid element.[13,14] While such evaluation is frequently sufficient for more proximal limb abnormalities, pathologic gait secondary to PTTD has profound effects on the complex interrelationships between the ankle, subtalar, and transverse tarsal joints. These abnormalities also have a significant effect on the more distal and proximal articulations of the foot.

The development of multisegmental foot and ankle models[15–20] has allowed for more precise quantitative clinical assessment of pathologic gait secondary to PTTD, as well as the precise effect of surgical intervention on the resultant gait. This chapter provides a quantitative characterization of patients with PTTD, including postoperative gait results, and compares both pre- and postoperative populations to a previously documented normal population.

12.2 POSTERIOR TIBIAL TENDON ANATOMY AND BIOMECHANICS

The posterior tibial muscle arises from the posterior aspect of the tibia, interosseous membrane, and fibula in the proximal leg and is contained in the deep posterior compartment with the flexor hallucis longus and flexor digitorum longus (FDL) muscles. It travels behind the medial malleolus and has its primary insertion on the navicular tuberosity, with secondary attachments to the cuneiforms and lesser metatarsals. The muscle serves as the primary inverter of the heel, with muscle contraction occurring from mid- to terminal stance (TSt). The muscular contraction allows the gastrocsoleus complex to shift to the medial side of the subtalar axis; when the gastrocsoleus complex contracts, it then becomes a powerful heel inverter. Heel inversion creates obliquity of the transverse tarsal (talonavicular, calcaneocuboid) joint, thereby creating a rigid midfoot during TSt, which allows efficient transfer of stored energy in the lower extremity for toe-off and the swing phase.

Dysfunction of the posterior tibial muscle results in less efficient gait, as the heel does not effectively medialize, and the gastrocsoleus complex requires greater excursion to become a heel inverter. In cases where the posterior tibial muscle no longer contracts, resting heel valgus may be accentuated as the gastrocsoleus complex becomes a deforming force, and its subsequent contraction creates an external valgus moment on the heel. In these cases, the supporting medial soft tissues become attenuated, further accentuating the resultant flatfoot deformity. Late changes with the pathologic flatfoot include lateral hindfoot bony impingement, sinus tarsi inflammation, peroneal tendonitis, equinus contracture, and eventual arthrosis.

12.3 PTTD CLASSIFICATION

Dysfunction of the posterior tibial tendon was first classified by Johnson and Strom,[21] with later modification by Myerson.[6] Stage I PTTD involves inflammation of the tendon with no functional deficiencies. Patients will have tenderness along the inframalleolar course of the tendon, in the "hypovascular zone" that exists 2 to 6 cm proximal to the insertion.[22] The hindfoot remains supple, and patients are able to perform both double and single heel raises. In Stage II PTTD, the hindfoot remains supple, as indicated by the ability to perform a double heel raise; however, patients are not able to perform a single heel raise, indicative of an incompetent tendon. The tendon may remain intact, but is no longer able to adequately contract. With Stage III PTTD, the tendon is incompetent, and the hindfoot is rigid, indicative of arthrosis. The patient is not able to invert the heel with a double heel raise. Myerson's classification modification includes a Stage IV, where there is additional deltoid ligament incompetence, resulting in varus tilt of the talus within the ankle mortise.

12.4 TREATMENT OPTIONS FOR PTTD

The treatment of patients with PTTD is determined by the severity of symptoms, duration, and stage of deformity and concomitant medical comorbidities. Initial treatment is designed to diminish symptoms with rest, immobilization, and rehabilitation. Immobilization may include the application of an ankle splint, boot brace, or casting in more severe cases. Once symptoms have improved, physical therapy is instituted, and the patient is gradually shifted from immobilization to an orthotic or brace, particularly for Stages II, III, and IV. Corticosteroid injection to the tendon is contraindicated, as it may lead to tendon disruption.

If tendon inflammation is not controlled by the above means, surgery is indicated, and the type of surgery is determined by stage of dysfunction and degree of deformity. Chronic Stage I inflammation requires tenosynovectomy of the PTT, and if there is concomitant heel valgus, the addition of a calcaneal osteotomy may be indicated. Stage II deformities require tendon substitution of the dysfunctional PTT, typically with the FDL, which is harvested from the medial plantar aspect of the midfoot, distal to the knot of Henry. The PTT is resected in its diseased portion, and a drill hole placed in the navicular tuberosity for transfer of the FDL. While this technique has been shown to relieve pain from the dysfunctional PTT, it does not restore the medial longitudinal arch, and patients frequently complain of continued deformity. For this reason, the addition of a calcaneal osteotomy has been advocated.[4,5]

Two such osteotomies are frequently utilized. The medial displacement calcaneal osteotomy (MDCO) is performed through the calcaneal tuberosity, and the inferior tuberosity displaced in a medial direction and transfixed with a screw.[3,5] This corrects heel valgus, improves the height of the medial longitudinal arch, and provides medialization of the insertion of the gastrocsoleus complex, thereby improving its biomechanical function. The osteotomy also provides a protective function for the concomitant FDL tendon transfer. A second type of osteotomy is performed through the lateral aspect of the calcaneus, either through the anterior process or through the calcaneocuboid joint.[1,2,12] This type of osteotomy is helpful to correct abduction deformities, as well as improve the medial longitudinal arch. Stage III deformities (by definition: an arthritic hindfoot) require a triple arthrodesis, involving the fusion of the subtalar, talonavicular, and calcaneocuboid joints. Stage IV deformities require hindfoot fusion, in combination with either deltoid ligament reconstruction or concomitant ankle fusion.

In an attempt to characterize the effects of PTTD on gait, as well as quantify the effects of surgical correction on postoperative gait, we have conducted pre- and postoperative gait analysis of patients with Stage II PTTD, and compared them to a previously reported normal gait population.

12.5 CURRENT INVESTIGATION OF PTTD GAIT

Twenty-seven (27) patients with Stage II PTTD were recruited from the Foot and Ankle Clinics at the Medical College of Wisconsin (23 females, 4 males; age 52.3 ± 9.9 yr). This constituted the preoperative PTTD gait population. Twelve patients (9 females, 3 males; age 52.9 ± 10.4 yr) underwent postoperative gait analysis at an average of 17.9 months postoperatively. Both populations were compared to a previously described normal population ("normal"; 12 females, 13 males; age 41.3 ± 12.5 yr).

Temporal-spatial and three-dimensional (3D) kinematic foot and ankle motion data for the PTTD population were obtained using a 15-camera Vicon Motion Analysis System (Vicon Motion Systems, Inc.; Lake Forest, CA). The Vicon system uses infrared strobes to illuminate reflective markers placed on key anatomic landmarks and reports the 3D positions of the markers within the laboratory. Marker position information was analyzed using the four-segment Milwaukee Foot Model (MFM; Figure 12.1), which calculates segment kinematics of four segments (tibia, hindfoot, forefoot, and hallux) in the sagittal, coronal, and transverse planes.[15,18-20] Segment motion is measured relative to the next most proximal segment, with tibial segment motion measured relative to the global coordinate system of the lab.

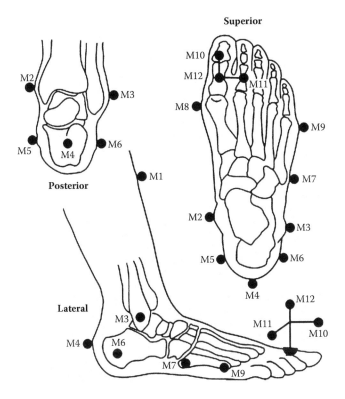

FIGURE 12.1 Placement of anatomical markers for the MFM.

Twelve reflective spherical markers (d = 16 mm) were placed on specific bony landmarks on the tibia, ankle, and foot and to define each of the four MFM segments (Figure 12.2a–b). Due to the limited size, the hallux was marked with a triad, which provides adequate marker separation. After marker placement, the subject stood comfortably and quietly while a static trial was collected to record the quiet standing position of the markers. A previously acquired tracing of foot position was used to facilitate repeatable posture and foot position. Walking trials were then collected while the subject walked at a self-selected speed. Video data was captured at 120 Hz.

Anterior–posterior, lateral, and modified hindfoot coronal alignment (Milwaukee view[23]) weight-bearing radiographs were obtained to relate marker position to underlying bone anatomy (Figure 12.3a–c). Indexing measurements were taken of all four foot segments in each of the three radiographic views.

12.5.1 Modified Hindfoot Coronal Alignment Radiograph (Milwaukee View)

This unique weight-bearing radiographic view demonstrates the "true" alignment of the calcaneus relative to the tibia.[23] The subject stands in a natural position, and tracings of both feet are drawn on a cardboard. A line is drawn, which bisects the

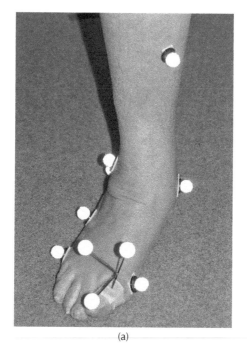

(a)

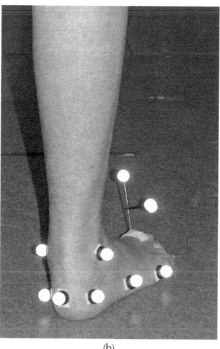

(b)

FIGURE 12.2 Oblique anterior (a) and posterior (b) views of patient foot instrumented with MFM markers.

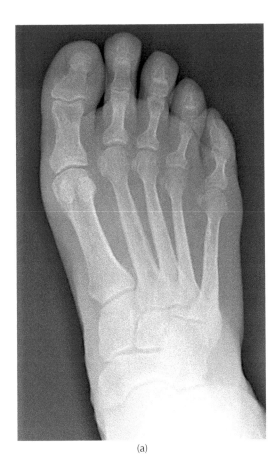

(a)

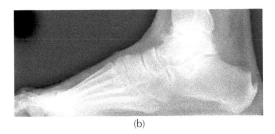

(b)

FIGURE 12.3 Weight-bearing A/P (a), lateral (b), and Milwaukee (c) views of foot used to index bony motion to MFM marker motion.

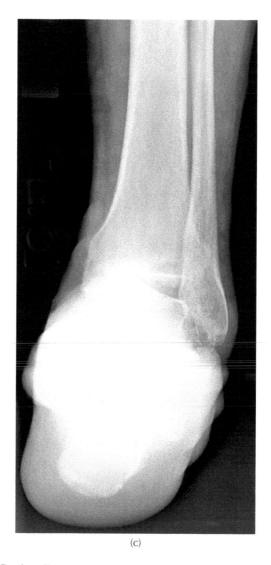

(c)

FIGURE 12.3 (Continued).

silhouette of the second toe and the heel. Another line is then drawn across the tips of the toes, which is perpendicular to the foot line. The foot tracings are then cut along this line. This tracing allows reproducibility of foot position, and assures that the foot is perpendicular to the x-ray plate. The subject stands on an x-ray stand with both feet positioned on the cardboard tracing. The x-ray beam is angled at 15 to 20° to the floor, while a posterior x-ray is taken with the cassette held at 90° to the floor. To measure the calcaneal/tibial alignment, an ellipse is superimposed over the posterior calcaneal tuberosity. The angle formed between the axis of the tibia and the axis of the ellipse is defined as the coronal hindfoot alignment (Figure 12.3c).

12.5.2 STATISTICAL ANALYSIS

Minimum, maximum, and range of motion (ROM) values were calculated for each subject during each of seven phases of gait. These seven phases, based on Perry's definitions,[24] were designated as load response (LR, 0 to 16% stance), mid-stance (MSt, 16 to 48% stance), TSt (48 to 81% stance), preswing (PSw, 81 to 100% stance), initial swing (ISw, 0 to 32% swing), midswing (MSw, 32 to 66% swing), and terminal swing (TSw, 66 to 100% swing). Temporal-spatial parameters (cadence, stride length, stance duration, and walking speed) were also calculated. For each segment in each plane, we tested the null hypothesis that the ROM measures were the same at each phase using unpaired nonparametric methods (Mann-Whitney U test). To adjust for multiple tests over the set of seven test points, a Bonferroni correction was used to achieve a family-wise 5% overall error rate. To maintain the overall error rate, we chose to make all comparisons of joint kinematics at a level of $p < .002$, and all comparisons of temporal-spatial parameters at a level of $p < .0125$ (slightly less than the levels needed).

12.6 RESULTS

12.6.1 TEMPORAL-SPATIAL PARAMETERS

Full temporal-spatial measures are provided in Table 12.1. The normal population exhibited a mean stride length of 1.2886 m, mean cadence of 104.23 steps/min, mean stance duration of 62.2619%, and mean walking speed of 1.1174 m/sec. The preoperative PTTD population exhibited a mean stride length of 0.9739 m, mean cadence of 94.8984 steps/min, mean stance duration of 63.0840%, and mean walking speed of 0.7812 m/sec. The postoperative PTTD population had a mean stride length of 1.1104 m, mean cadence of 101.1910 steps/min, mean stance percentage of 65.3279%, and mean walking speed of 0.9434 m/sec.

12.6.1.1 Comparison: Preoperative PTTD vs. Normal

Significant differences were recorded for stride length (0.9739 vs. 1.2886 m), stance duration (63.0840 vs. 62.2619%), and walking speed (0.7812 vs. 1.1174 m/sec). There was no significant difference seen in cadence.

12.6.1.2 Comparison: Postoperative PTTD vs. Preoperative PTTD

Significant improvements were seen in stride length (1.1104 vs. 0.9739 m), cadence (101.1910 vs. 94.8984 steps/min), and walking speed (0.9434 vs. 0.7812 m/sec). No significant improvement was seen in stance duration.

12.6.1.3 Comparison: Postoperative PTTD vs. Normal

Significant differences still remained postoperatively in stride length (1.1104 vs. 1.2886 m), percentage in stance (65.3279 vs. 62.619%), and walking speed (0.9434 vs. 1.1174 m/sec). No significant difference was seen in cadence.

TABLE 12.1
Temporal-Spatial Parameters for Normal vs. PTTD. Bolded *p*-Values Indicate Statistical Significance at *p* < .0125

Measure		Mean Values			*p* Values		
		Normal	PTTD Pre	PTTD Post	Pre vs. Norm	Post vs. Norm	Pre vs. Post
Stride length	(m)	1.2886 ± 0.1008	0.9739 ± 0.1606	1.1104 ± 0.1743	.0000	.0027	.0024
Cadence	(steps/min)	104.2300 ± 7.8593	94.8984 ± 20.3225	101.1910 ± 8.3487	.0140	.3061	.0122
Stance %	(%)	62.2619 ± 2.6138	63.0840 ± 12.3165	65.3279 ± 3.1544	.0004	.0124	.9697
Walking speed	(m/sec)	1.1174 ± 0.1009	0.7812 ± 0.2246	0.9434 ± 0.1992	.0000	.0041	.0015

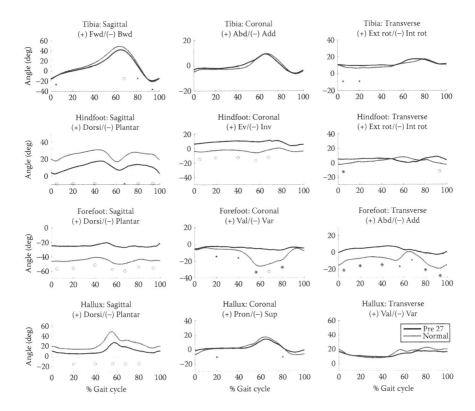

FIGURE 12.4 Segment kinematics for pre-op PTTD (pre27) vs. normal, compared during seven phases of the gait cycle. Asterisks (*) denote a significant difference in position during a phase. Circles (○) denote a significant difference in range of motion during a phase.

12.6.2 Kinematic Parameters

Changes noted as "significant" are statistically significant at $p < .002$ as described in *Statistical Analysis*. Additional changes, which are not noted as significant, represent apparent motion trends, which did not meet the criteria for statistical significance.

12.6.3 Preoperative PTTD vs. Normal (Figure 12.4)

12.6.3.1 Tibia

The tibia exhibits a significantly increased forward position during LR, along with a significantly more externally rotated position, which persists through MSt; a decreased sagittal plane ROM is also observed during ISw. Significant shifts toward a more neutral (vertical) position are also observed in MSw and TSw.

12.6.3.2 Hindfoot

Compared to normal, the hindfoot in the PTTD population demonstrates a position of reduced dorsiflexion and eversion throughout the gait cycle. However, this position difference only achieves statistical significance during ISw in the sagittal plane. Significant sagittal and coronal plane ROM deficits are present throughout the majority of the stride, and transverse plane ROM deficits are apparent during LR and TSw. The PTTD hindfoot is also significantly more externally rotated during LR.

12.6.3.3 Forefoot

Compared to normal, the PTTD forefoot demonstrates a position of reduced plantarflexion throughout the stride; however, this difference does not meet the threshold for statistical significance. Coronally, the PTTD forefoot maintains a position of slight varus, significantly different from normal from MSt through MSw. The PTTD forefoot also does not exhibit the varus thrust observed in the normal population from TSt through MSw. In the transverse plane, the PTTD forefoot maintains a position of significantly more abduction throughout the stance, approaching neutral in swing. Significant ROM deficits are apparent in all three planes throughout the stride.

12.6.3.4 Hallux

Hallux motion in the PTTD group is notable for a shift in sagittal plane motion toward a more neutral position. While this shift does not meet the threshold for statistical significance, the ROM observed from MSt through MSw in the PTTD group is significantly less than normal.

12.6.4   POSTOPERATIVE PTTD VS. PREOPERATIVE PTTD (FIGURE 12.5)

Following surgical correction of PTTD, several changes are apparent; however, few of these changes meet the criteria for statistical significance.

12.6.4.1 Tibia

In the tibia, motion patterns in both the coronal and the transverse planes demonstrated a shift away from normal and toward a more neutral position. These changes were most apparent in the portion of the cycle near toe-off.

12.6.4.2 Hindfoot

In the hindfoot, shifts toward the normal pattern were observed in the sagittal plane (increased dorsiflexion) and the coronal plane (increased inversion, closely matching that of the normal population). In addition, the transverse plane motion of the PTTD hindfoot shifted from its preoperative pattern to a pattern more in phase with normal.

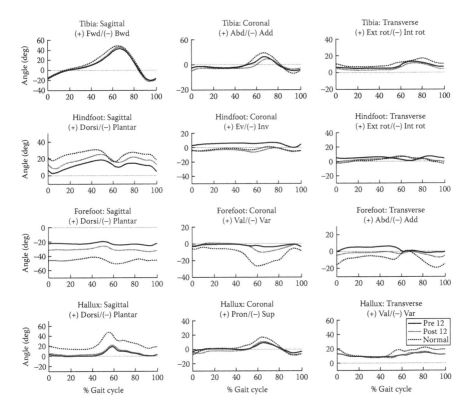

FIGURE 12.5 Segment kinematics for pre-op PTTD (pre12) vs. post-op PTTD (post12), compared during seven phases of the gait cycle. Asterisks (*) denote a significant difference in position during a phase. Circles (∘) denote a significant difference in range of motion during a phase. Kinematics for normal population also shown for reference.

12.6.4.3 Forefoot

Shifts toward normal were observed in all three planes in the PTTD forefoot. Increased plantarflexion was observed sagittally across the duration of the gait cycle. Minimal difference was observed in the coronal plane during early stance, but a restoration of the varus shift was observed in the late stance and swing. The transverse plane motion of the forefoot also demonstrated a shift toward normal, maintaining a position of neutral to slightly adducted over the course of the gait cycle.

12.6.4.4 Hallux

Minimal change was observed in the hallux postoperatively.

12.6.5 POSTOPERATIVE PTTD VS. NORMAL (FIGURE 12.6)

Significant differences from normal remained in the PTTD group following surgical intervention. The PTTD tibia maintained a position of significantly less external

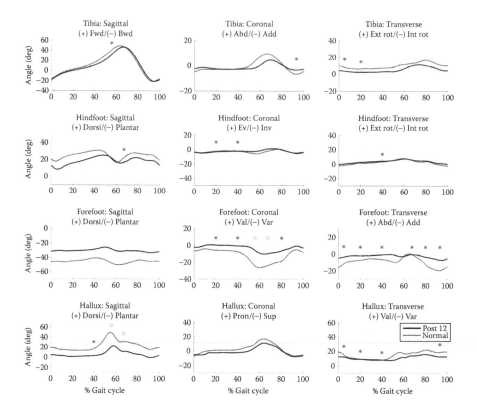

FIGURE 12.6 Segment kinematics for post-op PTTD (post12) vs. normal, compared during seven phases of the gait cycle. Asterisks (*) denote a significant difference in position during a phase. Circles (°) denote a significant difference in range of motion during a phase.

rotation (closer to neutral) during LR and MSt. The PTTD forefoot remained significantly more neutral in the coronal and transverse planes compared to normal. While the varus thrust in late stance and swing had been somewhat restored in the PTTD forefoot, the ROM in these phases was still significantly less than normal. Significant sagittal plane ROM deficits in the hallux were also apparent in PSw and ISw, and the transverse plane positioning was significantly more neutral from LR through TSt.

The sagittal plane motion of the PTTD hindfoot and forefoot demonstrated shifts toward normal patterns, and the differences between them were not statistically significant. Qualitative evaluation, however, revealed that the PTTD patterns still fell closer to neutral than the normal patterns.

12.7 DISCUSSION

The contribution of PTTD to pathologic pes planovalgus deformities is now well documented,[6,21,25] and the importance of the contribution of associated medial-sided soft tissue incompetence, especially the spring ligament and talonavicular capsule, has been identified in simulated gait models of cadaveric specimens.[26]

The contribution of the contracted gastrocsoleus complex is now recognized as a deforming force as well.

While several retrospective studies have evaluated the surgical outcomes from a functional and radiographic perspective,[2,4,7,9–11,25] only one *in vivo* study has evaluated the effect of the adult acquired flatfoot deformity on gait, as well as the subsequent effect of operative intervention on postoperative gait. Brodsky et al. evaluated a series of 12 patients that underwent FDL tendon substitution and MDCO for Stage II PTTD.[13] Single-segment foot and ankle kinematics were evaluated with a five-camera motion analysis system. One-year postoperative gait analysis was compared to preoperative analysis, and significant changes were seen in temporal parameters velocity, step length, and cadence. Single limb support time was actually increased, though not statistically significant. Maximum ankle joint power at push off increased significantly; however, there were no significant changes in lower limb kinematics of the hip or knee.

In our evaluation of 12 patients with Stage II PTTD, a similar surgical technique was utilized for most patients (two patients underwent subtalar and triple arthrodeses). Similar postoperative temporal results were seen in our population, with improvements noted in stride length, cadence, and walking speed. A similar increase of time spent in single limb stance was also noted. The postoperative population still recorded significant differences from normal in stride length, walking speed, and single stance percentage. However, stride length and walking speed demonstrated strong trends toward normal values, and it is expected that as the size of the postoperative population increases, these numbers will tend to normalize.

Based on video data from the 15-camera Vicon Motion Analysis System, the MFM provides additional information on triplanar motion of the tibia, hindfoot, forefoot, and hallux in the pre- and postoperative populations. In the preoperative PTTD population, the global position of the tibia was noted to be more forward during LR, and externally rotated during midstance. Decreased sagittal plane motion was also noted during ISw, and more vertical positioning was noted in mid- and TSw. All these deviations denote a more upright positioning attributed to a decreased walking speed and diminished ability for efficient toe-off.

Hindfoot kinematics were particularly interesting, given the previously noted effects of PTTD on calcaneal pitch and the perturbations affecting the talonavicular relationship. The decreased dorsiflexion and excessive eversion noticed throughout the gait cycle reflect decreased calcaneal pitch as well as the medial collapse of the longitudinal arch, and the increased external rotation reflects the increased heel valgus associated with PTTD. The patients' diminished stride length and walking speed are also reflected in the ROM deficits observed in the sagittal and coronal planes.

Forefoot segment differences include decreased plantarflexion throughout the stride cycle, reflecting the diminution of the medial longitudinal arch. This is consistent with the increase in forefoot abduction observed during stance phase. The lack of varus thrust from TSt through midswing is likely due to the lack of a rigid midfoot secondary to PTTD. This prevents energy transfer to the forefoot during TSt and toe-off. As with the hindfoot segment, the ROM deficits noted in all three planes are secondary to decreased stride length and speed. The hallux exhibits a similar ROM limitation in the sagittal plane from midstance through midswing, indicative of diminished toe-off.

Postoperative gait improvement was most noticeable in the hindfoot and forefoot segments. This is due to the restoration of the medial longitudinal arch and heel inversion secondary to medialization of the calcaneal tuberosity or lateral column lengthening, and improved inversion function from the FDL substitution. The motion pattern of the hindfoot segment shifted toward the normal pattern in the sagittal plane, as increased calcaneal pitch led to increased segment dorsiflexion throughout the stride. Improvement in the coronal plane reflects decreased eversion, as the postoperative PTTD pattern closely matches the normal pattern. Similar improvement is seen in the transverse plane, with a shift toward a pattern more in phase with normal.

Shifts in the forefoot motion pattern toward the normal pattern were seen in all three planes. Improvement in the sagittal plane indicates increased plantarflexion across the duration of the gait cycle, indicative of improvement in arch height. Coronal plane improvements include the restoration of varus shift in late stance and swing, denoting a more stable medial column. Similar improvements were noted in the transverse plane, as the forefoot assumed a position of neutral-to-slight adduction over the course of the gait cycle.

The gait patterns of patients after PTT reconstruction utilizing the FDL tendon substitution and calcaneal osteotomy tended to shift toward more normal gait patterns. This was particularly notable in the sagittal plane motion of the hindfoot and forefoot segments; these changes are attributed to increases in the calcaneal pitch and subsequent plantarflexion of the first ray. While the forefoot segment remained significantly more neutral in the coronal and transverse planes, varus thrust of the forefoot in late stance and swing was restored. Remaining ROM deficits were likely related to continued deficits in stride length and walking speed.

12.8 CONCLUSIONS

The MFM provides 3D analysis of gait of the pathologic flatfoot with a four-segment model, thus providing sophisticated evaluation of preoperative gait pathology and the effectiveness of operative intervention. Through such evaluation, it is hoped that surgeons will be able to more accurately predict the effects of operative intervention of PTTD and, as more results are evaluated, better stratify the gait differences seen in different PTTD patterns, as well as the effect of different combinations of tendon substitution and bony procedures.

REFERENCES

1. Evans D., "Calcaneo-valgus deformity," *J Bone Joint Surg Br*, 57:270–278, 1975.
2. Hintermann B., Valderrabano V., Kundert H.P., "Lengthening of the lateral column and reconstruction of the medial soft tissue for treatment of acquired flatfoot deformity associated with insufficiency of the posterior tibial tendon," *Foot Ankle Int*, 20:622–629, 1999.

3. Koutsogiannis E., "Treatment of mobile flat foot by displacement osteotomy of the calcaneus," *J Bone Joint Surg Br*, 53:96–100, 1971.

4. Manoli A.I., Beals T.C., Pomeroy G.C., "The role of osteotomies in the treatment of posterior tibial tendon disorders," *Foot Ankle Clin*, 2:309–317, 1997.

5. Marks R.M., "Posterior tibial tendon reconstruction with medial displacement calcaneal osteotomy," *Foot and Ankle Clin*, 1:295–313, 1996.

6. Myerson M.S., "Adult acquired flatfoot deformity: treatment of dysfunction of the posterior tibial tendon," *Instr Course Lect*, 46:393–405, 1997.

7. Pomeroy G.C., Manoli A. II, "A new operative approach for flatfoot secondary to posterior tibial tendon insufficiency: a preliminary report," *Foot Ankle Int*, 18:206–212, 1997.

8. Sangeorzan B.J., Smith D., Veith R., Hansen S.T. Jr., "Triple arthrodesis using internal fixation in treatment of adult foot disorders," *Clin Orthop Relat Res*, 299–307, 1993.

9. Toolan B.C., Sangeorzan B.J., Hansen S.T. Jr., "Complex reconstruction for the treatment of dorsolateral peritalar subluxation of the foot," *J Bone Joint Surg Am*, 81:1545–1560, 1999.

10. Fayazi A.H., Nguyen H.-V., Juliano P.J., "Intermediate term follow-up of calcaneal osteotomy and flexor digitorum longus transfer for treatment of posterior tibial tendon dysfunction," *Foot Ankle Int*, 23:1107–1111, 2002.

11. Myerson M.S., Corrigan J., Thompson F., Schon L.C., "Tendon transfer combined with calcaneal osteotomy for treatment of posterior tibial tendon insufficiency: a radiological investigation," *Foot Ankle Int*, 16:712–718, 1995.

12. Sangeorzan B.J., Mosca V., Hansen S.T. Jr., "Effect of calcaneal lengthening on relationships among the hindfoot, midfoot, and forefoot," *Foot Ankle*, 14:136–141, 1993.

13. Brodsky J.W., "Preliminary gait analysis results after posterior tibial tendon reconstruction: a prospective study," *Foot Ankle Int*, 25:96–100, 2004.

14. Brodsky J.W., Baum B.S., Pollo F.E., Shabat S., "Surgical reconstruction of posterior tibial tendon tear in adolescents: report of two cases and review of the literature," *Foot Ankle Int*, 26:218–223, 2005.

15. Abuzzahab F.S. Jr., Harris G.F., Kidder S.M., "Foot and ankle motion analysis system: instrumentation, calibration, and validation." In: Harris G.F., Smith P.A., eds. *Human Motion Analysis*. Piscataway, NJ, IEEE Press, 1996, pp. 152–166.

16. Carson M.C., Harrington M.E., Thompson N., O'Connor J.J., Theologis T.N., "Kinematic analysis of a multi-segment foot model for research and clinical applications: a repeatability analysis," *J Biomech*, 34:1299–1307, 2001.

17. Johnson J.E., Harris G.F., "Pathomechanics of posterior tibial tendon insufficiency," *Foot Ankle Clin*, 2:227–239, 1997.

18. Johnson J.E., Kidder S.M., Abuzzahab F.S. Jr., "Three-dimensional motion analysis of the adult foot and ankle," In: Harris G.F., Smith P.A., eds. *Human Motion Analysis*. Piscataway, NJ, IEEE Press, 1996, pp. 351–369.

19. Kidder S.M., Abuzzahab F.S. Jr., Harris G.F., Johnson J.E., "A system for the analysis of foot and ankle kinematics during gait," *IEEE Trans Rehabil Eng*, 4:25–32, 1996.

20. Myers K.A., Wang M., Marks R.M., Harris G.F., "Validation of a multisegment foot and ankle kinematic model for pediatric gait," *IEEE Trans Neural Syst Rehabil Eng*, 12:122–30, 2004.

21. Johnson K.A, Strom D.E., "Tibialis posterior tendon dysfunction," *Clin Orthop Relat Res*, 196–206, 1989.

22. Frey C., Shereff M., Greenidge N., "Vascularity of the posterior tibial tendon," *J Bone Joint Surgery Am*, 72:884–888, 1990.

23. Johnson J.E., Lamdan R., Granberry W.F., Harris G.F., Carrera G.F., "Hindfoot coronal alignment: a modified radiographic method," *Foot Ankle Int*, 20: 818–825, 1999.

24. Perry J., *Gait Analysis: Normal And Pathologic Function*. Thorofare, NJ: Slack Inc., 1992.

25. Mann R.A., Thompson F.M., "Rupture of the posterior tibial tendon causing flat foot. Surgical treatment," *J Bone Joint Surg Am*, 67:556–561, 1985.

26. Deland J.T., Arnoczky S.P., Thompson F.M., "Adult acquired flatfoot deformity at the talonavicular joint: reconstruction of the spring ligament in an in vitro model," *Foot Ankle*, 13: 327–332, 1992.

13 Hallux Valgus: A Pre- and Postoperative Analysis of Gait

Anne Gotstein Frea, Jason T. Long, Michael Khazzam, Richard M. Marks, and Gerald F. Harris

CONTENTS

13.1 INTRODUCTION

Hallux valgus is a lateral deviation of the great toe at the first metatarsal joint. It occurs almost exclusively in shoe-wearing cultures. Most notably, there is a high prevalence of hallux valgus in American women in their fourth to sixth decades of life,[5] with the female-to-male ratio of those affected reported as 9:1.[2,8,9] Extrinsically, the essential factor in the causation of hallux valgus is tight and constrictive footwear. Intrinsically, the condition can be caused by a multitude of factors including pronation of the hindfoot, pes planus, contracture of the Achilles' tendon, generalized joint laxity, hypermobility of the first metatarsocuneine joint, flaccid ligaments, poor musculature, neuromuscular disorders, congenital foot deformities, and rheumatic diseases. Heredity has also been implicated as a causal factor. Hardy and Clapham[8] discovered that of 91 hallux valgus cases, 63% had a positive family history of "bunions" compared to only 1% of the 84 control subjects. Certain anatomic variations in shape and stability of forefoot joint surfaces may predispose the foot to deforming forces from certain types of footwear.[9] Deformities associated with hallux valgus include metatarsus primus varus, pronation of the hallux, a prominent medial eminence, and second toe hammering.[6,9]

13.2 ANATOMY

The great toe differs from the lesser toes, in that the metatarsophalangeal joint has a sesamoid mechanism and a set of intrinsic muscles that provide strength and stability. The extensor hallucis longus and brevis pass centrally on the dorsal aspect of the great toe and insert into the distal and proximal phalanges, respectively; the long and short flexors pass on the plantar surface. The two tendons of the abductor and adductor hallucis pass medially and laterally, respectively.

The first metatarsal has a round, cartilage-covered head, which articulates with the elliptical, small, concave base of the proximal phalanx of the hallux. A fan-shaped ligamentous band, composed of the collateral ligaments of the metatarsophalangeal joint, originates from the medial and lateral metatarsal epicondyles. This band blends toward the plantar surface with the ligaments of the medial and lateral sesamoids while the sesamoid ligaments fan out in a plantar direction to the margins of the sesamoids and the plantar pad.

Two sesamoid bones are contained in the double tendon of the flexor hallucis brevis. The convex facets on their superior surfaces articulate with the corresponding longitudinal grooves on the inferior surface of the first metatarsal head. The two sesamoids are attached distally by the fibrous plantar pad to the base of the proximal phalanx. The sesamoid complex can therefore move in whatever direction the great toe moves, transmitting pressure from the skin to the head of the metatarsal and relieving the tendons of overloading.

13.3 PATHOANATOMY

The shape and stability of the joint surfaces of the forefoot may show anatomic variations that predispose the forefoot to deforming forces caused by various types of footwear. For instance, a rounded metatarsal head will be more prone to the development of a hallux valgus, whereas a flattened metatarsophalangeal articulation can resist deforming forces. Additionally, an oblique setting of the first metatarsal cuneiform joint may cause an increase in a metatarsal angle with subsequent hallux valgus, whereas a curved metatarsal cuneiform articulation or a lateral facet or exostosis on the basal lateral aspect of the first metatarsal may enhance the mobility of the metatarsal cuneiform joint and promote the tendency of the metatarsal to angle medially.[9]

Laterally, anatomical changes that may result from hallux valgus include joint capsule shrinking, lateral collateral ligament shortening, lateral sesamoid displacement, and shortening of the lateral head of the flexor hallucis brevis. From a medial aspect, pronounced fibrocartilaginous thickening of the capsule, displacement of the abductor tendon laterally and toward the plantar surface, and lateral displacement of the sesamoid can also occur.

When the metatarsophalangeal joint becomes unbalanced, the great toe is forced laterally by extrinsic deforming forces. The base of the proximal phalanx pushes the metatarsal head medially and there often is pronation of the metatarsal head. As the metatarsal head migrates medially, it attenuates the medial capsule. As this displacement occurs, the longitudinal ridges under the metatarsal head are gradually smoothed out, reducing bony resistance to this migration. The sesamoids are embedded in the adductor hallucis tendon and cannot drift medially with the metatarsal head. However, in severe cases, the lateral sesamoids may move to the lateral aspect of the metatarsal head and may eventually lie vertically above the medial sesamoids, which are articulating with the lateral facet of the first metatarsal. As the metatarsal head continues to migrate medially, the medial joint capsule is further stretched out, and the abductor hallucis tendon is pulled beneath the head, losing all power of abduction. The abductor hallucis has a splitting effect and pushes the first metatarsal toward the second metatarsal. The adductor hallucis opposes this action. As the metatarsal head moves medially, the base of the proximal phalanx is held laterally and forced to rotate along its longitudinal axis at the insertion of the adductor tendon. The two short flexor tendons are displaced laterally in relation to the metatarsal head and bowstring, so the force on the hallux is increased in the valgus direction. This is how pronation of the great toe occurs. Turan noted that significant pronation is regularly seen with hallux valgus deformities of 35° or more.[10]

If the hallux migrates into a more valgus position and the metatarsal deviates into a varus position, the only structure that affords medial stability is the medial ligamentous complex. Sesamoid subluxation occurs with increased angulation of the metatarsophalangeal joint.

13.4 CLINICAL PRESENTATION

Clinical symptoms revealed on physical exam include a lateral deviation of the hallux phalanx, often with impingement of the lesser toes, and a prominence of the medial eminence. Associated deformities include metatarsus primus varus, pronation of the hallux, and second toe hammering. Approximately 15 to 20% of patients have a pathologically dislocated second toe.[9] The splayed appearance of the forefoot is due to the first metatarsal escaping the control of the base of the proximal phalanx.[9] When evaluating for hallux valgus, a metatarsophalangeal angle greater than 15° or an intermetatarsal (IM) angle greater than 9° could be considered abnormal.[8] Hypermobility of the first ray and gastrocnemius equinus contracture may be present. Glasoe et al.[4] found that the mobility of the first ray was increased in the hallux valgus subjects, while a large IM angle may indicate increased dorsal mobility. Pain from hallux valgus is mostly caused by friction over the medial eminence due to tight and constrictive shoes. Radiographic measurements provide important classifying data by demonstrating increased hallux valgus and IM angles.

13.5 TREATMENT

Correction is necessary only when the bunion interferes with the patient's lifestyle. Initial treatment for this condition includes a variety of conservative measures dependent on the patient's symptoms and amount of deformity. Shoe modifications such as widening of the toe box and stretching shoes can help eliminate the friction over the medial eminence. Orthoses can help correct pes planus, which is commonly associated with hallux valgus. Stretching of the gastrocnemius can also be done to alleviate pain, if the soft tissue of the Achilles' tendon is contracted. Night bunion splints are also helpful for relief of symptoms, but rarely lead to significant change in the course of the deformity.

Operative treatment is recommended for those patients who have failed to see improvement from conservative treatment. Surgical options vary depending on the degree of deformity and radiographic appearance. Coughlin[5] has defined three levels of hallux valgus severity and the associated operative procedures (Table 13.1). The goal of surgical treatment is to obtain a stable, pain-free hallux, which improves functional capabilities. Results of surgical treatment are typically greater than 90% good-to-excellent results, with a recurrence rate below 5%.

Age is important in determining whether surgery is the appropriate means of treatment. In preadolescent children, surgical intervention should be postponed until the patient is more mature. If the hallux valgus is repaired and the underlying etiologic factor is still present, then a recurrence is probable. The modified McBride procedure can be used on patients as old as 70, but vascularity of the foot must be ensured. Additionally, if the skin is taut and atrophied, there is a high possibly that the surgery

TABLE 13.1
Hallux Valgus Severity Index

Severity	HVA	IMA	Sesamoid Subluxation	Surgical Options
Mild	< 20°	< 11°	< 50%	Chevron Akin Possible distal soft-tissue procedure (DSTP)
Moderate	20–40°	< 16°	50–75%	Chevron Akin Lapidus DSTP Proximal MT osteotomy w/DSTP
Severe	> 40°	< 16°	> 75%	Lapidus Proximal metatarsal osteotomy with DSTP

Source: Coughlin MJ. *J Bone Joint Surg Am* 78(6):932–966, 1996.

will fail. Certain congenital deformities such as increased webbing of the first web-space, congenital metatarsus adductus, severe pes planus with or without a tight heel cord, and neuromuscular disorders will prevent a satisfactory long-term result.

13.6 PREVIOUS STUDIES

Biomechanically, hallux valgus is associated with a decreased total arc of motion, marked limitations in plantar flexion, and moderate restriction of dorsiflexion.[6] Shereff noted that the range of motion limitations is likely due to capsule and ligamentous structure scarring in addition to articular degeneration. Patients spend a high percentage of time on their heel, mid-foot, and lateral metatarsal heads while walking. The degree of hallux loading at toe-off is decreased due to the greater reduced flexor activity.[6] This leads to gait pattern alterations ranging from antalgic gait and shortened stride length in mild cases to compensatory lower extremity rotatory misalignment in more severe cases. The gait alterations compensate for the reduced contact time on the lateral toes and first metatarsal head and may eventually lead to associated lower extremity and lower back problems.

Previous studies have analyzed different biomechanical aspects of the hallux valgus population. Blomgren et al.[3] found greater pressures in the small toe and tarsal regions during gait in 66 patients with hallux valgus prior to surgical inter-vention. Borton and Stephens[1] analyzed plantar loading and patient satisfaction before and after Chevron osteotomy for hallux valgus and found significant reduction in areas sustaining pressure > 5 kg/cm^2, an increased total foot contact area, and a higher percentage of forefoot contact area on heel raise. Conversely, Kernozek and Sterriker[7] discovered no change in contact area, contact time, or gait speed for a similar population. They concluded that although there was a decrease in perceived pain postsurgically, there was no increase in plantar loading of the medial forefoot or medial toe regions, as they had expected. They did find improvements in plantar flexion of the first metatarsophalangeal joint after surgery, but did not find improve-ments in force production in the MT region. Many of the studies utilizing plantar loading data are difficult to compare due to differences in sensor technology, sensor resolution, sampling rate, variables, and method of data collection.[7] There are cur-rently no published studies comparing hallux valgus patients before and after surgery on the basis of quantitative motion analysis.

Previous studies of plantar pressure distribution during gait show a shift in weight bearing to the lateral metatarsal heads and to the tarsals while decreasing the load on the hallux for patients with hallux valgus. These findings seem to correlate well with these results, which show that heel strike tended to begin with a more internally rotated hindfoot. It is possible that in order to compensate for this internal rotation and probable increased weight bearing on the lateral edge of the foot, the tibia abducts slightly in order to maintain balance, and forefoot abduction occurs as the foot rolls through the step. These changes in gait for the patients with hallux valgus are most likely due to the patients' efforts to keep weight off the painful hallux, which exhibits constant valgus positioning throughout the stride. This probable shift in weight to the lateral edge of the foot avoids excessive loading on the great toe.

Johnson et al.[11] have described normal motion of the foot and ankle during gait using the Milwaukee Foot Model (MFM).[12–16] The MFM is a four-segment bio-mechanical model, which subdivides the foot into the tibia, hindfoot (calcaneus), forefoot (proximal and distal tarsals), and hallux, and calculated joint motion in three planes during both stance and swing. From a population of healthy ambulatory adults, Johnson noted the following.

13.7 TIBIA

In the sagittal plane, the tibia has a negative angle at initial contact, as the knee is positioned behind the heel. This angle becomes steadily more positive as the tibia moves forward over the planted foot; the angle peaks just after foot-off and then decreases as the foot moves forward, in preparation for the next gait cycle. Coronally, the tibia moves from an adducted position (relative to the global reference frame) at initial contact to an abducted position in late stance. Following foot-off, the tibia returns to its adducted position. In the transverse plane, the tibia remains externally rotated (away from midline) throughout the entire gait cycle. While it does undergo some rotation in the internal direction, its position is never at or less than 0 (cutoff).

13.8 HINDFOOT

Sagittal plane motion of the hindfoot is measured with consideration for the "dor-siflexion offset," the angle between the tibia and calcaneus. During quiet standing, this angle is approximately 20 to 30° for a healthy adult; because of this offset, the hindfoot remains in a dorsiflexed position throughout the gait cycle. At initial contact during gait, the hindfoot is moving in a plantarflexion direction. This continues through midstance, when the motion reverses and the hindfoot begins dorsiflex. At the end of late stance (~50% cycle), the hindfoot begins to plantarflex again, in preparation for foot-off; dorsiflexion then increases again through swing phase, in preparation for the next foot strike.

Coronally, the hindfoot is relatively neutral from initial contact through most of the stance. The hindfoot inverts just prior to foot-off, and returns to neutral during swing phase. In the transverse plane, the hindfoot is internally rotated at initial contact. It steadily rotates externally throughout stance phase, approaching a neutral position just prior to foot-off. Following foot-off, the hindfoot reverses direction, rotating internally in preparation for the next gait cycle.

13.9 FOREFOOT

Similar to the dorsiflexion offset present in the hindfoot, the sagittal plane motion of the forefoot is measured with a plantarflexion offset, which accounts for the angle between the calcaneus and the first metatarsal. This angle is generally ~30° during quiet standing in healthy adults. The sagittal range of motion (ROM) of this segment is fairly small (generally less than 10°), with the majority of motion taking place just prior to foot-off. At this point, the segment quickly plantarflexes to a position it holds through midswing; it then gradually returns to its offset plantarflexed position.

In the coronal plane, the healthy forefoot maintains a slightly varus position from initial contact through the terminal stance; a rapid increase in varus occurs just prior to foot-off. During swing, the forefoot gradually moves back toward neutral, reaching its original varus positioning just prior to initial contact. In the transverse plane, the forefoot is in a slightly abducted position at initial contact. During load response, it moves quickly to a more abducted position, which is held for the remainder of the stance. Just after foot-off, the forefoot abducts even further; during midswing, it begins moving back toward neutral, and returns to its original position of slight abduction just prior to initial contact.

13.10 HALLUX

Sagittal pane motion of the hallux is measured with an established dorsiflexion offset; this represents the resting angle of the hallux relative to the first metatarsal (~15° for healthy adults). During gait, the hallux is in a position of neutral to slight dorsiflexion through midstance. During late stance, the hallux rapidly dorsiflexes in preparation for foot-off. Progressive plantarflexion is then observed during swing, as the hallux returns to its initial position.

In the coronal plane, the hallux moves from supinated to slightly pronated, during initial contact and load response. Pronation increases gradually through the terminal stance, then increases rapidly at foot-off. Peak pronation is seen in early swing, at which point the hallux steadily moves to a supinated position just prior to initial contact. In the transverse plane, the hallux maintains a valgus position with ~20° ROM throughout the stride. During early and midstance, the hallux moves in a varus direction, reversing direction at the end of the terminal stance and moving back to its original valgus position.

13.11 CASE EXAMPLES

Pre- and postoperative gait analysis sessions were conducted using a 15-camera Vicon 524 Motion Analysis System (Vicon Motion Systems, Inc., Lake Forest, CA). Multisegmental foot and ankle kinematics and temporal-spatial data were obtained using the MFM. The patient was instrumented with reflective markers placed over bony landmarks on the foot and ankle following the protocol specified by the MFM. Markers were secured with double-sided tape. Following a static orientation trial, the patient walked at a freely selected walking speed along the data collection corridor (length = 6 m). Each trial was subject to clinical screen; data collection continued until a minimum of three walking trials had been obtained for analysis. Case results from each visit are composed of three-dimensional joint kinematics during gait, as well as temporal-spatial parameters (cadence, stride length, stance/swing ratio, and walking speed).

13.11.1 PATIENT #1

B.K. is a 72-yr-old female who presented with a painful left hallux valgus deformity. The patient underwent conservative treatment for 2 yr using a shoe orthosis, which

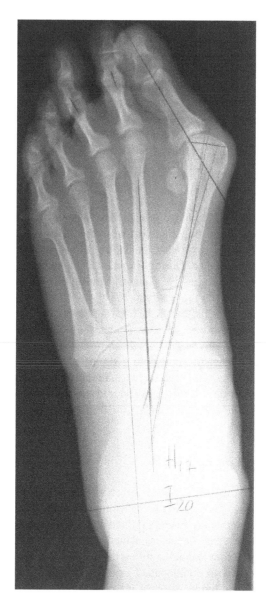

FIGURE 13.1 Preoperative A/P radiograph of patient B.K.

was helpful for approximately 2 yr. She now complains of problems with shoewear and limitations in activities of daily living. The patient has a previous history of hallux valgus correction (first MTP fusion) on the right foot several years ago. Physical examination of the left foot at this time reveals no hypermobility of the first metatarsal cuneiform joint and a hallux valgus deformity. Radiographic examination (Figure 13.1 and Figure 13.2) reveals a left hallux valgus angle of 47° with an IM angle of 20°; per Coughlin's criteria, hallux valgus is characterized as severe.

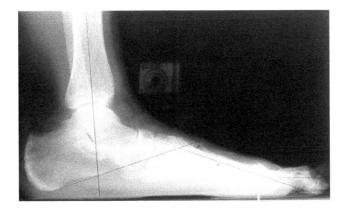

FIGURE 13.2 Preoperative lateral radiograph of patient B.K.

Following preoperative gait analysis, the patient underwent surgical correction of the left hallux valgus deformity using proximal metatarsal osteotomy and DSTP. One year following surgery, the patient underwent postoperative follow-up gait analysis.

13.11.1.1 Temporal-Spatial Results (Table 13.2)

The average preoperative walking speed for the patient was 0.87 m/sec, the average preoperative stride length was 1.08 m, the average preoperative cadence was 95.89 steps/min, and the average preoperative stance duration was 66.52%. The average postoperative walking speed was 1.01 m/sec, the average postoperative stride length was 1.09 m, the average postoperative cadence was 111.4 steps/min, and the average postoperative stance duration was 63.41%.

13.11.1.2 Kinematic Results (Figure 13.3)

13.11.1.2.1 Tibia
Preoperatively, the tibia demonstrated decreased dorsiflexion from load response throughout initial swing as compared to normal. The tibia also demonstrated an increase in abduction from midswing through terminal swing as compared to normal. Postoperatively, the tibia demonstrated a return to normal sagittal motion, but showed

---

TABLE 13.2
B.K. Temporal-Spatial Parameters

Visit	Stance Duration	Stride Length	Cadence	Walking Speed
Pre-op	66.52%	1.08 m	95.89 steps/min	0.87 m/sec
Post-op	63.41%	1.09 m	111.4 steps/min	1.01 m/sec

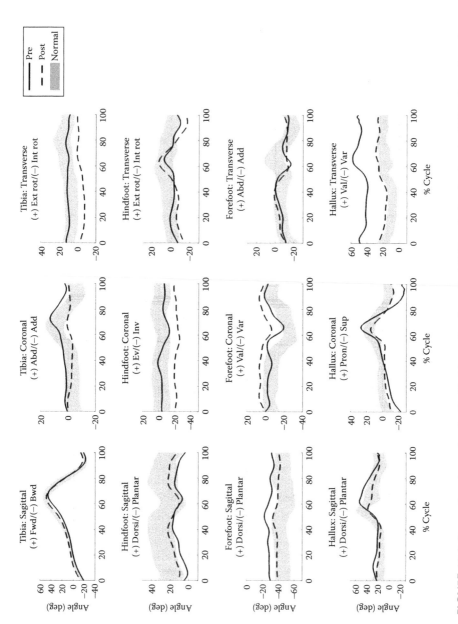

FIGURE 13.3 Pre- and postoperative foot/ankle kinematics for patient B.K., calculated using the MFM. Control results from healthy adult normals shown for comparison (mean ± 1 STD).

an increase in adduction (coronal plane motion) from the terminal stance through the midswing phase of the gait cycle as compared to preoperative and normal motion. Postoperative tibial motion in the transverse plane (external/internal rotation) was decreased throughout the gait cycle compared to normal.

13.11.1.2.2   Hindfoot

Preoperatively, the hindfoot demonstrated less dorsiflexion throughout the gait cycle compared to normal. Postoperatively, hindfoot sagittal motion (dorsiflexion/plantar flexion) demonstrated a return to motion, which was similar to normal. The hindfoot was more inverted throughout the gait cycle postoperatively compared to normal. The hindfoot demonstrated increased transverse (external/internal rotation) range of motion throughout the gait cycle postoperatively compared to preoperative and normal motion.

13.11.1.2.3   Forefoot

Preoperatively, the forefoot demonstrated decreased plantar flexion throughout the gait cycle compared to normal. Postoperatively, sagittal motion of the forefoot was similar to normal. The forefoot demonstrated increased valgus motion throughout the gait cycle postoperatively compared to normal.

13.11.1.2.4   Hallux

Preoperatively, the hallux demonstrated increased dorsiflexion from load response through the terminal stance and from the initial swing through midswing as compared to normal. Coronal plane (pronation/supination) range of motion was increased preoperatively throughout the gait cycle compared to normal. The hallux was in an increased valgus position throughout the gait cycle preoperatively as compared to normal.

Postoperative hallux motion in the sagittal plane (dorsiflexion/plantar flexion) was similar to normal. Coronal plane (pronation/supination) of the hallux postoperatively was less than what was seen preoperatively throughout the gait cycle. Transverse motion (valgus/varus) was less than what was seen preoperatively with positioning that more closely resembled normal.

13.11.2   PATIENT #2

M.M. is a 55-yr-old female who presented with left hallux valgus deformity. She had already undergone surgical correction (Chevron osteotomy with DSTP) of the right foot. She first noted bunions developing 3 to 4 yr earlier. She underwent conservative treatment for approximately 2 yr after the bunions worsened, including wide shoes and over-the-counter orthotics. She complains of increasing pain, which is no longer relieved by conservative measures. The patient's medical history is typical for any other medical problems. Physical examination during weightbearing reveals a neutral hindfoot with maintained longitudinal arch. On seated exam, there is left hallux valgus deformity with pain over the medial eminence bilaterally, along with bunionette deformity, which is tender to palpation. The patient is neurovascularly intact distally, with no hypermobility, transmetatarsalgia, or lesser toe hammering. Radiographic examination (Figure 13.4 and Figure 13.5) reveals hallux

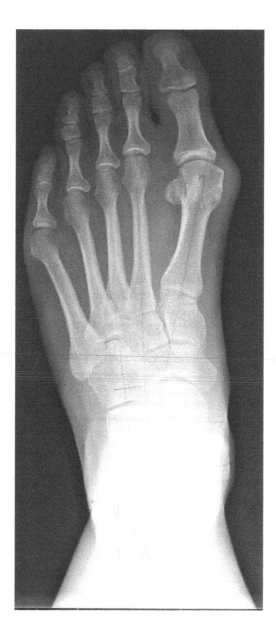

FIGURE 13.4 Preoperative A/P radiograph of patient M.M.

valgus and IM angles of 24° and 15°, respectively. Per Coughlin's criteria, hallux valgus is characterized as moderate.

Following preoperative gait analysis, the patient underwent surgical correction of the hallux valgus deformity with Chevron distal metatarsal osteotomy and DSTP. Nine months following the second surgery, the patient returned for postoperative gait analysis.

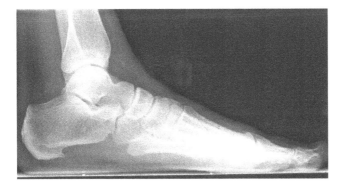

FIGURE 13.5 Preoperative lateral radiograph of patient M.M.

13.11.2.1 Temporal-Spatial Results (Table 13.3)

The average preoperative walking speed for M.M. was 1.04 m/sec, the average preoperative stride length was 1.12 m, the average preoperative cadence was 110.77 steps/min, and the average preoperative stance duration was 62.05%. The average postoperative walking speed was 1.03 m/sec, the average postoperative stride length was 1.15 m, the average postoperative cadence was 107.50 steps/min, and the average postoperative stance duration was 63.17%.

13.11.2.2 Kinematic Results (Figure 13.6)

13.11.2.2.1 Tibia

Tibial motion fell within the range of normal motion for all phases of gait in all three planes. Notably, the coronal plane ROM (abd/adduction) increased following surgery, and transverse plane motion shifted in an external rotation direction, even closer to a normal motion pattern.

13.11.2.2.2 Hindfoot

In the sagittal plane, preoperative hindfoot motion demonstrated reduced ROM with a slight plantarflexion shift from the normal motion pattern. Postoperatively, normal ROM has been restored, and the motion pattern demonstrates a dorsiflexion shift, which better follows the normal motion pattern. Coronally, the hindfoot falls within

TABLE 13.3
M.M. Temporal-Spatial Parameters

Visit	Stance Duration	Stride Length	Cadence	Walking Speed
Pre-op	62.05%	1.12 m	110.77 steps/min	1.04 m/sec
Post-op	63.17%	1.15 m	107.50 steps/min	1.03 m/sec

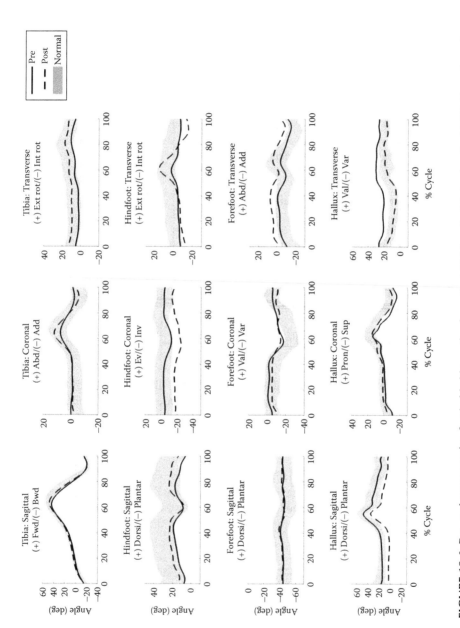

FIGURE 13.6 Pre- and postoperative foot/ankle kinematics for patient M.M., calculated using the MFM. Control results from healthy adult normals shown for comparison (mean ± 1 STD).

the normal range of motion preoperatively, maintaining a neutral to slightly inverted position throughout the stride. Postoperatively, an inversion shift is observed throughout the stride. In the transverse plane, the preoperative motion pattern shows slight external rotation throughout the stride. Postoperatively, increased ROM is observed, as the hindfoot moves from an externally rotated position to internally rotated (peaking around toe-off), then returning to a position of external rotation.

13.11.2.2.3   Forefoot

Forefoot motion tracks very close to normal in the sagittal plane for both the pre- and postoperative conditions, maintaining a plantarflexed position throughout the stride. Similar fidelity is observed in the coronal plane, where the only deviation from normal occurs in late stance when the forefoot does not move into as much varus as the normal population. This deviation is observed both pre- and postoperatively. In the transverse plane, preoperative gait falls close to normal motion; postoperatively, the forefoot becomes more abducted during stance.

13.11.2.2.4   Hallux

Preoperative motion of the hallux in the sagittal plane is in good agreement with the normal motion pattern. Postoperatively, ROM is maintained, albeit with a shift in the overall motion pattern to a slightly less dorsiflexed position. In the coronal plane, the hallux demonstrates fine ROM, with a slight supination shift from the normal motion pattern. Postoperatively, this shift is not observed, and the ROM motion falls well within the normal range. In the transverse plane, excessive valgus positioning with limited ROM is clearly seen throughout the stride during preoperative gait. Postoperatively, hallux motion closely follows normal motion, with increased ROM.

13.12   CONCLUSION

Quantified three-dimensional motion analysis of the foot and ankle during ambulation provides a useful means of assessing patient pathology preoperatively and evaluating intervention effectiveness postoperatively. The information gained through gait analysis with MFM may provide new insight into the disease state prior to conservative or surgical treatment, and provide a quantitative means of evaluating the effect of surgery on the foot and its function. Additional work could lead to a number of improvements in treatment; timing of surgical intervention, prescription of modified footwear, and rehabilitation methods following surgery could all be impacted by motion information. Integrated electromyography (EMG) and plantar pressure information would further augment the biomechanical picture provided by gait analysis, and may assist in translating laboratory measures to observations made during clinical exams. Further investigation to relate gait measures to functional level might also be warranted.

REFERENCES

1. Borton DC, Stephens MM. Basal metatarsal osteotomy for hallux valgus. *J Bone Joint Surg Br* 76(2):204–209, 1994.
2. Kernozek TW, Elfessi A, Sterriker SA. Clinical and biomechanical risk factors of patients diagnosed with hallux valgus. *J Am Podiatr Med Assoc* 93(2):97–103, 2003.
3. Blomgren M, Turan I, Agadir M. Gait analysis in hallux valgus. *J Foot Surg* 30(1):70–71, 1991.
4. Glasoe WM, Allen MK, Saltzman CL. First ray dorsal mobility in relation to hallux valgus deformity and first intermetatarsal angle. *Foot Ankle Int* 22(2):98–101, 2001.
5. Coughlin MJ. Hallux valgus. [Review] *J Bone Joint Surg Am* 78(6):932–966, 1996.
6. Shereff MJ. Pathophysiology, anatomy, and biomechanics of hallux valgus. Orthopedics 13(9):939–945, 1990.
7. Kernozek TW, Sterriker SA. Chevron (Austin) distal metatarsal osteotomy for hallux valgus: comparison of pre- and post-surgical characteristics. *Foot Ankle Int* 23(6):503–508, 2002.
8. Hardy RH, Clapham JC. Observations on hallux valgus. *J Bone Joint Surg Br* 33-B(3): 376–391, 1951.
9. Mann RA, Coughlin MJ. Hallux valgus — etiology, anatomy, treatment, and surgical considerations. *Clin Orthop Relat Res* 157:31–41, 1981.
10. Turan I. Normal and pathologic anatomy of hallux valgus. *J Foot Surg* 28(5):471–474, 1989.
11. Johnson JE, Kidder SM, Abuzzahab FS. Three-dimensional motion analysis of the adult foot and ankle. In: Harris GF, and Smith P eds., *Human Motion Analysis*. Piscataway, NJ, IEEE Press, 351–369.
12. Johnson JE, Harris GF. Pathomechanics of posterior tibial tendon insufficiency. *Foot Ankle Clin* 2(2):227–237, 1997.
13. Myers KA, Wang M, Marks RM, Harris GF. Validation of a multisegment foot and ankle kinematic model for pediatric gait. *IEEE Trans Neural Syst Rehabil Eng* 12(1):122–130, 2004.
14. Johnson JE, Lamdan, Granberry WF, Harris GF, Carrera GF. Hindfoot coronal alignment: a modified radiographic method. *Foot Ankle Int* 20(12):818–825, 1999.
15. Kidder SM, Abuzzahab FS, Harris GF. A system for the analysis of the foot and ankle kinematics during gait. *IEEE Trans Rehabil Eng* 4(1):25–32, 1996.
16. Abuzzahab FS, Harris GF, Kidder SM. Foot and ankle motion analysis system instrumentation, Calibration & Validation. In: Harris GF and P Smith P eds., *Human Motion Analysis*. Piscataway, NJ, IEEE Press, 152–166, 1996.

14 Hallux Rigidus: A Pre- and Postoperative Analysis of Gait

Joseph Schwab, Michael Khazzam, Jason T. Long, Richard M. Marks, and Gerald F. Harris

CONTENTS

14.1 INTRODUCTION

Hallux rigidus is characterized by osteoarthritis of the first metatarsophalangeal (MTP) joint, which leads to a restriction in motion about the joint. In particular, dorsiflexion of the joint is limited, often due to the formation of dorsal osteophytes. Following hallux valgus, hallux rigidus is the second most common pathologic condition associated with the first MTP joint. Symptoms associated with hallux rigidus include pain, rigidity, dorsal bunion, flexion deformity, and dorsal tilt of the first metatarsal head. These symptoms have led to a variety of names for the condition, including hallux flexus, hallux limitus, hallux dolorosus, metatarsus primus elevatus, and painful great toe. Kelikian has provided a thorough discussion of the history of hallux rigidus terminology.[6] Mann et al. summarize the proposed causes of the degenerative process, including poor footwear, a long narrow foot, pronated feet, osteochondritis dissecans, a long first metatarsal, hyperextension of the first metatarsal, an imperfect ball-and-socket relationship of the first MTP artic- ulation, abnormal gait, obesity, age, trauma, gender, and occupation.[10] Numerous surgical treatments for hallux rigidus have been suggested, including dorsal chei- lectomy, the Moberg wedge osteotomy, first MTP arthrodesis, distal oblique osteot- omy, and the Keller resection arthroplasty.[9–12,14] The success of these techniques has generally been measured by the postoperative arc of motion of the repaired hallux and the patient's own subjective pain assessment. There is limited kinematic infor- mation about the quantified effects of surgical hallux rigidus treatments on the patient's gait.

14.2 ANATOMY AND PATHOLOGY

The first MTP joint exhibits both rotational (ball-and-socket) motion and transla- tional (sliding) motion. As degenerative changes occur in the joint, multiple anatomic changes manifest, which lead to the clinical presentation of pain and limited range of motion (ROM). Formation of a dorsal osteophyte, typically found on the head of the first metatarsal, is one of the initial findings. As the disease progresses, this growth can extend to both the medial and lateral aspects of the metatarsal head, creating a U-shaped excrescence that prohibits full dorsiflexion. Osteophyte forma- tion is not limited to the metatarsal. In more severe presentations, osteophytes may also be noted on the proximal phalanx. As these excrescences develop, they give a flattened appearance to the first metatarsal head. In cases of severe bony proliferation, the mechanical blockage of dorsiflexion may be so complete that the toe is prevented from resting in a neutral position and remains partially plantarflexed. This deformity was the origin of the term "hallux flexus." Other anatomic changes to the joint include progressive joint space narrowing, periarticular sclerosis, cystic changes around the joint, and enlargement of the sesamoids.

14.3 ETIOLOGY

Multiple hypotheses exist as to the etiology of hallux rigidus. There is a bimodal age distribution for hallux rigidus, which may represent two distinct forms of the disease, or be a continuum of the same disease process.[10] The adolescent form of hallux rigidus is usually associated with osteochondritis dissecans, while the adult form often has no clear etiology. The existence of hallux rigidus in adults in the absence of other systemic arthritic conditions suggests pathology localized to the first MTP joint. Localized trauma that damages articular cartilage (stubbed toe, turf toe), abnormal anatomy (abnormally long first or second metatarsal), abnormal elevation of the first metatarsal (metatarsus primus elevatus), and previously asymp- tomatic osteochondritis dissecans have all been postulated as etiologic factors.[5] Contributing factors to this disease process include abnormal gait, poor footwear, and obesity. Similarly, metabolic disorders that mimic hallux rigidus, such as gout, may lead to similar degenerative patterns.[17]

14.4 CLINICAL PRESENTATION AND EVALUATION

Unilateral disease is the most common presentation.[10] The main presenting symptom of patients with hallux rigidus is pain about the first MTP joint. The pain is exacerbated by activities placing stress on the joint (walking, running, squatting, using footwear with high heels) and is relieved with rest. The pain is typically worse during terminal heel-rise immediately prior to toe-off. Subsequently, an antalgic gait often develops on the affected side. Patients may or may not describe any limitation of motion about the joint. There is often swelling and erythema around the joint, and a dorsal bony projection may be palpated. Lateral forefoot pain is a common complaint and most often results from a compensatory supinated gait. This type of gait is designed to relieve pressure on the great toe during heel-rise and toe-off by loading the lateral edge of the foot during stance phase. Patients may also externally rotate at the hip in order to shift toe-off pressure from the first metatarsal to the lesser metatarsals.

Both dorsal and plantar callous formation may occur. When the first ray is fixed in slight plantar flexion, stress is transferred to the plantar aspect of the first interphalangeal joint, which may lead to a plantar callous under this joint. Conversely, impingement of tissue between a dorsal osteophyte and the top of the toe-box of the shoe may lead to either dorsal callous formation or soft tissue inflammation and ulceration. Since the terminal branches of the deep peroneal nerve and the medial cutaneous branch of the superficial peroneal nerve travel over the dorsal aspect of the first ray, neuritic pain may occur if the dorsal prominence is impinged upon externally.

On clinical examination, there may be pain throughout the entire arc of motion of the first ray. Pain with plantar flexion usually occurs as the extensor hallucis longus tendon is irritated over the dorsal bony prominence. This pain may also occur as the result of inflamed synovium and joint capsule being stretched over the dorsal osteophyte. The patient may only complain of stiffness early in the disease process, or it may exist through the course of the disease. Both active and passive motion of the affected side are compared to the unaffected side whenever possible. Radiographic examination generally includes weight-bearing anteroposterior (A/P), lateral, and oblique views of the foot. These studies reveal the pathologic changes described above. Furthermore, fractures in the bony excrescences may lead to loose bodies within the joint space.

Several systems have been developed to evaluate the clinical effect of hallux rigidus. In 1994, the American Orthopaedic Foot and Ankle Society (AOFAS) created a clinical rating system designed to evaluate the hindfoot, midfoot, hallux, and lesser toes.[8] For evaluation of the hallux, scores on a scale of 1 to 100 are synthesized from subjective and objective data into quantified function (45 points), alignment (15 points), and pain (40 points) for the first metatarsal, MTP joint, proximal phalanx, distal phalanx, and interphalangeal joint. Coughlin and Shurnas proposed a clinical radiographic system for grading the severity of hallux rigidus (Table 14.1).[1] The system grades the severity of the disease from 0 through 4 and is based on a combination of quantified arc of motion, radiographic findings, and clinical findings. It is similar to previous grading systems but incorporates grades 0 and 4, which evaluate asymptomatic patients and advanced patients, respectively. Giannini et al.[4]

TABLE 14.1
Clinical Grading System for Hallux Rigidus Severity

Grade	Dorsiflexion	Radiographic Findings[a]	Clinical Findings
0	40–60° and/or 10–20% loss compared with normal side	Normal	No pain; only stiffness and loss of motion on examination
1	30–40° and/or 20–50% loss compared with normal side	Dorsal osteophyte; minimal joint-space narrowing; minimal periarticular sclerosis; minimal flattening of metatarsal head	Mild or occasional pain and stiffness; pain at extremes of dorsiflexion and/or plantarflexion on examination
2	10–30° and/or 50–75% loss compared with normal side	Dorsal, lateral, and, possibly, medial osteophytes giving flattened appearance to metatarsal head; no more than one fourth of dorsal joint space involved on lateral radiograph; mild-to-moderate joint-space narrowing and sclerosis; sesamoids not usually involved	Moderate-to-severe pain and stiffness that may be constant; pain occurs just before maximum dorsiflexion and maximum plantar flexion on examination
3	10° and/or 75–100% loss compared with normal side; notable loss of MTP plantar flexion (often 10° of plantar flexion)	Same as in Grade 2 but with substantial narrowing; possibly periarticular cystic changes; more than 1/4 of dorsal joint space involved on lateral radiograph; sesamoids enlarged, cystic, and/or irregular	Nearly constant pain; substantial stiffness at extremes of ROM but not at midrange
4	Same as in Grade 3	Same as in Grade 3	Same as in Grade 3 with definite pain at midrange of passive motion

[a]Based on weight-bearing A/P and lateral radiographs.

Source: Coughlin MJ, Shurnas PS. *J Bone Joint Surg Am* 85-A(11):2072–2088, 2003.

proposed a modified version of this classification based only on radiographic findings to help determine appropriate surgical intervention.

14.5 TREATMENT

The treatment for hallux rigidus is intended to provide relief of the symptoms described above. Conservative (nonoperative) treatment includes the use of nonsteroidal anti-inflammatory medications, modification of activities, and footwear alteration. The use of nonoperative treatment is almost always indicated as a first-line therapy for symptomatic hallux rigidus. Nonoperative treatment is intended to reduce the inflammatory processes involved in the disease, as well as the force across the joint during dorsiflexion. It should be noted that while conservative therapy can be successful in providing symptomatic relief, it does not alter the pathoanatomy or progression of the disease process. As the disease progresses, surgical intervention may be necessary to offer relief of symptoms.

Nonsteroidal anti-inflammatory medications may reduce the inflammation associated with first MTP synovitis. Activity modification can include the substitution of high-impact activities such as running with low-impact activities such as swimming or biking. Footwear alterations are varied and should be tailored to the specific complaint most concerning the patient. If dorsal osteophytes are being impinged upon by the toe-box of the shoe, causing irritation or skin breakdown, shoes with a higher toe-box should provide relief of pain and help avoid irritation. Sole modifications can be made to provide relief as well. Rocker-bottom soles can aid in push-off, relieving stress on the affected MTP joint. Pressure on the joint during gait can also be relieved by the use of firm materials such as spring steel, fiberglass, or carbon-reinforced material embedded within the sole of the shoe, or for use as an insole.

Patients who fail conservative treatment are eligible for operative treatment. There are multiple surgical options for the treatment of hallux rigidus, including cheilectomy, wedge osteotomy, oblique osteotomy, first MTP arthrodesis, joint-replacement arthroplasty, and resection arthroplasty, among others (Figure 14.1). Cheilectomy involves removal of the dorsal osteophytes followed by resection of 25 to 30% of the dorsal aspect of the metatarsal head. A number of different osteotomy techniques have been described, but the common aspect of this procedure is decompression of the joint space. This is achieved by the shortening and plantar displacement of the metatarsal head. Arthrodesis is intended to fuse the joint after resection of the metatarsal head and part of the proximal phalanx. To achieve proper joint fusion, the toe must be within 5 to 15° of valgus deviation, and in neutral position in the frontal plane. Total joint arthroplasty is intended to provide a prosthetic replacement for the joint following resection of the metatarsal head.

The indications for surgical intervention of hallux rigidus are pain refractory to conservative management and evidence of MTP joint degeneration. Giannini et al. suggest that the type of surgical procedure should be determined by the radiographic extent of MTP arthritis.[4] In a prospective study of 111 feet with hallux rigidus, they used a modified Coughlin and Shurnas classification that grades radiographic arthritis from Grade 0 through Grade 3 (Figure 14.2) to select different procedures indicated

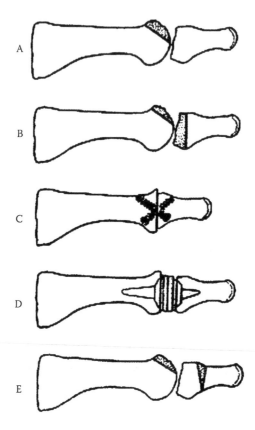

FIGURE 14.1 Various procedures commonly performed for correction of hallux rigidus: cheilectomy (A), Keller (B), arthrodesis (C), implant (D), and Moberg (E).

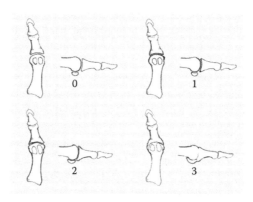

FIGURE 14.2 Radiographic classification of hallux rigidus. (See Table 14.1 for a description of the grades.) (From Giannini S, Ceccarelli F, Faldini C, Bevoni R, Grandi G, Vannini F. *J Bone Joint Surg* 86-A (Suppl 2):72–83, 2004. With permission.)

TABLE 14.2
Surgical Procedure(s) Indicated by Modified Coughlin/Shurnas Radiographic Classification

Grade	Procedure
0	Plantar release
1	Sliding decompressive oblique osteotomy; modified chevron decompressive osteotomy
2	Medial or dorsal approach cheilectomy
3	Arthrodesis; resection arthroplasty with bioabsorbable poly(DL-lactic acid) spacer

for increasing evidence of degenerative change (Table 14.2). They evaluated preoperative and postoperative AOFAS scores for motion about the hallux. Using this scale they noted a significant increase in the AOFAS score (correlated with an increase in function, correction of alignment, and decrease in pain), as well as an increase in mean ROM about the first MTP joint.

Postoperative complications in the Giannini study were noted in 20 of 111 feet. These complications included localized infection of an implant (one patient), inflammation around a Kirschner wire (five patients), deep venous thrombosis (four patients), and repeat surgery (ten patients). In Coughlin's study, reported complications included mild postoperative cellulitis (five patients), nonpainful fibrous unions (two patients undergoing arthrodesis), and repeat surgery (nine patients) for several reasons including painful hardware, rapid chondrolysis, and failed cheilectomy.[1] Coughlin reported no incidences of extensor hallucis longus scarring, concerns of foot cosmesis, neuritis, or hypertrophic dorsal scar.

14.6 PREVIOUS MOTION ANALYSIS STUDIES

A search of the literature reveals that there are few studies of quantified foot and ankle motion in hallux rigidus populations. While there are several studies examining the plantar pressure exhibited by the first ray during gait, there are not many studies that address the three-dimensional (3D) kinematics of the foot and ankle for hallux rigidus patients. DeFrino et al. prospectively analyzed a series of nine patients (ten feet) who were treated for symptomatic hallux rigidus with a first metatarsal arthrodesis.[2] Their kinematic gait analysis revealed a significantly shorter step length on the affected side, as well as decreased ankle plantar flexion during the toe-off phase. This study is limited by the lack of any preoperative gait analysis, the inclusion of only one surgical treatment, and the single-segment nature of the biomechanical model of the foot used for the analysis.

While there are not many kinematic gait analysis studies relating to hallux rigidus, there are several studies that develop models of gait analysis for the foot and ankle. Nawoczenski et al.[13] studied the motion of the hallux during gait using an electromagnetic tracking device that tracked sensors placed on anatomic landmarks. Kidder et al.[7] have described a system for 3D analysis of foot and ankle kinematics during gait using motion capture video to track reflective markers placed

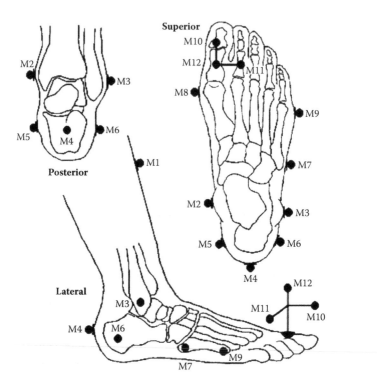

FIGURE 14.3 Schematic description of MFM, composed of 12 reflective markers (9 body-mounted, 3 on hallux-mounted triad).

at key anatomical landmarks (Figure 14.3). There have also been numerous cadaver studies to describe the motion about the hallux and forefoot. Shereff et al. described the instant centers of rotation about the first MTP joint and were able to compare normal subjects to cadaver subjects with existing hallux rigidus.[16]

14.7 CASE EXAMPLES

Pre- and postoperative gait analysis sessions were conducted using a 15-camera Vicon 524 Motion Analysis System (Vicon Motion Systems, Inc., Lake Forest, CA). Multisegmental foot and ankle kinematics and temporal-spatial data were obtained using the Milwaukee Foot Model (MFM).[18–23] The patient was instrumented with reflective markers placed over bony landmarks on the foot and ankle following the protocol specified by the MFM. Markers were secured with double-sided tape. Following a static orientation trial, the patient walked at a freely selected walking speed along the data collection corridor (length = 6 m). Each trial was subject to clinical screen; data collection continued until a minimum of three walking trials had been obtained for analysis. Case results from each visit comprise 3D joint kinematics during gait, as well as temporal-spatial parameters (cadence, stride length, stance/swing ratio, and walking speed).

14.7.1 PATIENT #1

S.S. is a 53-yr-old male complaining of left great toe pain for 6 months. The patient denied any injury, but stated that the toe has been stiff, sore, and swollen. The patient also complains of toe pain and irritation while exercising and while wearing dress shoes. On physical examination of the lower extremity, there is a dorsal prominence over the left great toe, which is tender to palpation. Motion of the left hallux metatarsalphalangeal joint is restricted with 45° of flexion and crepitus during motion. A/P and lateral radiographs (Figure 14.4 and Figure 14.5) of the

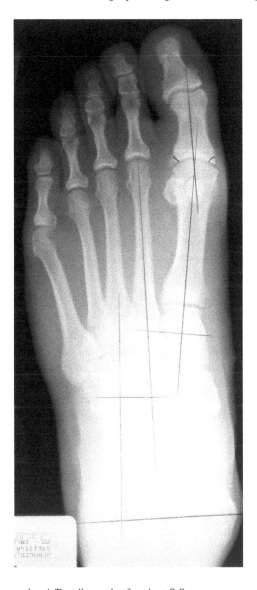

FIGURE 14.4 Preoperative A/P radiograph of patient S.S.

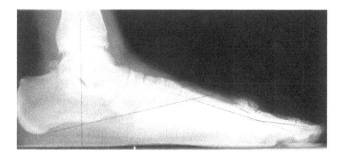

FIGURE 14.5 Preoperative lateral radiograph of patient S.S.

foot demonstrate narrowing of the joint space of the hallux metatarsalphalangeal joint with several dorsal osteophytes. The plantar aspect of the joint appeared to be preserved. Following preoperative 3D gait analysis, the patient underwent cheilectomy. One year following surgery he underwent a postoperative gait analysis.

14.7.1.1   Temporal-Spatial Results (Table 14.3)

The average preoperative walking speed for S.S. was 0.97 m/sec, the average pre-operative stride length was 1.27 m, the average preoperative cadence was 91.97 steps/min, and the average preoperative stance duration was 65.02%. The average postoperative walking speed was 1.08 m/sec, the average postoperative stride length was 1.30 m, the average postoperative cadence was 99.33 steps/min, and the average postoperative stance duration was 64.60%.

14.7.1.2   Kinematic Results (Figure 14.6)

14.7.1.2.1   Tibia

Sagittal motion (dorsiflexion/plantar flexion) was decreased preoperatively from midstance through the initial swing phase of the gait cycle as compared to normal. The tibia was in a more adducted position from the terminal stance through midswing phase and demonstrated decreased coronal (abduction/adduction) ROM throughout the gait cycle preoperatively as compared to normal. The tibia demonstrated less

TABLE 14.3
Temporal-Spatial Parameters (S.S.)

Visit	Stance Duration	Stride Length	Cadence	Walking Speed
Pre-op	65.02%	1.27 m	91.97 steps/min	0.97 m/sec
Post-op	64.60%	1.30 m	99.3 steps/min	1.08 m/sec

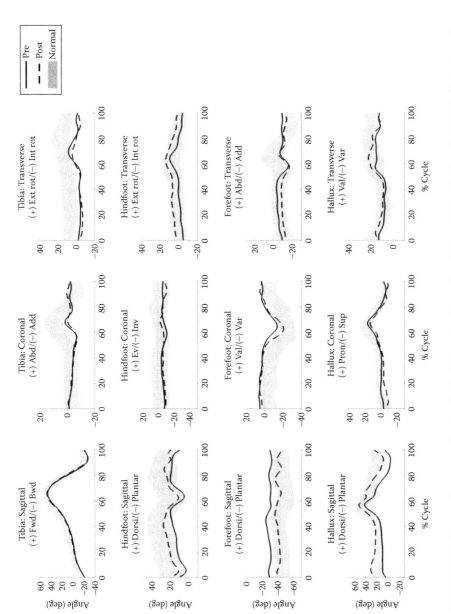

FIGURE 14.6 Pre- and postoperative foot/ankle kinematics for patient S.S., calculated using the MFM. Control results from healthy adult normals shown for comparison (mean ± 1 SD).

external rotation throughout the gait cycle preoperatively compared to normal. Postoperatively, motion and positioning of the tibia were unchanged compared to preoperative kinematics in the sagittal (dorsiflexion/plantar flexion), coronal (abduction/adduction), and transverse planes (external/internal rotation).

14.7.1.2.2 Hindfoot

Preoperatively, the hindfoot demonstrated decreased dorsiflexion throughout stance phase as compared to normal. Postoperatively, hindfoot motion returned to motion similar to normal in the sagittal (dorsiflexion/plantar flexion), coronal (eversion/inversion), and transverse planes (external/internal rotation) throughout the gait cycle.

14.7.1.2.3 Forefoot

Preoperatively, the forefoot demonstrated less plantar flexion throughout the gait cycle compared to normal. In the coronal plane (valgus/varus), the forefoot position was closer to neutral compared to normal (varus position) throughout the gait cycle. The forefoot demonstrated an increase in adduction at toe-off compared to normal. Postoperatively, forefoot coronal ROM was increased, compared to preoperative and normal motion throughout the gait cycle. Sagittal motion of the forefoot more closely resembled normal motion postoperatively.

14.7.1.2.4 Hallux

Preoperatively, the hallux demonstrated a decrease in dorsiflexion during swing phase, as compared to normal. Postoperatively, the hallux demonstrated increased dorsiflexion from load response through terminal stance and decreased pronation from load response through initial swing compared to preoperative and normal motion.

14.7.2 PATIENT #2

N.L. is a 58-yr-old female who has had pain in the right hallux for 2 yr, with an increase in pain over the past 6 months. She had multiple injuries to the toe in the past and is now bothered by it on a daily basis. In particular, pain increases when she wears shoes with even minimal heel elevation and when the hallux moves into a dorsiflexed position. She wears flat shoes to keep the foot in a comfortable position, and occasionally takes Advil for the pain. Physical exam while weight-bearing reveals a neutral hindfoot with maintained arch. Seated exam reveals a dorsal prominence over the hallux MTP joint with tenderness, as well as severely restricted hallux MTP joint ROM (20° compared to 70° on the left). There is no pain secondary to axial tension/compression of the hallux. A/P and lateral radiographs (Figure 14.7 and Figure 14.8) show dorsal osteophytes of the metatarsal head and the base of the proximal phalanx. Mild joint space narrowing is also observed. Following preoperative gait analysis, the patient underwent cheilectomy. Seven months following surgery, she underwent postoperative gait analysis.

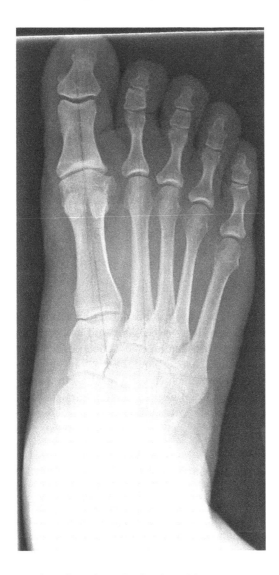

FIGURE 14.7 Preoperative A/P radiograph of patient N.L.

14.7.2.1 Temporal-Spatial Results (Table 14.4)

The average preoperative walking speed for N.L. was 0.080 m/sec, the average preoperative stride length was 0.99 m, the average preoperative cadence was 97.24 steps/min, and the average preoperative stance duration was 67.25%. The average postoperative walking speed was 0.92 m/sec, the average postoperative stride length was 1.07 m, the average postoperative cadence was 102.63 steps/min, and the average postoperative stance duration was 66.26%.

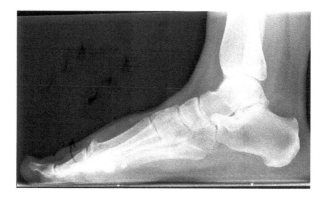

FIGURE 14.8 Preoperative lateral radiograph of patient N.L.

14.7.2.2 Kinematic Results (Figure 14.9)

14.7.2.2.1 Tibia

In the sagittal plane, both pre- and postoperative tibia motion fall fairly close to a normal pattern, with a slight delay in peak forward motion in terminal stance/pre-swing. In the coronal plane, an abnormal adduction positioning is noted preoperatively from late stance through midswing. Postoperatively, this adduction is still present, but it is reduced and much closer to neutral. In the transverse plane, the preoperative data show significant internal rotation throughout the stride. Postoperatively, this motion moves closer to neutral, falling much closer to a normal internally rotated pattern.

14.7.2.2.2 Hindfoot

Hindfoot motion fell mostly within normal bounds in the sagittal and coronal planes. Sagitally, a small increase in plantarflexion at toe-off was seen postoperatively. Coronally, the hindfoot moved to a more neutral position from midstance through midswing, more closely mimicking normal motion. In the transverse plane, slightly excessive external rotation was observed from midstance through terminal swing; this remained the same following surgery.

14.7.2.2.3 Forefoot

Forefoot motion in the sagittal plane improved following surgery, moving to a slightly more plantarflexed position within the range of normal motion. Coronally,

TABLE 14.4
Temporal-Spatial Parameters (N.L.)

Visit	Stance Duration	Stride Length	Cadence	Walking Speed
Pre-op	67.25%	0.99 m	97.24 steps/min	0.80 m/sec
Post-op	66.26%	1.07 m	102.63 steps/min	0.92 m/sec

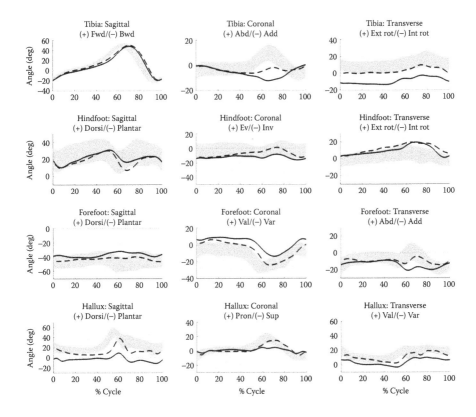

FIGURE 14.9 Pre- and postoperative foot/ankle kinematics for patient N.L., calculated using the MFM. Control results from healthy adult normals shown for comparison (mean ± 1 SD).

the preoperative motion pattern revealed stance phase valgus and swing phase varus. A varus shift was observed postoperatively, as the entire pattern moved closer to the normal range. A slight delay was observed in peak varus position both pre- and postoperatively; this is likely due to the patient's prolonged stance phase duration. In the transverse plane, postoperative motion revealed a shift toward neutral in initial and midswing, moving away from the preoperative adducted position. All other aspects of pre- and postoperative motion in the transverse plane closely follow the normal pattern.

14.7.2.2.4   Hallux

Hallux motion in the sagittal plane exhibits severely restricted ROM preoperatively (~10°, compared to ~35° for normal motion). Postoperatively, ROM increased to near-normal values, and the entire motion pattern underwent a dorsiflexion shift to move closer to the normal pattern. In the coronal plane, preoperative motion fell within normal bounds for all phases of the cycle except for initial swing, when it remained near neutral. Postoperatively, a pronation shift was restored during this phase of the cycle. In the transverse plane, a hallux valgus shift was observed between the preoperative and postoperative conditions, as the subject more closely mimicked a normal pattern following surgery.

14.8 CONCLUSION

Quantified 3D motion analysis of the foot and ankle during ambulation provides a useful means of assessing patient pathology preoperatively and evaluating intervention effectiveness postoperatively. In both cases presented, the MFM analysis found improved walking speeds postoperatively, due to increases in both stride length and cadence. Analysis of hallux motion found improved positioning and ROM postoperatively, particularly for patient N.L. Surgery also served to shift the motion patterns of other foot segments into a more normal range, as evidenced by the sagittal plane differences between pre- and postoperative patterns.

The information gained through gait analysis with the MFM may provide new insight into the disease state prior to conservative or surgical treatment and provide a quantitative means of evaluating the effect of surgery on the foot and its function. Additional work could lead to a number of improvements in treatment; timing of surgical intervention, prescription of modified footwear, and rehabilitation methods following surgery could all be impacted by motion information. Integrated electromyography (EMG) and plantar pressure information would further augment the biomechanical picture provided by gait analysis and may assist in translating laboratory measures to observations made during clinical exams. Further investigation to relate gait measures to functional level might also be warranted.

REFERENCES

1. Coughlin MJ, Shurnas PS. Hallux rigidus: grading and long-term results of operative treatment. *J Bone Joint Surg Am* 85-A(11):2072–2088, 2003.
2. DeFrino PF, Brodsky JW, Pollo FE, Crenshaw SJ, Beischer AD. First metatarsophalangeal arthrodesis: a clinical, pedobarographic and gait analysis study. *Foot Ankle Int* 23(6):496–502, 2002.
3. Easley ME, Davis WH, Anderson RB. Intermediate to long-term follow-up of medial-approach dorsal cheilectomy for hallux rigidus. *Foot Ankle Int* 20(3):147–152, 1999.
4. Giannini S, Ceccarelli F, Faldini C, Bevoni R, Grandi G, Vannini F. What's new in surgical options for hallux rigidus? *J Bone Joint Surg* 86-A (Suppl 2):72–83, 2004.
5. Horton GA, Hallux Rigidus. In: Myerson MS ed. *Foot and Ankle Disorders*. Philadelphia: WB Saunders Company, 289–307, 2000.
6. Kelikian, H. *Hallux Valgus, Allied Deformities of the Forefoot and Metatarsalgia*. Philadelphia: WB Saunders Company, 262–281, 1965.
7. Kidder SM, Abuzzahab FS, Harris GF, Johnson JE. A system for the analysis of foot and ankle kinematics during gait. *IEEE Trans Rehabil Eng* 4(1):25–32, 1996.
8. Kitaoka HB, Alexander IJ, Adelaar RS, Nunley JA, Myerson MS, Sanders M. Clinical rating systems for the ankle-hindfoot, midfoot, hallux, and lesser toes. *Foot Ankle Int* 15(7):349–353, 1994.
9. Lombardi CM, Silhanek AD, Connolly FG, Dennis LN, Keslonsky AJ. First metatarsophalangeal arthrodesis for treatment of hallux rigidus: a retrospective study. *J Foot Ankle Surg* 40(3):137–143, 2001.

10. Mann RA, Coughlin MJ, DuVries HL. Hallux rigidus: a review of the literature and a method of treatment. *Clin Orthop Relat Res* (142):57–63, 1979.

11. Mann RA, Clanton TO. Hallux rigidus: treatment by cheilectomy. *J Bone Joint Surg Am* 70(3):400–406, 1988.

12. Moberg E. A simple operation for hallux rigidus. *Clin Orthop Relat Res* (142):55–56, 1979.

13. Nawoczenski DA, Baumhauer JF, Umberger BR. Relationship between clinical measurements and motion of the first metatarsophalangeal joint. *J Bone Joint Surg* 81-A(3):370–376, 1999.

14. Ronconi P, Monachino P, Baleanu PM, Favilli G. Distal oblique osteotomy of the first metatarsal for the correction of hallux limitus and rigidus deformity. *J Foot Ankle Surg* 39(3):154–160, 2000.

15. Roukis TS, Jacobs PM, Dawson DM, Erdmann BB, Ringstrom JB. A prospective comparison of clinical, radiographic, and intraoperative features of hallux rigidus. *J Foot Ankle Surg* 41(2):76–95, 2002.

16. Shereff MJ, Bejjani FJ, Kummer FJ. Kinematics of the first metatarsophalangeal joint. *J Bone Joint Surg* 68(3):392–398, 1986.

17. Shereff MJ, Baumhauer JF. Hallux Rigidus and osteoarthrosis of the first metatarsal phalangeal joint. *J Bone Joint Surg* 80-A(6):898–908, 1998.

18. Johnson JE, Kidder SM, Abuzzahab FS. Three-dimensional motion analysis of the adult foot and ankle. In: Harris GF and Smith P eds., *Human Motion Analysis*. Piscataway, NJ, IEEE Press, 351–369.

19. Johnson JE, Harris GF. Pathomechanics of posterior tibial tendon insufficiency. *Foot Ankle Clin* 2(2):227–237, 1997.

20. Myers KA, Wang M, Marks RM, Harris GF. Validation of a multisegment foot & ankle kinematic model for pediatric gait. *IEEE Trans Neural Syst Rehabil Eng* 12(1):122–130, 2004.

21. Johnson JE, Lamdan R, Granberry WF, Harris GF, Carrera GF. Hindfoot Coronal Alignment: A Modified Radiographic Method. *Foot Ankle Int* 20(12):818–825, 1999.

22. Kidder SM, Abuzzahab FS, Harris GF. A system for the analysis of the foot & ankle kinematics during gait. *IEEE Trans Rehabil Eng* 4(1):25–32, 1996.

23. Abuzzahab FS, Harris GF, Kidder SM. Foot and ankle motion analysis system instrumentation, calibration and validation. In: Harris GF and Smith P eds., *Human Motion Analysis*. Piscataway, NJ, IEEE Press, 152–166, 1996.

15 Preoperative and Postoperative Gait Analysis of the Rheumatoid Forefoot

Kristen Maskala, Jason T. Long, Richard M. Marks, and Gerald F. Harris

CONTENTS

15.1 INTRODUCTION

The effective treatment of rheumatoid forefoot deformity and functional impairment in the arthritic patient continues to present a challenging problem. While follow-up studies of forefoot correction generally report acceptable surgical results, none to date has addressed the more rigorous and perhaps meaningful combination of clinical, radiological, and biomechanical outcomes. To more accurately assess the results of treatment and to compare treatments requires adequate measures of physical function and outcomes of interventions. Various clinical and radiographic measures of outcomes have been proposed. While valuable, these measures lack assessment of function in terms of quantitative motion (gait). This study combines three-dimensional (3D) gait metrics with radiographic and clinical assessment tools in order to investigate the correlation of these measures as they pertain to rheumatoid patients undergoing forefoot reconstruction.

15.2 BACKGROUND AND SIGNIFICANCE

Rheumatoid arthritis is a systemic condition that can lead to disabling conditions in multiple joints throughout the body. Rheumatoid arthritis primarily causes a chronic, proliferative synovitis, which ultimately invades and destroys the joint as well as the ligamentous support of the joint.[23] This is particularly devastating when rheumatoid arthritis involves the foot, as there are many joints within the foot that can be destroyed and rendered incapable of withstanding the stresses of weight bearing. It has been reported that 80 to 90% of rheumatoid patients will develop arthritis of the forefoot.[34] The deformity most commonly includes a hallux valgus deformity, as well as lesser toe metatarsophalangeal (MTP) subluxation/dislocation and hammertoe or claw toe deformity. In addition, as the hammertoe or claw toe deformity occurs in the interphalangeal joint, the plantar fat pad is pulled distally, allowing the subluxed or dislocated metatarsal heads to assume a more superficial plantar position.[6,9,23] These prominent metatarsal heads can cause pain with every step the patient takes, leading to an antalgic gait. Indeed, the mechanics of the patient's gait can be severely altered as he/she tries to avoid weight bearing on the painful foot. Conservative measures can be attempted to provide the patient with some relief, including shoe wear modifications, but eventually the deformity often requires surgical correction.

15.3 TREATMENT

There are many techniques that have been described in the literature for the correction of the deformities of the rheumatoid forefoot. For treatment of the hallux valgus in the rheumatoid patient, surgical options that have been described include resecting the first metatarsal head,[2,3,5,25] fusion of the first MTP joint,[11,22–24] and resecting the proximal phalanx.[2,3,21] Several options also have been published for correction of the MTP joint subluxation or dislocation. These options include resecting the metatarsal heads,[2,3,4,14,18,23,35] excising the base of the proximal phalanx,[28,29] and resecting both the base of the proximal phalanx and the metatarsal head.[5,10,15,23,24] The hammertoe deformity is surgically corrected in the rheumatoid forefoot usually with partial proximal phalangectomy[3,12,26,28,29,36] or resection of the distal condyles of the proximal phalanx;[7,8,22] however, a closed osteoclasis has also been described.[8,23,24,29]

Recently, Coughlin[7] published his comprehensive long-term follow-up of rheumatoid forefoot correction with reports of 96% good-to-excellent results. This is similar to the results of Mann and Schakel,[23] who reported 95% good-to-excellent results. Both of these studies combined first MTP arthrodesis with lesser metatarsal head excision and hammertoe correction. The results have not been as favorable when the first metatarsal head is simply excised.[13,35] In this study, all patients will have had a first metatarsal fusion combined with lesser metatarsal head resection and correction of hammertoe deformity.

15.4   CRITICAL STUDIES

While there are many procedures described for the correction of the rheumatoid forefoot deformity, there have been few critical preoperative and postoperative studies evaluating these procedures. Coughlin[7] proposed various clinical and radiographic measures to assess outcome in his recently published retrospective study of his rheumatoid forefoot surgeries. This evaluation, while providing very thorough clinical and radiographic evaluation, does not provide gait analysis of patients prior to or after their procedures.

Previous pedobarographic data on patients with rheumatoid forefoot has been published.[27,32,33] A prospective study by Stockley et al. looked at patients before and after excisional arthroplasty of all metatarsal heads.[32] In their study, they found that after excision, the load bearing was shifted to the first metatarsal. They also found that during gait, heel strike and forefoot contact occurred almost simultaneously, deviating from the normal rolling pattern of the foot.[32] Stockley et al.[33] also published their study of patients with concomitant valgus hindfoot deformity, and found that these patients were more likely to have abnormally high forefoot pressures.

Previous 3D analysis of patients with rheumatoid forefoot deformity has been limited. A report by Siegel et al.[30] evaluated several patients with rheumatoid arthritis using the Vicon Motion Analysis System (Vicon Motion Systems, Inc. Lake Forest, Ca.). Of the four patients with rheumatoid arthritis, two were described as having isolated forefoot arthritis. The findings from the data collected on all four rheumatoid patients suggested that the period of foot-flat is prolonged, heel rise at toe-off was decreased, dorsiflexion (DF) at the ankle was prolonged, and plantar flexion at toe-off was diminished.[30] Again, these combined data included rheumatoid patients with various foot deformities and did not isolate or investigate the data of the patients with isolated forefoot involvement.

Reviewing the literature, there are currently no published studies that seek to compare patients with rheumatoid arthritis on the basis of clinical, radiographical, and gait analysis data. Nor are there studies in which a detailed 3D segmental foot model has been used to describe motion. This study combines these entities in a prospective evaluation, which will provide new information regarding the effects of a standard surgical procedure with published high rates of good-to-excellent results.[13] In particular, the comparison of the preoperative and postoperative gait analysis of these patients will allow further understanding of the overall effect of this surgical procedure on the patients' gait.

15.5   TEST METHODS

Nine patients were selected for the study based on the following inclusion criteria:

1. Independent ambulators with pain and deformity of the forefoot.
2. Patients with documented rheumatoid arthritis.

Patients with the following criteria were excluded:

1. Previous surgery for their forefoot deformity.
2. Patients with pain or documented arthritis in any other joint in the affected lower extremity being tested.
3. Medical contraindications to surgery.

All subjects received informed consent as approved by the Institutional Review Board (IRB) at the Medical College of Wisconsin. Nine patients who met the above criteria were enrolled in the study. Each of the nine patients (11 feet) underwent forefoot reconstruction, which consisted of first MTP fusion, lesser metatarsal head resection, and lesser hammertoe correction. Seven of the eleven feet also had lengthening of the extensor hallucis longus tendon to reduce dynamic hallux valgus.

The radiographic assessment performed preoperatively and postoperatively included evaluation and comparison of the hallux valgus angle (HVA), the first intermetatarsal angle (IMA), the angle of DF at the first MTP joint, and the number of subluxed and/or dislocated lesser toes. Also, fusion of the first MTP joint postoperatively was determined, as was maintenance of the lesser toe correction.

The Milwaukee Foot Model (MFM) was used to evaluate the subjects' gait for both pre- and postoperative analysis.[1,16,17,20] The MFM has been developed at the Medical College of Wisconsin as a four-segment kinematic model of the foot and ankle (FANDA). The model measures 3D motion of the tibia, hindfoot, forefoot, and hallux. Motion is measured in the three clinical planes, during both stance and swing of an entire stride. As part of the dynamic measurement process, radiographs (anteroposterior, lateral, and modified coronal views) are used to index foot motion to underlying bony landmarks. The MFM incorporates 12 reflective markers placed over specific bony landmarks on the subject's foot. These markers are tracked by a 15-camera Vicon Motion Analysis System, which captures video data at 120 Hz. The video data are then synchronized to provide 3D coordinates of each marker within the lab collection space.

Each patient underwent preoperative gait analysis as well as postoperative analysis at a minimum of six months after surgery. The results of these patients were then graphically compared to a normal asymptomatic adult population previously described using the same gait analysis system.[1,16,17,20] Analysis was performed on the minimum and maximum values for the range of motion in each segment. These metrics were then averaged and the pre- and postoperative values compared using two sample techniques ($p < .05$).

Temporal parameters, which included stride length, cadence, stance percent, and swing percent, were also recorded. Averaged values were computed from the trials both preoperatively and postoperatively and then compared ($p < .05$). Comparison of the patient metrics to the normal population was also done ($p < .05$).

Each patient was then surveyed for subjective evaluation. Patients rated their result as excellent, good, fair, or poor. A rating of excellent means the patient has minimal or no pain, walks without difficulty, and is very satisfied with the result. A rating of good means minimal pain is present, the patient walks with minimal or no difficulty, and is satisfied with the result. A rating of fair means the patient has moderate residual foot pain, walks with some difficulty, and has reservations regarding the effectiveness of the procedure. A rating of poor means the patient continues to have foot pain, walks with difficulty, and has regrets about the procedure. All patients were asked if they would be willing to undergo the procedure again and if they would recommend the procedure to someone with a similar condition.

15.6 RESULTS

Of the 9 patients (11 feet) tested, the average patient age was 52.5 yr. All patients tested were female. Time from surgery to postoperative testing averaged 365 d. Average time between preoperative and postoperative gait analysis was 372 d.

The radiographic parameters were measured and compared (Table 15.1). Average HVA postsurgery was 19.7°. The average correction of the hallux valgus was 12°. The IMA was corrected an average of 1.7°. Average IMA postoperatively was 9.8°. The DF angle of fusion was also noted to be an average of 15.8°. Radiographic evaluation showed fusion of the first MTP in 9 of 11 cases (82%).

The measured temporal parameters of gait were compared between the normal population and the preoperative state (Table 15.2), the normal population and the postoperative state (Table 15.3), and between the preoperative and postoperative states (Table 15.4).

Significant differences were found between all temporal parameters when comparing the normal population to the preoperative and postoperative states except for cadence. Stride length was the only temporal parameter significantly altered between the preoperative and postoperative states. Dynamic range of motion was then determined for all four segments of the foot in both the swing and stance phases (Table 15.5).

TABLE 15.1
Radiographic Parameters

	HVA		IMA			
Patient	Pre-Op	Post-Op	Pre-Op	Post-Op	DF Fusion Angle	MTP Fusion
1.	36	18	18	18	16	+
2.	22	26	12	6	20	*
3.	22	24	12	12	12	+
4.	22	15	8	8	24	+
	14	8	5	4	14	+
5.	44	33	18	16	11	*
6.	50	28	13	10	10	+
	42	15	10	6	22	+
7.	38	16	12	12	24	+
8.	38	24	12	9	9	+
9.	15	10	7	7	12	+

Note: * denotes fibrous union.

TABLE 15.2
Temporal Data

	Pre	Normal	p-Value
Stride length (m)	1.01	1.29	< .0001
Cadence (steps/min)	107.01	104.31	.440
Stance %	66.07	61.76	< .0001
Swing %	33.93	38.24	< .0001

TABLE 15.3
Temporal Data

	Normal	Post-Op	p-Value
Stride length (m)	1.29	1.05	< .0001
Cadence (steps/min)	104.31	106.76	.512
Stance %	61.76	65.47	< .0001
Swing %	38.24	34.53	< .0001

For each motion segment, the following sign and term conventions were applied (Figure 15.1).

For the tibia, in the sagittal plane, a positive value indicated a position in which the knee is anterior to the ankle, whereas a negative value showed that the ankle is in front of the knee. For tibial coronal motion, a positive value indicated abduction or the ankle moving laterally with respect to the knee, while a negative value indicated adduction or the ankle moving medial to the knee. For transverse motion of the tibia, a positive value indicated more external rotation of the tibia whereas a negative value indicated more internal rotation.

The hindfoot is described in terms of its relation to the tibia. In the sagittal plane, a positive value indicated DF and a negative value indicated plantarflexion. In the

TABLE 15.4
Temporal Data

	Pre	Post	p-Value
Stride length (m)	1.01	1.05	.004
Cadence (steps/min)	107.01	106.76	.891
Stance %	66.07	65.47	.570
Swing %	33.93	34.53	.570

TABLE 15.5
Range of Motion

Segment	Plane	Phase	p-Value
Tibia	Sagittal	Stance	.120
		Swing	.060
	Coronal	Stance	.830
		Swing	.640
	Transverse	Stance	.210
		Swing	.190
Hindfoot	Sagittal	Stance	< .001
		Swing	.003
	Coronal	Stance	.006
		Swing	.520
	Transverse	Stance	< .001
		Swing	< .001
Forefoot	Sagittal	Stance	< .001
		Swing	.039
	Coronal	Stance	.750
		Swing	.970
	Transverse	Stance	.280
		Swing	.670
Hallux	Sagittal	Stance	.034
		Swing	.007
	Coronal	Stance	.580
		Swing	.390
	Transverse	Stance	.290
		Swing	.060

coronal plane, a positive described eversion of the hindfoot while a negative described inversion. In the transverse plane, a positive value indicated external rotation of the hindfoot away from the midline and a negative value indicated internal rotation of the hindfoot toward the midline.

The forefoot was described in relation to the hindfoot. In the sagittal plane, a positive value indicated DF and a negative plantarflexion of the forefoot. In the coronal plane, a positive value indicated valgus of the forefoot and a negative for varus position. In the transverse plane, a positive value described more abduction of the forefoot and a negative described more adduction.

Hallux motion was described with respect to the forefoot. In the sagittal plane, a positive value indicated DF and a negative value was indicative of plantarflexion. In the coronal plane, positive values indicated pronation and negative values indicated supination. In the transverse plane, a positive value indicated a valgus position of the hallux while a negative indicated a varus position.

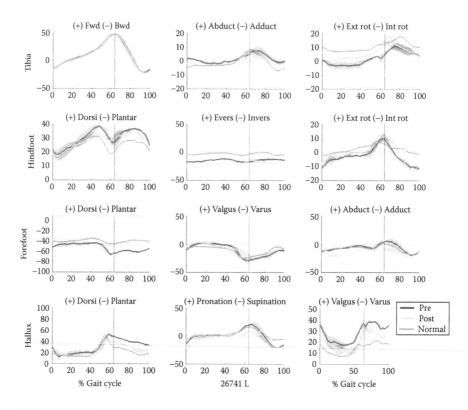

FIGURE 15.1 Segment kinematics for pre- and postoperative states and normal population. Plots represent average angle ± 1 SD.

No significant changes in range of motion were noted in the tibia. The hindfoot range of motion was significantly affected in the sagittal and transverse planes and in the coronal plane in stance phase. The forefoot and hallux range of motion were significantly affected in the sagittal plane throughout the gait cycle. The positions of the four segments at heel strike and toe-off were determined (Table 15.6 and Table 15.7).

TABLE 15.6
Heel Strike

	Sagittal			Coronal			Transverse		
	Pre	Post	*p*-Value	Pre	Post	*p*-Value	Pre	Post	*p*-Value
Tibia	−13.44	−15.06	.11	−0.90	−2.12	.38	6.74	3.91	.20
Hindfoot	14.88	11.79	.17	−4.74	−5.94	.53	−3.47	−3.56	.93
Forefoot	−40.78	−40.41	.88	−5.24	−6.93	.42	−7.57	−8.21	.82
Hallux	13.50	14.56	.85	−8.48	−5.49	.29	33.37	23.02	.027

TABLE 15.7
Toe-Off

	Sagittal			Coronal			Transverse		
	Pre	**Post**	**p-Value**	**Pre**	**Post**	**p-Value**	**Pre**	**Post**	**p-Value**
Tibia	44.68	48.70	.006	5.58	0.26	.019	9.93	8.01	.48
Hindfoot	22.00	15.63	.03	−4.09	−5.07	.62	3.24	6.66	.03
Forefoot	−42.40	−39.24	.26	−15.63	−18.88	.08	−0.41	−0.13	.92
Hallux	21.03	16.86	.73	18.44	19.73	.63	33.66	23.21	.02

These positions were compared between the preoperative and postoperative states and gait trends were noted. Significant changes were noted in the tibia in the sagittal and coronal planes at toe-off. Significant changes were noted in the hindfoot at toe-off in the sagittal and transverse planes. The hallux was noted to have significant changes in position in the transverse plane at both heel strike and toe-off.

Subjective evaluation was recorded for each of the nine patients using the previously described ratings. This subjective evaluation was done on an average of 656 d (21.8 months) postoperatively. Four patients reported an excellent result, four patients a good result, and one a poor result. Eight of nine patients stated they would undergo the surgery again, and all of the patients said they would recommend this procedure to someone with a similar condition.

15.7 DISCUSSION

Forefoot pathology in rheumatoid patients is a particularly disabling condition. Successful clinical results have been documented with the use of first MTP fusion combined with lesser metatarsal head resection and hammertoe correction.[7] Radiographic results of this study compare favorably to previous published data, following a similar procedure for forefoot reconstruction.[13,23]

In these series, the average correction of the HVA was 30° and 18°. The average reduction of the first-second IMA was 3° in both and the DF angle of fusion was 22° and 21°. In the present series, average reduction of the HVA was 12°, average reduction of the first-second IMA was 1.7°, and the DF angle of fusion was 15.8°. The average postoperative HVA in this study was 19.7° and the first-second IMA was 9.8°, similar to the average postoperative HVA and first-second IMAs reported by Coughlin of 20° and 8°.[7] The rate of first metatarsal fusion in the current study was 82%, which is comparable to that reported in the literature.[13,23,24]

Reoperation rate has been reported to be as high as 36% after rheumatoid forefoot reconstruction.[7] Recurrent plantar callosities are also a common complaint after reconstruction of the forefoot, and range from 6 to 36%.[7,36] In this study, one patient required a second operation, 18 months after the forefoot reconstruction, for removal of a rheumatoid nodule.

In this study, eight of nine (89%) patients reported their results as good or excellent. One patient reported the outcome as poor (patient no. 4) and no patient reported his or her outcome as fair. In Coughlin's article, 96% of feet were rated as good or excellent and others have shown similarly high patient satisfaction rates between 89 and 93%.[23,24] Eight patients said they would have the surgery again, and all said they would recommend the procedure to a friend or family member with a similar condition.

Temporal gait parameters of patients with rheumatoid arthritis were previously reported in a pedobarographic study.[27] Stride length in these patients was measured at 0.65 m and cadence at 82 steps per min. In the current study, stride length was measured preoperatively at 1.01 m and postoperatively at 1.05 m. This difference was significant and did move toward the stride length of the normal population used in this study (1.29 m). Cadence in this group of patients was not significantly lower in both preoperative and postoperative testing from the normal population. The cadence decreased after surgery and moved toward the cadence of the normal population, but this change was not significant. Importantly, patients spent less time in stance phase after surgery (65%) and moved toward the percentage of stance phase for the normal population (61.7%), although this value did not reach significance.

Three-dimensional gait analysis showed certain trends postoperatively as compared to the preoperative state. First in heel strike, the hindfoot tended to be less dorsiflexed and in a more inverted position. The forefoot was more commonly in a varus position at heel strike while the hallux tended to assume a less valgus position. At toe-off, the hindfoot tended to be more dorsiflexed, more inverted, and more externally rotated. Also at toe-off, the forefoot was in a more varus position while the hallux tended to be less dorsiflexed and in a less valgus position. The tibia was more externally rotated at toe-off and more internally rotated at heel strike.

Stockley et al.[32] felt that the importance of hindfoot valgus in forefoot surgery was under-recognized. They emphasized that excessive pronation of the forefoot occurred after heel strike when the hindfoot was in more than 10° of valgus, and this could lead to poor outcomes in forefoot reconstruction surgeries. Spiegel and Spiegel[31] noted that 25% of patients had abnormal hindfoot valgus on weight bearing. Cracchiolo[9] proposed that loss of articular cartilage and erosions of the subtalar and talonavicular joints gave a persistent valgus to the hindfoot, which caused increased pronation of the forefoot and increased medial overload. In this study, patients at heel strike showed less pronation of the forefoot and less eversion of the hindfoot. This would tend to diminish the high medial forefoot pressures that Stockley et al.[32] described as excessive pronation of the forefoot just after heel strike.

Keenan et al.[19] analyzed the gait of patients with rheumatoid arthritis with varying degrees of hindfoot valgus. They concluded that the valgus deformity of the foot is due to excessive pronation forces on the subtalar joint. They felt that the alterations in the gait of rheumatoid patients were due to symmetrical muscle weakness and the patients' efforts to walk with less pain. They also noted excessive external rotation of the lower limb during weight bearing to diminish pain under the metatarsal heads.

Using gait analysis, Siegel[30] reported that rheumatoid arthritis involvement of the foot and ankle caused increased valgus deformity of the heel during loading, increased DF of the ankle joint, delayed heel rise, a shortened step length, and decreased walking velocity. There have been no previous published reports detailing the actual dynamic changes that occur following rheumatoid forefoot reconstruction. This study is the first to examine the complex relationship that correction of the forefoot deformity has on the other motion segments of the foot and ankle. It is important to recognize and document that significant changes in motion occur in the hindfoot, forefoot, and hallux following forefoot surgery (Table 15.5).

It is also important to analyze the position that each segment assumes at various phases in the gait cycle. Only then can any determination be made regarding the effect that forefoot correction has on the overall gait pattern of the rheumatoid patient. In this study, several pertinent findings were made through the use of gait analysis:

- Patients had significant improvements in stride length toward a more normal value.
- Range of motion was improved in the hindfoot, forefoot, and hallux throughout the gait cycle.
- Following forefoot correction, the forefoot exhibited less pronation at heel strike, the heel was in less valgus at heel strike, and the hallux was in significantly less valgus at both toe-off and heel strike.

These improvements would seem to benefit the overall function of patients with rheumatoid arthritis, who can become plagued by recurrent hallux valgus, as well as by acquired hindfoot valgus with resultant excessive forefoot pronation and medial overload.

The limitations of this study include the small number of feet evaluated. The follow-up time from surgery was relatively short, although Coughlin[7] reported duration of follow-up did not significantly affect outcomes in his patients with an average of 74 months follow-up. Gait analysis in the future on this same set of patients would be helpful to assess if there were any longer-term changes in the motion segments of the foot and ankle. At this length of follow-up, it appears that forefoot correction consisting of first MTP fusion, lesser metatarsal head resection, and lesser hammertoe correction with or without extensor hallucis longus lengthening provides satisfactory outcomes when assessed radiographically, subjectively, and with 3D (MFM) gait analysis.

REFERENCES

1. Abuzzahab FS, Harris GF, Johnson JE, and Nery J. Foot and Ankle Motion Analysis System Instrumentation Calibration and Validation in Human Motion Analysis. In: Harris GF, ed. Piscataway, NJ: IEEE Press, 1996:152–166.
2. Amuso SJ, Wissinger HA, Margolis HM, Eisenbeis CH Jr, and Stolzer BL. Metatarsal Head Resection in the Treatment of Rheumatoid Arthritis. *Clin Orthop Relat Res* 1971; 74:94–100.
3. Barton NJ. Arthroplasty of the Forefoot in Rheumatoid Arthritis. *J Bone Joint Surg Br* 1973; 55(1):126–133.
4. Brattstrom H and Brattstrom M. Resection of the Metatarsophalangeal Joints in Rheumatoid Arthritis. *Acta Orthop Scand* 1970; 41:213–224.

5. Clayton ML. Surgery of the Lower Extremity in Rheumatoid Arthritis. *J Bone Joint Surg Am* 1963; 45:1517–1536.

6. Coughlin MJ. The Rheumatoid Foot. In: Chapman, MW, ed. *Operative Orthopedics.* Philadelphia: J.B. Lippincott, 1993:2311–2322.

7. Coughlin MJ. Rheumatoid Forefoot Reconstruction. *J Bone Joint Surg* Am 2001; 82(3):322–341.

8. Cracchiolo A. Management of the Arthritic Forefoot. *Foot Ankle* 1982; 3:17–23.

9. Cracchiolo A. Rheumatoid Arthritis of the Forefoot. In: Gould JS, ed. *Operative Foot Surgery.* Philadelphia: W.B. Saunders, 1994:141–159.

10. Craxford AD, Stevens J, and Park C. Management of the deformed rheumatoid forefoot. A Comparison of Conservative and Surgical Methjods. *Clin Orthop Relat Res* 1982; 166:121–126.

11. Dwyer AH Correction of Severe Toe Deformities. *J Bone Joint Surg Br* 1970; 52(1):192.

12. Fowler AW. A Method of Forefoot Reconstruction. *J Bone Joint Surg Br* 1959; 41(3):507–513.

13. Goldie L, Bremmel T, Althoff B, and Irstam L. Metatarsal Head Resection in the Treatment of the Rheumatoid Forefoot. *Scand J Rheumatol* 1983; 12:106–112.

14. Gould N. Surgery of the Forepart of the Foot in Rheumatoid Arthritis. *Foot Ankle* 1982; 3:173–180.

15. Hasselo LG, Willkens RF, Toomey HE, Karges DE, and Hansen ST. Forefoot Surgery in Rheumatoid Arthritis: Subjective Assessment of Outcome. *Foot Ankle* 1987; 8:148–151.

16. Johnson J and Harris GF. Pathomechanics of Posterior Tibial Tendon Insufficiency. *Foot Ankle Clin* 1997; 2:227–239.

17. Johnson J, Kidder S, and Abuzzahab F. Three-Dimensional Motion Analysis of the Adult Foot and Ankle in Human Motion Analysis. In: Harris GF, ed. Piscataway, NJ: IEEE Press, 1996:351–369.

18. Kates A, Kessel L, and Kay A. Arthroplasty of the Forefoot. *J Bone Joint Surg Br* 1967; 49(3):552–557.

19. Keenan ME, Peabody TD, Gronley JK, and Perry J. Valgus Deformities of the Feet and Characteristics of Gait in Patients who have Rheumatoid Arthritis. *J Bone Joint Surg Am* 1991; 2:237–247.

20. Kidder SM, Harris GF, Abuzzahab FS, and Johnson JE. A Biomechanical Model for Foot and Ankle Motion Analysis. In: Harris GF, ed. *Human Motion Analysis.* Piscataway, NJ: IEEE Press, 133–150.

21. Lipscomb PR. Surgery for Rheumatoid Arthritis—Timing and Techniques: Summary. *J Bone Joint Surg Am* 1968; 50:614–617.

22. MacClean CR and Silver WA. Dwyer's Operation for the Rheumatoid Forefoot. *Foot Ankle* 1981; 1:343–347.

23. Mann RA and Schakel ME. Surgical Correction of Rheumatoid Forefoot Deformities. *Foot Ankle Int* 1995; 16:1–6.

24. Mann RA and Thompson FM. Arthrodesis of the First Metatarsophalangeal Joint for Hallux Valgus in Rheumatoid Arthritis. *J Bone Joint Surg Am* 1984; 66:687–692.

25. Marmor L. Resection of the Forefoot in Rheumatoid Arthritis. *Clin Othop Relat Res* 1975; 108:223–227.

26. McGarvey SR and Johnson KA. Keller Arthroplasty in Combination with Resection Arthroplasty of the Lesser Metatarsophalangeal Joints in Rheumatoid Arthritis. *Foot Ankle* 1988; 9:75–80.

27. Minns RJ and Craxford AD. Pressure under the Forefoot in Rheumatoid Arthritis. *Clin Orthop Relat Res* 1984; 187:235–242.
28. Newman RJ and Fitton JM. Conservation of Metatarsal Heads in Surgery of Rheumatoid Arthritis of the Forefoot. *Acta Orthop Scand* 1983; 54:417–421.
29. Saltzman CL, Johnson KA, and Donnelly RE. Surgical Treatment for Mild Deformities of the Rheumatoid Forefoot by Partial Phalangectomy and Syndactylization. *Foot Ankle* 1993; 14:325–329.
30. Siegel KL, Kepple TM, O'connell PG, and Stanhope SJ. A Technique to Evaluate Foot Function During the Stance Phase of Gait. *Foot Ankle Int* 1985; 16 (12):764–770.
31. Spiegel TN and Spiegel JS. Rheumatoid Arthritis in the Foot and Ankle—Diagnosis, Pathology and Treatment. *Foot Ankle* 1982; 2:318–324.
32. Stockley I, Betts RP, Rowley DI, Getty CJ, and Duckworth T. A Prospective Study of Forefoot Arthroplasty. *Clin Orthop* 1989; 248:213–218.
33. Stockley I, Betts RP, Rowley DI, Getty CJ, and Duckworth T. The Importance of the Valgus Hindfoot in Forefoot Surgery in Rheumatoid Arthritis. *J Bone Joint Surg Br* 1990; 72(4):705–708.
34. Vainio K. Rheumatoid Foot. Clinical Study with Pathological and Roentgenological Comments. *Ann Chir Gynaecol Fenn Suppl* 1956; 45:1–107.
35. van der Heijden KW, Rasker JJ, Jacobs JW, and Dey K. Kates Forefoot Arthroplasty in Rheumatoid Arthritis. A Five-Year Follow-Up Study. *J Rheumatol* 1992; 19:1545–1550.
36. Watson MS. A Long-Term Follow-Up of Forefoot Arthroplasty. *J Bone Joint Surg Br* 1974; 56(3):527–533.

16 Foot and Ankle Motion Analysis of Patients with Ankle Arthritis

Michael Khazzam, Jason T. Long, Richard M. Marks, and Gerald F. Harris

CONTENTS

16.1 INTRODUCTION

Quantitative gait analysis evolved from a need to address musculoskeletal and neurologic impairments of the lower extremities. Classic techniques measure joint kinematics in three dimensions at the hip, knee, and ankle, modeling each limb (pelvis, thigh, shank, and foot) as a single rigid segment. These methods have been demonstrated to provide important information for surgical decision-making, and can assist in the measurement of outcomes following treatment. However, the rigid foot segment incorporated into most of the lower extremity models is insufficient for appropriately modeling the multiple articulations that take place distal to the ankle joint; in most cases, no distinction is made between the two articulations that make up the ankle (talocrural and subtalar joints).

To date, there has been limited information available concerning dynamic foot and ankle motion in patients with foot and ankle pathology. Advances in technology and the development of multisegmental foot and ankle models have created new tools for quantitative clinical assessment. These tools are available to the practicing orthopedic surgeon treating foot and ankle pathology, and can be incorporated directly into the clinical practice.

This chapter offers a paradigm for applying these techniques to patients suffering from ankle arthritis before and after treatment. We present a brief description of ankle anatomy, followed by a review of ankle arthritis and its treatment options. Motion analysis case studies from two patients are presented to clarify the clinical efficacy and usefulness of multisegmental foot and ankle gait analysis.

16.2 ANKLE ANATOMY AND BIOMECHANICS

The ankle (talocrural) joint consists of three articulations: the tibiotalar, tibiofibular, and fibulotalar joints. These articulations make up the ankle mortise,[7] which is composed of the following bony relationships: the articulation of the tibial plafond (distal tibia) and the dorsal surface (trochlear surface) of the talus, as well as the medial and lateral malleolar articulations with the medial and lateral talar facets, respectively (Figure 16.1). Several ligamentous structures aid in the stabilization of the ankle joint. The deltoid ligament, which consists of both superficial and deep segments, provides medial stability. The anterior talonavicluar, the tibiocalcaneal, and the tibiotalar ligaments make up the superficial deltoid ligament. The deep deltoid ligament attaches from the tip of the medial malleolus to the talus, and has anterior and posterior segments. Lateral ankle stability is provided by the anterior talofibular ligament, fibulocalcaneal ligament, and the posterior talofibular ligament (Figure 16.2).[7,30]

Ankle joint motion occurs in the sagittal (dorsiflexion/plantarflexion), coronal (abduction/adduction), and transverse (external/internal rotation) planes. Triplanar motion of the ankle joint occurs simultaneously as a result of the cone-shaped trochlea with its apex directed medially and the larger surface anteriorly. The cone-shaped dorsal surface of the talus, together with the position and orientation of the joint axis, results in abduction and external rotation of the ankle during dorsiflexion and adduction and internal rotation during plantar flexion.[7-9,30]

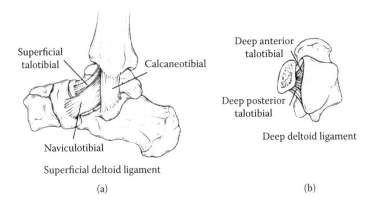

Superficial talotibial

Calcaneotibial

Deep anterior talotibial

Deep posterior talotibial

Deep deltoid ligament

Naviculotibial

Superficial deltoid ligament

(a)

(b)

FIGURE 16.1 The medial collateral ligament of the ankle. (a) The superficial fibers connecting the medial malleolus to the talus, calcaneus, and navicular have a roughly triangular appearance and suggest the name deltoid. (b) The much more important deep fibers run nearly transversely from the posterior colliculus to the talus posterior to its medial articular facet. [Reprinted from *Skeletal Trauma* (3rd ed.), BD Browner, pp. 2308–2313, Copyright (2003), with permission from Elsevier.]

Although it is difficult to determine the contribution of motion of the subtalar joint, specifically during gait analysis, it is important to have a complete understanding of the anatomy and biomechanics that occur at this joint when analyzing gait. The subtalar joint consists of the articulation between the talus and the calcaneus. The talus articulates with the calcaneus at three facets (anterior, middle, and posterior). At the anterior and middle facets, the calcaneus rotates around the talus; at the

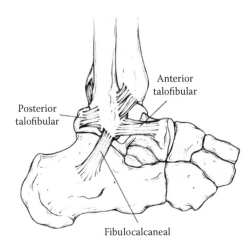

Anterior talofibular

Posterior talofibular

Fibulocalcaneal

FIGURE 16.2 The three components of the lateral collateral ligament are the anterior and posterior talofibular ligaments, and, between them, the fibulocalcaneal ligament, which crosses the talus. [Reprinted from *Skeletal Trauma* (3rd ed.), BD Browner, pp. 2308–2313, Copyright (2003), with permission from Elsevier.]

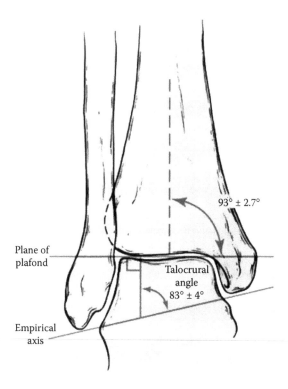

FIGURE 16.3 The tibiotalar articular surface (plafond) usually has a slight lateral tilt, averaging 3°. The empirical axis is in a relatively varus position, as indicated by the talocrural angle, formed by the intersection of a line perpendicular to the plafond with the empirical axis. This averages 83 ± 4° and is a reliable radiographic indicator of the relationship among malleoli and plafond. It should be similar to that of the opposite ankle. [Reprinted from *Skeletal Trauma* (3rd ed.), BD Browner, pp. 2308–2313, Copyright (2003), with permission from Elsevier.]

posterior facet, the talus glides on the calcaneus.[7–10,30,31] The axis of the subtalar joint has an oblique orientation, which provides simultaneous triplanar motion (Figure 16.3).[7,30,31] Motion of the subtalar joint occurs in the sagittal (dorsiflexion/plantarflexion), coronal (inversion/eversion), and transverse (internal/external rotation) planes. The ankle and subtalar joints act in conjunction during sagittal plane motion of the foot and ankle, and are clinically indistinguishable.[7–10]

16.3 ANKLE ARTHRITIS

Abnormal ankle joint biomechanics, frequently secondary to trauma (intra-articular fracture), are the most common cause of ankle arthritis. Less common causes are primary osteoarthritis or inflammatory arthropathies, neuropathic (Charcot) arthropathy, infection, and tumor. These pathologies cause irreversible destruction of tibiotalar articular cartilage, chronic cartilage overloading from articular incongruity, and eventual destruction of the joint space. The progressive nature of the disease results in increasing deformity and pain, especially during weight-bearing.[1–6] Severe symptoms develop because of restricted/painful range of motion and varus or valgus joint deformities.

16.4 CLINICAL ASSESSMENT

Patients with ankle arthritis present with a history of pain, swelling, and decreased mobility. Antalgic gait in these patients is a result of a fixed deformity and/or pain associated with weight-bearing. Patients with isolated talocrural joint arthritis will frequently retain more function because of the adaptive and energy-absorbing nature of the subtalar joint, especially on uneven surfaces.[6,8,10] Thorough evaluation of active and passive range of motion, strength of surrounding muscles, presence of callosities, and abnormal shoe wear and gait in conjunction with a detailed history of the presenting problem aid in the selection of the appropriate treatment modality. History should include details of previous treatment (conservative and surgical) as well as mechanism of injury in patients with posttraumatic arthritis. Selective use of local anesthetic blocks to adjacent joints may help clarify the origin point of pain (i.e., injecting the subtalar joint with 5 ml of 1% lidocaine may rule out pathology of this joint contributing to pain).

Radiographic evaluation should include weight-bearing anteroposterior (AP) and lateral views of the entire foot and ankle as well as a mortise view of the ankle. Identification of joint space narrowing, osteophytes, subchondral sclerosis, talar subluxation within the ankle mortise, talar bone loss, and the presence of any existing hardware will help determine the degree of arthritis present. Computed tomography is also a useful study that provides a more detailed assessment of joint surface defects, degenerative joint changes, location of osteophytes, and status of adjacent joints.

16.5 TREATMENT

The goal of treatment of patients with end-staged ankle arthritis is to create a pain-free, stable, plantigrade foot. Current treatment options include both conservative (anti-inflammatory medications, orthotic devices, footwear modifications, and activity modification in conjunction with weight loss if necessary) and surgical [debridement, arthrodesis, and total ankle replacement (TAR)] modalities. If a patient fails nonoperative therapy and the disease is limited to the tibiotalar joint, surgery should be considered as a viable treatment option.

16.6 SURGICAL TREATMENT

Several surgical options are available; these include arthroscopic debridement, anterior cheilectomy, supramalleolar osteotomy, distraction ankle arthroplasty, allograft surface replacement, arthrodesis (fusion), and TAR.[1–3,5,6,11,28,29] Extent of ankle arthritis, age, and activity level of the patient will determine the appropriate surgical treatment option. A complete discussion of all surgical treatment modalities is beyond the scope of this text; we will focus specifically on arthrodesis and TAR, as these were the techniques identified for our population of patients with end-stage ankle arthritis.

16.7 ARTHRODESIS

Ankle arthrodesis is defined as fusion of the tibia to the talus.[5] Functionally disabling ankle joint pain and stiffness are the most common indications for ankle arthrodesis. Ankle arthrodesis is indicated for treatment when the patient presents with pain and deformity secondary to posttraumatic osteoarthritis, previous infection, osteochondral defects, osteonecrosis of the talus, primary osteoarthritis, inflammatory arthropathies, rheumatoid arthritis, and failed TAR.[1–3,5,6,11] Additionally, the bone of the subtalar complex should be without arthritic changes and in normal alignment.[3] The optimal position for fusion is neutral plantarflexion, 0 to 5° hindfoot and ankle valgus, and 5 to 10° external rotation.[1,3,5,6,12] Several surgical techniques (arthroscopic, "mini open" arthrotomy, or open arthrotomy) and stabilization methods (external fixation, internal fixation with screws or internal fixation with blade plate) are available.[1–3,5,6,11] In this study, we performed an ankle arthrodesis using a transfibular approach, with an anterior incision and two canulated screws for fixation.[3–6]

In most published studies,[12–18] results of ankle fusion demonstrate a good functional outcome. Although the majority of these studies rely on subjective criteria based on physical examination and radiographic analysis, several studies[12,17,18] have provided objective assessment based on gait analysis data.

16.8 TAR

A detailed description of TAR would examine the various devices available for implantation, the many methods for implanting them, and the numerous controversies arising from the lack of long-term follow-up results of the currently used systems (second-generation TAR). Such a description is beyond the scope of this text. While criteria for the ideal TAR patient are still being developed, several contraindications have been clearly defined. The use of TAR is not recommended in the presence of active or recent infection, peripheral vascular disease, vascular impairment, neuropathic joint disease (Charcot), neurologic dysfunction, severe malalignment, severe osteoporosis, osteonecrosis of the talus, compromised soft tissue envelope, or severe joint laxity. In addition, the procedure is not recommended for young active patients.[3–6,20]

In this study, we performed a TAR using the Agility Total Ankle System (DePuy Orthopaedics, Inc., Warsaw, IN). This is a second-generation total ankle arthroplasty, and consists of a two-component design, which provides complete articular surface replacement of the medial, lateral, and superior articular surfaces of the ankle joint. The implant is placed in 20° of external rotation relative to the tibia, which allows external rotation during dorsiflexion and reproduction of normal joint kinematics.[3–6,20]

16.9 PREVIOUS INVESTIGATIONS

Numerous studies have provided descriptions of foot and ankle motion during gait, using such varied techniques as mathematical modeling, cadaveric specimen analysis, and lower extremity gait analysis. Most of these studies treat the ankle–joint complex as a single articulation, and many exclude other foot segments.

Stauffer et al.[21] investigated motion analysis in normal, diseased, and prosthetic ankle joints, using foot switches to obtain temporal parameters, and used high-speed video to track reflective tape applied to the medial malleolus and tibia. Reduced cadence and ankle range of motion in the sagittal plane were observed in the diseased and prosthetic groups. Mazur et al.[17] examined 12 patients following ankle arthrodesis using three markers to model the ankle–foot complex as part of a standard whole body gait analysis; motion data were obtained using a three-camera system. The authors reported decreased sagittal plane range of motion and decreased walking speed in the fused ankles compared to normal, with cadence unchanged from normal. Both of these studies ignored motion distal to the ankle joint, and only addressed motion in the sagittal plane.

Buck et al.[12] analyzed the gait patterns of 19 patients following ankle arthrosis using three-dimensional electrogoniometers attached to braces, mounted on the distal tibia and heel of the shoe. Foot switches were also used to obtain temporal parameters. The authors reported reduced sagittal range of motion during gait following ankle arthrodesis, as well as diminished varus-valgus motion in the coronal plane.

Demottaz et al.[19] examined the motion of the ankle–joint complex during gait in 21 ankles following TAR. Subjects were filmed during both barefoot and shod ambulation, and the film was digitized to obtain kinematic and temporal-spatial parameters. The TAR group demonstrated decreased walking speed, cadence, and stride length. In contrast to the Buck study, these subjects demonstrated increased range of motion in the sagittal plane, but abnormal motion patterns were observed (increased plantarflexion at heel strike, and decreased dorsiflexion during swing).

Wu et al.[18] examined foot and ankle motion following ankle arthrodesis using a three-segment model (tibia/fibular, hindfoot/midfoot, and forefoot). This study compared the gait data acquired from ten patients following ankle arthrodesis with ten normal subjects. Three-dimensional joint motion was obtained using a three-segment rigid body foot model, and temporal-spatial parameters were obtained using foot switches attached to the heel, first and fifth metatarsals, and hallux. The results of this study agreed with the previously reported findings in studies examining gait following ankle fusion, with increased stance phase and generalized decreased range of motion in the sagittal, coronal, and transverse planes.

16.10 CURRENT INVESTIGATION

Two patients with end-stage ankle arthritis underwent three-dimensional gait analysis using a 15-camera Vicon 524 Motion Analysis System (Vicon Motion Systems, Inc., Lake Forest, CA). Multisegmental foot and ankle kinematics and temporal-spatial data were obtained using the Milwaukee Foot Model (MFM);[22–27] patients were tested one week prior to surgery and one year following surgery (arthrodesis or TAR).

For each testing session, patients were instrumented with reflective markers placed over bony landmarks on the foot and ankle. Markers were secured with double-sided tape following the protocol specified by the MFM. Following a static orientation trial, subjects ambulated at a freely selected walking speed along the data collection corridor (length = 6 m). Each trial was subject to clinical screening; data collection continued until a minimum of three walking trials had been obtained for analysis.

16.11 CASE EXAMPLES

For each patient, results of pre- and postoperative gait analysis are detailed. Each result set comprises three-dimensional joint kinematics during gait, and temporal-spatial parameters (cadence, stride length, stance/swing ratio, and walking speed). Patient results were compared to results from a population of normal adults ($n = 25$).

16.11.1 Subject One

L.M. is a 32-yr-old female who presented with a history of a painful right ankle, which had been worsening for 3 yr. The patient has a history of right ankle fracture following a fall, which was surgically repaired by open reduction and internal fixation with screws 8 yr prior to presentation. Since the time of injury, the patient has complained of decreased motion, stiffness, difficulty with ambulation, and pain. Past surgical history was significant for open reduction internal fixation (ORIF) right ankle fracture, hardware removal 1 yr following surgery, and arthroscopic right ankle debridement 2 yr prior to presentation for osteophytes removal. The patient has failed numerous conservative treatment modalities including corticosteroid injection, orthotics, and anti-inflammatory medication. On examination, her right foot was in a pes planus position without hindfoot deformity; ankle range of motion was limited, with dorsiflexion only to neutral. Plain radiographs of the foot and ankle demonstrated moderate degenerative ankle joint changes with multiple medial osteophytes and calcifications. There was no evidence of degenerative changes to adjacent joints visualized radiographically. Following preoperative gait analysis, she underwent right ankle (tibiotalar) fusion (Figure 16.4). One year following surgery, she underwent a postoperative gait analysis.

16.11.2 Temporal-Spatial Results (Table 16.1)

The average preoperative walking speed for this patient was 0.95 m/sec, the average preoperative stride length was 1.1 m, the average preoperative cadence was 103.85 steps/min, and the average preoperative stance duration was 65.62%. The average postoperative walking speed was 0.91 m/sec, the average postoperative stride length was 1.04 m, the average postoperative cadence was 105.11 steps/min, and the average postoperative stance duration was 67.15%.

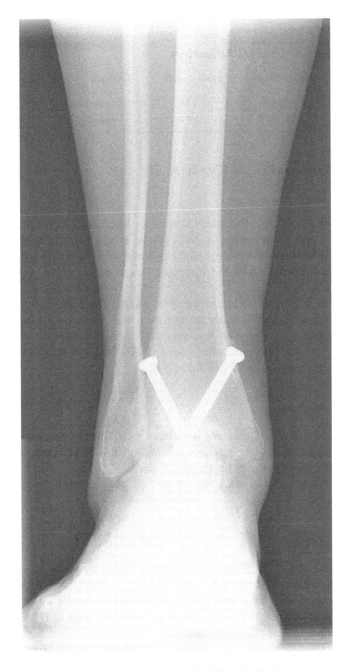

FIGURE 16.4 Coronal plane view of ankle mortise S/P ankle fusion.

TABLE 16.1
L.M. Temporal-Spatial Parameters

Visit	Stance Duration	Stride Length	Cadence	Walking Speed
Pre-op	65.62%	1.10 m	103.85 steps/min	0.95 m/sec
Post-op	67.15%	1.04 m	105.11 steps/min	0.91 m/sec

16.11.3 Kinematic Results (Figure 16.5)

16.11.3.1 Tibia

Preoperatively, there was decreased motion of the tibia in the sagittal plane at load response and from midstance through the initial swing phase. There was also decreased motion in the coronal (abduction/adduction) and transverse (external/internal rotation) planes with the tibia in a position of reduced abduction and external rotation.

Postoperative sagittal motion of the tibia also demonstrated decreased motion at load response and from midstance through the initial swing phase; range of motion (ROM) appeared to be less than that observed during preoperative gait analysis. Postoperative coronal and transverse motion of the tibia appeared to be improved compared to preoperative motion in these planes.

16.11.3.2 Hindfoot

Preoperative motion of the hindfoot was found to be decreased in all three planes throughout the gait cycle. The hindfoot appeared in a more plantarflexed, inverted, and externally rotated position. Postoperative hindfoot motion, although not normal, demonstrated improvements in the sagittal, coronal, and transverse planes throughout the gait cycle.

16.11.3.3 Forefoot

Preoperative motion of the forefoot was decreased throughout the gait cycle in the sagittal (dorsiflexion/plantar flexion), coronal (valgus/varus), and transverse planes (abduction/adduction). The forefoot demonstrated a less plantar flexed, neutral or less varus, adducted position. Postoperatively, the overall range of motion exhibited minimal change, but overall positioning of the segment was altered in the sagittal (increased plantar flexion), coronal (increased varus), and transverse (increased abduction) planes.

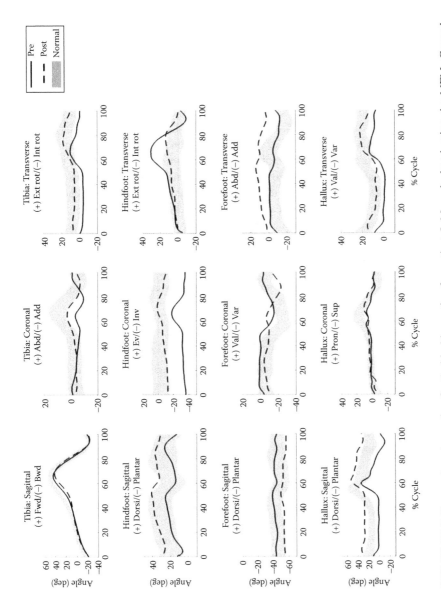

FIGURE 16.5 Pre- and postoperative foot/ankle kinematics for patient L.M., calculated using the MFM. Control results from healthy adult normals shown for comparison (mean ± 1 STD).

16.11.3.4 Hallux

Preoperative hallux motion was decreased throughout the gait cycle in all three planes. Postoperative motion demonstrated triplanar improvements.

16.11.4 SUBJECT TWO

A.D. is a 54-yr-old female who presented with a history of a painful right ankle for the past 10 yr. The patient's history is remarkable for ankle fracture following a fall (20 yr prior, treated by cast immobilization) and primary osteoarthritis. Past surgical history was significant for several bone graft procedures of the ankle 15 yr ago. The patient experienced a second falling incident 4 yr ago; she fell off a horse and sustained a pelvic fracture, which was treated by Open Reduction Internal Fixation (ORIF). Since that time she has had increasing ankle pain with movement and weight-bearing activities.

On examination, there was no hindfoot angular deformity. Ankle range of motion was severely limited to only 10 to 20° of dorsiflexion/plantarflexion, and the patient was unable to dorsiflex the foot to neutral (5 to 10°). In addition, there was tenderness to palpation of the anteromedial and anterolateral aspects of the tibiotalar joint. Plain radiographic examination of the foot and ankle revealed degenerative changes of the tibiotalar joint with anterior osteophytes and cystic changes. Slight collapse and flattening of the talar dome were also observed. The patient had not been responsive to immobilization and physical therapy. Following preoperative gait analysis, she underwent right TAR (Figure 16.6). One year following surgery she underwent a postoperative gait analysis.

16.11.5 TEMPORAL-SPATIAL RESULTS (TABLE 16.2)

The average preoperative walking speed for this patient was 1.01 m/sec, the average preoperative stride length was 1.12 m, the average preoperative cadence was 108.83 steps/min, and the average preoperative stance duration was 60.45%. The average postoperative walking speed was 1.12 m/sec, the average postoperative stride length was 1.23 m, the average postoperative cadence was 110.54 steps/min, and the average postoperative stance duration was 61.65%.

16.11.6 KINEMATIC RESULTS (FIGURE 16.7)

16.11.6.1 Tibia

Preoperative range of motion of the tibia was decreased in the coronal plane (abduction/adduction) from terminal stance through midswing phase. Tibial motion was also decreased preoperatively in the transverse plane (external/internal rotation) from load response through terminal stance and from initial swing through terminal swing. Postoperative motion of the tibia was improved in all three planes.

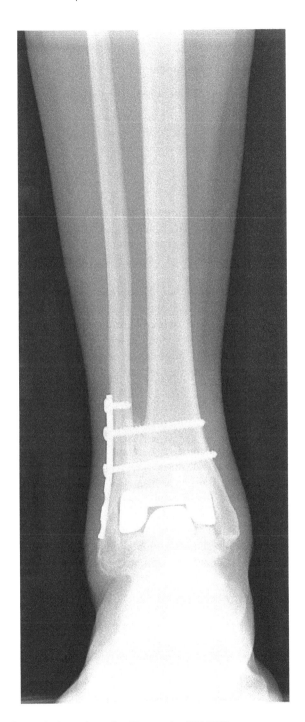

FIGURE 16.6 Coronal plane view of ankle mortise S/P TAR.

TABLE 16.2
A.D. Temporal-Spatial Parameters

Visit	Stance Duration	Stride Length	Cadence	Walking Speed
Pre-op	60.45%	1.12 m	108.83 steps/min	1.01 m/sec
Post-op	31.65%	1.23 m	110.54 steps/min	1.12 m/sec

16.11.6.2   Hindfoot

Preoperatively, the hindfoot was in a position of greater inversion as compared to normal throughout the gait cycle. The hindfoot also demonstrated increased range of motion in the transverse plane (external/internal rotation) as compared to normal and specifically greater magnitude of external rotation from midstance through midswing.

Postoperative hindfoot motion in the coronal plane was improved when compared with preoperative motion, but demonstrated increased eversion from terminal stance through the initial swing phase compared to normal. Transverse plane hindfoot motion demonstrates a decrease in overall range of motion compared to preoperative and normal motion and was still maintained in a position of increased external rotation throughout the gait cycle, but with less dynamic range of motion.

16.11.6.3   Forefoot

Preoperatively, the forefoot appeared to maintain a valgus position throughout the gait cycle, which was greater than normal. Overall, forefoot range of motion was decreased in the sagittal and transverse planes as compared to normal throughout the gait cycle. Postoperative forefoot motion demonstrated a decrease in overall motion in the coronal plane (valgus/varus) throughout the gait cycle compared to preoperative and normal motion. Both sagittal and transverse excursion/positioning of the forefoot more closely resemble normal motion postoperatively, and range of motion in the transverse plane appears similar to normal.

16.11.6.4   Hallux

Preoperatively, the hallux maintained a position of dorsiflexion throughout the gait cycle, which was greater than normal. Postoperative hallux motion demonstrates similar range of motion to normal throughout the gait cycle in the sagittal, coronal, and transverse planes.

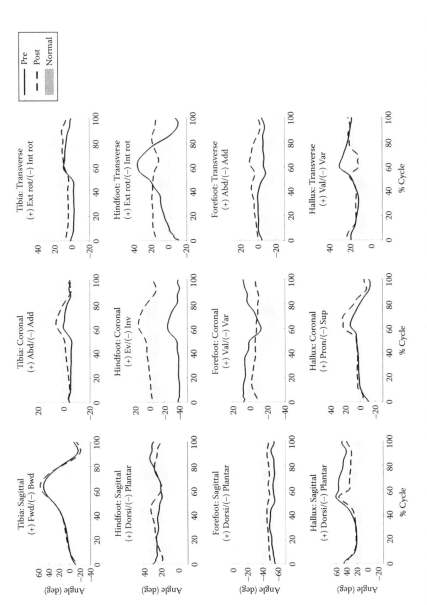

FIGURE 16.7 Pre- and postoperative foot/ankle kinematics for patient A.D., calculated using the MFM. Control results from healthy adult normals shown for comparison (mean ± 1 STD).

16.12 CONCLUSION

The quantitative assessment of multisegmental foot and ankle motion during gait is an important clinical tool for the outcomes' assessment following treatment. As illustrated in the case studies, the application of this methodology provides a detailed evaluation of motion at the tibia, hindfoot, forefoot, and hallux. In our examination of these two patients, we found a decrease in temporal-spatial parameters preoperatively, which was found to improve following surgery in both cases. Kinematically, both subjects had similar triplanar motion alterations preoperatively. Postoperatively, it appears that both subjects' motion was improved, and that mode of treatment (fusion or TAR) did not impact the magnitude of improvement overall. Noteworthily, the subject that received a TAR demonstrated greater improvement in range of motion of the hindfoot in the coronal plane. Further study will be required to clarify the nature of this finding.

This information may be clinically useful for preoperative assessment of disease severity, as well as providing a means for quantifying progression of pathology. Further investigation may lead to indications for the appropriate timing of surgical intervention, similar to the application of lower extremity gait analysis techniques to the pediatric cerebral palsy population. The integration of additional elements such as electromyogram (EMG) and plantar pressure assessment may also provide a more complete picture of foot and ankle biomechanics during gait and help relate quantified measures to clinical presentation. Additional study of a larger patient population should provide evidence as to the clinical utility of multisegmental foot and ankle motion analysis as an objective clinical outcomes' assessment tool.

REFERENCES

1. Thomas RH, Daniels TR. Ankle Arthritis: Current Concepts Review. *J Bone Joint Surg Br* 2003; 85A(5):923–936.
2. Demetriades L, Strauss E, Gallina J. Osteoarthritis of the Ankle. *Clin Orthop Relat Res* 1998; 1(349):28–42.
3. Abidi NA, Gruen GS, Conti SF. Ankle Arthrosis: Indications & Techniques. *J Am Acad Orthop Surg* 2000; 8(3):200–209.
4. Hansen ST. Posttraumatic and Degenerative Problems in the Joints. *Functional Reconstruction of the Foot and Ankle*. Philadelphia: Lippincott Williams & Wilkins, 2000:145–186.
5. Mann RA. Arthrodesis of the Foot and Ankle. In: Mann RA, ed. *Surgery of the Foot*. 7th ed. St. Louis: CV Mosby, 1999:651–699.
6. Quill GE. An Approach to the Management of Ankle Arthritis. In: Myerson MS, ed. *Foot and Ankle Disorders*. Philadelphia: Saunders, 2000:1059–1084.
7. Donatelli RA. Normal Anatomy and Biomechanics. In: Donatelli RA, ed. *The Biomechanics of the Foot and Ankle*. 1st ed. Philadelphia: F.A. Davis Company, 1990:3–31.
8. Harris GF. Analysis of Ankle & Subtalar Motion During Human Locomotion. In: Stiehl JB, ed. *Inman's Joints of the Ankle*. 2nd ed. Baltimore: Williams & Wilkins, 1991:75–84.
9. Castro MD. Ankle Biomechanics. *Foot Ankle Clin* 2002; 7:679–693.

10. Mann RA. Biomechanics of the Foot and Ankle. In: Mann RA, ed. *Surgery of the Foot*. 7th ed. St. Louis: CV Mosby, 1999:2–35.

11. Thordarson DB. Fusion in Posttraumatic Foot and Ankle Reconstruction. *J Am Acad Orthop Surg* 2004; 12:322–333.

12. Buck P, Morrey BF, Chao EYS. The Optimum Position of Arthrodesis of the Ankle: A Gait Study of The Knee and Ankle. *J Bone Joint Surg* 1987; 69A(7):1052–1062.

13. Chen YJ, Huang TJ, Shih HN, Hsu KY, Hsu RW. Ankle Arthrodesis with Cross Screw Fixation. Good Results in 36/40 Cases Following 3–7 Years. *Acta Orthop Scand* 1996; 67:473–478.

14. Mann RA, Rongstad KM. Arthrodesis of the Ankle: A Critical Analysis. *Foot Ankle Int* 1998; 19:3–9.

15. Morgan C, Henke JA, Bailey RW, Kaufer H. Long-term Results of Tibiotalar Arthrodesis. *J Bone Joint Surg* 1985; 67A:546–549.

16. Takaura Y, Tanaka Y, Sugimoto K, Akiyama K, Tamai S. Long-term Results of Arthrodesis for Osteoarthritis of the Ankle. *Clin Orthop Relat Res* 1999; 361:178–185.

17. Mazur JM, Schwartz E, Simon SR. Ankle Arthrodesis: Long Term Follow-Up with Gait Analysis. *J Bone Joint Surg* 1979; 61A(7):964–975.

18. Wu WL, Su FC, Cheng YM, Huang PJ, Chou YL, Chou CK. Gait Analysis After Ankle Arthrodesis. *Gait Posture* 2000; 11(1):54–61.

19. Demottaz JD, Mazur JM, Thomas WH, Sledge CB, Simon SR. Clinical Study of Total Ankle Replacement with Gait Analysis. *J Bone Joint Surg* 1979; 61A(7):976–988.

20. Easley ME, Vertullo CJ, Urban WC, Nunley JA. Total Ankle Arthroplasty. *J Am Acad Orthop Surg* 2002;10:157–167.

21. Stauffer RN, Chao EYS, Brewster RC. Force and Motion Analysis of the Normal, Diseased, & Prosthetic Ankle Joint. *Clin Orthop* 1977; 127:189–196.

22. Johnson JE, Kidder SM, Abuzzahab FS. Three-Dimensional Motion Analysis of the Adult Foot & Ankle. In: Harris GF, Smith P, eds. *Human Motion Analysis*. Piscataway, NJ: IEEE Press, 351–369.

23. Johnson JE, Harris GF. Pathomechanics of Posterior Tibial Tendon Insufficiency. *Foot Ankle Clin* 1997; 2(2):227–237.

24. Myers KA, Wang M, Marks RM, Harris GF. Validation of a Multisegment Foot & Ankle Kinematic Model for Pediatric Gait. *IEEE Trans Neural Syst Rehabil Eng* 2004; 12(1):122–130.

25. Johnson JE, Lamdan, Granberry WF, Harris GF, Carrera GF. Hindfoot Coronal Alignment: A Modified Radiographic Method. *Foot Ankle Int* 1999; 20(12):818–825.

26. Kidder SM, Abuzzahab FS, Harris GF. A System for the Analysis of the Foot & Ankle Kinematics during Gait. *IEEE Trans Rehabil Eng* 1996; 4(1):25–32.

27. Abuzzahab FS, Harris GF, Kidder SM. Foot & Ankle Motion Analysis System Instrumentation, Calibration and Validation. In: Harris GF, Smith P, eds. *Human Motion Analysis*. Piscataway, NJ: IEEE Press, 1996:152–166.

28. Kim CW, Jamali A, Tontz W, Convery FR, Brage ME, Bugbee W. Treatment of Post-Traumatic Ankle Arthritis with Bipolar Tibiotalar Osteochondral Shell Allografts. *Foot Ankle Int* 2002; 23(12):1091–1102.

29. Tontz WL, Bugbee WD, Brage ME. Use of Allografts in the Management of Ankle Arthritis. *Foot Ankle Clin* 2003; 8(2):361–373.

30. Resch S. Functional Anatomy and Topography of the Foot and Ankle. In: Myerson MS, ed. *Foot and Ankle Disorders*. Philadelphia: Saunders; 2000:25–49.

31. Perry J. Anatomy and Biomechanics of the Hindfoot. *Clin Orthop* 1983; 177:9–15.

17 Total Ankle Arthroplasty: A Pre- and Postoperative Analysis of Gait*

James W. Brodsky, Fabian E. Pollo, and Brian S. Baum

CONTENTS

17.1 INTRODUCTION

Total ankle arthroplasty has been in a renaissance over the last decade. This second generation of ankle replacement prostheses appears to be more successful in providing pain relief for arthritic conditions while maintaining at least some of the function of the ankle joint (Figure 17.1 and Figure 17.2). Early and intermediate results of second-generation prostheses have been promising, pointing to trends of greater longevity than the earlier two generations of ankle arthroplasty, which were plagued by subsidence and mechanical failures.[3,6,7,9] The mechanical demands on the tibiotalar joint are tremendous. This is a function of the small size of the weight-bearing surface of the talus, the complex motions of the ankle and the hindfoot, and the mechanical effect of deformities and arthritis in the hindfoot and midfoot on the ankle. The latter consideration is an important and complex influence and is expressed primarily as deformities of some or all of the "triple joints" (subtalar, calcaneocuboid, and talonavicular joints), or of fixed deformities of the midfoot. Further mechanical difficulties of total ankle arthroplasty are related to the limited anatomic structures available for balancing and correction of severe deformities.

---

* Disclaimer: The original work contained in this Chapter was submitted for publication to a peer-reviewed journal prior to the publication of this book.

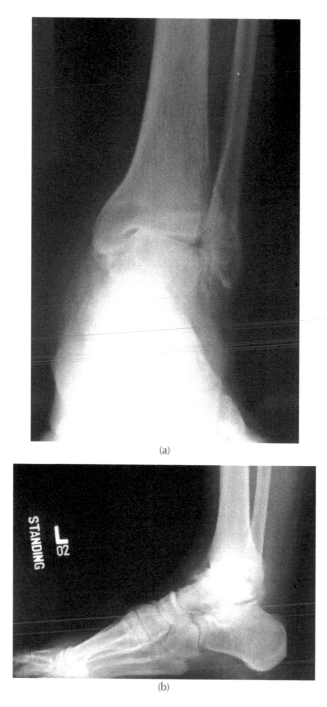

(a)

(b)

FIGURE 17.1 (a) AP radiograph of patient with primary arthritis of the tibiotalar joint in a position of varus deformity. (b) Lateral radiograph of this patient. Note the varus position of the hindfoot as well.

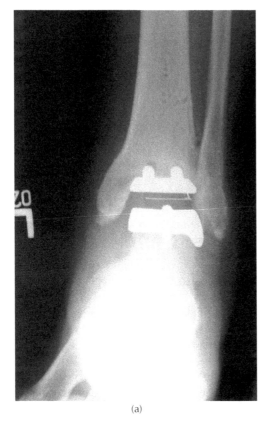

(a)

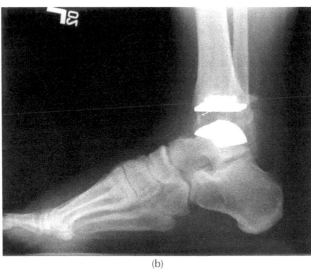

(b)

FIGURE 17.2 (a) AP radiograph of the patient postoperatively after a total ankle arthroplasty. (b) Lateral postoperative radiograph.

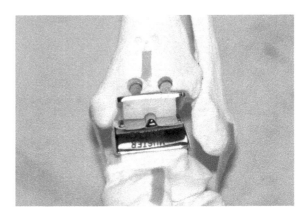

FIGURE 17.3 Model of STAR prosthesis. Note the mobile polyethylene bearing between the tibial plate and talar component. Note also that the talar component covers medial and lateral facets of the talar dome.

Recent studies[4,10] have shown that large coronal plane deformities, i.e., varus or valgus (greater than 12°), were more likely to result in early mechanical failure of total ankle arthroplasty. Techniques for reconstruction have included balancing soft tissue releases together with the use of a larger polyethylene spacer, or lateral ligament reconstruction using the peroneal tendons.[8]

The conventional clinical wisdom on total ankle arthroplasty has been that the procedure can be effective for relief of pain, but that it does not produce improvement in range of motion. Significant controversy still remains regarding the indications and relative advantages and disadvantages of total ankle arthroplasty to ankle arthrodesis. However, total ankle replacement is gaining in acceptance and popularity in Europe, the U.S., and around the world. A number of new prosthetic designs have been introduced in recent years. Most of these have employed a mobile bearing model, as does the Scandinavian Total Ankle Replacement (STAR) prosthesis (Figure 17.3). Mobile bearings are considered to reduce the strain on the polyethylene component of the prosthesis.[2] They have been used widely in total knee arthroplasty for the main purpose of reducing polyethylene wear and enhancing range of motion.

Other complicating factors with regard to total ankle arthroplasty include existing concomitant or secondary arthritis of the hindfoot and midfoot joints both before and after replacement surgery. This prospective study was designed to investigate the hypothesis that total ankle arthroplasty is effective in improving objective parameters of gait in patients with unilateral tibiotalar arthritis.*

17.2 MATERIALS AND METHODS

17.2.1 PATIENT DEMOGRAPHICS

A prospective gait analysis study was performed on 49 patients (11 males and 38 females) who were enrolled in a Food and Drug Administration (FDA) clinical trial of the STAR.

---

* This chapter presents the preliminary data of this study.

Patients were recruited on a consecutive basis as they presented to the lead author's clinic and they met the inclusion criteria of the study. Patient inclusion criteria included:

Moderate or severe pain, loss of mobility, and loss of function of the ankle (Buechel–Pappas Scale total score of less than 50 and Buechel–Pappas pain score of 20 or less)[2]

Primary arthritis, posttraumatic arthritis, or rheumatoid arthritis

At least 6 months of conservative treatment for severe ankle conditions, confirmed by the patient's medical history, radiograph studies, and medication record

Patients meeting any of the following criteria were excluded from the study:

Active or prior deep infection in the ankle joint or adjacent bones

Prior arthrodesis at the involved site

Obesity (weight greater than 250 lb)

Hindfoot malpositioned by more than 35° or forefoot malalignment, which would preclude a plantigrade foot

Avascular necrosis of the talus

Insufficient ligament tissue, which would preclude ligament reconstruction when indicated

Motor dysfunction due to neuromuscular impairment, insulin-dependent diabetes, peripheral neuropathy, or Charcot changes

Once each patient met the inclusion/exclusion criteria, they gave informed consent before participation.

The 49 patients had an average height of 164.5 ± 8.7 cm, weight of 79.7 ± 19.8 kg, and age of 60.9 ± 11.2 yr (range: 37–80 yr) at the time of surgery. Unilateral STAR total ankle arthroplasty was performed on each patient. Three of the patients had a diagnosis of rheumatoid arthritis, and the remainder had a diagnosis of advanced primary osteoarthritis or posttraumatic arthritis of the tibiotalar joint. All had failed a trial of nonoperative therapy of a minimum of 6 months, although the mean duration of arthritic symptoms was 8 yr, with a range of 2 to 30 yr.

17.3 SURGICAL PROCEDURE

The surgical technique has been described and is basically as follows.[1] The ankle was approached through an anterior vertical incision, developing the interval between the tibialis anterior and extensor hallucis longus tendons. The neurovascular bundle was retracted laterally. A vertical, midline capsulotomy of the ankle joint was performed. Subperiosteal dissection was performed on the distal portion of the anterior tibia and continued over the ankle joint. The anterior tibial osteophytes were removed with osteotomes.

Positioning of the tibial jigs for the arthroplasty was done under fluoroscopic control in the anteroposterior (AP) and medial–lateral planes. The horizontal cuts to remove the articular surface of the distal tibia and the top of the talar dome were performed with a large straight power saw and osteotomes. Preparation for the talar component was done by creating a series of chamfered cuts on the medial–lateral and anterior–posterior portions of the talar body. Both the tibial and talar saw cuts are designed to remove a minimal amount of bone.

The talar component has a central fin that fits into a sagittally oriented slot created in the body of the talus. The talar component is designed with a metallic undersurface for bone ingrowth. It was inserted first. The tibial component has a flattened metallic surface with a similar surface for bony ingrowth. It is inserted into the distal tibia from the anterior aspect of the ankle and depends upon two parallel barrel-shaped slots for fixation in the distal tibial metaphysis.

The last major step of the procedure requires the sizing and placement of the polyethylene mobile bearing. This has a flat superior and curved inferior surface to match the contour of the corresponding tibial and talar metallic components, respectively. There is a groove in the undersurface of the mobile bearing to correspond with a sagittally oriented, raised ridge in the center of the talar component.

A suction drain was placed after closure of the joint capsule. The lower limb was placed in a bulky, soft, sterile dressing and fiberglass splint for the first 10 to 14 d postoperatively. Cast immobilization was then continued for another 2 to 3 weeks. The patient then was placed into a removable walking boot and allowed to weight-bear, beginning at approximately 1 month after surgery. This was followed by a course of physical therapy.

17.4 GAIT ANALYSIS

Three-dimensional gait analysis was performed between 1 and 2 weeks prior to the ankle replacement surgery and then again at 1 yr after surgery. These tests were repeated on successive anniversaries of the original surgery up to 5 yr following surgery. Gait analysis data are reported for the most recent postoperative findings for each patient (average of 2.40 ± 1.23 yr postoperatively, range: 0.71–5.13 yr), comparing these to each patient's preoperative values.

Pre- and postoperative gait analyses were collected at 100 Hz using a 12-camera Vicon Motion Capture System (Vicon Peak, Lake Forest, CA). Kinetic parameters were collected with 2 AMTI OR6-5 force platform (Advanced Medical Technology, Inc., Newton, MA) recordings at 1000 Hz, which were embedded in the center of a 12-m walkway. Inverse dynamics were used to derive kinetic information from the kinematic and ground reactive force data. Prior to testing, 14-mm passive reflective markers were secured to anatomic locations with double-sided adhesive tape using a modified Helen Hayes Marker configuration.[5] Markers were placed bilaterally on the anterior superior iliac spine, posterior superior iliac spine, lateral thigh, lateral epicondyle of the knee, anterior and lateral tibia, lateral malleolus, heel, and second metatarsal head. Extra markers were placed during a static trial on the medial knee epicondyle and the medial malleolus.

Subjects were requested to walk barefoot at a self-selected pace up and down this walkway. Ten trials were collected for averaging and further statistical analysis.

17.4.1 GAIT ANALYSIS RESULTS

Temporal-spatial parameters collected, including velocity, cadence, stance phase percentage, stride length, and step width, are summarized in Table 17.1. On average, patient

TABLE 17.1
Temporal-Spatial Parameters

	Velocity (cm/sec)	Cadence (steps/min)	Support Time (% gait cycle)	Stride Length (cm)	Step Width (cm)
Pre-Op	81.2 ± 17.5	101.9 ± 11.2	63.1 ± 3.2	95.2 ± 16.8	14.3 ± 3.9
Post-Op	104.8 ± 16.4	112.9 ± 8.3	62.1 ± 2.1	111.2 ± 13.7	15.2 ± 4.8
p-Value	< 0.0001*	< 0.0001*	0.017	< 0.0001*	.0.25

*Statistically significant differences between pre- and postoperative values.

cadence, stride length, and, consequently, velocity significantly increased postoperatively ($p < .0001$ for all). Total support time decreased significantly but step width was unchanged postoperatively.

The most notable effects were demonstrated at the operated ankle itself. The study patients preoperatively had an ankle range of motion during gait of $14.0 \pm 4.9°$, while at the last follow-up visit, ankle range of motion increased by an average of over 3° or 23% ($p < 0.0001$; Figure 17.4). Most of this increase in range of

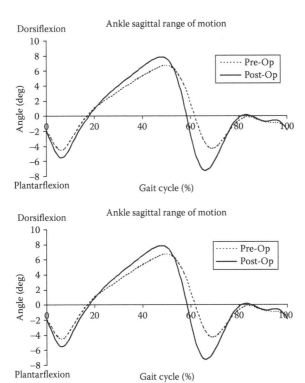

FIGURE 17.4 Average ankle sagittal range of motion pre- and postoperatively during the gait analysis.

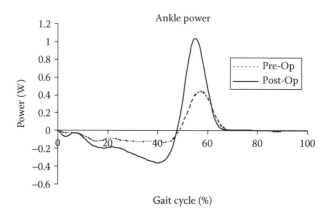

FIGURE 17.5 Average ankle push-off power pre- and postoperatively during the gait analysis.

motion came from an increase in plantar flexion motion near terminal stance and initial swing.

Peak external ankle dorsiflexion moment significantly increased postoperatively by 20% ($p = 0.0002$). Maximum sagittal ankle joint power (Figure 17.5) at push-off also significantly increased by 75%, from 0.68 ± 0.42 W before surgery to 1.19 ± 0.43 W after surgery ($p < 0.0001$).

17.5 DISCUSSION

The preliminary data of this study are presented. Although there is a relatively short follow-up, the study showed a number of interesting and unanticipated results. The unanticipated result was the unequivocal demonstration of improvement in sagittal range of motion of the ankle following total ankle arthroplasty. As noted above, this difference was statistically significant. Statistical significance, of course, does not equate to clinical significance and the improvement of a few degrees of range of motion may be of uncertain clinical meaning.

It is interesting to note that while a small amount of improvement occurred in dorsiflexion, the majority of improvement in range of motion occurred in plantar flexion. These are patients who had very limited range of motion preoperatively, with the average being $14 \pm 5°$ prior to surgery. The increase of 3° was an increase of almost 25%, although even by this measure, this is still a rather limited range of motion.

The improvement in ankle power was less surprising. This clearly showed improvement in the patient's ability to push off in the later stages of the stance phase of gait.

What is less certain is the relationship of the improved range of motion and the increased ankle power with the other objective temporal-spatial parameters of gait. The patients had increased gait velocity. Of course, velocity is the product of stride length and cadence, both of which were independently increased at statistically significant levels. The step width did not diminish, but the support time as a percentage of the gait cycle did decrease at a statistically significant, although smaller, amount.

The most important unanswered question raised by this study regards the source of the patient's improved gait, i.e., pain relief vs. biomechanical change. These data cannot afford a conclusive insight into this question. The improvement in gait could be a function of the improved mechanical function of the ankle itself. On the other hand, it would be highly likely to be influenced by the patient's diminished pain. All gait studies examining the ankle and foot in this fashion have faced this dilemma to a greater or lesser extent. This is particularly true, given the past treatment of the foot and ankle in gait analysis as a single unit or "black box." Current and future strides in segmental motion analysis of the foot and ankle, as discussed in other chapters of this book, hold important promise for our understanding and discrimination of other factors that will hopefully help to address this question.

This study is also limited to a single surgical technique. Total ankle arthroplasty addresses only one of the two major sets of joints, referred to in layman's terms as "the ankle region," viz. the tibiotalar joint. But many patients have arthritic involvement or sustain injury to both the tibiotalar and the "triple joints."

In some of our patients, concomitant, persistent, or even worsening disease of the hindfoot joints can occur. This limits subtalar function and may be a prominent or dominant source of pain and thus could limit the clinical effectiveness of isolated total ankle arthroplasty. On the other hand, while many of our patients did have concomitant hindfoot arthritis, it is encouraging that objective gait improvement was achieved even while addressing only the tibiotalar component of arthritis.

All photos and tables in this chapter are copyrighted by James W. Brodsky, MD.

REFERENCES

1. Anderson, T., Montgomery, F., et al. (2004). "Uncemented STAR total ankle prostheses." *J Bone Joint Surg Am* 86-A Suppl 1(Pt 2):103–111.
2. Buechel, F.F., Sr. Buechel, F.F. Jr., et al. (2003). "Ten-year evaluation of cementless Buechel-Pappas meniscal bearing total ankle replacement." *Foot Ankle Int* 24(6):462–472.
3. Easley, M.E., Vertullo, C.J., et al. (2002). "Total ankle arthroplasty." *J Am Acad Orthop Surg* 10(3):157–167.
4. Haskell, A., Mann, R.A., (2004). "Perioperative complication rate of total ankle replacement is reduced by surgeon experience." *Foot Ankle Int* 25(5):283–289.
5. Kadaba, M.P., Ramakrishnan, H.K., et al. (1990). "Measurement of lower extremity kinematics during level walking." *J Orthop Res* 8(3):383–392.
6. Kitaoka, H.B., Patzer, G.L., et al. (1996). "Clinical results of the Mayo total ankle arthroplasty." *J Bone Joint Surg Am* 78(11):1658–1664.
7. Kitaoka, H.B., Patzer, G.L., et al. (1994). "Survivorship analysis of the Mayo total ankle arthroplasty." *J Bone Joint Surg Am* 76(7):974–979.
8. Kofoed, H. (2004). "Scandinavian total ankle replacement (STAR)." *Clin Orthop* 424:73–79.
9. Valderrabano, V., Hintermann, B., et al. (2004). "Scandinavian total ankle replacement: a 3.7-year average followup of 65 patients." *Clin Orthop Relat Res* 424:47–56.
10. Wood, P.L., Deakin, S. (2003). "Total ankle replacement. The results in 200 ankles." *J Bone Joint Surg* Br 85(3):334–341.

18 Dynamic Poly-EMG in Gait Analysis for the Assessment of Equinovarus Foot

Alberto Esquenazi

CONTENTS

18.1 INTRODUCTION

Limb deformities and gait dysfunction are common consequences of the upper motor neuron syndrome (UMNS), which is seen commonly after neurological injuries of the central nervous system. Such injuries may result from a stroke, traumatic brain injury, cerebral palsy, anoxia, spinal cord diseases, and other degenerative processes of the brain or spinal cord. UMNS is characterized by impaired motor control in the sensorimotor action system, in combination with impaired production and control of voluntary movement due to muscle paresis and spasticity.[4, 18–20]

A net imbalance of muscle forces across joints can lead to dynamic (muscle overactivity), static (changes in rheologic features of viscous, elastic, and plastic properties of muscle), and contractural changes (permanently shortened length of a muscle-tendon system), resulting in ankle-foot joint deformities that produce an equinovarus foot deformity and resulting gait dysfunction.[3–5,17] Physiotherapy, bracing, serial casting, chemodenervation, and surgery have been used to treat this foot deformity and attempt to restore joint balance through stretching and muscle-specific weakening and strengthening. Surgical procedures attempt to restore the balance of forces across the joint through selective muscle lengthening, tendon transfer, and release or selective denervation of the deforming muscles.[12,16] Clinical examination and observational gait analysis have been the mainstays of evaluation for most physicians treating this type of patient.[1] However, these clinical techniques provide limited and often insufficient diagnostic methods in the evaluation of UMNS limb deformities and the resulting gait abnormalities. For example, an equinovarus foot deformity results from the combined potential action of multiple muscles crossing the ankle that may be spastic and/or weak. For this reason, standard clinical examination and observational gait assessment have been identified as inadequate diagnostic methods in the evaluation of gait abnormalities.[7–10,13–15,24] This is particularly important when treatments with botulinum toxin or surgery are contemplated.[4,6,26]

Instrumented gait analysis utilizes dynamic electromyographic, kinetic, and kinematic data to help characterize movement disorders (Figure 18.1). The objective of dynamic poly-EMG and gait analysis is to assess muscle activity patterns, select specific muscles that may be contributing to the deformity and those that may be playing a compensatory role, and to predict the functional behavior after treatment intervention.

Despite the logic behind instrumented gait analysis, its practical contribution to surgical decision making is not well understood. Many authors are now reporting the contributions of instrumented gait analysis in providing valuable diagnostic information, altering treatment considerations, and improving outcomes.[7–12,21,22,29]

Multiple muscle agonists and antagonists acting for all the joint movements in the upper and lower limbs exist. This redundancy of motor control is very valuable in normal physiology, but when a central nervous system injury with resulting UMNS takes place, the source of the functional impairment may be difficult to localize.[4,27,28,31]

The equinovarus ankle-foot posture may result from various sources. A muscle-specific treatment approach that identifies the deformity-generating forces or the presence of contracture produces the best outcomes when treating the equinovarus spastic foot. Dynamic-EMG of the selected musculature is necessary to determine

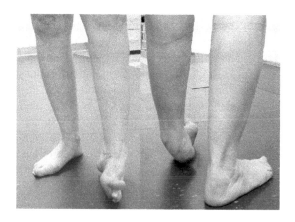

FIGURE 18.1 A patient's abnormal ankle-foot posture during standing A–P and P–A.

the muscles that produce the deformity and to appropriately implement treatment strategies.[3,5,7,8,12]

18.2 METHODOLOGY

At our institution, gait analysis is performed routinely for most patients with gait dysfunction who are under consideration for treatment intervention (chemodenervation or surgical reconstruction) of complex ankle-foot deformities. Gait studies for these patients utilize a standard protocol and are performed by experienced staff. A physical examination is performed first to determine anthropometric measurements, passive joint motion, muscle strength, motor control, muscle tone, and spasticity.[3–5,7,9,11]

Gait studies collect kinetic and kinematic data using a bilateral CODA mx1 optoelectronic active marker system (Charnwood Dynamics), two force platforms (Bertec), and dynamic EMG data with recording surface and wire electrodes (Motion Lab). Surface and wire electrodes are two practical means of obtaining skeletal muscle electrical responses, which can determine the timing of activation during gait. Surface electrodes are placed over the superficial leg muscles, while Teflon® coated bipolar wire electrodes made in our laboratory (as described by Basmajian[1]) are inserted into the deeper leg muscles. Nine muscle-tendon units crossing the ankle are commonly included in this clinical protocol: tibialis anterior and posterior, extensor hallucis and digitorum longus, peroneus longus, flexor hallucis and digitorum longus, gastrocnemius, and soleus. The moment arms for the muscles crossing the ankle have been described to help understand the contribution of each muscle to equinovarus posturing. The patient completes at least ten gait cycles during the examination, and at least five representative cycles are included in the printed report and contrasted to velocity-matched normative data for analysis.

For each limb segment abnormality, the clinical questions of interest regarding each muscle include the following: (1) Does the patient have voluntary control over the given muscle? (2) Is the muscle activated dyssynergically (i.e., in antagonism to movement or with cocontraction) when the patient attempts to move the relevant joint? (3) Is the muscle resistive to passive stretch (i.e., spastic)? (4) Does the given muscle have fixed shortening (i.e., contracture)?[5,7,10] These questions are answered in part by the dynamic poly-EMG data. Dynamic poly-EMG identifies which muscles are causing or contributing to a deformity. Combined use of dynamic poly-EMG with three-dimensional (3D) motion data can differentiate spasticity (an excessive reaction to a quick stretch stimulus) from dyssynergy (a response in an antagonist muscle to the action of an agonist muscle) by showing the timing of the muscle activity in relation to the movements and forces across a joint. Motion and force data (joint moments and powers) can help to identify muscle strength and weakness, which is critical to planning surgical treatment.

In the equinovarus foot, over 20 possible muscle combinations are apparent and can be considered for chemodenervation treatment with botulinum toxin (Botox®, Allergan) or surgical intervention (tendon lengthening, transfer, or release). Soft tissue reconstruction is considered possible, if the deformity has no restrictions to bony motion and the forces can be rebalanced.[25,30,31]

18.3 EQUINOVARUS FOOT

The equinovarus foot deformity is the most common lower limb pathologic posture seen in the UMNS. The foot and ankle are in a toe-down (equinus) and inverted (varus) position. The patient frequently develops a painful bursa in the lateral aspect of the foot, particularly in the area of the base of the fifth metatarsal. During ambulation, initial contact of the foot with the ground occurs at the forefoot, and weight is borne primarily on the lateral border. Toe flexion is typically present.[4,5,7]

Equinovarus is frequently maintained throughout stance phase and inversion may increase, causing ankle instability as weight bearing is applied. Limited dorsiflexion during early and midstance prevents the appropriate forward advancement of the tibia over the stationary foot, which frequently promotes knee hyperextension. Impairment in dorsiflexion range of motion in the late stance and preswing phases interferes with push-off and forward propulsion, resulting in significant reduction in ankle joint power generation. During swing phase, the equinus posture of the foot may result in limb clearance impairment, whereas the lack of adequate posture of the foot in stance phase may result in stance phase instability of the body as a whole. Under these circumstances, correction of this problem is essential even for limited ambulation (Figure 18.2).[4,5,7,9,16,19]

Dynamic poly-EMG recordings often demonstrate prolonged activation of the gastrocnemius and soleus complex as well as the long toe flexors as the most common causes of plantar flexion. Occasionally, the gastrocnemius and soleus may activate differentially, and treatment interventions must take this into consideration. Inversion is the result of the overactivation of the tibialis posterior and anterior in combination with the gastrocnemius, soleus, and, at times, the extensor hallucis longus (EHL).

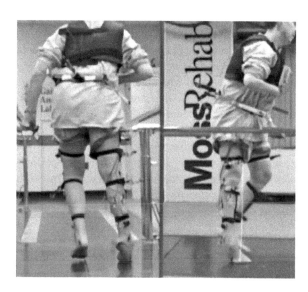

FIGURE 18.2 Example of a patient with equinovarus ankle foot posture with abnormal force application (A–P and P–A views).

If the tibialis posterior and anterior are both contributing to the varus deformity, a decision has to be made about which one of the two muscles is the main contributor. Two approaches are possible. The first one is to use the joint powers obtained as part of the kinematic data in routine gait analysis. The second consideration is a diagnostic posterior tibial nerve block with lidocaine or other short-lasting local anesthetic.[4,5,12,15–17,22]

Surgical lengthening of the Achilles tendon is indicated when the patient's foot and ankle position is not adequately controlled by an orthosis, or when attempting to make the patient brace-free. Because equinus and toe curling usually accompany the varus deformity, a lengthening of the Achilles tendon should be performed first and the toe flexor tendons divided. When calf weakness is evident by ankle plantar flexor powers, the flexor digitorum longus (FDL) tendon can be transferred to the heel to increase plantarflexion strength. When dynamic EMG has documented the tibialis anterior to be the cause of varus, a split anterior tibial tendon transfer (SPLATT) is done to correct the foot inversion. The SPLATT maintains half of the tendon on the medial aspect of the foot and transfers the other half to the lateral side of the foot (cuboid). When spasticity of the tibialis posterior muscle is present, a myotendinous lengthening of the tendon is performed posterior and slightly proximal to the medial malleolus.

In striated toe or hitchhiker's toe, the great toe is held in extension throughout the gait cycle. Ankle equinus and varus may accompany this foot posture. At times, lesser toe flexion is also noted. Dynamic poly-EMG can elucidate the contribution of an overactive gastroc–soleus group or underactive tibialis anterior to this deformity, because the EHL may be overactive in an effort to compensate for the lack of dorsiflexion in swing phase. Many of these patients complain of shoe wear problems with discomfort from pressure of the hallux against the top of the shoe box. An overactive EHL muscle can be fractionally lengthened by transecting the tendon as it overlies the muscle belly, or it can be transferred to the midfoot to assist in the balanced dorsiflexion of the foot.[7,11,12,18,22] Symptomatic plantar fasciitis may also become evident after interventions to reduce ankle plantar flexor spasticity are carried out and the patient increases his or her walking.

In a recent study, patients with equinovarus foot deformities were evaluated by two surgeons before and after laboratory gait analysis, and a surgical plan was formulated.[7] Overall a change was made in 64% of the surgical plans after the gait study was made available to them for review. The frequency of changing the surgical plan was not significantly different between the more and less experienced surgeons. The agreement between surgeons increased from 0.34 to 0.76 ($p = 0.009$) after the gait study data were made available to them. The number of surgical procedures planned by each surgeon became more similar after the gait studies. In this study, correction of the equinovarus foot deformity was seen in all patients who underwent surgical treatment based on the gait analysis results.

Sample of the EMG recordings from selected muscles normalized to the gait cycle is depicted in Figure 18.3. The vertical line approximately at 70% of the gait cycle indicates the end of stance time and the beginning of swing phase.

Note the electromyographic representation of clonus in the FDC, gastrocnemius, and soleus muscles for this case. Although the tibialis posterior has prolonged

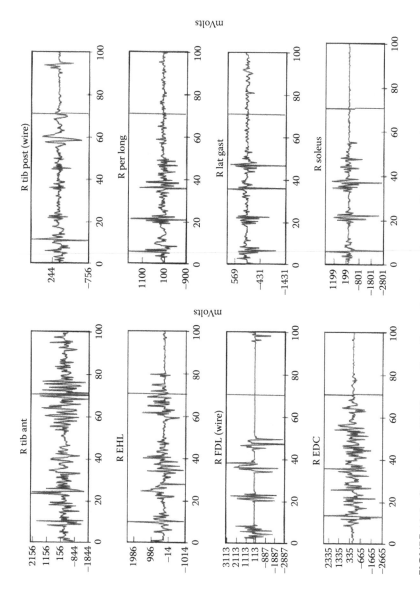

FIGURE 18.3 Sample of the EMG recordings from selected muscles normalized to the gait cycle. The vertical line at approximately 70% of the gait cycle indicates the end of stance time and the beginning of swing phase.

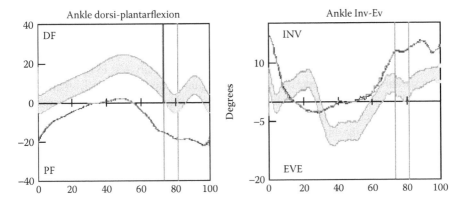

FIGURE 18.4 Sample of kinematic and kinetic data normalized to the gait cycle. The vertical line at approximately at 70% of the gait cycle indicates the end of stance time and the beginning of swing phase.

activation in stance phase, it is the abnormal activity of the tibialis anterior with some overactivity of the EHL that are the likely culprits of the inversion in the swing phase.

The clonus during stance represents a stretch response consistent with spasticity. A sample of the kinematic and kinetic data normalized to the gait cycle is depicted in Figure 18.4. The vertical line approximately at 70% of the gait cycle indicates the end of stance time and the beginning of swing phase. Table 18.1 shows a sample list of the potential deforming muscle combinations.

TABLE 18.1
Sample List of the Potential Deforming Muscle Combinations for Equinovarus Foot

G–S, TA	G–S, FHL, EHL
G–S, TP	G–S, FHL, TA, TP
G–S, TA, TP	G–S, FHL, TA, TP, EHL
G–S, TA, TP, EHL	G–S, FHL, FDL, TA
G–S, TP, EHL	G–S, FHL, FDL, TP
G–S, EHL	G–S, FHL, FDL, TA, TP
G–S, FHL , TA	G–S, FHL, FDL, TA, EHL
G–S, FHL, TP	G–S, FHL, FDL, TA, TP, EHL

Note: G-S = gastrocnemius-soleus; TA = tibialis anterior; TP = tibialis posterior; EHL = extensor hallucis longus; FHL = flexor hallucis longus; FDL = flexor digitorum longus

---

18.4 CONCLUSIONS

Gait dysfunction resulting from spasticity and contracture, and impaired motor control after upper motor neuron injury can be quite complex. Dynamic poly-EMG as a component of instrumented gait analysis is a necessary test to optimize some of the available treatment interventions for the equinovarus foot deformity that results from UMNS. It is important to clearly identify the muscles involved by a combination of focused clinical examination and evaluation in the Gait and Motion Analysis Laboratory, with the intent to improve care of the patient with UMNS. Improved knowledge of the causes of a limb deformity can only improve the outcome of treatment in this patient population.

REFERENCES

1. Basmajian JV. Muscles Alive, Chapter 2, pp. 32–37. Williams and Wilkins: Baltimore, 1979.
2. Botte, MJ, Abrams, RA, Keenan, MA, Mooney, V. Limb rehabilitation in stroke patients. *J Muscoskel Med* 9:66–78, 1992.
3. Esquenazi, A. Talaty, M. Gait analysis: technology and clinical application. In: Braddom RL, ed. Physical Medicine and Rehabilitation. 2nd ed. Philadelphia, PA: WB Saunders Co., 2000:93–108.
4. Esquenazi, A, Mayer, NH, Keenan, MA. Dynamic polyelectromyography, neurolysis, and chemodenervation with botulinum toxin A for assessment and treatment of gait dysfunction. *Adv Neurol* 87:321–31, 2001.
5. Esquenazi, A. Computerized gait analysis for rehabilitation and surgical planning in upper motor neuron syndrome. *Eura Medicophys* 35:111–118, 1999.
6. Etnyre, B, Chambers, CS, Scarborough, N, Cain, TE. Preoperative and postoperative assessment of surgical intervention for equinus gait in children with cerebral palsy. *J Pediatr Orthop* 13:24–31, 1993.
7. Fuller, DA, Keenan MA, Esquenazi, A, Whyte, J, Mayer, N, Fidler-Sheppard, R. The impact of instrumented gait analysis on surgical planning: treatment of spastic equinovarus deformity of the foot and ankle. *Foot Ankle Int* 22(8):738–743, 2002.
8. Gage, JR. Surgical treatment of knee dysfunction in cerebral palsy. *Clin Orthop Relat Res* 45–54, 1990.
9. Keenan, MA, Creighton, J, Garland, DE Moore, T. Surgical correction of spastic equinovarus deformity in the adult head trauma patient. *Foot Ankle* 5:35–41, 1984.
10. Keenan, MA. Surgical decision making for residual limb deformities following traumatic brain injury. *Orthop Rev* 17:1185–1192, 1988.
11. Keenan, MA, Lee, GA, Tuckman, AS, Esquenazi, A. Improving calf muscle strength in patients with spastic equinovarus deformity by transfer of the long toe flexors to the os calcis. *J Head Trauma Rehabil* 14:163–175, 1999.
12. Keenan, MA, Esquenazi, A, Mayer, NH. Surgical treatment of common patterns of lower limb deformities resulting from upper motoneuron syndrome. *Adv Neurol* 87:333–346, 2001.
13. Keenan, MA, Perry, J. Evaluation of upper extremity motor control in spastic brain-injured patients using dynamic electromyography. *J Head Trauma Rehabil.* 5:13–22, 1990.

14. Kerrigan, DC, Gronley, J, Perry, J. Stiff-legged gait in spastic paresis. A study of quadriceps and hamstrings muscle activity. *Am J Phys Med Rehabil* 70:294–300, 1991.

15. Kerrigan, DC, Annaswamy, TM. The functional significance of spasticity as assessed by gait analysis. *J Head Trauma Rehabil* 12:29–39, 1997.

16. Lee, GA, Keenan, MA. Management of lower extremity deformities following stroke and brain injury. In: *Chapman's Orthopaedic Surgery* (Chapman, MW.3201–43). Philadelphia: Lippincott, Williams & Wilkins Publishers, 2001.

17. Mayer NH, Esquenazi, A, Wannstedt, G. Surgical planning for upper motoneuron dysfunction: the role of motor control evaluation. *J Head Trauma Rehabil* 11:37–56, 1996.

18. Mayer, NH, Esquenazi, A, Keenan, MA, Fuller, DA. Approach to management of motor dysfunction after acquired brain injury. *Arab Medico* 18:65–70, 2000.

19. Mayer, NH, Esquenazi, A, Keenan, MA. Analysis and management of spasticity, contracture, and impaired motor control. In: Horn LJ, Zasler, ND, eds. *Medical Rehabilitation of Traumatic Brain Injury.* Philadelphia: Hanley & Belfus, 1996: 411–458.

20. Mayer, NH, Esquenazi, A, Keenan, MA. Patterns of upper motoneuron dysfunction in the lower limb. *Adv Neurol* 87:311–9, 2001.

21. Miller, F, Cardoso Dias, R, Lipton, GE, Albarracin, JP, Dabney, KW, Castagno, P. The effect of rectus emg patterns on the outcome of rectus femoris transfers. *J Pediatr Orthop* 17:603–607, 1997.

22. Molteni. Clinical and kinematic gait modifications after surgical correction of equino-varus foot deformity in hemiplegic adults. Archives paper.

23. Perry, J, Waters, RL, Perrin, T. Electromyographic analysis of equinovarus following stroke. *Clin Orthop Relat Res* 47–53, 1978.

24. Perry, J. Distal rectus femoris transfer. *Dev Med Child Neurol* 29:153–158, 1987.

25. Perry, J. Determinants of muscle function in the spastic lower extremity. *Clin Orthop Relat Res* 288:10–26, 1993.

26. Piccioni, L, Keenan, MA. Surgical management of the spastic equinovarus foot deformity. *Oper Tech Orthop* 2:146–150, 1992.

27. Pinzur, MS, Sherman, R, DiMonte-Levine, P, Kett, N, Trimble, J. Adult-onset hemi-plegia: changes in gait after muscle-balancing procedures to correct the equinus deformity. *J Bone Joint Surg Am* 68:1249–57, 1986.

28. Pinzur, MS. Surgical correction of lower extremity problems in patients with brain injury. *J Head Trauma Rehabil* 44:69–77, 1996.

29. Sutherland, DH, Santi, M, Abel, MF. Treatment of stiff-knee gait in cerebral palsy: a comparison by gait analysis of distal rectus femoris transfer verses proximal rectus release. *J Pediatr Orthop* 10:433–441, 1990.

30. Waters, RL, Frazier, J, Garland, D, Jordan, C, Perry, J. Electromyographic gait analysis before and after treatment for hemiplegic equinus and equinovarus deformity. *J Bone Joint Surg Am* 64A:284–288, 1982.

31. Young, S, Keenan, MA, Stone, LR. The treatment of spastic planovalgus foot defor-mity in the neurologically impaired adult. *Foot Ankle* 10:317–324, 1990.

19 The Challenge of the Diabetic Foot

Michael S. Pinzur

CONTENTS

19.1   THE PROBLEM AND THE CHALLENGE

The American Diabetes Association estimates that over 60,000 lower extremity amputations are performed yearly on the 16 to 18 million individuals with diabetes in the U.S.[1–3] Three to four percent of diabetic individuals will have a foot ulcer at any point in time. Fifteen percent will develop a foot ulcer or foot infection at some point in their lifetime. Eighty-five percent of diabetes-associated amputations are preceded by the development of a foot ulcer. The development of a foot ulcer in individuals with diabetes is currently appreciated as the risk-associated marker for lower extremity amputation.

The primary risk factor for the development of a diabetic foot ulcer is peripheral neuropathy, as measured by insensitivity to the Semmes–Weinstein 5.07 (10 g) monofilament (Figure 19.1).[4–8] When diabetic patient populations are screened, one in four is insensate to the monofilament.[9,10] Other associated risk factors include peripheral vascular disease; history of ipsilateral partial; contralateral partial or total foot amputation; history or presence of foot ulcer or infection; and bony/mechanical deformity, i.e., hammertoes, bony prominences, etc.

In an era of evidence-based medicine, it appears that programs that combine the preventive strategies of foot-specific patient education, prophylactic skin and nail care, and therapeutic footwear have become well-accepted methods capable of decreasing the risk for the development of diabetic foot ulcers and lower extremity amputations.[3,9–12] These health science data take on even more importance when one understands that following lower extremity amputation, individuals with diabetes experience a significant negative impact on health-related quality of life, are at increased risk for

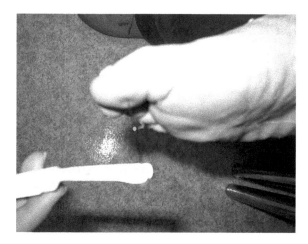

FIGURE 19.1 The Semmes–Weinstein 5.07 (10 g) monofilament is applied to areas at risk for the development of a diabetes-associated foot ulcer (under the pulps of the toes or the plantar surface underlying the metatarsal heads) with sufficient force to deform the filament (corresponding to 10 g of direct pressure). Individuals who are incapable of identifying the 10 g of applied pressure have lost protective sensation and are at substantially increased risk for developing diabetes-associated foot morbidity.

undergoing amputation of the contralateral limb, and have an accelerated risk for death at an earlier age.[13–15]

The pathophysiology responsible for the development of diabetic foot ulcers and the design of preventive and protective devices present many challenges to the bioengineering community. Paul Brand, in his studies of Hansen's Disease (leprosy), showed that repetitive shear forces applied to the skin overlying bony prominences are responsible for the tissue failure/ulceration in insensate individuals.[16] The normal human foot is a remarkable terminal organ of weightbearing, which is composed of 26 linked bones and a cushioned underlayer composed of muscle, uniquely differ-entiated connective tissue, and durable skin. The linked motion between these small bones is minimal and occurs in multiple planes. Engineering load transmission between and through the individual bones is also very complex and difficult to measure (Figure 19.2). The goal of this discussion is to present the beauty and the challenge of the adult diabetic foot to the bioengineering community. The disciplines of medicine and bioengineering will need to work together to develop methods, both internal and external, to tackle this epidemic problem that faces our community.

19.2 THE NORMAL ADULT FOOT

Inman's classic studies in the 1950s gave us a model of foot biomechanics that has been scientifically substantiated over time.[17,18] The axis of motion of the ankle joint is directed approximately 15° (5 to 25°) outward from the forward line of walking progression (Figure 19.3). The arc of normal motion at the ankle joint is from

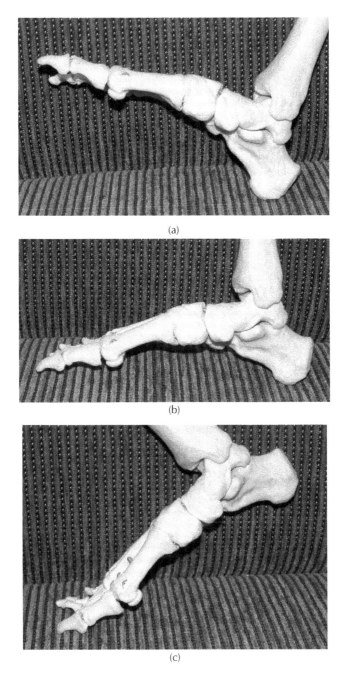

FIGURE 19.2 The positions of the joints of the foot and the loads applied to the bones and joints are appreciably different, depending on the period of the gait cycle: (a) heel strike, or initial loading response, (b) foot flat, or (c) push-off, propulsion phase. Within each of these phases, the loading forces change appreciably during the deceleration associated with initial loading or the acceleration during push-off.

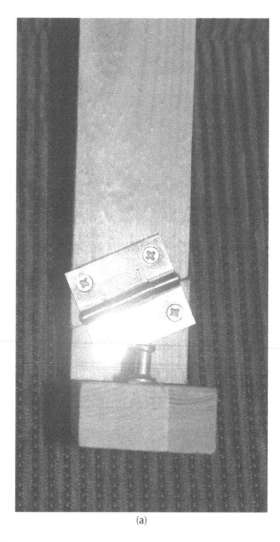

(a)

FIGURE 19.3 The axis of motion of the ankle joint is directed approximately 15° outward from the line of walking progression. (a) Neutral ankle position that occurs during midswing phase and foot-flat segment of stance phase. (b) External rotation plane of ankle motion achieved with ankle dorsiflexion.

approximately 30 to 40°of dorsiflexion to 30° of plantarflexion. The plane of motion of the hindfoot (talocalcanealnavicular and subtalar joint complex) occurs at an angle of approximately 45° to the plane of motion of the ankle joint (Figure 19.4). The arc of motion in this joint complex is substantially less, and rotates about a central axis during the stance phase of gait. The motion of these two important joint complexes is linked, so that the normal foot assumes a preload position of supination coupled with dorsiflexion of the ankle at heel-strike (initial loading). As loading progresses from heel-strike to foot-flat to push-off, the foot rotates, i.e., pronates about a central axis.

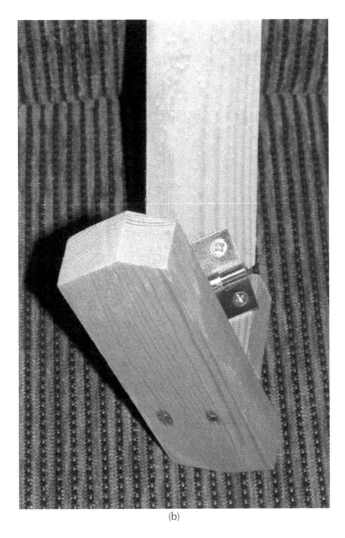

(b)

FIGURE 19.3 (Continued).

While this complex-linked motion is occurring during the stance phase of gait, an intricate load shift occurs at the tarsal–metatarsal joint. It has long been held that the medial three metatarsals are stable, with motion occurring at the more mobile fourth and fifth tarsal–metatarsal joints. It appears that the kinetic activity at this joint complex is much more complex than earlier understood. The arc of dorsiplantar flexion, which occurs at this joint complex, is approximately 6°. During the early stance phase, there is a shift of load from the stable medial tarsal–metatarsal junction laterally to the fourth and fifth tarsal–metatarsal joints. This allows the efficient transfer of a great deal of loading force during midstance, without the necessity of a great deal of motion (Figure 19.5).[19]

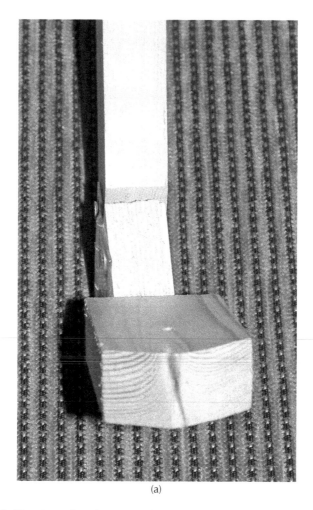

(a)

FIGURE 19.4 The plane of motion of the hindfoot (subtalar joint complex) occurs approximately 45° to the plane of motion of the ankle joint.

The coordinated muscle activity that controls this highly tuned load transfer apparatus acts to provide a mechanically locked (pronated) and stable foot at terminal stance. This allows the quadriceps muscle complex of the thigh to extend the knee against a stable foot and ankle complex to achieve push-off/walking propulsion.

Another unique loading characteristic of the foot and ankle is the eccentric loading of the foot. The weightbearing loading vector of the hip is directly applied across the hip joint from the acetabulum to the femoral head. Likewise, the tibia is directly loaded by the femur, and the talus by the tibia. This is not true with the talocalcaneal joint, where the talus overlies the medial aspect of the calcaneus, creating eccentric loading of the calcaneus (Figure 19.6).

In summary, normal walking requires a complex coordination of joint motion and bony stability, complex load transfer, and dynamic motor control. The magnitude

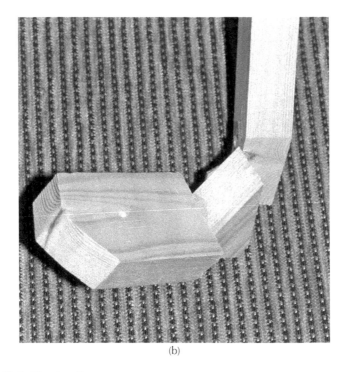

(b)

FIGURE 19.4 (Continued).

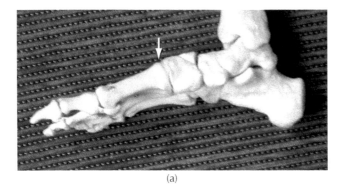

(a)

FIGURE 19.5 (a) There is only a 6° vertical arc of motion at the tarsal–metatarsal joint. (b) During this small arc of motion that occurs as the foot is positioned in plantarflexion for push-off, the load is shifted from the medial side of the five joint complex to the lateral joints.

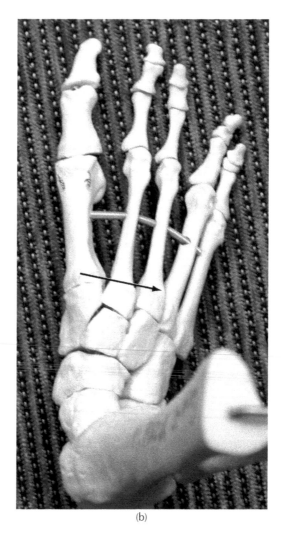

(b)

FIGURE 19.5 (Continued).

of each of these kinetic activities is small, and current available technology is relatively cumbersome and inadequate to determine the small magnitudes of change.

19.3 PATHOPHYSIOLOGY OF DIABETIC FOOT ULCERS

The development of diabetes-associated foot ulcers is due to multiple related factors. The objective designation of risk status is based on lack of protective sensation as measured by insensitivity to the Semmes–Weinstein 5.07 (10 g) monofilament (Figure 19.1). It has long been thought that sensory peripheral neuropathy simply identified a loss of protective sensation. If this were true, other individuals with a simple lack of protective sensation would develop tissue breakdown/ulceration at

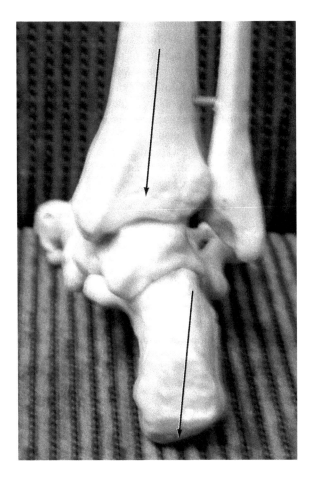

FIGURE 19.6 Most joints are directly loaded by the joint above. In the ankle, the force of body mass is loaded through the tibia, but is accepted by the calcaneus. This creates a bending moment in the linkage between tibia and calcaneus.

the same rate as the diabetic. This is simply not the case. Identification of sensory peripheral neuropathy highlights the associated presence of both motor and vasomotor peripheral neuropathies.

Peripheral neuropathy affects smaller motor nerves before it affects larger motor nerves. Foot and ankle dorsiflexor muscles are smaller; hence their efferent motor nerves are smaller and are affected earlier in the disease process than the larger plantarflexor muscles and nerves. This leads to dynamic ankle equinus/plantarflexion loading during stance phase. Not surprisingly, it has been shown that this increased loading leads to increased forefoot loading under the heads of the metatarsals, and bony failure at the midfoot leading to the development of Charcot foot arthropathy.[20,21] As the sensory and motor neuropathies are developing, a concurrent vasomotor neuropathy affects vessel tone and the ability to return venous fluid. This development of chronic soft-tissue swelling makes the tissues less able to tolerate the shear and pressure forces applied during walking. Morbid obesity appears to magnify these loads, increasing the potential for tissue failure.[22] In addition, there are differences in the quality and durability of the connective tissues covering the bones, which possess differences in stiffness (elastic modulus). This multitude of factors leads to tissue failure and skin ulceration.

Once the skin fails and ulcerates, the ability of the diabetic to mount an immune/healing response is impaired by the disease process.[23] The end result of the associated effects of diabetes is cumulative shear and pressure loading of tissues with underlying static bony and dynamic motor deformities that are not capable of withstanding these otherwise normally applied forces. Hence, the affected diabetic individual host is not capable of withstanding the normally applied loads that occur during walking.

19.4   PREVENTION OF DIABETIC FOOT ULCERS

The current strategy for preventing the development of diabetic foot ulcers is a combination of foot-specific patient education, prophylactic professional skin and nail care, and the use of therapeutic/protective footwear. Current technology allows us simply to accommodate for the structural deficiencies of the foot with footwear that attempts to dissipate the pathologic loading forces. These devices are very restrictive and do not allow for altered accommodation during high-stress periods of walking (Figure 19.7). When the deformities become worse, our current solution is to add more structural immobility with cumbersome protective orthoses (Figure 19.8).

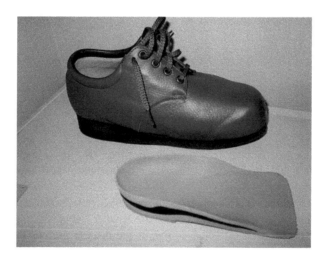

FIGURE 19.7 Commercially available therapeutic footwear used to prevent the development of diabetes-associated foot morbidity. The depth inlay shoe is composed of soft leather that will accommodate for deformity with its high toe box and accommodate volume fluctuation/swelling by its lacing capacity. The custom accommodative foot orthosis is composed of pressure-dissipating materials that dissipate point loading to bony prominences over a large surface area, as well as lessening the shear forces applied to the foot.

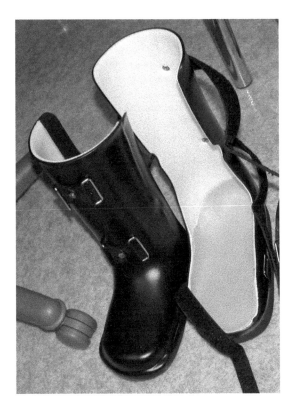

FIGURE 19.8 Charcot Restraint Orthotic Walker (CROW). This device is custom fabricated and lined with pressure and shear-dissipating materials. It tends to be very cumbersome but affords some element of protection. (From Morgan, JM, Biehl III, WC, and Wagner, FWW Jr. *Clin Orthop* 1993; 296:58–63.)

When these devices become incapable of protecting the diabetic foot with deformity due to Charcot arthropathy, we attempt surgical correction (Figure 19.9). While generally successful in correcting the deformity, surgical successes are achieved by corrective osteotomy and fusion. While a stable and plantargrade foot can be achieved, this "success" is achieved at the cost of motion. This now makes the role of accommodative/protective footwear even more crucial.

19.5 THE CHALLENGE OF THE DIABETIC FOOT

In this discussion, the factors that contribute to the development of diabetes-associated foot morbidity and the current low-tech strategies that are used in treatment have been highlighted. The challenges to the bioengineering community are great. The motion segments that need to be evaluated are anatomically small and their motion segment excursions are of a very small magnitude. The transmission of loading force is very complex and is intimately related to the position of the foot

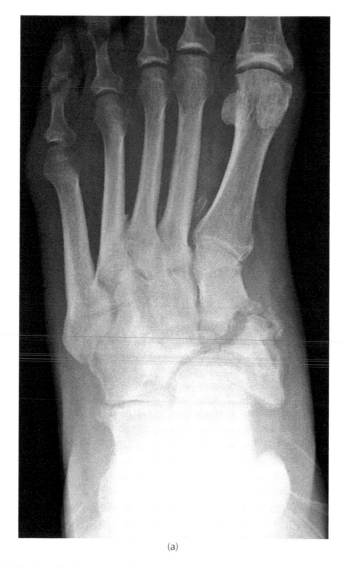

(a)

FIGURE 19.9 (a,b) Radiographs of a patient who failed at nonoperative accommodative care. (d) Radiograph following successful surgical stabilization (c).

and the temporal timeline of the gait cycle. The greatest challenge may be in evaluating the actual forces that lead to tissue breakdown, with shear being the greatest culprit and the most difficult force to measure.

Our current methods of treatment afford protection to the diabetic foot externally by accommodative immobilization or internally by surgical stabilization, and are

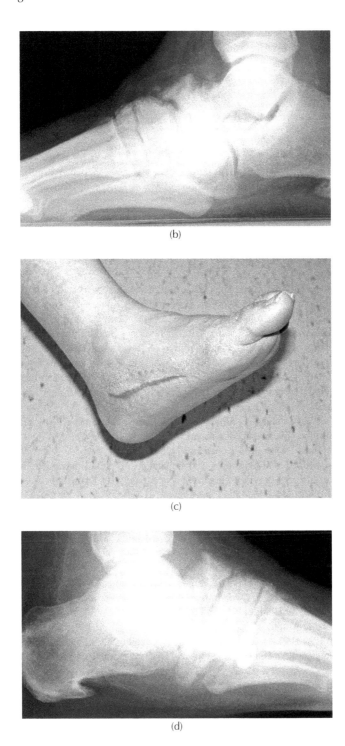

(b)

(c)

(d)

FIGURE 19.9 (Continued).

both achieved at the cost of eliminating normal motion. The challenge issued to the bioengineering community is to develop methods to measure the small motion segments of the foot, better understand the method of force transmission therein, and measure the pathologic forces leading to tissue failure.

REFERENCES

1. National Diabetes Fact Sheet. United States Department of Health and Human Services. Washington, DC. http://www.cdc.gov/diabetes/pubs/pdf/ndfs_2003.pdf.
2. Reiber, GE, Lipsky, BA, and Gibbons, GW. The Burden of Diabetic Foot Ulcers. *Am J Surg* 1998; 176(2A suppl):5S–10S.
3. Mason, J, et. al. A Systematic Review of Foot Ulcer in Patients with Type 2 Diabetes Mellitus. Prevention and Treatment. *Diabet Med* 1999; 16:801–812.
4. Apelqvist, J, Agardh, CD. The Association Between Clinical Risk Factors and Outcome of Diabetic Foot Ulcers. *Diabetes Res Clin Pract* 1992; 18:43–53.
5. McNeeley, MJ, Boyko, EJ, Ahroni, JH, Stensel, VL, Reiber, GE, Smith, DG, and Pecoraro, RF. The Independent Contributions of Diabetic Neuropathy and Vasculopathy in Foot Ulceration. *Diabetes Care* 1995; 18:216–219.
6. Rith-Najarian, SJ, Stolusky, T, and Gohdes, DM. Identifying Diabetic Patients at High Risk for Lower Extremity Amputation in a Primary Health Care Setting. A Prospective Evaluation of Simple Screening Criteria. *Diabetes Care* 1992; 15:1386–1389.
7. Veves, A, Uccioli, L, Manes, C, Van Acker, K, Komninou, H, Philippides, P, and Katsilambros, N. Comparison of Risk Factors for Foot Problems in Diabetic patients Attending Teaching Hospital Outpatient Clinics in Four Different European States. *Diabet Med* 1994; 11:709–713.
8. Olmos, PR, Cataland, S, O'Dorisio, TM, Casey, CA, Smead, WL, and Simon, SR. The Semmes–Weinstein Monofilament as a Potential Predictor of Foot Ulceration in Patients with NonInsulin-Dependent Diabetes. *Am J Med Sci* 1995; 309:76–82.
9. Pinzur, MS, Kernan-Schroeder, D, Emmanuele, NV, and Emmanuele, MA. Development of a Nurse-Provided Health System Strategy for Diabetic Foot Care. *Foot Ank Int* 2001; 22:744–746.
10. Pinzur, MS, Slovenkai, MP, and Trepman, E. Guidelines for Diabetic Foot Care. *Foot Ank Int* 1999; 20:695–702.
11. Malone, JM, Snyder, M, Anderson, G, Bernhard, VM, Holloway, GA, and Bunt, TJ. Prevention of Amputation by Diabetic Education. *Am J Surg* 1989; 158:520–525.
12. Larsen, J, Apelqvist, J, Agardh, CD, and Steinstrom, A. A Decreasing Incidence of Major Amputation in Diabetic Patients: A Consequence of a Multidisciplinary Foot Care Team Approach. *Diabet Med* 1995; 12:770–776.
13. Lavery LA, VanHoutum WH, and Harkless LB. In-Hospital Mortality and Disposition of Diabetic Amputees in The Netherlands. *Diabet Med* 1996; 13:192–197.
14. Gregg EW, Beckles GL, Williamson DF, Leveille SG, Langlois JA, Engelgau MM, and Narayan KM. Diabetes and Physical Disability among Older U.S. Adults. *Diabetes Care* 2000; 23:1272–1277.
15. Pinzur MS, Gottschalk F, Smith D, Shanfield S, Shanfield S, deAndrade R, et al. Functional Outcome of Below-Knee Amputation in Peripheral Vascular Insufficiency: A Multicenter Review. *Clin Orthop* 1990; 286:247–249.
16. Brand, PW. Repetitive Stress in the Development of Diabetic Foot Ulcers. In: Levin, ME, O'Neil, LW, eds. *The Diabetic Foot.* 4th Edition. St. Louis: CV Mosby, 1988:83–90.

17. Saunders, JBM, Inman, VT, and Eberhart, HD. The Major Determinants in Normal and Pathologic Gait. *J Bone Joint Surg* 1953; 35A:543–558.
18. Inman, VT, Ralston, HJ, and Todd, F. *Human Walking*. Baltimore: Williams and Wilkins, 1981.
19. Lakin, RC, DeGnore, LT, and Pienkowski, D. Contact Mechanics of Normal Tarsal-metatarsal Joints. *J Bone Joint Surg Am* 2001; 83A(4):520:520–528.
20. Mueller, MJ, Sinacore, DR, Hastings, MK, Strube, MJ, and Johnson, JE. Effect of Achilles Tendon Lengthening on Neuropathic Plantar Ulcers. *J Bone Joint Surg* 2003; 85A:1436–1445.
21. Pinzur, MS, Sage, R, Stuck, R, Kaminsky, S, and Zmuda, A. A Treatment Algorithm for Neuropathic (Charcot) Midfoot Deformity. *Foot Ankle* 1993; 14:189–197.
22. Pinzur, MS, Freeland, R, and Juknelis, D. The Association between Body Mass Index and Diabetic Foot Disorders. *Foot Ank Int* 2005; 26:375–377.
23. Bibbo, C, Lin, SS, Beam, HA, and Behrens, FF. Complications of Ankle Fractures in Diabetic Patients. *Orthop Clin North Am* 2001; 32:113–133.
24. Morgan, JM, Biehl III, WC, and Wagner, FWW Jr. Management of Neuropathic Arthropathy with the Charcot Restraint Orthotic Walker. *Clin Orthop* 1993; 296:58–63.

20 The Biomechanics of the Diabetic Foot

William Ledoux

CONTENTS

20.1 INTRODUCTION

Diabetes mellitus is a progressive disease that can have deleterious effects on the foot and ankle, most notably ulceration, infection, and subsequent amputation. Ulcers can be neuropathic, vascular (ischemic), or mixed (neuroischemic) in etiology.[79] Complications of diabetes in the lower extremity include arterial insufficiency or peripheral vascular disease, peripheral neuropathy, and musculoskeletal abnormalities, each of which has been associated with the development of foot ulcers.[13,73] Reduced blood flow can lower tissue oxygenation and decrease wound healing, both of which can contribute to ulceration. However, increasingly the role of foot biomechanics in the

317

development of ulcers is being appreciated. Peripheral neuropathy can result in an insensitive foot with altered structure and function, and musculoskeletal abnormalities (including foot deformities, stiffer soft tissue, and reduced joint range of motion) can lead to aberrant loading conditions (compression or shear) on the soft tissues of the foot. The resulting neuropathic ulcer is caused by mechanical insult to the insensate foot.[20.] A critical triad of neuropathy, minor foot trauma, and foot deformity has been found to occur in greater than two thirds of the causal pathways to ulceration.[64]

The purpose of this chapter is to explore the effect of diabetes mellitus on the biomechanics of the foot. We will begin with an overview of the etiology of diabetic neuropathic foot ulcers, which are more common than ischemic ulcers.[20,79] We will also review the effects of diabetes on soft-tissue characteristics, gait patterns, joint range of motion, Ground Reaction Force (GRFs), and foot deformities. Finally, we will describe how foot structure relates to plantar pressure and ulceration, and how aberrant loading (normal and shear) is related to plantar ulceration.

20.2 ETIOLOGY OF DIABETIC NEUROPATHIC ULCERATION

20.2.1 PERIPHERAL VASCULAR DISEASE

Among people in the U.S. older than 40 yr of age, peripheral vascular disease is more than twice as prevalent in people with diabetes than without (10 vs. 5%).[59] Lack of an adequate blood supply decreases tissue resilience, causes rapid tissue death, and interferes with normal wound healing.[73] Wound healing is disrupted because the tissues are not receiving enough oxygen, nutrients, or soluble mediators critical to the repair process.[71] Multifactorial studies have found that arterial insufficiency was a positive risk factor for the development of ulcers.[13,79] However, despite the clear role in ulcer development, arterial insufficiency is not often sufficient in and of itself for diabetic neuropathic ulceration; rather, other factors must be present as well.

20.2.2 PERIPHERAL NEUROPATHY

Although it is well accepted that peripheral neuropathy consists of deficits in all three components of the peripheral nervous system (sensory, motor, and autonomic), it is often the case that sensory neuropathy is emphasized.[17] While sensory neuropathy plays a very important role in the development of neuropathic ulcers, there are also motor and autonomic neuropathic components that should be considered as well.

Peripheral *sensory neuropathy* can lead to loss of light-touch feeling, vibration perception, and protective sensation.[27] Indications of sensory neuropathy to the patient can be paresthesia (tingling), thermal and touch insensitivity, and numbness.[27] Sensory neuropathy can be disastrous to the diabetic patient; due to absent protective sensation, accidental mechanical or thermal trauma to the foot may occur unbeknownst to the patient. This trauma can lead to inflammation, tissue breakdown, ulceration, and infection.[22]

Sensory neuropathy, as quantified using several different measures, has been found to be an independent predictor of ulcers in several multifactorial studies.[1,13,66,79] Rith-Najarian et al. and Boyko et al. found positive relationships between insensitivity to Semmes–Weinstein 5.07 mm (10 g) monofilament and ulcers[13,66] Abbott et al. determined that there was a positive relationship for both vibration perception threshold and a reflex/muscle strength score and ulcers,[1] while Walters et al. associated absent light-touch sensation with ulceration.[79]

Motor neuropathy can affect both the intrinsic and extrinsic musculature of the lower extremity. Andersen et al. found a significant decrease in muscle strength when comparing 56 Type 1 diabetic neuropathic patients with gender-, age-, and BMI (body mass index)-matched healthy controls.[6] The diabetic patients had a 21% reduction in both ankle dorsiflexor and ankle plantar flexor strengths. In 1997, the same group also examined 8 diabetic neuropathic patients, 8 diabetic nonneuropathic patients, and 16 healthy subjects matched for age, gender, and BMI using magnetic resonance imaging (MRI).[4] They found that the neuropathic patients had 41% of the ankle dorsiflexor and plantar flexor strengths of the nonneuropathic patients. Furthermore, using stereological imaging techniques, the neuropathic patients had a 32% reduction in the volume of the nonneuropathic patients. Bus et al. used MRIs of frontal plane sections to explore how diabetic neuropathy affects the intrinsic musculature.[17] They determined that there was a 73% decrease in the muscle cross-sectional area between the diabetic neuropathic subjects and the controls. Intrinsic muscle weakness can lead to extrinsic muscles that function earlier and for a longer period of time without the stabilizing influence of the intrinsics; this results in "extensor substitution," also known as the "intrinsic minus foot." This imbalance has been associated with toe deformities (claw and/or hammer toes), prominent metatarsal heads, equinus contractures, and/or a varus hindfoot[11,73] although some recent studies have contradicted this notion (see below).[17,77] Motor neuropathy can also lead to an altered gait pattern that may lead to aberrant pressures and subsequent ulcer formations.[22]

Loss of autonomic control can indirectly lead to ulceration. The process begins by simply causing a loss of sweating in the foot, which can lead to dry, cracked skin that serves as an entry point for infection.[27,67] This is often the key symptom for indicating autonomic neuropathy.

20.2.3 MUSCULOSKELETAL ABNORMALITIES

Since this chapter deals with the biomechanics of the diabetic foot, musculoskeletal abnormalities are a central component of this review. As such, we will go into much greater detail on how diabetes causes altered tissue properties (e.g., stiffer plantar soft tissue), aberrant foot mechanics (e.g., reduced joint range of motion), and specific deformities (e.g., hammer/claw toes) later in the chapter. For now, suffice to say that diabetes greatly alters the lower extremity musculoskeletal system.

20.2.4 ABERRANT LOADING

The musculoskeletal abnormalities discussed in this chapter all result in increased loading through the soft tissue in the foot. Aberrant loading can be normal to the skin surface (compressive) or tangential (shear); both types of forces have been associated with ulcer development.[12,25,78] Mechanical stresses are closely related to the development of neuropathic ulcers as diabetic neuropathic foot trauma may occur in three ways.[11] Constant pressure over a period of hours may exacerbate vascular problems and lead to ischemic ulcers. High, localized pressure due to a foreign body (a nail or a stone) in a shoe can cause immediate damage. Lastly, repetitive moderate stress (probably the most common cause in neuropathic patients) can lead to inflammatory autolysis.

Brand recognized that most wounds to insensitive feet are not caused by ischemia from continuous pressure or traumatic injury, but rather due to moderate stresses repeated again and again on the same location on the foot.[14] As such, he studied the effect of repetitive moderate loading levels by conducting animal experiments. Rat feet were stimulated with repetitive pressures of 137 kPa; the footpads could withstand 10,000 repetitions a day without apparent damage. Hyperemia, edema, and an increased temperature were noted, but all subsided with rest. If, however, the same test were repeated the next day on the same foot, the swelling occurred earlier and subsided slower. After a week, the inflamed areas of the footpad became ulcerated and necrotic. In additional experiments, with less cycles (8000) and with weekends to rest, the loading patterns did not lead to ulcer development, but the footpad became hypertrophic.

Peripheral vascular disease, peripheral neuropathy (sensory, motor, and autonomic), foot deformity, and aberrant soft-tissue loading are all important etiologic considerations in the development of diabetic neuropathic foot ulcers.

20.3 THE EFFECT OF DIABETES ON SOFT-TISSUE CHARACTERISTICS

20.3.1 PLANTAR SOFT TISSUE

Several studies have demonstrated that diabetes mellitus can alter the mechanical characteristics of the plantar soft tissue. This is important because stiffer, less compliant tissue will not properly distribute loads, which can lead to abnormally high normal and shear stresses. Hsu et al. compared 20 age-matched healthy subjects with 21 patients with Type 2 diabetes.[37,38] Using an ultrasound-based device, the authors loaded and unloaded the plantar tissues and generated stress–strain plots (Figure 20.1). They found that diabetic tissue had increased energy absorption and a decrease in the rate of tissue recovery in diabetic heel pads. Also using an ultrasound device, other researchers have shown that the plantar soft tissues were stiffer and thinner in four older diabetic subjects, as compared to four young, nondiabetic tissues.[81] It should be noted that the effects of age and diabetes could not be easily separated in this study. Another group has used an indentor system (consisting of a load cell mounted on a three-dimensional measurement device) to study the plantar tissue beneath the metatarsal heads of 20 diabetic subjects with peripheral neuropathy and a history of ulcers and 20 control subjects matched for age, gender, and BMI.[44] They determined that the diabetic tissue was stiffer than the control tissue. It has also been demonstrated that the plantar soft tissue of diabetic neuropathic patients is harder than the tissue of age-matched diabetic nonneuropathic or control subjects.[62] Diabetic plantar soft tissue has been shown to

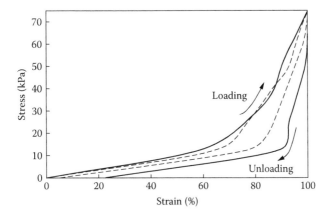

FIGURE 20.1 The stress–strain curve for the plantar soft tissue of a 60-yr-old healthy person (dashed line) and a 58-yr-old patient with Type 2 diabetes (solid line). The difference between the area under the loading curve and the area under the unloading curve is the energy absorption. Diabetic subjects have increased energy absorption. (Reproduced from Hsu TC, Lee YS, Shau YW. *Clin Biomech* (Bristol, Avon) 17(4):291–296, 2002. With permission.)

be thinner beneath the heel and the first and second metatarsals (Table 20.1).[33] Others have shown that in the high-risk diabetic neuropathic foot peak plantar pressure at the metatarsal heads is inversely proportional to soft-tissue thickness.[2]

The alterations in diabetic plantar soft-tissue characteristics seen at the macroscopic level also have corresponding changes that occur at a cellular/microscopic level as well. Dysvascular plantar soft tissue has been shown to have decreased adipose cell size as well as more numerous, thicker, and fragmented elastic septa.[39]

TABLE 20.1

The Thickness of the Plantar Soft Tissue beneath the Heel and Metatarsal Heads

	Heel (n = 48/76)	Met 1 (n = 48/75)	Met 2 (n = 48/76)	Met 3 (n = 48/76)	Met 4 (n = 46/76)	Met 5 (n = 47/76)
Control subjects	18.62 ± 0.36	12.92 ± 0.42	14.17 ± 0.26	13.56 ± 0.29	12.91 ± 0.34	11.47 ± 0.27
Diabetic subjects	17.33 ± 0.29[a]	11.60 ± 0.29[a]	12.70 ± 0.29[a]	13.06 ± 0.24	12.10 ± 0.26	10.70 ± 0.23

[a]Statistically significantly different from control subjects.

Met = metatarsal head; n = number of controls/number of diabetic subjects.

Source: Reproduced from Gooding GA, Stess RM, Graf PM, Moss KM, Louie KS, and Grunfeld C. *Invest Radiol* 21:45–48, 1986. With permission.

These morphometric changes were quantified in a later study that found a 30% smaller mean cell area, a 16% smaller mean cell diameter, and septal walls that were 75% wider than normal.[18] Collagen fibrils in septal walls of diabetic heel pads appear distorted and fragmented, as they are no longer arranged in parallel with band periodicity.[37] Biochemical changes have been found with diabetic tissue as several parameters obtained via MRI have demonstrated differences between older, diabetic and younger, nondiabetic tissue that are consistent with increased amounts of collagen in diabetic tissue.[41] (Note that it is possible that the effects of diabetes were compounded with changes due to specimen age.)

20.3.2 Plantar Fascia

Researchers have explored how diabetes can alter the characteristics of the plantar fascia using both ultrasound[24,32] and computer tomography (CT) scans (Table 20.2A, B).[10] When compared to 21 healthy controls, diabetic patients without neuropathy ($n = 27$), diabetic patients with neuropathy ($n = 19$), and diabetic patients with neuropathy and a history of ulceration ($n = 15$) were found to have significantly thicker plantar fascia.[24,32] Similarly, Bolton et al. examined the plantar aponeurosis of 16 diabetic neuropathic subjects in contrast with the plantar aponeurosis of ten age-matched healthy subjects.[10] As with the other study, the plantar fascia was significantly thicker with the diabetic subjects.

The plantar fascia has an important role in the biomechanics of the foot, in particular, the windlass mechanism first described by Hicks, whereby the arch height can be increased when the great toe extends and pulls on the hallux.[35] It was thought

---

TABLE 20.2A

The Demographics and Plantar Fascia Thickness (n or Mean $\pm$ SD) of Control Subjects, Diabetic Subjects, Diabetic, Neuropathic Subjects, and Diabetic Neuropathic Subjects with a History of Ulcers

	Control ($n = 21$)	Diabetic ($n = 27$)	Diabetic Neuropathic ($n = 19$)	Diabetic Neuropathic with Ulcer History ($n = 15$)
Gender (M/F)	13/8	19/8	10/9	10/5
Age (yr)	56.6 ± 11.8	52.7 ± 12.7	53.7 ± 10.4	57.3 ± 9.6
BMI (kg/cm²)	25.0 ± 3.1	25.3 ± 3.4	27.0 ± 4.9	27.5 ± 4.1
Plantar fascia thickness (mm)	2.0 ± 0.5	2.9 ± 1.2[a]	3.0 ± 0.8[a]	3.1 ± 1.0[a]

[a]Significantly different ($p < .05$) from control subjects.

M/F = male/female; BMI = body mass index.

Source: Reproduced from D'Ambrogi E, Giurato L, D'Agostino MA, Giacomozzi C, Macellari V, Caselli A, and Uccioli L. *Diabetes Care* 26:1525–1529, 2003. With permission.

TABLE 20.2B
The Demographics and Plantar Fascia Thickness (*n* or Mean ± SD)
of Control and Diabetic Subjects

	Control (*n* = 10)	Diabetic Neuropathic (*n* = 16)
Gender (M/F)	8/2	12/4
Age (yr)	53.8 ± 9.1	55.2 ± 10.5
BMI (kg/cm²)	37.0 ± 8.6	31.7 ± 7.6
Plantar fascia thickness (mm)	3.6 ± 0.8	4.2 ± 0.9[a]

[a]Significantly different ($p < .05$) from control subjects.

M/F = male/female; BMI = body mass index

Source: Reproduced from Bolton NR, Smith KE, Pilgram TK, Mueller MJ, and Bae KT. *Clin Biomech* (Bristol, Avon) 20:540–546, 2005. With permission.

that alterations in the mechanics of the plantar aponeurosis can affect the function of the windlass mechanism; specifically, a thicker plantar fascia can result in an early onset of the windlass mechanism, resulting in a stiffer foot with reduced range of motion.[23]

Diabetic plantar soft tissue has been found to be stiffer, absorb more energy, recover more slowly, and be harder and thinner than healthy tissue. These macroscopic characteristics are also manifested with changes at the cellular level. These alterations in the plantar soft tissue can lead to the aberrant distribution of force beneath the foot. The plantar fascia is another lower extremity soft tissue that is affected by diabetes in a manner that can have biomechanical consequences. This tissue has been shown to be thicker in diabetic subjects and is thought to result in an early onset of the windlass mechanism, resulting in a stiffer foot.

20.4 THE EFFECT OF DIABETES ON THE KINEMATICS AND KINETICS OF GAIT

20.4.1 GAIT PATTERNS

Research has shown that changes in sensory perception due to peripheral neuropathy could cause changes in gait patterns.[42,51,52,65] Katoulis et al. studied 20 healthy controls, 20 diabetic non-neuropathic subjects, and 20 diabetic neuropathic subjects who were matched for age, gender, and BMI.[42] They found that diabetic neuropathic subjects walked slower than the other groups, which they acknowledge could potentially confound their results. They also found that the diabetic neuropathic subjects had smaller sagittal plane knee angles and a larger frontal plane ankle joint moment. Meier et al. compared 15 subjects with Type 2 diabetes and polyneuropathy with 15 control subjects who were matched for age, gender, and BMI.[51] They investigated gait termination and found that the diabetic neuropathic patients approached the stopping line

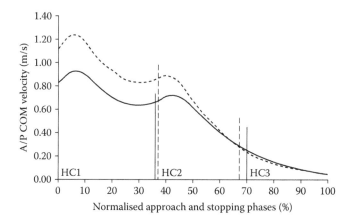

FIGURE 20.2 The mean anterior/posterior (A/P) center of mass (COM) velocity profile during the approach and stop phase. The bottom axis is normalized from the first heel contact (HC1) to velocity < 0.05 m/sec. The dashed curve is the elderly mean, while the solid line is the diabetic mean. The vertical lines represent heel contact. Diabetic subjects had a reduced velocity when approaching the stopping line. (Reproduced from Meier MR, Desrosiers J, Bourassa P, and Blaszczyk J. *Diabetologia* 44(5):585–592, 2001. With permission.)

with less velocity (Figure 20.2), had a weaker braking force, and took longer to develop the force. Using three-axis accelerometers mounted to the head and pelvis, Menz et al. studied the gait of 30 diabetic neuropathic patients and 30 age-matched controls.[52] The diabetic neuropathic patients walked slower and had a reduced cadence and step length. Those subjects also had decreased peak accelerations and a less rhythmic gait pattern than the control subjects. Richardson et al. conducted comparisons between older women matched for age and BMI ($n = 12$) with and without neuropathy ($n = 12$) while walking in standard and "challenging" environments.[65] The authors demonstrated that a challenging environment affected both control and neuropathic subjects, but that the neuropathic subjects' gait was slower, less efficient, and more variable than the control subjects'.

Alterations in gait patterns could also be generated in healthy subjects by simulating neuropathy. Eils et al. examined the effect of reduced plantar sensation via an ice immersion technique on plantar pressure during gait for 40 healthy subjects.[29] (Since they employed a first-step protocol, gait velocity was not reported.) Their results indicated a shift in the plantar pressure distribution from the heel and toes to the central and lateral forefoot and the lateral mid-foot. In 2004, the same group also found that simulated sensory neuropathy via an ice immersion technique on 20 healthy subjects caused a "cautious" walking pattern with significant changes in lower limb electromyography (EMG) patterns and ankle, knee, and hip kinematics and kinetics.[28] The specific changes included a delay in the timing of the braking force (Figure 20.3); a decreased push-off vertical force (Figure 20.3); and reduced ankle, knee, and hip angles, particularly in push-off, all indicative of an apropulsive, "cautious" walking pattern.

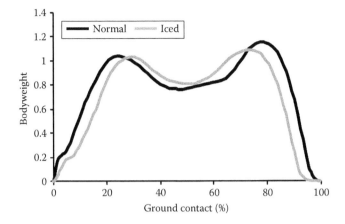

FIGURE 20.3 The GRF of normal and iced (simulating neuropathy) subjects; the peak braking force was delayed and the propulsive force was decreased with the iced subjects. (Reproduced from Eils E, Behrens S, Mers O, Thorwesten L, Volker K, and Rosenbaum D. *Gait Posture* 20:54–60, 2004. With permission.)

It is not clear that all of the changes in gait are due to loss of sensation.[26,61] Dingwell and Cavanagh examined 14 patients with severe peripheral neuropathy and compared them to 12 gender-, age-, and BMI-matched controls.[26] They found that neuropathic patients were slower and exhibited increased locomotion variability. However, they determined that the increased variability was linked to decreased self-selected velocity rather than neuropathy. The importance of velocity rather than neuropathy is supported by a recent study that compared the gait characteristics of 16 controls and 15 Type 2 diabetic subjects without neuropathy during linear walking and in turns of 0.33 and 0.66 m in diameter.[61] They found that compared to the control group, the diabetic non-neuropathic subjects walked at a slower velocity with a wider base of support for both linear walking and turning. Furthermore, the diabetic subjects also had increased flexion/extension and lateral movement at the hip, knee, and ankle compared to the control group.

Whether the changes in gait patterns seen in diabetic patients are caused by diabetic neuropathy or by the decreased velocity of the diabetic neuropathic subjects is a point of contention. Nevertheless, the data demonstrate that diabetic neuropathic patients walk differently than age-, gender-, and BMI-matched controls. Specifically, the diabetic subjects walked slower, stopped moving differently, had altered lower extremity joint kinematics, and had gait patterns that were more cautious, less efficient, and more variable.

20.4.2 Joint Range of Motion

Researchers have shown that the ankle joint's passive characteristics are altered with diabetes.[75] Trevino et al. used a single degree of freedom device to measure ankle torque while rotating the foot through dorsiflexion and plantar flexion. They used this device to study the passive ankle joint motion of 42 diabetic adults and

TABLE 20.3
The Ankle Joint Passive Characteristics (Mean ± SD) for Control and Diabetic Subjects

	Control (*n* = 41)	Diabetic (*n* = 42)
Range of motion (°)	64 ± 14	65 ± 12
Hysteresis (Nm-°)	91 ± 47	162 ± 66[a]
Stiffness, plantar flexion (Nm/°)	0.3 ± 0.1	0.7 ± 0.33[a]
Stiffness, dorsiflexion (Nm/°)	0.4 ± 0.1	0.9 ± 0.33[a]

[a]significantly different (*p* < 0.05) from control subjects.

Source: Reproduced from Trevino SG, Buford WL, Jr., Nakamura T, John Wright A, and Patterson RM. Foot Ankle Int 25:561–567, 2004. With permission.

41 age-matched subjects without diabetes. The diabetic feet had an increased hysteresis (i.e., they absorbed more energy) and were stiffer in the terminal regions of both dorsiflexion and plantar flexion (Table 20.3).

Furthermore, limited joint mobility has been associated with plantar pressures in subjects with diabetic neuropathy.[24,30,32,69,82] Fernando et al. examined diabetic patients with and without joint mobility, along with control subjects who were matched for age and gender.[30] The authors determined if limited joint mobility was present in the foot by examining the subtalar joint and first metatarsophalangeal joint. Plantar pressure was significantly higher in patients with limited joint mobility, and there was a strong negative correlation between joint mobility and plantar pressure. Sauseng and Kastenbauer explored the relationship between the range of motion at the ankle joint and first metatarsophalangeal joint, and the pressure beneath the metatarsal heads for 50 Type 1 diabetic subjects and 44 age-matched nondiabetic controls.[69] They found a significant correlation between the ankle joint range of motion and the pressure beneath the second to fifth metatarsal heads, as well as between the first metatarsophalangeal joints and the pressure beneath the fourth and fifth metatarsal heads. Zimny et al. examined ankle and first metatarsophalangeal joint mobility in 70 Type 1 or Type 2 diabetic subjects, half with neuropathy, and 30 controls subjects who were matched for age, gender, and BMI.[82] The authors found that joint mobility was severely reduced for the diabetic neuropathic patients compared to the diabetic controls and the healthy controls, and that joint mobility was strongly inversely related to the pressure time integral (a measure of pressure dosage). Another group studied the relationship between plantar fascia thickness, Achilles tendon thickness, and flexion/extension of the first metatarsophalangeal joint for 61 diabetic subjects and 21 age-, gender-, occupation-, and BMI-matched controls.[24,32] (The results of the soft-tissue thickness analysis are discussed elsewhere in this chapter.) They found that the first metatarsophalangeal joint range of motion was significantly reduced in diabetic neuropathic patients, and that this parameter was strongly related to increased vertical force.

Diabetic subjects have been found to have altered joint mechanics compared to healthy subjects. These changes included increased ankle joint hysteresis and stiffness in plantar flexion as well as dorsiflexion. It has also been shown that patients with diabetes have limited joint mobility at the ankle, subtalar, and first metatarsal joints, and that limited joint mobility was strongly associated with increased plantar pressure or increased vertical force.

20.4.3 GRFs and Pressures

In addition to motion analysis, several groups have also examined the effect of diabetes on the vertical and shear GRFs and pressures. Shaw et al. examined a wide cross section of 181 subjects, found that a subset (diabetic neuropathic subjects with previous ulcers) had increased GRFs when compared to speed-, gender-, age-, and weight-matched controls, primarily due to increased weight acceptance.[70] Conversely, Katoulis et al. (see above for study details; subjects were age-, gender-, and BMI-matched, and diabetic neuropathic patients walked slower) found that diabetic neuropathic patients had a decreased vertical component of the vertical GRF when compared to healthy controls or diabetic controls.[42] They also found that diabetic neuropathic patients had a decreased anteroposterior shear force compared to the diabetic controls. Despite this apparent discrepancy, it should also be noted that both of these studies employed force plates and reported the resultant GRFs. In other words, there was no understanding of how the forces were distributed to the various areas of the foot.

Two groups have addressed this issue by developing force platforms that were able to measure vertical and shear forces distributed beneath the foot.[31,60,76] Perry et al. employed a custom built 16 transducer array based on strain gage technology; the 4×4 array includes sensors that were 2.5 cm^2 and flush with the floor.[60] They examined 12 subjects with diabetes mellitus and loss of protective sensation. The sensor array was large enough to capture the metatarsal heads and toes. The largest vertical pressure (189 kPa) was found beneath the medial metatarsal heads, while the greatest shear (33 kPa) was located at the lateral metatarsal heads. However, no direct comparison to healthy subjects was provided. A second group examined the distributed vertical and shear forces beneath the feet of diabetic neuropathic patients and controls by rigidly attaching a pressure platform to a force plate.[31,76] This allowed for the measurement of the resultant GRF (vertical, shear, free moment, and center of pressure) and the pressure distribution, from which the local shear forces can be calculated by assuming that the local normal and shear forces are proportional. Diabetic neuropathic patients with a history of ulcers had decreased heel and big toe pressures, but increased metatarsal head pressures when compared to the controls (Table 20.4A, B, and C and Figure 20.4). Comparing diabetic neuropathic patients with a history of ulcers to controls, the anterior shear forces were smaller at the heel, while posterior, medial, and lateral forces were smaller at the hallux. However, lateral forces were greater beneath the metatarsals for diabetic neuropathic patients with a history of ulcers. The authors also found that the diabetic neuropathic patients had a significantly longer loading pattern and a reduced center of pressure excursion.

TABLE 20.4A
The Vertical GRF (Mean ± SD) of Control Subjects, Diabetic Subjects, Diabetic Neuropathic Subjects, and Diabetic Neuropathic Subjects with a History of Ulcers

	Control (n = 21)	Diabetic (n = 27)	Diabetic Neuropathic (n = 19)	Diabetic Neuropathic with Ulcer History (n = 15)
Total foot (%BW)	108.8 ± 5.2	106.8 ± 5.3	107.4 ± 5.7	107.0 ± 9.1
Heel (%BW)	93.8 ± 8.4	91.3 ± 9.0	87.3 ± 8.4[a]	83.1 ± 11.1 [a,b]
Metatarsals (%BW)	89.9 ± 6.3	93.9 ± 6.7	96.0 ± 7.0 [a]	97.5 ± 7.0 [a]
Hallux (%BW)	21.9 ± 9.2	17.1 ± 7.7 [a]	14.0 ± 6.2 [a]	10.7 ± 6.4 [a,b]

[a]Significantly different ($p < 0.05$) from control subjects.

[b]Significantly different ($p < 0.05$) from diabetic subjects.

Source: Reproduced from Uccioli L, Caselli A, Giacomozzi C, Macellari V, Giurato L, Lardieri L, and Menzinger G. *Clin Biomech* (Bristol, Avon) 16:446–454, 2001. With permission.

TABLE 20.4B
The Anteroposterior GRF (Mean ± SD) of Control Subjects, Diabetic Subjects, Diabetic Neuropathic Subjects, and Diabetic Neuropathic Subjects with a History of Ulcers

	Control (n = 21)	Diabetic (n = 27)	Diabetic Neuropathic (n = 19)	Diabetic Neuropathic with Ulcer History (n = 15)
Forward Peak				
Total foot (%BW)	15.9 ± 3.9	15.2 ± 3.3	13.3 ± 3.9[a]	13.3 ± 3.8[a]
Heel (%BW)	15.3 ± 3.6	14.8 ± 3.4	12.5 ± 3.5[a,b]	11.8 ± 3.7[a,b]
Metatarsals (%BW)	3.3 ± 1.5	2.6 ± 1.4	2.7 ± 1.9	3.0 ± 1.5
Hallux (%BW)	0.4 ± 0.7	0.5 ± 0.6	0.4 ± 0.5	0.7 ± 1.2
Backward Peak				
Total foot (%BW)	18.5 ± 3.1	16.6 ± 3.7	15.3 ± 3.7[a]	15.2 ± 3.5[a]
Heel (%BW)	0.5 ± 0.9	0.4 ± 0.8	0.9 ± 1.3	1.0 ± 1.0
Metatarsals (%BW)	13.4 ± 2.5	13.2 ± 3.3	12.6 ± 3.2	13.5 ± 3.4
Hallux (%BW)	5.3 ± 2.4	3.8 ± 2.0[a]	3.1 ± 1.9[a]	2.4 ± 1.7[a]

[a]Significantly different ($p < 0.05$) from control subjects.

[b]Significantly different ($p < 0.05$) from diabetic subjects.

Source: Reproduced from Uccioli L, Caselli A, Giacomozzi C, Macellari V, Giurato L, Lardieri L, and Menzinger G. *Clin Biomech* (Bristol, Avon) 16:446–454, 2001. With permission.

TABLE 20.4C
The Mediolateral GRF (Mean ± SD) of Control Subjects, Diabetic Subjects, Diabetic Neuropathic Subjects, and Diabetic Neuropathic Subjects with a History of Ulcers

	Control (n = 21)	Diabetic (n = 27)	Diabetic Neuropathic (n = 19)	Diabetic Neuropathic with Ulcer History (n = 15)
Medial Peak				
Total foot (%BW)	4.4 ± 2.4	3.4 ± 1.6	3.3 ± 1.7	3.9 ± 1.8
Heel (%BW)	4.4 ± 2.4	3.4 ± 1.7	3.3 ± 1.7	3.9 ± 1.8
Metatarsals (%BW)	0.5 ± 0.6	0.4 ± 0.5	0.4 ± 0.6	0.4 ± 0.7
Hallux (%BW)	0.8 ± 0.7	0.4 ± 0.5 [a]	0.2 ± 0.3 [a]	0.3 ± 0.4 [a]
Lateral Peak				
Total foot (%BW)	5.0 ± 2.3	5.0 ± 2.2	5.2 ± 2.3	6.2 ± 3.1
Heel (%BW)	3.4 ± 1.8	3.5 ± 1.9	3.6 ± 1.7	3.5 ± 1.6
Metatarsals (%BW)	3.9 ± 2.1	4.3 ± 2.0	4.4 ± 2.1	5.8 ± 3.0 [a]
Hallux (%BW)	0.9 ± 0.6	0.7 ± 0.5	0.7 ± 0.5	0.5 ± 0.4 [a]

[a] Significantly different ($p < 0.05$) from control subjects.

[b] Significantly different ($p < 0.05$) from diabetic subjects.

Source: Reproduced from Uccioli L, Caselli A, Giacomozzi C, Macellari V, Giurato L, Lardieri L, and Menzinger G. *Clin Biomech* (Bristol, Avon) 16:446–454, 2001. With permission.

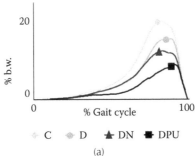

(a)

FIGURE 20.4 The (a) vertical (hallux), (b) anteroposterior (heel), and (c) mediolateral (metatarsals) GRFs for control (C), diabetic (D), diabetic neuropathic (DN), and diabetic neuropathic with previous ulceration (DPU). For the vertical hallux force, the GRF was significantly reduced for DPU, DN and D vs. C and DPU vs. D; for the anteroposterior heel force, the GRF was reduced for DPU and DN vs. D and C; for the mediolateral metatarsal force, the lateral GRF was greater for the DPU compared to C. b.w. = body weight. (Reproduced from Uccioli L, Caselli A, Giacomozzi C, Macellari V, Giurato L, Lardieri L, and Menzinger G. *Clin Biomech* (Bristol, Avon) 16:446–454, 2001. With permission.)

Anteroposterior GRF component: heel

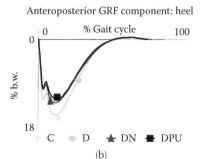

(b)

Mediolateral GRF component: metatarsals

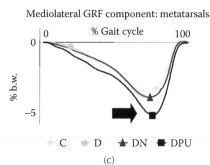

(c)

FIGURE 20.4 (Continued).

Other researchers have used plantar pressure measurement devices to study the normal pressure distribution without considering shear stresses.[68,72] Sarnow et al. used an F-Scan system to measure in-shoe pressures of 44 diabetic neuropathic patients and 65 controls who were matched for age, weight, race, and gender to determine the effect of wearing shoes on foot pressure.[68] They found significantly lower pressures on the foot for all groups when shoes were worn as compared to when walking with socks alone. They also determined that diabetic subjects exhibited higher peak pressures than the control group for all regions of the foot when socks were worn alone. Stess et al. used an EMED pressure platform to measure the peak pressures in the forefoot.[72] They considered diabetic patients without neuropathy (diabetic controls), diabetic patients with neuropathy but no history of ulcers, and diabetics with neuropathy along with a history of ulcers; the diabetic ulcer group was statistically significantly heavier than the diabetic control group. Compared with the diabetic controls, the diabetic ulcer group had higher peak pressures beneath the fourth and fifth metatarsal heads and increased pressure time integrals (a measure of pressure dosage) at all the metatarsal heads. As with Sarnow et al., this work indicates diabetic neuropathic subjects have aberrant plantar pressures.

There seems to be some debate as to whether changes in the distributed force are due to diabetes or neuropathy. A recent study by Pataky et al. compared the plantar pressure beneath the heel, first, third, and fifth metatarsals, and the great toe between 15 diabetic nonneuropathic patients and 15 nondiabetic controls who were matched for age, gender, and BMI.[58] They found that peak force decreased for the diabetic subjects beneath the heel but increased beneath the fifth metatarsal and the big toe, while remaining unchanged at the first and third metatarsals. These data seem to indicate that neuropathy is not necessary to see changes in the distributed GRF.

While analyses comparing vertical GRFs using just force plates have conflicting results, others have used specialized sensors to measure distributed pressure and shear stresses. They have found diabetic neuropathic patients with a history of ulcers had decreased plantar pressure and shear stresses beneath the heel and hallux, but increased plantar pressure and shear stresses beneath the metatarsal heads.

20.5   THE EFFECT OF DIABETES ON FOOT DEFORMITIES

There are many foot deformities that have been associated with musculoskeletal imbalances (i.e., either overpulling or underpulling on a particular muscle tendon). Some of these imbalances and their possible etiologies include: the pes planus deformity caused by posterior tibial tendon dysfunction;[49] the pes cavus deformity related to a tight Achilles tendon; a weak tibialis anterior and a normal tibialis posterior and peroneus longus;[50] the clawed hallux deformity, which is caused by overactive extensor hallucis longus, flexor hallucis longus, and/or peroneus longus;[57] and the hammer/claw toe deformity, which can be due to an imbalance between the foot extrinsic muscles (which have normal strength) and foot intrinsic muscles (which are weak).[56] Although all of these deformities can arise with diabetic subjects, it is the hammer/claw toe deformity that we will emphasize.

The plantar surface of the foot is well protected with thick fat pads that normally dissipate applied forces; problems arise, however, when these pads are displaced or atrophied.[73] One common musculoskeletal imbalance seen with diabetic subjects, which can cause displacement of the fat pads, is the hammer/claw toe deformity.[15] (Hammer toes are defined as extended metatarsophalangeal joints, flexed proximal interphalangeal joints, and extended distal interphalangeal joints, while claw toes are defined as extended metatarsophalangeal joints, flexed proximal interphalangeal joints, and flexed distal interphalangeal joints; the two have similar etiologies and are often lumped together in the literature as one deformity of the lesser toes. In the hallux, a claw toe is possible extended metatarsophalangeal joints and flexed interphalangeal joint, but a hammer toe is not; hence, the term "clawed hallux" is used, but "hammer hallux" is not.) The primary cause for this deformity has been thought to be imbalance[11,43,56,74] between the intrinsic foot muscles (the lumbricals and interosseus muscles), which are normally responsible for holding the proximal phalanx against the ground, and the extrinsic foot muscles that insert on the distal phalanx (the extensor digitorum longus and the flexor digitorum longus), which extend and flex the toes, respectively. Although all lower extremity muscles are affected by motor neuropathy in the diabetic neuropathic foot, the more distally located intrinsic muscles are affected before the extrinsic muscles are;[5] when the intrinsic muscles are weakened, it is theorized that they are overpowered by the extrinsic muscles. This is exacerbated by dorsiflexion of the metatarsophalangeal joint, which causes the moment arm of the interosseous tendons to decrease, further reducing their ability to keep the proximal phalanx plantar flexed.[9]

However, two recent studies using MRI to quantify intrinsic muscle atrophy in diabetic neuropathic subjects have raised important questions with this hypothesis.[5,17] Bus et al.'s work has been summarized elsewhere in this chapter; briefly, they found a 73% decrease in muscle cross-sectional area when comparing diabetic neuropathic patients to controls.[17] Similarly, Andersen et al. conducted a study to examine intrinsic muscle volume.[5] They considered 15 neuropathic diabetic patients, 8 non-neuropathic diabetic patients, and 23 control subjects matched for age, gender, and BMI. They found that neuropathic patients had a little more than 50% of the intrinsic muscle volume of the non-neuropathic diabetic or the control subjects. However, Bus et al. noted that only two of the eight neuropathic patients that they studied had toe deformities. They concluded that the lack of toe deformity in a representative diabetic neuropathic population suggested that intrinsic muscle atrophy may not be the primary causative factor as once thought.[17] None of Andersen et al.'s 15 diabetic neuropathic patients had a significant foot or toe deformity, which they stated "supports the notion that loss of foot muscles precedes development of toe abnormalities."[5]

In support of Bus et al. and Andersen et al.'s conclusions, Van Schie et al. pointed out "while it is commonly accepted that specific foot deformities in diabetes are the result of a muscle imbalance between intrinsic and extrinsic musculature, the relationship has not received much scientific attention to date."[77] They aimed to address this potential shortcoming in the literature by studying nerve conduction velocity, muscle weakness, and foot deformity in diabetic men, as well as the relationship between muscle weakness, foot deformities, and sensory neuropathy in diabetic men with or without motor neuropathy or foot ulceration. While the authors found a relationship between motor nerve conduction deficit and muscle weakness, they were unable to determine if muscle weakness caused foot deformities or if foot deformities caused muscle weakness. They noted that prominent metatarsal heads and toe deformities have similar etiologies and that deficiencies in the plantar aponeurosis, joint capsules, and intrinsic musculature are all likely to lead to an extended proximal phalanx.

Regardless of the specific etiology of hammer/claw toes, other research has shown that the fat pads of diabetic neuropathic subjects are displaced distally[15] and that subjects with hammer/claw toes have elevated plantar pressures.[16] Bus et al. examined 13 diabetic neuropathic subjects with toe deformity, 13 age- and gender-matched neuropathic subjects without deformity, and 13 age- and gender-matched control subjects.[15] They found that neuropathic patients with deformities had significantly thinner plantar soft tissue beneath the metatarsal heads but thicker soft tissue beneath the phalanges, indicating a distal displacement of the fat pad. In 2005, the same group also reported the plantar pressure from diabetic neuropathic subjects with ($n = 13$) and without ($n = 13$) toe deformities.[16] It was determined that feet with toe deformities had higher pressures beneath the metatarsal heads, in addition to the thinner fat pads (Figure 20.5).

The hammer/claw toe deformity is often seen with diabetic subjects. The cause is thought to be a muscle imbalance between the extrinsic and intrinsic muscles of the foot. However, recent work has shown that subjects with intrinsic muscle atrophy

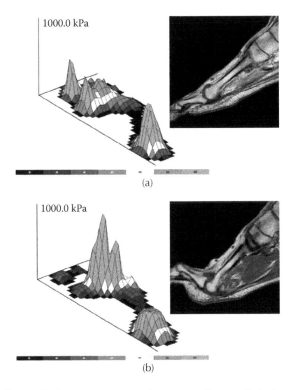

FIGURE 20.5 The peak plantar pressures and corresponding sagittal plane MRI scans for two matched subjects, one with a normally aligned toe and one with a hammer/claw toe. The foot with the deformity has a much higher pressure and a reduced fat pad thickness. (Reproduced from Bus SA, Maas M, de Lange A, Michels RP, and Levi M. *J Biomech* 38:1918–1925, 2005. With permission.)

do not have hammer/claw toes, calling the well-accepted etiology into question. It has been shown that hammer/claw toes (regardless of etiology) do have higher plantar pressures due to displaced fat pads beneath the metatarsal heads.

20.6 THE RELATIONSHIP BETWEEN FOOT STRUCTURE AND PLANTAR PRESSURE

Cavanagh et al. measured various x-ray parameters and peak plantar pressures from 50 healthy adult subjects.[21] From standard lateral and anterior/posterior radiographs, 27 measurements, i.e., static parameters, were obtained. The peak plantar pressures during walking from regions beneath the same feet were taken as dynamic functional measures. A stepwise regression was employed to determine what percentage of the variability in the peak pressure at the heel and first metatarsal head could be explained with the radiographic parameters. Only 31 and 38% of the variance in plantar pressure beneath the heel and first metatarsal, respectively, were explainable with the radiographic parameters. The authors concluded that the dynamics of gait are a major influence on plantar pressures.

Morag and Cavanagh broadened the above study by correlating both structural and functional parameters to the functional outcome of peak plantar pressure.[53] The potential predictor variables included physical characteristics, anthropometric data, passive joint ranges of motion, radiographic parameters, plantar soft-tissue mechanical properties, stride parameters, three-dimensional foot motion, and EMG data. Peak pressure values were obtained for the heel, midfoot, first metatarsal head, and hallux. A best subset regression was performed in order to limit the number of variables in the regression and to preserve physical meaning for the final models. For each of the four areas, approximately 50% of the variance could be explained by the measured structural and functional parameters, indicating that there are additional parameters that the authors have not yet considered. Nevertheless, this represented an improvement from static radiographic parameters considered alone. It should be noted that neither of the studies from Cavanagh's group concentrated on diabetic feet. However, these papers are germane to the topic because of the importance of foot structure and plantar pressure on ulcer development.

Ahroni et al. conducted an extensive study of diabetic foot pressures and their relation to a large number of possible factors, including, but not limited to, weight, neuropathic status, various foot deformities, insulin use, and history of ulceration.[3] They performed 1017 pressure recordings from 517 subjects using an F-scan in-shoe pressure sensor. Both univariate and multiple regression analyses were performed on the data; the discussion here will be limited to the parameters relevant to foot architecture. The specific foot deformities studied were hallux valgus, hallux limitus, hammer/claw toes, prominent metatarsal heads, and Charcot foot. With the univariate analysis, there was significantly increased hallux pressure with hallux valgus or hallux limitus, and significantly decreased pressure with hammer/claw toes or prominent metatarsal heads. The metatarsal head peak pressure was significantly higher with hammer/claw toes or prominent metatarsal heads, and significantly lower with hallux limitus. Finally, the peak pressure at the heel was significantly larger when hallux limitus was present. When a multivariate analysis was conducted, the peak hallux pressure was proportional to hallux limitus and hallux valgus and inversely related to hammer/claw toes; the peak metatarsal head pressure was related to prominent metatarsal heads and inversely related to hallux limitus; the peak heel pressure was not related to any biomechanical variables. These results demonstrate a relationship between foot structure and peak plantar pressure.

To determine which structural parameters best predicted forefoot plantar pressure, Mueller et al. enrolled 20 diabetic subjects with peripheral neuropathy and 20 people without diabetes who were age-, gender-, and BMI matched.[54] Their measures of foot structure were taken primarily from a CT scan of the foot (Figure 20.6), while plantar pressure was obtained with an F-Scan system. They used a hierarchical multiple regression analysis to predict peak plantar pressure at the great toe and five metatarsal heads. There were able to account for 47 to 71% of the variance for the diabetic group, with the metatarsophalangeal joint being the most important variable. For the healthy subjects, they were able to predict 52 to 83% of the variance, with

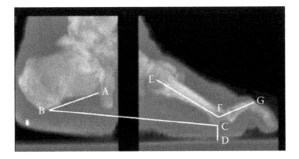

FIGURE 20.6 A lateral CT scan through the second metatarsal of a subject with diabetes mellitus. Angle ABC was a measure of calcaneal inclination, line CD was a measure of soft-tissue thickness, and angle EFG is a measure of hammer/claw toe deformity. (Reproduced from Mueller MJ, Hastings M, Commean PK, Smith KE, Pilgram TK, Robertson D, and Johnson J. *J Biomech* 36:1009–1017, 2003. With permission.)

soft-tissue thickness, hallux valgus angle, and forefoot arthropathy having the most influence.

With increasing sophistication, researchers have used various static and some dynamic measurements to predict the variance of peak plantar pressures. Recently, approximately three quarters of the plantar pressure variance has been predicted beneath the metatarsal heads of diabetic and healthy subjects.

20.7   THE RELATIONSHIP BETWEEN FOOT STRUCTURE AND ULCERATION

Several studies have either directly or indirectly investigated the relationship between foot structure and ulcer development.[8,46,55] Mueller et al. explored the relationship between foot deformity and ulcer location by retrospectively examining 42 feet with existing ulcers and foot deformity, which were classified as: (1) Charcot foot, (2) compensated forefoot varus, or (3) uncompensated forefoot varus or forefoot valgus.[55] By dividing the plantar mid-foot and forefoot into three regions, they were able to demonstrate that Charcot feet were more likely to have mid-foot ulcers (six of seven), feet with compensated forefoot varus had ulcers under the second, third, or fourth metatarsal heads (9 of 18), while feet with uncompensated forefoot varus or forefoot valgus had ulcers under the first or fifth metatarsal heads (15 of 17), thus demonstrating that ulcer location is related to the structure of the foot (i.e., foot deformity).

Bevans has demonstrated that diabetic neuropathic ulcerations may be related to biomechanical foot alignment by studying the relationship between static calcaneal stance position and the location of ulcers in diabetic subjects.[8] In this study, 28 feet from 19 patients with either active or recently healed neuropathic ulcerations were examined. All were associated with abnormal hindfoot alignment. He also noted that an everted calcaneus was associated with ulcers under the medial metatarsal heads and an inverted calcaneus was associated with ulcers under metatarsal

TABLE 20.5

Demographic, Foot Type, and Foot Deformity Variables (Mean ± SD or Percentage) by Ulcer Outcome and Odds Ratios and *p*-Values Calculated from Logistic Regressions of Ulcer Outcome on These Variables

	No Ulcer (n = 722)	Ulcer (n = 26)	OR (95% CI): Ulcer vs. None	*p*-Value
Gender (%Male)	76.3	88.5	2.38 (0.71, 7.99)	0.2
Mean age (yr)	62.3 ± 10.1	65.8 ± 10.5	1.43[a] (0.95, 2.16)	0.09
Mean BMI (kg/m²)	33.0 ± 7.0	30.9 ± 6.3	0.78[b] (0.56, 1.07)	0.1
Duration of DM >10 y (%)	42.9	53.9	1.55 (0.71, 3.38)	0.3
Neuropathy (%)	55.0	88.5	6.28 (1.88, 21.0)	0.003
Foot type (%)				0.7
Neutrally aligned	51.0	50.0	1.00	
Pes planus	29.2	34.6	1.25[c,d] (0.53, 2.98)	0.6
Pes cavus	19.8	15.4	0.77[c,d] (0.25, 2.37)	0.7
Hallux valgus (%)	23.6	42.3	1.97[c] (0.90, 4.31)	0.09
Hammer/claw toes (%)				0.001
None	53.2	38.5	1.00	
Supple	36.8	23.1	0.68[c,e] (0.25, 1.87)	0.5
Fixed	10.0	38.5	3.91[c,e] (1.57, 9.71)	0.003
Hallux limitus (%)	23.1	53.9	3.02[c] (1.37, 6.66)	0.006

[a]Per 10-yr increase.

[b]Per 5 kg/m² increase.

[c]Adjusted for neuropathy.

[d]Vs. neutrally aligned foot type.

[e]Vs. none

Source: Reproduced from Ledoux WR, Shofer JB, Smith DG, Sullivan K, Hayes SG, Assal M, and Reiber GE. *J Rehabil Res Dev* 42(5):665–672, 2005. With permission.

heads 4 and 5 (*r* = .87, *p* < .001). This investigation indicates that biomechanical foot alignment may play a major role in the development (i.e., occurrence and location) of diabetic foot complications.

More recently, Ledoux et al. examined the relationship between foot type, foot deformity, and ulceration in a group of high-risk diabetic subjects.[46] Foot type was associated with foot deformity (pes planus feet and hallux valgus or hallux limitus and pes cavus feet and hammer/claw toes), but not with ulcer outcome (Table 20.5). However, fixed hammer/claw toes and hallux limitus were associated with ulcer occurrence, affirming the relationship between foot deformity and ulceration.

Several groups have explored how foot structure is related to ulceration by demonstrating that certain foot deformities are more likely to develop ulcers in specific locations.

20.8 THE RELATIONSHIP BETWEEN PLANTAR PRESSURE AND ULCERATION

Boulton et al. studied 41 diabetic neuropathic subjects with and without a history of ulceration ($n = 22$ feet and $n = 59$ feet, respectively), 41 diabetic subjects without neuropathy ($n = 81$ feet), and 41 nondiabetic controls ($n = 82$ feet).[12] All groups were matched for age and gender. The authors noted that 100% of the neuropathic feet with previous ulcers had aberrant peak pressures (defined as greater than 11 kg/cm^2) underneath the metatarsal heads at the site of ulceration (Table 20.6). In comparison, high plantar pressures were found in 31% of the diabetic neuropathic feet without a history of ulceration, 17% of the diabetic controls, and 7% of the nondiabetic subjects. This retrospective study indicates a strong link between plantar pressure and ulcer development.

In a prospective study, Veves et al. studied diabetic patients ($n = 86$) who were neuropathic ($n = 58$) or non-neuropathic ($n = 28$).[78] They measured plantar pressures during walking as a baseline and followed the subjects for a mean period of 30 months (range of 15 to 34 months) and noted the incidence of neuropathic ulceration. Of all the patients, 43 subjects (31 neuropathic and 12 non-neuropathic) exhibited high pressures (defined as greater than 12.3 kg/cm^2) at baseline. Fifteen (35%) of the diabetic patients (14 of 31 neuropathic and 1 of 12 non-neuropathic) developed plantar ulcers (Table 20.7); all of these patients had aberrantly high pressures at baseline. In contrast, none of the patients with normal baseline pressures developed ulcers. These results demonstrate that plantar pressure is highly predictive of subsequent plantar ulceration. However, it should be noted that 17 out of 31 diabetic neuropathic patients who had high foot pressures did not develop neuropathic ulceration, suggesting that while both abnormal peak plantar pressure and insensitivity are necessary for ulceration to occur, these factors in and of themselves are not sufficient to predict ulcer development. Also, the authors did not explore if the location of the high baseline pressure was related to the location of the eventual ulcer.

Recently, a prospective study on the relationship between plantar pressure and ulceration was completed by Ledoux et al. as part of the Seattle Diabetic Foot

---

TABLE 20.6
Percentages of Feet with Abnormally High Pressures for the Four Groups

	No. Feet	% Abnormal
Diabetic subjects with neuropathy and a history of foot ulceration	22	100
Diabetic subjects with neuropathy	59	31
Diabetic subjects	81	17
Control subjects	82	7

Source: Reproduced from Boulton AJ, Hardisty CA, Betts RP, Franks CI, Worth RC, Ward JD, and Duckworth T. *Diabetes Care* 6:26–33, 1983. With Permission.

TABLE 20.7
Foot Pressure Measurements and Plantar Ulceration

	Diabetic ($n = 86$)	Neuropathic Subgroup ($n = 58$)	Non-Neuropathic Subgroup ($n = 28$)
Baseline peak pressure (mean ± SD, kg/cm²)	11.2 ± 5.4	12.2 ± 5.8	9.0 ± 3.9
Number of patients with high foot pressures at baseline	43 (50%)	31 (53%)	12 (43%)
Number of patients with plantar ulceration and high pressures at baseline	15 (35%)	14 (45%)	1 (8%)

Source: Reproduced from Veves A, Murray HJ, Young MJ, and Boulton AJ. *Diabetologia* 35:660–663, 1992. With permission.

Study.[45] Diabetic subjects ($n = 549$) were enrolled from a single VA hospital and five trials of in-shoe plantar pressure were collected on both feet using an F-Scan system. A mask was applied to each trial to separate pressure data into eight areas: heel, lateral mid-foot, medial mid-foot, first metatarsal head, second through fourth metatarsal heads, fifth metatarsal head, hallux, and other toes. During follow-up (2.5 ± 1.7 yr), 42 subjects developed plantar ulcers. Without adjusting for ulcer site, the peak pressure was significantly higher (mean ± standard error) in sites where ulcers developed (214.7 ± 18.2 kPa) than in sites where there were no ulcers (193.9 ± 1.2, $p = .0001$). In the analyses that considered whether plantar pressure differed within each foot site by foot ulcer occurrence, no significant differences were seen for peak pressure (mean difference –3.1 kPa, $p = .6$). If, however, only the metatarsal ulcers were considered, then there was a strongly significant relationship, i.e., the locations that ulcerated experienced higher pressures (333.7 ± 43.0 vs. 242.7 ± 2.0, $p < .0001$). This analysis demonstrates the importance of accounting for ulcer location when associating plantar pressure and diabetic foot ulceration.

Studies have shown retrospectively and prospectively that high-peak plantar pressure is associated with plantar ulceration. Recent work has found that it is also important to consider the location of the plantar pressure when assessing how pressure is related to ulcer occurrence.

20.9 THE RELATIONSHIP BETWEEN SHEAR STRESS AND ULCERATION

Several authors have postulated that shear stress is an important component of ulcer development.[14,34,40] While it is known from force plate analyses that there are medial/lateral and anterior/posterior shear components of the GRF, there is little known about the actual distribution of this force during daily activities, nor about the role that shear plays in causing plantar ulceration.[19] It has been suggested that the effects of shear and pressure on damaging deeper soft tissue are additive.[47] In the mid-thigh region, pressure and shear components, resulting in internal compressive stress of deep tissue, have been shown to have equal effects on reducing blood flow.[80] Elsewhere, at the thenar eminence, blood flow occlusion has been shown to be affected by shear stress.[7]

Unlike vertical pressure, which has been linked both retrospectively and prospectively to ulceration,[12,45,78] shear stress has not been clearly associated with ulcer development. Only one study retrospectively measured shear forces at the location of recently heeled ulcers. Pollard and Le Quesne studied seven ulcerated feet from six diabetic subjects and found that ulcers occurred at the areas of highest vertical and shear stress.[63] However, positioning and holding the sensor in place was accomplished by taping the sensor to the subject's skin. This method of transducing shear forces could have caused elevated forces while attempting to measure them. Further study with a larger number of subjects and a less obtrusive sensor is required.

Recently, Lord and Hosein have employed a magnetoresistive-type shear sensor to study ten asymptomatic (mean 34.3 yrs of age) and six not age-matched diabetic (mean 65.3 yrs of age) subjects.[36,47] Peak vertical pressure was also measured with an F-Scan system. The shear sensors, which are embedded in a Plastazote–Poron insole, have been described and used previously.[48] Due to size constraints, only the heel and two metatarsal heads could be measured at one time. Therefore, two insoles were made; one measured the heel and the second and fourth metatarsals, while the other measured the heel and the first and third metatarsals. Over all areas, the maximum shear stress of the asymptomatic (87 kPa) did not differ from the diabetic (73 kPa). The diabetic subjects did demonstrate lower magnitudes on the third and fourth metatarsal heads (51/39 vs. 86.5/71 kPa, respectively) as well as higher magnitudes on the first and second metatarsal heads (73/64 vs. 35/31 kPa, respectively), indicating a medial shift of the loading. A corresponding relationship was not seen with the pressure data. Additionally, the six diabetic patients had nine previous ulcers, eight beneath the first or second metatarsal heads, and one beneath the fifth. Although not a direct correlation, the location of the ulcers is suggestive of a relationship between increased shear and ulceration. It should be noted that the study groups were not age matched nor was foot architecture considered. Thus, the medial shift in loading could possibly be explained by the fact that the older group may have had flatter feet.

High-shear stress is thought to play a role in plantar ulcer development, but the evidence is not as direct as with peak pressure. Higher shear stresses have been found after ulcers have healed, but the sensor itself may have contributed to the stress.

20.10 SUMMARY

Peripheral vascular disease, peripheral neuropathy (sensory, motor, and autonomic), foot deformity, and aberrant soft-tissue loading are all important etiologic considerations in the development of diabetic neuropathic foot ulcers.

Diabetic plantar soft tissue has been found to be stiffer, absorb more energy, recover more slowly, and be harder and thinner than healthy tissue. These macroscopic characteristics are also manifested with changes at the cellular level. These alterations in the plantar soft tissue can lead to the aberrant distribution of force beneath the foot. The plantar fascia is another lower extremity soft tissue that is affected by diabetes in a manner that can have biomechanical consequences. This tissue has been shown to be thicker in diabetic subjects and is thought to result in an early onset of the windlass mechanism, resulting in a stiffer foot.

Whether the change in gait patterns seen in diabetic patients is caused by diabetic neuropathy or by the decreased velocity of the diabetic neuropathic subjects is a point of contention. Nevertheless, the data demonstrate that diabetic neuropathic patients walk differently than age-, gender-, and BMI-matched controls. Specifically, the diabetic subjects walked slower; stopped moving differently; had altered lower extremity joint kinematics; and had gait patterns that were more cautious, less efficient, and more variable. Diabetic subjects have been found to have altered joint mechanics compared to healthy subjects. These changes included increased ankle joint hysteresis and stiffness in plantar flexion as well as dorsiflexion. It has also been shown that patients with diabetes have limited joint mobility at the ankle, subtalar, and first metatarsal joints, and that limited joint mobility was strongly associated with increased plantar pressure or increased vertical force.

While analyses comparing vertical GRFs using just force plates have conflicting results, others have used specialized sensors to measure distributed pressure and shear stresses. They have found diabetic neuropathic patients with a history of ulcers had decreased plantar pressure and shear stresses beneath the heel and hallux, but increased plantar pressure and shear stresses beneath the metatarsal heads.

The hammer/claw toe deformity is often seen with diabetic subjects. The cause is thought to be a muscle imbalance between the extrinsic and intrinsic muscles of the foot. However, recent work has shown that subjects with intrinsic muscle atrophy do not have hammer/claw toes, calling the well-accepted etiology into question. It has been shown that hammer/claw toes (regardless of etiology) do have higher plantar pressures due to displaced fat pads beneath the metatarsal heads. With increasing sophistication, researchers have used various static and some dynamic measurements to predict the variance of peak plantar pressures. Recently, approximately three-quarters of the plantar pressure variance has been predicted beneath the metatarsal heads of diabetic and healthy subjects.

Several groups have explored how foot structure is related to ulceration by demonstrating that certain foot deformities are more likely to develop ulcers in specific locations. Studies have shown retrospectively and prospectively that high-peak plantar pressure is associated with plantar ulceration. Recent work has found that it is also important to consider the location of the plantar pressure when assessing how pressure is related to ulcer occurrence. High shear stress is thought to play a role in plantar ulcer development, but the evidence is not as direct as with peak pressure. Higher shear stresses have been found after ulcers have healed, but the sensor itself may have contributed to the stress.

REFERENCES

1. Abbott CA, Vileikyte L, Williamson S, Carrington AL, and Boulton AJ. Multicenter study of the incidence of and predictive risk factors for diabetic neuropathic foot ulceration. *Diabetes Care* 21:1071–1075, 1998.
2. Abouaesha F, van Schie CH, Griffths GD, Young RJ, and Boulton AJ. Plantar tissue thickness is related to peak plantar pressure in the high-risk diabetic foot. *Diabetes Care* 24:1270–1274, 2001.
3. Ahroni JH, Boyko EJ, and Forsberg RC. Clinical correlates of plantar pressure among diabetic veterans. *Diabetes Care* 22:965–972, 1999.
4. Andersen H, Gadeberg PC, Brock B, and Jakobsen J. Muscular atrophy in diabetic neuropathy: a stereological magnetic resonance imaging study. *Diabetologia* 40:1062–1069, 1997.
5. Andersen H, Gjerstad MD, and Jakobsen J. Atrophy of foot muscles: a measure of diabetic neuropathy. *Diabetes Care* 27:2382–2385, 2004.
6. Andersen H, Poulsen PL, Mogensen CE, and Jakobsen J. Isokinetic muscle strength in long-term IDDM patients in relation to diabetic complications. Diabetes 45:440–445, 1996.
7. Bennett L, Kavner D, Lee BK, and Trainor FA. Shear vs pressure as causative factors in skin blood flow occlusion. *Arch Phys Med Rehabil* 60:309–314, 1979.
8. Bevans JS. Biomechanics and plantar ulcers in diabetes. *The Foot* 2:166–172, 1992.
9. Bojsen-Moller F. Anatomy of the forefoot, normal, and pathologic. *Clin Orthop Relat Res* 142:10–18, 1979.
10. Bolton NR, Smith KE, Pilgram TK, Mueller MJ, and Bae KT. Computed tomography to visualize and quantify the plantar aponeurosis and flexor hallucis longus tendon in the diabetic foot. *Clin Biomech (Bristol, Avon)* 20:540–546, 2005.
11. Boulton AJ. The diabetic foot. *Med Clin North Am* 72:1513–1530, 1988.
12. Boulton AJ, Hardisty CA, Betts RP, Franks CI, Worth RC, Ward JD, and Duckworth T. Dynamic foot pressure and other studies as diagnostic and management aids in diabetic neuropathy. *Diabetes Care* 6:26–33, 1983.
13. Boyko EJ, Ahroni JH, Stensel V, Forsberg RC, Davignon DR, and Smith DG. A prospective study of risk factors for diabetic foot ulcer. The Seattle Diabetic Foot Study. *Diabetes Care* 22:1036–1042, 1999.
14. Brand PW: Repetitive stress in the development of diabetic foot ulcers. In: ME Levin ME, O'Neal LW, eds. *The Diabetic Foot, 4th ed.* St. Louis: C. V. Mosby, 83–90, 1988.
15. Bus SA, Maas M, Cavanagh PR, Michels RP, and Levi M. Plantar fat-pad displacement in neuropathic diabetic patients with toe deformity: a magnetic resonance imaging study. *Diabetes Care* 27:2376–2381, 2004.
16. Bus SA, Maas M, de Lange A, Michels RP, and Levi M. Elevated plantar pressures in neuropathic diabetic patients with claw/hammer toe deformity. *J Biomech* 38:1918–1925, 2005.
17. Bus SA, Yang QX, Wang JH, Smith MB, Wunderlich R, and Cavanagh PR. Intrinsic muscle atrophy and toe deformity in the diabetic neuropathic foot: a magnetic resonance imaging study. *Diabetes Care* 25:1444–1450, 2002.
18. Buschmann WR, Jahss MH, Kummer F, Desai P, Gee RO, and Ricci JL. Histology and histomorphometric analysis of the normal and atrophic heel fat pad. *Foot Ankle Int* 16:254–258, 1995.
19. Cavanagh P, Ulbrecht JS, and Capulo GM. The biomechanics of the foot in diabetes mellitus. In: Bokwer JH, Pfeifer MA, eds. *The Diabetic Foot.* St. Louis: 125–196, 2001.

20. Cavanagh PR, Lipsky BA, Bradbury AW, and Botek G. Treatment for diabetic foot ulcers. *Lancet* 366:1725–1735, 2005.

21. Cavanagh PR, Morag E, Boulton AJM, Young MJ, Deffner KT, and Pammer SE. The relationship of static foot structure to dynamic foot function. *J Biomech* 30:243–250, 1997.

22. Coleman WC: Foot care and lower extremity problems of diabetes mellitus. In: Haire-Joshu D, ed. *Management of Diabetes Mellitus: Pespectives of Care Across the Life Span*. Calsbad, CA: C.V. Mosby, 309–339, 1996.

23. D'Ambrogi E, Giacomozzi C, Macellari V, and Uccioli L. Abnormal foot function in diabetic patients: The altered onset of Windlass mechanism. *Diabet Med* 22:1713–1719, 2005.

24. D'Ambrogi E, Giurato L, D'Agostino MA, Giacomozzi C, Macellari V, Caselli A, and Uccioli L. Contribution of plantar fascia to the increased forefoot pressures in diabetic patients. *Diabetes Care* 26:1525–1529, 2003.

25. Delbridge L, Ctercteko G, Fowler C, Reeve TS, and Le Quesne LP. The aetiology of diabetic neuropathic ulceration of the foot. *Br J Surg* 72:1–6, 1985.

26. Dingwell JB, Cavanagh PR. Increased variability of continuous overground walking in neuropathic patients is only indirectly related to sensory loss. *Gait Posture* 14:1–10, 2001.

27. Edmonds ME, Watkins PJ. Plantar neuropathic ulcer and Charcot joints: Risk factors, presentation, and management. In: Dyck PJ, Thomas PK, eds. *Diabetic Neuropathy*. Philadelphia: W. B. Saunders, 560, 1999.

28. Eils E, Behrens S, Mers O, Thorwesten L, Volker K, and Rosenbaum D. Reduced plantar sensation causes a cautious walking pattern. *Gait Posture* 20:54–60, 2004.

29. Eils E, Nolte S, Tewes M, Thorwesten L, Volker K, and Rosenbaum D. Modified pressure distribution patterns in walking following reduction of plantar sensation. *J Biomech* 35:1307–1313, 2002.

30. Fernando DJ, Masson EA, Veves A, and Boulton AJ. Relationship of limited joint mobility to abnormal foot pressures and diabetic foot ulceration. *Diabetes Care* 14:8–11, 1991.

31. Giacomozzi C, Caselli A, Macellari V, Giurato L, Lardieri L, and Uccioli L. Walking strategy in diabetic patients with peripheral neuropathy. *Diabetes Care* 25:1451–1457, 2002.

32. Giacomozzi C, D'Ambrogi E, Uccioli L, and Macellari V: Does the thickening of Achilles tendon and plantar fascia contribute to the alteration of diabetic foot loading? *Clin Biomech (Bristol, Avon)* 20:532–539, 2005.

33. Gooding GA, Stess RM, Graf PM, Moss KM, Louie KS, and Grunfeld C. Sonography of the sole of the foot. Evidence for loss of foot pad thickness in diabetes and its relationship to ulceration of the foot. *Invest Radiol* 21:45–48, 1986.

34. Habershaw GM, Chzran J. Biomechanical considerations of the diabetic foot. In: Kozak GP, ed. *Management of Diabetic Foot Problems*. Philadelphia: W. B. Saunders, 53–65, 1995.

35. Hicks JH. The mechanics of the foot II. The plantar aponeurosis and the arch. *J Anat* 88:25–31, 1954.

36. Hosein R, Lord M. A study of in-shoe plantar shear in normals. *Clin Biomech (Bristol, Avon)* 15(1):46–53, 2000.

37. Hsu TC, Lee YS, Shau YW. Biomechanics of the heel pad for type 2 diabetic patients. *Clin Biomech (Bristol, Avon)* 17(4):291–296, 2002.

38. Hsu TC, Wang CL, Shau YW, Tang FT, Li KL, and Chen CY. Altered heel-pad mechanical properties in patients with Type 2 diabetes mellitus. *Diabet Med* 17:854–859, 2000.

39. Jahss MH, Michelson JD, Desai P, Kaye R, Kummer F, Buschman W, Watkins F, and Reich S. Investigations into the fat pads of the sole of the foot: Anatomy and histology. *Foot Ankle* 13(5):233–242, 1992.

40. Jenkin WM, Palladino SJ. Environmental stress and tissue breakdown. In: Frykberg RG, ed. *The High Risk Foot in Diabetes Mellitus.* New York: Churchill Livingston, 103–123, 1991.

41. Kao PF, Davis BL, and Hardy PA. Characterization of the calcaneal fat pad in diabetic and non-diabetic patients using magnetic resonance imaging. *Magn Reson Imaging* 17(6):851–857, 1999.

42. Katoulis EC, Ebdon-Parry M, Lanshammar H, Vileikyte L, Kulkarni J, and Boulton AJ. Gait abnormalities in diabetic neuropathy. *Diabetes Care* 20:1904–1907, 1997.

43. Kelikian H. Hallux valgus. *Allied Deformities of the Forefoot and Metatarsalgia.* Philadelphia: W. B. Saunders, 292, 1965.

44. Klaesner JW, Hastings MK, Zou DQ, Lewis C, and Mueller MJ. Plantar tissue stiffness in patients with diabetes mellitus and peripheral neuropathy. *Arch Phys Med Rehabil* 83:1796–1801, 2002.

45. Ledoux WR, Cowley MS, Ahroni JH, Forsberg RC, Stensel VL, Shofer JB, and Boyko EJ. No relationship between plantar pressure and diabetic foot ulcer incidence after adjustment for ulcer location. 65th Annual Scientific Sessions of the American Diabetes Association. San Diego, CA: 2005.

46. Ledoux WR, Shofer JB, Smith DG, Sullivan K, Hayes SG, Assal M, and Reiber GE. The relationship between foot type, foot deformity and ulcer occurrence in the high risk diabetic foot. *J Rehabil Res Dev* 42(5):665–672, 2005.

47. Lord M, Hosein R. A study of in-shoe plantar shear in patients with diabetic neuropathy. *Clin Biomech* 15:278–283, 2000.

48. Lord M, Hosein R, and Williams RB. Method for in-shoe shear stress measurement. *J Biomed Eng* 14:181–186, 1992.

49. Mann RA, Thompson FM. Rupture of the posterior tibial tendon causing flat foot. Surgical treatment. *J Bone Joint Surg Am* 67(4):556–561, 1985.

50. McCluskey WP, Lovell WW, and Cummings RJ. The cavovarus foot deformity. Etiology and management. *Clin Orthop Relat Res* (247):27–37, 1989.

51. Meier MR, Desrosiers J, Bourassa P, and Blaszczyk J. Effect of type II diabetic peripheral neuropathy on gait termination in the elderly. *Diabetologia* 44(5):585–592, 2001.

52. Menz HB, Lord SR, St George R, and Fitzpatrick RC. Walking stability and sensorimotor function in older people with diabetic peripheral neuropathy. *Arch Phys Med Rehabil* 85:245–252, 2004.

53. Morag E, Cavanagh PR. Structural and functional predictors of regional peak pressures under the foot during walking. *J Biomech* 32(4):359–370, 1999.

54. Mueller MJ, Hastings M, Commean PK, Smith KE, Pilgram TK, Robertson D, and Johnson J. Forefoot structural predictors of plantar pressures during walking in people with diabetes and peripheral neuropathy. *J Biomech* 36:1009–1017, 2003.

55. Mueller MJ, Minor SD, Diamond JE, and Blair VP, 3rd. Relationship of foot deformity to ulcer location in patients with diabetes mellitus. *Phys Ther* 70:356–62, 1990.

56. Myerson MS, Shereff MJ. The pathological anatomy of claw and hammer toes. *J Bone Joint Surg Am* 71(1):45–49, 1989.

57. Olson SL, Ledoux WR, Ching RP, and Sangeorzan BJ. Muscular imbalances resulting in a clawed hallux. *Foot Ankle Int* 24:477–485, 2003.

58. Pataky Z, Assal JP, Conne P, Vuagnat H, and Golay A. Plantar pressure distribution in Type 2 diabetic patients without peripheral neuropathy and peripheral vascular disease. *Diabet Med* 22:762–767, 2005.

59. Paulose-Ram R, Gu Q, Eberhardt M, Gregg l, and Engelgau M. Lower extremity disease among persons aged > or = 40 years with and without diabetes—United States, 1999–2002. *MMWR Morb Mortal Wkly Rep* 54(45):1158–1160, 2005.

60. Perry JE, Hall JO, and Davis BL. Simultaneous measurement of plantar pressure and shear forces in diabetic individuals. *Gait Posture* 15:101–107, 2002.

61. Petrofsky J, Lee S, and Bweir S. Gait characteristics in people with type 2 diabetes mellitus. *Eur J Appl Physiol* 93:640–647, 2005.

62. Piaggesi A, Romanelli M, Schipani E, Campi F, Magliaro A, Baccetti F, and Navalesi R. Hardness of plantar skin in diabetic neuropathic feet. *J Diabetes Complications* 13(3):129–134, 1999.

63. Pollard JP, Le Quesne LP. Method of healing diabetic forefoot ulcers. *Br Med J (Clin Res Ed)* 286(6363):436–437, 1983.

64. Reiber GE, Vileikyte L, Boyko EJ, del Aguila M, Smith DG, Lavery LA, and Boulton AJ. Causal pathways for incident lower-extremity ulcers in patients with diabetes from two settings. *Diabetes Care* 22:157–162, 1999.

65. Richardson JK, Thies SB, DeMott TK, and Ashton-Miller JA. A comparison of gait characteristics between older women with and without peripheral neuropathy in standard and challenging environments. *J Am Geriatr Soc* 52(9):1532–1537, 2004.

66. Rith-Najarian SJ, Stolusky T, and Gohdes DM. Identifying diabetic patients at high risk for lower-extremity amputation in a primary health care setting. A prospective evaluation of simple screening criteria. *Diabetes Care* 15:1386–1389, 1992.

67. Sammarco GJ, Stephens MM. Diabetic foot function. In: Sammarco GJ, Malvern PA, eds. *The Foot in Diabetes*. Philadelphia: Lea & Febiger, 36–53 1991.

68. Sarnow M, Veves A, Giurini J, Rosenblum B, Chrzan J, and Habershaw G. In-shoe foot pressure measurements in diabetic patients with at-risk feet and in healthy subjects. *Diabetes Care* 17:1002–1006, 1994.

69. Sauseng S, Kastenbauer T. Effect of limited joint mobility on plantar pressure in patients with type 1 diabetes mellitus]. *Acta Med Austriaca* 26(5):178–181, 1999.

70. Shaw JE, van Schie CH, Carrington AL, Abbott CA, and Boulton AJ. An analysis of dynamic forces transmitted through the foot in diabetic neuropathy. *Diabetes Care* 21:1955–1959, 1998.

71. Singer AJ, Clark RA. Cutaneous wound healing. *N Engl J Med* 341:738–746, 1999.

72. Stess RM, Jensen SR, and Mirmiran R. The role of dynamic plantar pressures in diabetic foot ulcers. *Diabetes Care* 20:855–858, 1997.

73. Sumpio BE. Foot ulcers. *N Engl J Med* 343:787–793, 2000.

74. Taylor RG. The treatment of claw toes by multiple transfers of the flexors into extensor tendons. *J Bone Joint Surg* 33–B:539–542, 1951.

75. Trevino SG, Buford WL, Jr., Nakamura T, John Wright A, and Patterson RM. Use of a Torque-Range-of-Motion device for objective differentiation of diabetic from normal feet in adults. *Foot Ankle Int* 25:561–567, 2004.

76. Uccioli L, Caselli A, Giacomozzi C, Macellari V, Giurato L, Lardieri L, and Menzinger G. Pattern of abnormal tangential forces in the diabetic neuropathic foot. *Clin Biomech* (Bristol, Avon) 16:446–454, 2001.

77. van Schie CH, Vermigli C, Carrington AL, and Boulton A. Muscle weakness and foot deformities in diabetes: relationship to neuropathy and foot ulceration in caucasian diabetic men. *Diabetes Care* 27:1668–1673, 2004.

78. Veves A, Murray HJ, Young MJ, and Boulton AJ. The risk of foot ulceration in diabetic patients with high foot pressure: A prospective study. *Diabetologia* 35:660–663, 1992.

79. Walters DP, Gatling W, Mullee MA, and Hill RD. The distribution and severity of diabetic foot disease: A community study with comparison to a non-diabetic group. *Diabet Med* 9:354–358, 1992.

80. Zhang M, Turner-Smith AR, and Roberts VC. The reaction of skin and soft tissue to shear forces applied externally to the skin surface. *Proc Inst Mech Eng* 208:217–222, 1994.

81. Zheng YP, Choi YK, Wong K, Chan S, and Mak AF. Biomechanical assessment of plantar foot tissue in diabetic patients using an ultrasound indentation system. *Ultrasound Med Biol* 26(3):451–456, 2000.

82. Zimny S, Schatz H, and Pfohl M. The role of limited joint mobility in diabetic patients with an at-risk foot. *Diabetes Care* 27:942–946, 2004.

21 Three-Dimensional Finite Element Analysis of the Fifth Metatarsal Jones Fracture

Eric S. Rohr, Jeffrey E. Johnson, Linping Zhao, and Gerald F. Harris

CONTENTS

21.1 INTRODUCTION

Fractures of the fifth metatarsal (MT) of the human foot are among those most commonly observed by orthopedic surgeons.[1-3] Fracture occurrence is associated with running and sports activities such as recreational basketball. One anatomical characteristic of the fifth MT is the strong ligamentous capsule surrounding the base, which binds it to the cuboid and fourth MT. This coupling makes it easier to fracture

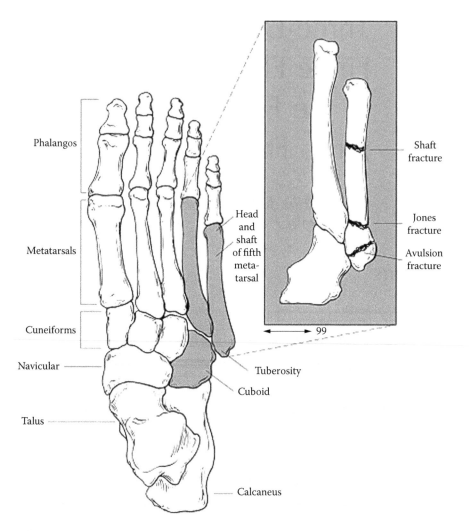

Phalangos

Metatarsals

Cuneiforms

Navicular

Talus

Head
and
shaft
of fifth
meta-
tarsal

Shaft
fracture

Jones
fracture

Avulsion
fracture

99

Tuberosity

Cuboid

Calcaneus

FIGURE 21.1 Anatomy of the foot and fractures of the fifth MT. (Illustration by Sally Cummings, Shriners Hospitals for Children, Chicago, IL.)

the fifth MT than to rupture the powerful ligaments.[1] Both proximal metaphyseal avulsion-type fractures and Jones fractures occur near the base of the fifth MT[4,5] (Figure 21.1). Jones fractures occur typically at the junction of the metaphysis with the diaphyseal segment of the proximal fifth MT at least 1.5 cm distal to the styloid process. By definition, these fractures do not enter the tarsometatarsal joint.[6–10]

Jones fractures can occur when the forefoot experiences high loads, creating an acute injury, or it can develop from repetitive loading, resulting in a stress fracture.[10–12] Conservative (nonoperative) treatment is reported to be more successful when subjects do not weight bear until clinical evidence of union is achieved.[13,14] This period may take from 2 to 12 months. This delay makes surgical treatment more desirable for some patients, including athletes who want to return to their sports more rapidly. Operative treatment includes bone grafting and intramedullary screw fixation. With operative treatment, over 80% of the patients achieved union within 6 to 12 weeks.[13–16]

The Jones fracture is thought to result from forcible inversion of the foot, with the ankle in plantar flexion. This places a medial force over the base of the fifth MT.[4,6,10] Activities associated with Jones fractures include falls, jumping, turning or pivoting, and stepping on uneven surfaces.[8–10,17–19] There have been a lot of postulations on the causation of Jones fractures, but disagreement exists on whether inversion is necessary and what role the muscle forces play on the fracture.[3,6,8,12,19] These studies have focused on observations, cadaveric testing, and investigating the means of injury. Only two studies have investigated the internal stresses in the fifth MT in regard to Jones fractures. Roca et al., in 1980,[20] provided evidence (with a photoelastic model) that the peroneus brevis (PB) contributes to stresses that may result in Jones fractures. However, this model could only describe the changes in stress qualitatively and not quantitatively. Arangio et al., in 1997,[21] conducted a quantitative analysis of stress distribution on the fifth MT using beam theory. They found that the fifth MT is most susceptible to fracture when the foot is inverted 30 to 60° and the forces are above the levels of normal walking, suggesting Jones fractures are stress fractures. This study, however, was limited to a simplified loading condition (a single force at the fifth MT head) and did not include muscle forces or accurate real-life ground reaction forces (GRFs). Further comprehensive models, which incorporate muscle forces, ligament forces, bone density, and dynamic analysis of normal locomotion, are needed to better understand the biomechanical conditions that result in a stress fracture in the proximal fifth MT, and how these affect the condition that may lead to difficulties in healing Jones fractures. Recently, the finite element (FE) approach has been employed to simulate the motions, forces, and stresses of the foot,[22–24] but no studies have been reported on the Jones fracture.

As a preliminary approach toward the comprehensive and systematic investigation, we developed a hypothesis that Jones fracture location correlates with the von Mises stress concentration in an anatomic model to an accuracy of 1 mm. The objectives of the present work were to develop an anatomically correct three-dimensional (3-D) FE model of the fifth MT that accurately incorporates muscular forces, GRFs, and ligamentous attachments. An analysis of stress distribution throughout the bone is done to determine where the fifth MT is most susceptible to fracture. The model is also used to systematically alter muscular forces to determine their sensitivity and contribution in the development of stress concentrations throughout the fifth MT.

21.2 MATERIALS AND METHODS

21.2.1 SUBJECT SELECTION

A case-specific analysis of the bare right foot was conducted in this study. Magnetic Resonance Imaging (MRI) were obtained, according to Institutional Review Board (IRB) approval and informed consent procedures. The subject was an adult male (age 23, height 175 cm, and weight 78 kg) and had no history of injury or pain to the extremities. Scans were obtained using a General Electric (GE) 1.5 T whole-body

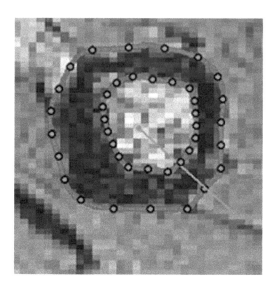

FIGURE 21.2 Identifying the outlines of the cortical and cancellous bone from MRI scans using an edge detection program.

MRI scanner (General Electric Medical Systems, Milwaukee, WI), with the following protocol: 256×256 acquisition matrix, 9 cm field of view, and 70° flip angle. A slice interval of 1 mm resulted in approximately 70 slices containing information on the fifth MT. The scan was limited to the foot from mid-calcaneus to a point approximately 2 cm distal to the head of the fifth MT.

21.2.2 FE Modeling

A custom edge detection program[25] was used to process the MRI and to identify the outer boundary of the bone and the cortical–cancellous interface, as shown in Figure 21.2.

The model consisted of an outer layer of cortical bone covering the interior cancellous bone, with the intramedullary canal being modeled as cancellous bone. This assumption was necessary, as the MRI could not clearly identify the canal. The effect of this assumption (i.e., cancellous vs. hollow canal) was not tested. Using ANSYS FE software (ANSYS Inc., Houston, PA) the cortical and cancellous bone were meshed with 20-node, solid brick elements (Solid95). Due to the irregular shape of the bone, refinement of the mesh is difficult. Therefore, the ANSYS p-method analysis was performed to determine the convergence of the model. This method does not require a refined mesh, as it solves the model at increasing polynomial levels of the FE element shape functions to better approximate the real solution. Global strain energy and displacement were used with a tolerance of 5% to determine convergence criteria. Based upon the results of the convergence tests on the mesh size and the mesh order, the final mesh consisted of 3072 elements (Figure 21.3).

Both the cortical and the trabecular bones were modeled as homogenous, linear elastic materials with isotropic properties. The values of Young's modulus and Poisson's

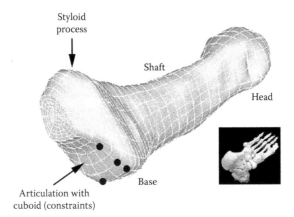

FIGURE 21.3 Plantar view of the meshed right fifth MT and the constraint system used. Four additional constraints were applied symmetrically over the joint surface, but are not shown, as they were located on the back side of the model (dorsal surface).

ratio assigned to the bone were obtained from the literature.[26–28] The cortical bone was modeled with a Young's modulus of 15,000 MPa and Poisson's ratio of 0.3, while the cancellous bone used a Young's modulus of 300 MPa and Poisson's ratio of 0.3.

21.2.3 Motion Analysis

A six-camera VICON (Oxford, England) motion analysis system was used to obtain foot and ankle motion data (kinematic and kinetic).[29] A force plate was used to measure the GRF, and a Tekscan pressure mat (87 × 70 array) of force sensors (Tekscan Inc., Boston, MA) was used to obtain the plantar pressure data. These systems were synchronized to quantify the 3-D of the bare right foot and ankle and GRFs throughout the gait cycle.

The subject underwent 15 trials, in which the right bare foot and ankle were analyzed. The subject ambulated at a normal cadence while traversing the capture volume and walking over the force plate and pressure mat. The force plate was used to determine the normal forces and the medial–lateral and anterior–posterior shear forces. The pressure mat was used to measure the plantar pressure distribution under the foot. The maximum pressure under the head of the fifth MT was identified to determine the frame of interest for the foot position and force generation. Using the pressure mat data, the total vertical force and the force of the fifth MT head were calculated, to determine what percentage of the overall force occurred at the fifth MT head.

This percentage was multiplied by the measured force plate data to determine the force at the fifth MT head:

$$F_{\text{5th metatarsal (force plate)}} = \left(\frac{F_{\text{5th metatarsal (press mat)}}}{F_{\text{total force (press mat)}}} \right) \left(F_{\text{total force (force plate)}} \right) \tag{21.1}$$

The shear forces generated by the fifth MT were determined using the same index. The average values of the vertical and shear forces over the 15 trials were used in the FE model.

The four-segment Milwaukee Foot Model (MFM)[29] was used to determine the kinematic foot position. Using the frame of interest determined by the pressure mat, the orientation of the fifth MT was determined. As two markers were placed on the fifth MT (base and head), the sagittal and transverse plane orientations were calculated. As only two markers were placed on this rigid body, the rotation had to be assumed. The assumption supported by cadaveric dissection and literature was that the apex of the styloid process was orientated at an angle of 35° from the horizontal plane.[30] Furthermore, the markers at the ankle and over the foot were used to determine the line of action of the muscle forces.

21.2.4 ANATOMIC MUSCLE FORCE MODEL

The muscle force model uses five muscles that insert into or originate from the fifth MT: PB, peroneus tertius (PT), dorsal interosseous (DI), plantar interosseous (PI), and flexor digiti minimi brevis (FDMB). The muscle and GRFs were modeled as distributed forces over their insertion or origin sites.

MRI was used to define the origin and insertion sites of these muscles and ligaments on the fifth MT using bony landmarks. The line of action was determined using the MFM markers to determine the orientation of the muscle bodies. The PB and PT muscles are multijoint muscles and were modeled with their forces acting from their insertion to their wraparound points at the ankle. The lines of action for the FDMB, DI, and PI were modeled as straight lines from origin to insertion.

The physiologic cross-sectional area (PCSA) of each muscle was determined from the literature and used to estimate the maximum muscle force.[31–34] A force-generating capacity of 25 N/cm² was multiplied by the PCSA to obtain the muscle forces. The magnitudes of muscle forces are listed in Table 21.1, while muscle forces and GRFs are illustrated in Figure 21.4.

The current model does not include the lateral band of the plantar fascia that inserts into the base of the fifth MT. While the lateral band may contribute to stress development, the stresses of the fascia during normal walking are assumed to be small when compared to the GRFs.

TABLE 21.1
Magnitudes of the Muscle Forces Used in the FE Model

Muscle	PCSA (cm²)	Force (N)
FDMB	2.00	50.0
PI	1.38	34.5
DI	2.72	68.0
PB	11.5	287.5
PT	3.10	77.5

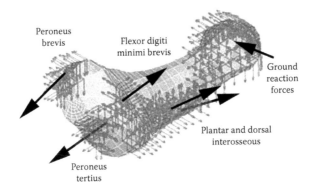

FIGURE 21.4 The five muscle forces and resultant GRFs as applied to nodes corresponding to their respective insertion, origin, or contact areas (GRFs). The forces are applied as x, y, and z force components in the FE model coordinate system at each node of interest.

In performing the static FE analyses, the GRFs and muscle forces were applied to the fifth MT. The analyses applied the measured GRFs, and each muscle was maximally activated to present a worst case scenario.

21.2.5 BOUNDARY CONDITIONS

The FE model of the fifth MT was constrained at the tarsometatarsal joint to prevent rigid body motion. Eight nodes at the base of the fifth MT were fixed in all three degrees of freedom (Figure 21.3). These constraints were based on physiologic criteria and simulated the interaction between the bordering bones and ligamentous attachments that limit the motion of the bone. The joint reaction forces were calculated in the FE solution.

These eight nodes were selected for constraints after a perturbation study was conducted using 2, 4, 5, 8, and 14 nodal constraints. The study indicated that the rigid fixation did not effect the computed stress distribution over the region of the Jones fracture site.

21.2.6 FE ANALYSIS

The fifth MT was analyzed with an FE model using ANSYS. The model was used to systematically alter muscle forces to determine their influence on the stress distribution throughout the fifth MT. Simulations were done to monitor the effect of altered magnitude ($\pm 25\%$) and orientation ($\pm 15°$) of muscle forces. A total of 33 simulations were conducted in the current model.

The von Mises stress and principal stresses were studied. The von Mises stress is an equivalent stress that combines the effects of the stress in all directions, and is used to determine failure probability and fracture propagation. Therefore, a von Mises stress concentration indicates a possible fracture location. The principal stresses reveal the local stress state, where tensile stress is more deleterious to osseous structures.

21.3 RESULTS

21.3.1 KINEMATIC/KINETIC CALCULATIONS

Figure 21.5 provides an illustration of the GRFs from the force plate and the force curve from the pressure mat for a typical trial. The vertical line represents the frame where the maximum force over the fifth MT head was recorded. This point was selected for the FE model. The average peak values of measured and calculated parameters from 15 trials are summarized in Table 21.2. These values were selected and applied to the FE model to describe the maximum force that the fifth MT experienced in the gait cycle as a worst case scenario.

The maximum force on the head of the fifth MT occurred at 40.2% of the gait cycle when the foot was in stance phase and single limb support (Figure 21.5). Terminal stance occurred from 30 to 50% of the gait cycle beginning with heel rise and continuing until the other foot struck the ground. From the pressure mat measurements, the total foot vertical force was 841.3 N, while the vertical force at the

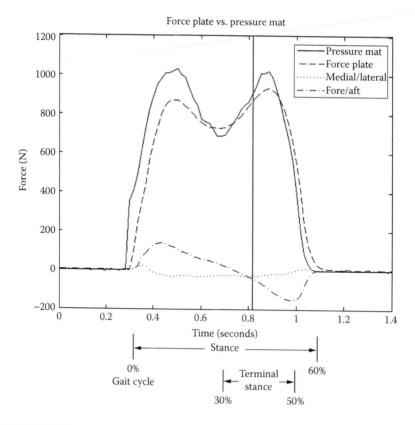

FIGURE 21.5 The normal and shear forces calculated by the pressure mat and force plate for a typical trial. The vertical line indicates the frame where the maximum force on the fifth MT was recorded.

TABLE 21.2
Average Maximum GRFs and Pressures

Instrument	Parameter	Mean	Standard Deviation
Pressure mat	Percentage of gait cycle	40.2%	3.5%
Pressure mat	Total foot vertical force	841.3 N	91.7 N
Pressure mat	Vertical force at fifth MT	101.8 N	27.5 N
Calculated	Percentage of GRF at fifth MT	12.0%	2.6%
Force plate	Foot vertical force	802.4 N	59.9 N
Force plate	A–P foot shear force	–32.0 N	15.3 N
Force plate	M–L foot shear force	–39.9 N	5.8 N
Calculated	Vertical force at fifth MT	97.2 N	25.2 N
Calculated	A–P shear force at fifth MT (N)	–3.9 N	2.2 N
Calculated	M–L shear force at fifth MT (N)	–4.8 N	1.2 N

fifth MT was 101.8 N. This resulted in 12% of the GRF acting on the head of the fifth MT. Thus, the calculated vertical force from the force plate at the fifth MT head was 97.2 N, the A–P shear force was 3.9 N in the aft direction and the M–L shear was 4.8 N in the lateral direction (Table 21.2).

The orientation of the fifth MT was determined at 40.2% of the gait cycle using the MFM, specifically the markers placed on the head and base of the fifth MT. A transformation matrix was then calculated to transform the motion analysis orientation into the FE model orientation, which was determined by the MR images. Using the transformation matrix and the other markers of the MFM, the muscle orientations were calculated to apply the muscle forces to the FE model along the muscles line of action.

21.3.2 FE MODEL EVALUATION

To evaluate the performance of the FE model, the effect of the mesh density was analyzed using the p-method convergence criteria. The global strain energy and displacement with a tolerance of 5% were chosen. In both cases, the model converged at the third iteration (third-order polynomial). In comparing the stress development, the patterns of stress concentration did not change and the magnitude of the stress over the fracture region changed by less than 2%. This indicated that the mesh density used in this study was sufficient to perform the analysis.

In addition, the constraint system was perturbed to understand its overall influence on the stress distribution of the model. Models in which 2, 4, 5, and 14 nodes were constrained over the articulation surface of the base of the fifth MT were compared to the model with 8 nodes constrained. When only two constraints were chosen, the fifth MT was not rigidly constrained, and no solution was possible. The remaining models showed that the overall stress distribution pattern did not change throughout the bone, except at the nodes directly surrounding the constraints. At these nodes, the stress decreased as more constraints were applied. The only place the stress changed due to the constraints over the Jones fracture region occurred on

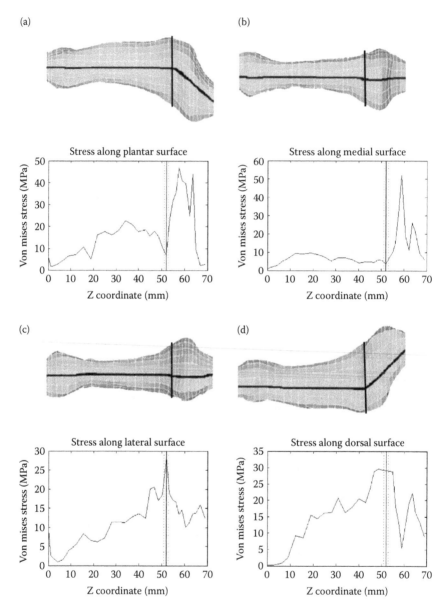

FIGURE 21.6 Von Mises stress distribution for the right fifth MT on (a) plantar surface; (b) medial surface; (c) lateral surface; and (d) dorsal surface. The vertical black line indicates the predicted location where Jones fractures occur, while the dotted band represents the reported location in which Jones fractures occur according to the literature. (From Jones, R. *Ann Surg*, 35, 697–701, 1902; Byrd, T. *South Med J*, 85, 748–750, 1992; Kavanaugh, J.H., Brower, T.D., and Mann, R.V. *J Bone Joint Surg*, 60-A, 776–782, 1978; Sammarco, G.J. *Phys Sportsmed*, 113, 353–360, 1991; Carp, L. Fracture of the fifth metatarsal bone. With special reference to delayed unions, *Ann Surg*, 86, 308–320, 1927.)

the dorsal surface when 4 or 5 nodes were constrained. Under these conditions, an increase in the stress concentration of approximately 18% developed, when compared to models in which 8 and 14 nodes were constrained. Using eight constraints was a conservative choice as it produced a smaller stress over the region than a less-constrained model, and provided the same stress distribution pattern as that of the other three models.

21.3.3 Analysis of von Mises Stress

The von Mises stress distribution over the fifth MT is shown in Figure 21.6. The stress was plotted along a path over the plantar, dorsal, medial, and lateral surfaces. The vertical black line is 16 mm from the proximal joint surface of the fifth MT, and the red lines mark the region in which Jones fractures can occur. The error of the exact point in which Jones fractures occur (15 mm distal from the proximal joint surface) is approximately 1 mm as the actual joint surface identification can be off by at least 1 mm due to the spacing of the MR slices.

The high stress concentrations in the plantar and medial surfaces occurring between 58 and 66 mm occur at a constrained node or a node bordering a constraint. As constraints produce a discontinuity in the stress, this high stress is considered insignificant. Of interest are the peak stresses that occur on the lateral and dorsal surfaces over the region in which Jones fractures occur. This stress concentration indicates a vulnerable location for fracture initiation and propagation.

21.3.4 Principal Stresses on the Cross Section

Contour plots as shown in Figure 21.7 demonstrate the cross section in which Jones fractures occur. The maximum principal stress (principal stress 1) ranged from 9 to 18 MPa, with the highest stresses located over the lateral and dorsal surfaces. The medium principal stress (principal stress 2) demonstrated tensile stresses of 3 to 9 MPa existing over the plantar surface near the tip of the styloid process. The minimum principal stress (principal stress 3) was primarily compressive, as shown in Figure 21.7, with a region over the plantar surface measuring a small tensile stress of 2 MPa. All three stress components produced a tensile stress over the plantar and lateral surfaces of the fifth MT (denoted by arrows in Figure 21.7). However, the greatest tensile stress state is noted over the dorsal and lateral regions in the fifth MT (depicted in Figure 21.7, principal stress 1), which is in agreement with the maximum von Mises stress state, and indicates a region in which the fifth MT is susceptible to fracture initiation and propagation.

21.3.5 Effect of Muscles

Individual muscle forces were increased or decreased by 25%, while the remaining muscles were held constant to investigate the parametric effects each muscle has on the stress contribution. The maximum von Mises stress over the fracture site

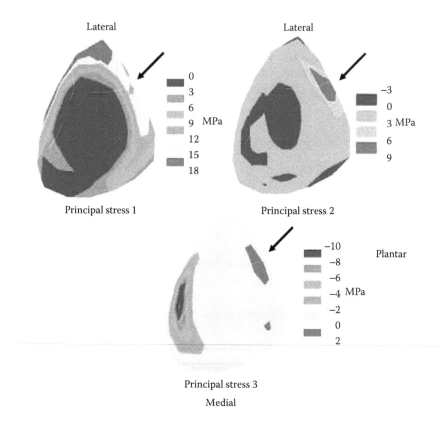

FIGURE 21.7 Contour plots of the three principal stresses through the cross section in which Jones fractures occur. The black arrow points to the site where a 3-D tensile stress state occurs.

for the normal FE model occurred along the dorsal surface and was 45% of the stress necessary to fracture the fifth MT. Over the lateral surface, a stress of 42% of the ultimate stress was recorded (Figure 21.8). Alterations to the PB force resulted in the most prominent changes to the stress distribution throughout the proximal half of the fifth MT along the lateral surface (Figure 21.8). The maximum increase in the von Mises stress was 11% and occurred 16 mm distal to the styloid process. This is the location where the Jones fracture has been described.[6–10] The FDMB, PT, DI, and PI muscles had no obvious influence on the stress distribution along the lateral surface (Figure 21.8). Over the dorsal surface, an increase in the PB muscle force resulted in a 7% increase in stress over the Jones fracture region (data not shown). Alterations in the other muscle force magnitudes were either insensitive or created a smaller influence on the change of the stress concentration. Alterations of the muscle force line of action were also smaller and then the magnitude changed; therefore, only the lateral influence of the PB muscle magnitude was shown in these results.

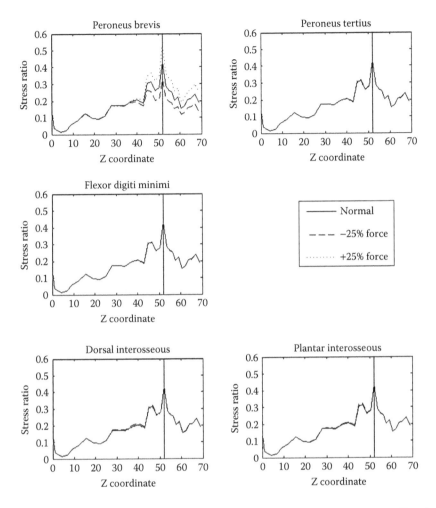

FIGURE 21.8 Ratio of the von Mises stress along the lateral surface of the fifth MT to the ultimate stress of the femur. The black vertical line represents the prediction of the current FE model, while the dotted band represents the reported location where the Jones fracture occurs. (From Jones, R. *Ann Surg*, 35, 697–701, 1902; Byrd, T. *South Med J*, 85, 748–750, 1992; Kavanaugh, J.H., Brower, T.D., and Mann, R.V. *J Bone Joint Surg*, 60-A, 776–782, 1978; Sammarco, G.J. *Phys Sportsmed*, 113, 353–360, 1991; Carp, L. Fracture of the fifth metatarsal bone. With special reference to delayed unions, *Ann Surg*, 86, 308–320, 1927.)

21.4 DISCUSSION

Since Sir Robert Jones first discovered the Jones fracture in 1902,[6] numerous cases have been reported.[10–12,19,35] Jones fractures can occur when the forefoot experiences sufficient loads in the region of the fifth MT. Injuries generally occur in persons older than 21 yr and are equally prevalent in males and females.[9] Jones fractures are clinically noted with increased activity levels.[9,17,18] The fractures are difficult to treat due to a high incidence of delayed union, nonunion, and refracture, if treated conservatively (nonoperatively).[10–12] Eighty percent of the fractures occur in athletes.[9] It has been noted, in some studies, that nonoperative treatment can be successful if the subject does not bear weight until clinical evidence of union is achieved.[13,14] This period may take from 2 to 12 months, again making surgical treatment an attractive option. Operative techniques include bone grafting, intramedullary screw fixation, and combinations of both, where success rates in excess of 80% are noted.[13–16]

The results of this work demonstrated stress concentration at the fifth MT base approximately 1.5 cm distal to the styloid process.[6] The study also demonstrated that with normal gait GRFs and reasonable muscle forces, a stress concentration existed with a localized 3D tensile stress state in the region of reported Jones fractures. This study advanced previous knowledge as it shows that muscular activity along with GRFs can act together to form regions of stress concentrations deleterious to fracture over the Jones region.

The hypothesis of this project has been shown to be true. That is, von Mises stress distribution correlated with known locations of the Jones fracture. In our study, we found von Mises stress concentrations on the lateral and dorsal regions of the fifth MT in the areas of reported Jones fractures. It should be noted, however, that this study did not conduct a combinational examination of alterations to these forces. Each individual change in the model inputs (force magnitude and orientation) demonstrated a change to the stress concentration. Examining a combinational effect may produce a more detrimental stress distribution not investigated in this study. Furthermore, a less rigorous constraint system where bordering bones and ligaments are modeled may produce a better understanding of what the stress distribution is due to muscular and GRFs. Also, it is still not understood whether inversion is a necessary element in fracture development; so future work investigating this effect is necessary. Finally, the findings of this study suggest that the PB muscle is a primary contributor to this fracture; however, this study focused on loads associated with walking. If activities such as running, turning, or pivoting along with inversion control are analyzed, greater understanding of what causes Jones fractures may be evident.

We have also noted a 3D tension stress state that may suggest a delay in fracture union without appropriate activity level controls. Persistent tension stress at the fracture site will delay healing.[36] Surgical intervention employs intramedullary screw fixation and bone grafting to promote compression at the fracture site. The degree and magnitude of change from tension to compression with fixation, however, are beyond the scope of this study.

Control of the rehabilitative activity environment offers one means for reducing fracture occurrence. Results from the current study demonstrated the influence of the GRF and muscle forces (PB) and supported the results of Roca et al. that PB increased the stress concentration in the fifth MT.[20]

ACKNOWLEDGMENT

We gratefully acknowledge the support from the Orthopaedic and Rehabilitation Engineering Center at the Medical College of Wisconsin and Marquette University.

REFERENCES

1. Watson-Jones, R. *Fractures and Joint Injuries*, Churchill Livingstone, New York, 1982.
2. Clapper, M.F., O'Brien, T.J., and Lyons, P.M. Fractures of the fifth metatarsal. Analysis of a fracture registry, *Clin Orthop Relat Res*, 315, 238–241, 1995.
3. Morrison, G.M. Fractures of the bones of the feet, *Am J Surg*, 38, 721–726, 1937.
4. Dameron, T.B. Fractures and anatomical variations of the proximal portion of the fifth metatarsal, *J Bone Joint Surg*, 57-A, 788–792, 1975.
5. Torg, J.S. et al. Fractures of the base of the fifth metatarsal distal to the tuberosity. Classification and guidelines for non-surgical and surgical management, *J Bone Joint Surg*, 66-A, 209–214, 1984.
6. Jones, R. Fracture of the base of the fifth metatarsal bone by indirect violence, *Ann Surg*, 35, 697–701, 1902.
7. Byrd, T. Jones Fracture: relearning an old injury, *South Med J*, 85, 748–750, 1992.
8. Kavanaugh, J.H., Brower, T.D., and Mann, R.V. The Jones fracture revisited, *J Bone Joint Surg*, 60-A, 776–782, 1978.
9. Sammarco, G.J. Be alert for Jones fractures, *Phys Sportsmed*, 113, 353–360, 1991.
10. Carp, L. Fracture of the fifth metatarsal bone. With special reference to delayed unions, *Ann Surg*, 86, 308–320, 1927.
11. Lichtblau, S. Painful nonunion of a fracture of the 5th metatarsal, *Clin Orthop Relat Res*, 59, 171–175, 1968.
12. Peltier, L.F. Eponymic Fractures: Robert Jones and Jones's fracture, *Surgery*, 71, 522–526, 1972.
13. Zelko, R.R., Torg, J.S., and Rachun, A. Proximal diaphyseal fractures of the fifth metatarsal — treatment of the fractures and their complications in athletes, *Am J Sports Med*, 7, 95–101, 1979.
14. Josefsson, P.O. et al. Jones fracture: surgical versus nonsurgical treatment, *Clin Orthop Relat Res*, 299, 252–255, 1994.
15. Mann, R.A. and Coughlin, M.J. *Surgery of the Foot and Ankle*, Mosby, St. Louis, 1993.
16. Pearson, J.R. Combined fracture of the base of the fifth metatarsal and the lateral malleolus, *J Bone Joint Surg*, 43-A, 513–516, 1961.
17. Spector, F.C. et al. Lesser metatarsal fracture. Incidence management and review, *J Am Podiatry Assoc*, 74, 259–264, 1984.
18. Delee, J.C., Evans, J.P., and Julian, J. Stress fracture of the fifth metatarsal, *Am J Sports Med*, 11, 349–353, 1983.
19. Stewart, I.M. Jones's fracture: fracture of base of fifth metatarsal, *Clin Orthop Relat Res*, 16, 190–198, 1960.
20. Roca, J. et al. Stress fractures of the fifth metatarsal, *Acta Orthop Belg*, 46, 630–636, 1980.
21. Arangio, G.A., Xiao, D., and Salathe, E.P. Biomechanical study of stress in the fifth metatarsal, *Clin Biomech*, 12, 160–164, 1997.
22. Camacho, D.L.A. et al. A three-dimensional, anatomically detailed foot model: a foundation for a finite element simulation and means of quantifying foot-bone position, *J Rehabil Res Dev*, 39, 401–410, 2002.
23. Asai, T. and Murakami, H. Development and evaluation of a finite element foot model, in *Proceedings of Proc. of the 5th Symposium on Footwear Biomechanics*, Zurich/Switzerland, 2001, 10–11.

24. Beillas, P. et al. Foot and ankle finite element modeling using CT-scan data, in *Proceedings of 43rd STAPP Car Crash Conference*, San Diego, CA., 1999, 217–242.

25. Todd, B.A. and Wang, H. A visual basic program to pre-process MRI data for finite element modeling, *Comput Biol Med*, 26, 489–495, 1996.

26. Reilly, D.T. and Burstein, A.H. The elastic and ultimate properties of compact bone tissue, *J Biomech*, 8, 393–405, 1975.

27. Tannous, R.E. et al. A three-dimensional finite element model of the human ankle: development and preliminary application to axial impulsive loading, *Aerosp Eng*, 1996.

28. Van Buskirk, W.C. and Ashman, R.B. The elastic moduli of bone, *Transaction of American Society of Mechanical Engineering*, 45, 131–143, 1981.

29. Kidder, S.M. et al. A system for the analysis of foot and ankle kinematics during gait, *IEEE Trans Rehabil Eng*, 4, 25–32, 1996.

30. Seireg, A. and Arvikar, R. *Biomechanical Analysis of the Musculoskeletal Structure for Medicine and Sports*, Hemisphere Publishing Corporation, New York, 1989.

31. Wickiewicz, T.L. et al. Muscle architecture of the human lower limb, *Clin Orthop Relat Res*, 179, 275–283, 1983.

32. Brand, R.A., Pedersen, D.R., and Friederich, J.A. The sensitivity of muscle force predictions to changes in physiologic cross-sectional area, *J Biomech*, 19, 589–596, 1986.

33. Friederich, J.A. and Brand, R.A. Muscle fiber architecture in the human lower limb, *J Biomech*, 23, 91–95, 1990.

34. Kura, H. et al. Quantitative analysis of the intrinsic muscles of the foot, *Anat Rec*, 249, 143–151, 1997.

35. Wilson, E.S. and Katz, F.N. Stress Fractures: an analysis of 250 consecutive cases, *Radiology*, 92, 481–486, 1969.

36. Carter, D.R. et al. Mechanobiology of skeletal regeneration, *Clin Orthop*, 355S, S41–S55, 1998.

Part 2

Technical Developments and Emerging Opportunities

Section C

Foot and Ankle Modeling

22 A System for the Analysis of Foot and Ankle Kinematics during Gait*

Steven M. Kidder, Faruk S. Abuzzahab,
Gerald F. Harris, and Jeffrey E. Johnson

CONTENTS

22.1 INTRODUCTION

The foot is the final segment in the locomotor chain, providing support to the body by distributing gravitational and inertial loads. Abnormalities of the foot and ankle can cause irregular loading and pain in more proximal parts of the body.[1] Current methods of foot and ankle analysis include a combination of physical exam, observation, and radiographs. Clinical studies frequently model the foot as a single rigid body.[2–8] More descriptive models require recognition and definition of the major segments and articulations. Although these methods have been used to describe motion of the pelvis, hip, knee, and ankle, there are no reports of foot segment tracking during the stance and swing phases of gait.[3,4,7,9]

Many of the articulations of the foot do not act as simple hinge joints, but rather possess more complex characteristics reflective of the multiplanar contact at the joint surfaces.[10,11] Scott and Winter have reported that a single-axis characterization of the ankle in the sagittal plane lacks accuracy at initiation and termination of stance phase.[11] A series of cadaveric motion studies by Engsberg[12] and later by Siegler et al.[13] also concluded that ankle and subtalar joint motion was multiplanar.[12,13] These results were again confirmed by Lundberg[5] in studies of adult humans with implanted ratioopaque markers using stereoradiography and a stationary test apparatus.[5]

* © 1996 IEEE. Reprinted, with permission, from *IEEE Trans Rehab Eng.*, 4:1, 25–32, 1996.

The talonavicular joint was also examined by Lundberg and shown to possess multiplanar motion characteristics.[5] Rotation of the foot from a plantarflexed to neutral position has demonstrated shape changes in the longitudinal arch affecting the position between the hindfoot and forefoot, as well as changes in the transverse plane orientation.[5]

In order to better describe the complex intersegmental motion patterns of the foot during gait, an analysis system should accurately capture multisegmental data during both swing and stance phases.[14] A video-based system capable of capturing intersegmental foot motion during stance phase was described by Alexander and Campbell.[15] It was used to track motion between the tibia, calcaneus, forefoot, and hallux.[15] D'Andrea et al.[16] reported on three-dimensional (3-D) motion patterns of a single adult subject during stance using a video-based system.[16] In this study, we report on a system designed to track 3-D motion of the tibia, hindfoot, forefoot, and hallux segments during both stance and swing phases of the gait cycle.[17–22]

22.2 MATERIALS AND METHODS

A five-camera Vicon (Oxford Metrics, Oxford, England) motion analysis system was used to collect and process foot and ankle motion analysis data. Stereophotogrammetric methods were employed to describe the positions of markers placed on the foot and ankle.[23,24]

A rectangular capture volume was defined with appropriate dimensions for obtaining stance and swing phase data.[25] It measured 0.5 m (width) by 0.6 m (height) by 2.4 m (length). For calibration, brass spheres (15.9 mm diameter) were attached to lengths of brass ball-chains suspended at the corners of the capture volume. Four markers were mounted to each chain at 200 mm intervals. A fifth identification marker was affixed at a 30 mm interval to the lower end of three of the chains and at the upper end of the fourth. This ensured unique camera views of the volume. Calibration marker positions were measured with a vernier micrometer (accuracy ± 0.02 mm). An average of three measurements was used to determine the marker positions within ± 0.1 mm of tolerance. The tolerance was established by the index gradation spacing on the micrometer scale (0.02 mm per division). A plumb bob was used to accurately locate the point of intersection between each vertical corner of the capture volume and the horizontal walkway. The four intersection points were remeasured in the horizontal plane of the floor to assure that each corner of the capture volume was accurately positioned. The intersection points were measured and cross-checked trigonometrically to lie within 0.5 mm of their design locations.

A linearization process reduced error due to system characteristics, including lens curvature and deformation, focal length, aperture setting, changes due to thermal expansion/contraction, and nonlinearities inherent in video scanning.[26] The known locations of a matrix of 600 discs (12 mm diameter) were compared to those measured by the video system and used to construct a correction matrix. Each disc was 12 mm in diameter and was placed in a linear pattern separated from adjacent discs by 7 cm in the vertical and horizontal directions.

System resolution was calculated from the results of both static and dynamic testing.[9,26] In the static tests, two 15.9 mm diameter target markers were mounted to the ends of a rigid steel rod at a distance of 132.80 ± 0.02 mm. Marker separation was measured with a vernier micrometer (± 0.02 mm tolerance). The static test marker separation corresponded approximately to the intersegmental distances of the biomechanical foot model. The rod was oriented along the laboratory X-axis at one corner of the capture volume as marker images were sampled for a period of 4 sec (240 images of each marker). This procedure was repeated with alignment along the Y- and Z-axes as well, and at each corner and at the center of the capture volume. System resolution was calculated as

$$R = \left| D - \frac{1}{n}\sum_{i=0}^{n-1} d_i \right| \pm t\left(\frac{s}{\sqrt{n}} + \varepsilon_r + \varepsilon_m\right) \tag{22.1}$$

where D = measured (empirical) distance; di = computed distance; n = total number of samples; s = sample standard deviation; t = t-test coefficient; ε_r = round-off error; and ε_m = measurement error, based on micrometer resolution (± 0.02 mm).

T-test coefficients were obtained from statistical tables.[27]
Roundoff error was computed as

$$\varepsilon_r = \frac{5}{10^m} \tag{22.2}$$

where m = the number of significant digits.
In application, values were rounded to 0.01 nm, resulting in $\varepsilon_r = 0.05$.
Accuracy was determined as

$$A = \left(1 - \frac{\left| x_w - \frac{1}{n}\sum_{i=0}^{n-1} d_i \right|}{\frac{1}{n}\sum_{i=0}^{n-1} d_i}\right) \times 100\% \tag{22.3}$$

where A = system accuracy as a percentage; x_w = "worst" data point.

Because of measurement error, the average value of the computed distances was used as an estimate of the true distance.[28]

In order to define dynamic resolution and accuracy, a pendulum was developed using two brass spheres covered with reflective tape and connected by a thin cable at a distance of $\pm$ 594.0 mm. The physical characteristics of the pendulum were chosen to provide a known output displacement as a function of time. This information was then used to cross-check displacement obtained with the system against known (calculated) displacements. The pendulum was placed in the center of the capture volume for independent testing of sagittal (XZ) and coronal (YZ) plane motion. For each test, the lower marker was perturbed from a rest position and allowed to swing freely in the plane of interest. Data were captured for 4 sec at a sampling rate of 60 Hz, yielding 240 total samples, which were analyzed to determine dynamic resolution and accuracy.

Spectral analysis of static marker position data was performed with a single marker placed in the center of the capture volume on a wooden stand. The center of the capture volume was chosen because this position is equally distant from the defining outer surfaces of the capture volume. Cartesian vector components defining the position of the center marker were spectrally analyzed after acquiring 4 sec of data at 60 sp/sec (240 samples). A Fast Fourier Transform (FFT) was performed on the mean difference between the magnitude of each vector component and the overall mean vector magnitude (where the ith vector component of vector Xq is described as x_{qi}). In order to eliminate offset factors corresponding to the time average of the signal, the mean difference is computed at each sample point as

$$X_{qi} - \frac{\sum_{r=1}^{N} \sqrt{x_{r_1}^2 + x_{r_2}^2 + x_{r_3}^2}}{N} \tag{22.4}$$

where $i = 1, 2, 3$; $q = 1...N$.

A four-segment rigid body model without joint constraints was developed to describe the kinematics of the foot and ankle during ambulation. The segments were (Figure 22.1) (1) tibia and fibula (segment #1); (2) calcaneus, talus, and navicular

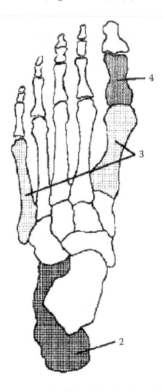

FIGURE 22.1 Four model segments: hindfoot (2), forefoot (3), hallux (4), and tibia/fibula (1), not depicted.

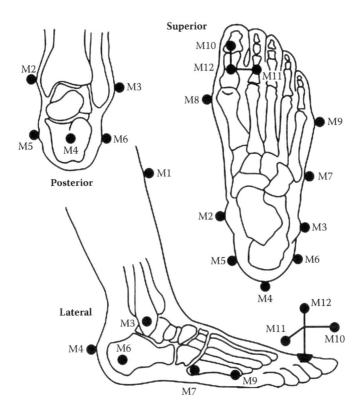

FIGURE 22.2 Twelve retroreflective marker positions.

(segment #2); (3) cuneiforms, cuboid, and metatarsals (segment #3); and (4) proximal phalanx of the hallux (segment #4). A total of 12 markers were required for the four-segment model (Figure 22.2, Table 22.1). Lightweight nylon markers covered with reflective tape were used in this study. A 15.9 mm marker diameter was selected because it offered an adequate reflective surface for identification without obscuring neighboring markers. Due to the small size of the hallux, a marker triad was constructed to achieve adequate marker separation. To minimize motion errors from inertial artifacts, the triad was constructed of a small metal base with three 1.60 mm diameter wires fixed to the markers (Figure 22.2). It should also be noted that other deviations from the rigid body assumptions can result in error (skin motion, segment distortion, etc.).

A clinical method for expressing a distal segment orientation relative to the next proximal segment was used in this study.

Partly due to widespread clinical acceptance in whole body gait applications, and following analysis of other methods of 3-D orientation description (Grood and Suntay, helical axis, direction cosines),[29,30] an Euler system was selected for this study.[29] The order of rotations selected was sagittal, coronal, and then transverse.

TABLE 22.1
Anatomic Marker Positions with AMASS Designations

Segment #	Marker #	AMASS Designations	Anatomical Location
1	1	MSAT	Medial surface of the anterior tibia
1	2	MAL	Medial malleolus
1	3	LMAL	Lateral malleolus
2	4	TCAL	Tuberosity of the calcaneus
2	5	MCAL	Medial calcaneus
2	6	LCAL	Lateral calcaneus
3	7	T5ML	Tuberosity of the 5th metatarsal laterally
3	8	MH1M	Medial head of the 1st metatarsal
3	9	LH5M	Lateral head of the 5th metatarsal
4	10	XHAL	Anteriorly directed hallux marker
4	11	YHAL	Laterally directed hallux marker
4	12	ZHAL	Superiorly directed hallux marker

The assembled rotation matrix R was expressed as $R = R_z R_x R_y$:

$$R = \begin{bmatrix} cy\ cz + sx\ sy\ sz & cx + sz & -sy\ cz + sx\ cy\ sz \\ -cy\ sz + sx\ sy\ cz & cx\ cz & sy\ sz + sx\ cy\ cz \\ cx\ sy & -sx & cx\ cy \end{bmatrix} \qquad (22.5)$$

where c_i is the cosine of the rotation about the ith axis and si is the sine of the rotation about the ith axis.

The three Eulerian angles, y, x, and z, were calculated using arcsin terms to return angular values, $-\pi/2 \leq \theta \leq \pi/2$.

Segment rotation matrices are described with respect to the global laboratory system. For a given vector q, referenced to the global coordinate system, the following relationship can be demonstrated:

$$\begin{bmatrix} q_x \\ q_y \\ q_z \end{bmatrix} = A \begin{bmatrix} r_{Ax} \\ r_{Ay} \\ r_{Az} \end{bmatrix} \quad and \quad \begin{bmatrix} q_x \\ q_y \\ q_z \end{bmatrix} = B \begin{bmatrix} r_{Bx} \\ r_{By} \\ r_{Bz} \end{bmatrix} \qquad (22.6)$$

where A and B are 3×3 rotation matrices, and r_A and r_B are vectors of q expressed in their relative coordinate systems.

Therefore

$$Ar_A = Br_B$$

or

$$r_A = A^T Br_B$$

where

$$A^T A = [I].$$ (22.7)

Marker coordinates were used to construct segment rotation matrices referenced to the lab coordinate system. The method of construction for the tibial body coordinate system is described below. Similar constructions are used for the other segments. The origin of the tibial body coordinate system is located midway between markers 2 and 3, with vector (t) defined

$$t = \begin{bmatrix} \dfrac{m_{2x} + m_{3z}}{2} \\[2ex] \dfrac{m_{2y} + m_{3y}}{2} \\[2ex] \dfrac{m_{2z} + m_{3z}}{2} \end{bmatrix}$$ (22.8)

The unit vector, t_2', is defined as pointing laterally from the origin of t to marker 3 for the left foot (marker 2 for the right):

$$t_2' = \begin{bmatrix} m_{3x} - t_x \\ m_{3y} - t_y \\ m_{3z} - t_z \end{bmatrix} \qquad t_2' = \begin{bmatrix} m_{2x} - t_x \\ m_{2y} - t_y \\ m_{2z} - t_z \end{bmatrix}$$

$$\text{(left foot)} \qquad\qquad \text{(right foot)}$$ (22.9)

The unit vector t_1' is formed by crossing t_2' with the unit vector from the origin of t to marker 1:

$$t_1' = t_2' \times \begin{bmatrix} m_{1x} - t_x \\ m_{1y} - t_y \\ m_{1z} - t_z \end{bmatrix}$$ (22.10)

Unit vector t_3' is formed by t_1' crossed with t_2':

$$t_3' = t_1' \times t_2'$$ (22.11)

The rotation matrix (T) for the tibial segment is constructed from the three unit vectors

$$T = [t_1' t_2' t_3']$$ (22.12)

The initial orientation of embedded model segment coordinate systems is determined by the location of the target markers. Consequently, without correction for anthropometric considerations, the relative orientations of the model segments would not be correlated with the position of the underlying bony structures. To provide this correlation by aligning the marker-based coordinates with underlying bony anatomy, a correction rotation matrix was determined with the use of radiographic data.

22.2.1 SUBJECT TEST PROTOCOL

The subject was instrumented and instructed to assume a comfortable, stable stance near the center of the capture volume. Several frames of data were captured to determine the original position of the markers. The position and loading conditions of the foot and ankle during the "snapshot" were not intended to simulate loading conditions during gait. The rigid body model used in this study to represent the foot and ankle structure is sensitive to loads as they affect the orientation of the various

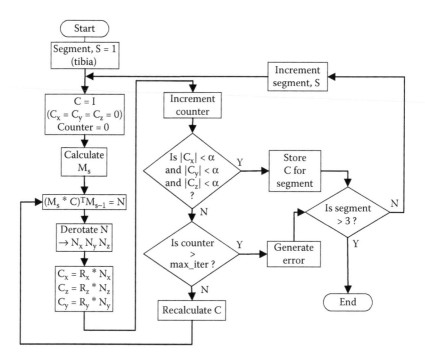

FIGURE 22.3 Procedure for calculation of matrices to realign marker-based coordinate systems with radiographic alignment. S: Segment counter, 0 to 4 (0 is the lab, 1-tibia, 2-hindfoot, 3-forefoot, and 4-hallux). C_s: Correction matrix for model of S. C_x, C_y, C_z: Euler rotations, which make up C. M_s: Uncorrected rotation matrix for the Sth model segment. N: Relative rotation matrix between the Sth and $(S - 1)$th segment. N_x, N_y, N_z: Euler rotations determined by N. R_{sx}, R_{sy}, R_{sz}: Relative rotations between segments S and $S - 1$ as determined from radiographs. α: Error term, maximum absolute difference accepted between the calculated angle, C_q, and the desired angle, R_q ($q = x$, y, or z). I: Identity matrix. max_iter: Maximum number of iterations allowed.

segments. Although indexed during quiet standing at body weight, the system will track the markers and the underlying bony anatomy of the rigid body model during dynamic foot loading and unloading. Foot position was recorded on graph paper and used to duplicate the foot position during the subsequent radiographic session. This allowed measurement of the maker positions relative to the underlying bony anatomy in a stable, repeatable posture. Three radiographic views were taken: anterior–posterior view, lateral view, and a hindfoot alignment view. An iterative process was used to construct correction matrices based upon x-ray measurements. The correction matrix procedure is detailed in a flowchart, as shown in Figure 22.3. Before calculation of relative segment orientation, segment coordinate systems (as determined from marker positions) are rotated into anatomical positions using the correction matrices.

Some measurements are difficult to obtain even with radiographic views. Coronal plane rotations of the hallux and forefoot are difficult to determine radiographically or clinically. No radiographic view exists, which would allow determination of coronal forefoot angle. Transverse plane tibial and hindfoot rotations are determined clinically.

An adult male subject (25-yr-old, 175 cm height, 60 Kg mass) without any prior surgery or pathology was tested at a freely selected cadence.[4] Data were acquired during five to ten unilateral walking trials. The exclusion criterion eliminated any trials with ten or more successive (60 Hz) frames of missing data. These usually occurred on the medial side of the foot during contralateral foot swing. Marker dropout was minimized through adherence to the linearization and calibration protocols and by optimizing camera position.

22.3 RESULTS

The residual was defined as the difference between the least-squares average of the measured and computed marker locations. While large residual values may indicate errors in the calibration procedure or faulty instrumentation, zero-value residuals reflect quixotic conditions. Commercial system residual values usually do not exceed 0.1% of the largest dimension of the capture volume.[31] Residual values in this study were under 2.0 mm or 0.083% of the largest capture volume dimension, 2400 mm.

Static computations required identification of the least accurate (computed) separation distance between target markers. This was accomplished through an automated sorting routing, which examined the computed target marker distances, d_i. Accuracy was expressed as a percentage in Equation 22.3. A synopsis of results is provided in Table 22.2. For statistical comparison, the t-test coefficient used in the static resolution expression was computed at the 0.05 and 0.01 levels of significance. Marker separation distance for the dynamic tests was determined within 0.5 mm of accuracy (ε_m) as shown in Table 22.3.

The most notable frequency component observed in the spectral analysis was found at 30 Hz. The x-component position vector demonstrated a uniform spectral appearance. The y-component was characterized by several spectral peaks, most notably at 30 Hz. This frequency was also noted in the z-component spectral analysis.

TABLE 22.2
Static Resolution and Accuracy Results
Computed at the $p = .05$ and $p = .01$ Levels
of Significance

Plane	Resolution (mm)	Accuracy	p-Value
Sagittal	0.1 ± 0.89	99.4%	.05
	0.1 ± 1.20	99.4%	.01
Coronal	0.6 ± 0.82	99.5%	.05
	0.6 ± 1.10	99.5%	.01

Data from a normal adult subject are illustrated in Figure 22.4, depicting relative orientations of the hindfoot, forefoot, and hallux model segments. Tibial orientation is presented relative to the global laboratory coordinate system. Hindfoot, forefoot, and hallux segment motions are presented relative to the next most proximal model segment. Mean data plus and minus one standard deviation are presented for three trials collected for the sagittal plane hindfoot motion as shown in Figure 22.5.

TABLE 22.3
Dynamic Resolution and Accuracy Results Computed at the (a) $p = 0.05$ and (b) $p = 0.1$ Levels of Significance

Location	X-Axis Resolution (mm)	X-Axis Accuracy Percentage	Y-Axis Resolution (mm)	Y-Axis Accuracy Percentage	Z-Axis Resolution (mm)	Z-Axis Accuracy Percentage
1	0.43 ± 0.06	99.1	0.88 ± 0.06	98.8	1.27 ± 0.08	99.3
2	0.78 ± 0.08	99.1	1.11 ± 0.08	99.0	0.13 ± 0.18	98.7
3	0.64 ± 0.07	99.0	0.81 ± 0.10	98.8	1.42 ± 0.15	98.3
4	0.47 ± 0.08	98.8	0.44 ± 0.08	98.8	0.73 ± 0.04	99.7
5	0.92 ± 0.06	98.7	1.49 ± 0.10	98.8	1.33 ± 0.05	99.2

Location	X-Axis Resolution (mm)	X-Axis Accuracy Percentage	Y-Axis Resolution (mm)	Y-Axis Accuracy Percentage	Z-Axis Resolution (mm)	Z-Axis Accuracy Percentage
1	0.43 ± 0.08	99.1	0.88 ± 0.08	98.8	1.27 ± 0.11	99.3
2	0.78 ± 0.10	99.1	1.11 ± 0.10	99.0	0.13 ± 0.23	98.7
3	0.64 ± 0.09	99.0	0.81 ± 0.13	98.8	1.42 ± 0.19	98.3
4	0.47 ± 0.10	98.8	0.44 ± 0.10	98.8	0.73 ± 0.05	99.7
5	0.92 ± 0.08	98.7	1.49 ± 0.13	98.8	1.33 ± 0.07	99.2

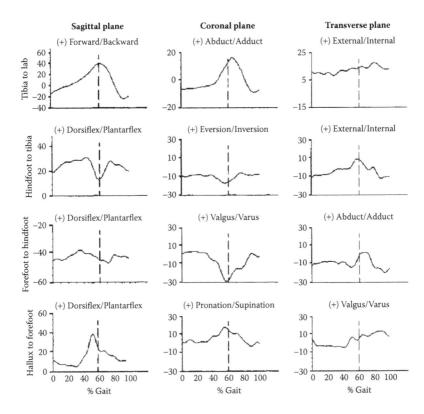

FIGURE 22.4 Kinematic data for a single trial. Data are presented from heelstrike to heel-strike (0 to 100% gait cycle). The vertical dashed lines indicates foot-off. Columns represent sagittal, coronal, and transverse motion, respectively.

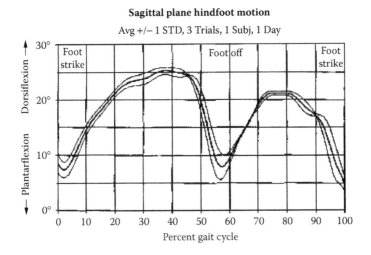

FIGURE 22.5 Sagittal plane hindfoot motion. Data presented for three trials, mean ± 1 STD.

22.4 DISCUSSION

Error in marker location reconstruction was reduced through cameral linearization, which provided a contour map of lens distortion for each camera. This process also reduced incidence of marker dropout. Poorly reflecting markers were replaced prior to each data-capture session. Slight changes in marker separation occurred during dynamic tests due to elastic properties of the pendulum. Thus, there was some error in assuming a constant marker separation. The use of a rigid foot frame is suggested for further system validation (static and dynamic). The double-edge detection routine used to calculate the centroid of each marker required a spherical marker. The markers may have the double edge located at different scan lines between cameras, adding variability to the computed marker location.

Resolution in the sagittal plane exceeded that of the coronal and transverse planes. This effect could be altered through reorientation of one or more cameras. Television video screens consisting of 525 horizontal lines are normally scanned at 30 Hz to compose a single frame. Each 30 Hz frame is composed of two alternating 60 Hz "half frames." The system alternatively scans half of the horizontal lines (the odd field) and then a second set of horizontal lines (the even field). Although close, these fields do not lie exactly between one another, which results in an image vibration seen in the vertical component of the camera image plane, coupled to the alternating scan rate (30 Hz). The spectral peak at 30 Hz was likely due to the interlace characteristic (odd/even frame), which was most prominent along the vertical plane of the camera.

During periods of marker dropout, an interpolation algorithm was used. This procedure used prior and subsequent curve histories and was effective for all stance and swing phase events except heel strike (initial contact) and foot-off (initial swing). These events present high accelerations and rapid displacement slope reversals, which cannot be accurately interpolated. If data were missing during these events, the trial was discarded.

Clinical results from system application are illustrated in Figure 22.4. The range of motion of knee flexion of 55 to 70° reported in previous work is similar to the change in tibial angle from toe-off to heel strike of approximately 75° (+ 55 to 20°).[3,32] The coronal plane motion of the tibia demonstrates an increase in abduction during swing phase. Shortly after heel strike and through stance, there is a return to a more neutral position and a period of adduction shortly before toe-off. Direct comparison to other work is difficult, but these motions seem to correlate with the current understanding of the events of the gait cycle.[9,32] The tibia remains externally rotated throughout the gait cycle and does not reach a neutral position even during early stance phase. This pattern agrees with previously reported motion of the tibia with relative internal rotation of the entire limb beginning at toe-off and continuing through the loading response.[9]

The sagittal plane hindfoot motion pattern shows dorsiflexion during swing phase. The hindfoot begins to plantarflex during late swing and this plantarflexion increases after heel strike. At the beginning of midstance, the hindfoot motion reverses and begins to dorsiflex until late stance, when the hindfoot plantarflexes during toe-off. The patterns and ranges of motion obtained for the sagittal plane in this study agree with previous work.[3,9,33–36] Motion of the hindfoot in the coronal plane shows an increase in inversion at toe-off, which moves to a relative neutral or slightly everted position shortly before heel strike. Through most of the stance phase, a relatively neutral position is maintained. These patterns and ranges agree with reported normal data.[16,33,34] Transverse plane hindfoot motion shows a steady movement into internal rotation throughout the swing phase to the beginning of midstance. At midstance, the hindfoot begins external rotation, which continues through toe-off. There are no reports for direct comparison of transverse hindfoot patterns.

Sagittal plane forefoot motion demonstrates relative plantar flexion at toe-off, which changes to a more dorsiflexed position approaching heel strike. The total range of motion of this segment is small, measuring less than 10°. Little data are available for this motion segment. D'Andrea et al. reported a similar motion pattern but recorded greater ranges of motion.[16] Coronal plane forefoot motion shows forefoot varus rotation at toe-off, with rotation toward a forefoot valgus position occurring steadily to midstance. A sudden increase in forefoot varus rotation occurs at toe-off. There are no known reports of this motion for comparison. Transverse plane forefoot motion demonstrates a near-neutral position at toe-off with an abduction motion occurring in early swing followed by adduction of the forefoot that increases through heel strike. There are no known reports of this motion for comparison.

Sagittal plane hallux motion shows dorsiflexion at toe-off with a progressive plantarflexion movement to a more neutral position at midstance. A rapid transition back to dorsiflexion is seen in the late stance phase and toe-off. These data correlate well with Delozier et al.[34] and D'Andrea et al.[16] Coronal plane hallux motion shows that from midswing to heel strike, there is an increase in hallux supination. At heel strike, the motion changes to pronation, increasing gradually throughout the stance phase. Transverse plane hallux motion is in a varus direction from heel strike through midstance, with a rapid movement back to valgus at toe-off. The hallux remains in a relative valgus position throughout the swing phase. There are no known reports of these motions for direct comparison.

22.5 SUMMARY

We have presented a system designed to track and quantify 3-D motion characteristics of the tibia, hindfoot, forefoot, and hallux segments of the distal lower extremity. The system requires the use of radiographs to index the reflective markers and underlying bony anatomy. Clinical data gathered during the testing phase of our study were collected from a single adult subject, which limits the clinical significance of these findings. Further work will be necessary to characterize the clinical reliability of the system. Normal kinematic patterns could then be examined in a large population to better understand the dynamic characteristics of the foot and ankle structure during ambulation. Possible rehabilitative and clinical/surgical applications could include treatment of diabetic neuropathy, characterization of pathological motion patterns, hallux valgus, posterior tibial tendon insufficiency, calcaneal reconstruction, pedothic management, prosthetic design and application, and therapeutic treatment.

REFERENCES

1. Radin, E.L., Yang, K.H., Riegger, C., Kish, V.L., O'Connor, J.J., "Relationship between lower limb dynamics and knee joint pain," *J. Orthop. Res.,* 9:398–405, 1991.
2. Dul, J., Johnson, G.E., "A kinematic model of the human ankle," *J. Biomed. Eng.,* 7:137–143, 1985.
3. Kadaba, M.P., Ramakrishnan, H.K., Wooten, M.E., "Measurement of lower extremity kinematics during level walking," *J. Orthop. Res.,* 8:383–392, 1990.
4. Kadaba, M.P., et al., "Repeatability of kinematic, kinetic, and electromyographic data in normal adult gait," *J. Orthop. Res.,* 7: 849–860, 1989.
5. Lundberg, A., "Kinematics of the ankle and foot: In vivo roentgen stereophotogrammetry," *Acta Orthopaedica Scandinavica — Supplementum,* 233:1–24, 1989.
6. [6] Nissan, M., Whittle, M.W., "Initiation of gait in normal subjects: a preliminary study," *J. Biomed. Eng.,* 12:165–171, 1990.
7. Ounpuu, S., Gage, J.R., Davis, R.B., "Three-dimensional lower extremity joint kinetics in normal pediatric gait," *J. Pediatr Orthop.,* 11:341–349, 1991.
8. White, S.C., Yack, H.J., Winter, D.A., "A three-dimensional musculoskeletal model for gait analysis. Anatomical variability estimates," *J. Biomech.,* 22:885–893, 1989.
9. Kadaba, M.P., Wootten, M.E., Ramakrishnan, H.K., Hurwitz, D., Cochran, G.V.B., "Assessment of human motion with VICON," *ASME Biomechan. Symp.,* 84:335–338, 1987.
10. Scott, S.H., Winter, D.A., "Biomechanical model of the human foot: kinematics and kinetics during the stance phase of walking," *J. Biomech.,* 26:1091–1104, 1993.
11. Scott, S.H., Winter, D.A., "Talocrural and talocalcaneal joint kinematics and kinetics during the stance phase of walking," *J. Biomech.,* 24:743–752, 1991.
12. Engsberg, J.R., "A biomechanical analysis of the talocalcaneal joint in vitro," *J. Biomech.,* 20:429–442, 1987.
13. Siegler, S., Chen, J., Schneck, C.D., "The three-dimensional kinematics and flexibility characteristics of the human ankle and subtalar joints — Part 1: kinematics," *J. Biomech. Eng.,* 110:364–373, 1988.
14. Harris, G.F., "Analysis of ankle and subtalar motion during human locomotion," In *Inman's Joints of the Ankle,* 2nd ed., J. Stiehl, Ed. Baltimore, MD: Williams and Wilkins, 75–84, 1991.
15. Alexander, I.J., Campbell, K.R., "Dynamic assessment of foot mechanics as an adjunct to orthotic prescription," In *The Biomechanics of the Foot and Ankle,* Donatelli, R., Ed., Philadelphia: F.A. Davis, 148–152, 1990.
16. D'Andrea, S., Tylkowski, C., Losito, J., Arguedas, W., Bushman, T., Howell, V., "Three dimensional kinematics of the foot," In *Proc. 8th Annu. East Coast Clin. Gait Lab. Conf.,* Rochester, MN, 109–110, May 5–8, 1993.
17. Abuzzahab, F.S., Harris, G.F., Kidder, S.M., Johnson, J.E., "A clinical system for foot and ankle motion analysis," *Proc. Annu. Conf. IEEE Eng. Med. Biol. Soc.,* San Diego, CA, Oct. 28–31, 1993, vol. 15, no. 3, pp. 1067–1068, 1993.
18. Abuzzahab, F.S., Hams, G.F., Kidder, S.M., Johnson, J.E., "A clinical system for foot and ankle motion analysis during gait," In *Proc. 8th Annu. East Coast Clin. Gait Lab. Conf.,* Rochester, MN, 137–138, May 5–8, 1993.
19. Abuzzahab, F.S., Harris, G.F., Kidder, S.M., Johnson, J.E., Alexander, I.J., DeLozier, G.S., "Development of a system for dynamic 3-D analysis of foot and ankle motion," In *Proc. Annu. Conf. IEEE Eng. Med. Biol. Soc.,* Paris, France, vol. 14, 110–111, 1992.

20. Kidder, S.M., Harris, G.F., Abuzzahab, F.S. Jr., Johnson, J.E., "A four-segment model for clinical description of foot and ankle motion," In *Proc. Annu. Conf. IEEE Eng. Med. Biol. Soc.,* San Diego, CA, Oct. 28–31, vol. 15, no. 3, 1065–1066, 1993.

21. Kidder, S.M., Harris, G.F., Johnson, J.E., Abuzzahab, F.S., "A kinematic model for clinical description of foot and ankle motion," In *Proc. Eighth Annu. East Coast Gait Conf.,* Rochester, MN, May 5–8, 111–112, 1993.

22. Kidder, S.M., Harris, G.F., Wynarski, G.T., Johnson, J.E., Alexander, I., DeLozier, G., Abuzzahab, F.S., "A four-segment model for clinical description of foot and ankle motion," In *Proc. Annual Conf. IEEE Eng. Med. Biol. Soc.,* Paris, France, vol. 14, 52–53, 1992.

23. Abdel-Aziz, Y.I., Karara, H.M., "Direct linear transformation from comparator coordinates into object space coordinates in close-range photogrammetry," In *ASP Symp. Close-Range Photogrammetry,* Amer. Soc. Photogrammetry, Falls Church, VA, 1971.

24. Antonsson, E.K., "A three dimensional kinematic acquisition and intersegmental dynamic analysis system for human motion," Ph.D. dissertation, Massachusetts Inst. Technol., Cambridge, MA, June 1982.

25. Whittle, M.W., *Gait Analysis: An Introduction.* Oxford, England: Butterworth-Heinemann Ltd., 136, 1991.

26. Whittle, M.W., "Calibration and performance of a 3-dimensional television system for kinematic analysis," *J. Biomech.,* 15, 185–196, 1982.

27. Ott, L., *An Introduction to Statistical Methods and Data Analysis.* Boston, MA: PWS-Kent, A5, 1988.

28. Nachtigal, C.H., *Instrumentation and Control: Fundamentals and Applications.* New York: Wiley, 62, 1990.

29. Goldstein, H., *Classical Mechanics.* New York: Addison-Wesley, 2nd ed., 1980.

30. Grood, E.S., Suntay, W.J., "A joint coordinate system for the clinical description of three-dimensional motions: Application to the knee," *J. Biomech.,* 105, 136–144, 1983.

31. "AMASS: ADiTECH Motion Analysis Software System," ADTECH,

32. Perry, J., Gait Analysis: Normal and Pathological Function, 1992. Thorofare, NJ: Slack Incorporated.

33. Apkarian, J., Naumann, S., Carins, B., "A three-dimensional kinematic model of the lower limb," *J. Biomech.,* 22, 143–155, 1989.

34. DeLozier, G.S., Alexander, I.J., Narayanaswamy, R., "A method for measurement of integrated foot kinematics," In *Proc. 1st Int. Symp. Three-Dimensional Anal. Human Motion,* Montreal, P.Q., Canada, July, 1991.

35. Lundberg, A., Goldi, I., Kalin, B., Selvik, G., "Kinematics of the ankle/foot complex: plantarflexion and dorsiflexion," *Foot Ankle,* 9(4), 194–200, 1989.

36. Stauffer, R.N., Chao, E.Y.S., Brewster, R.C., "Force and motion analysis of the normal, diseased, and prosthetic ankle joint," *Clin. Orthop.,* 127, 189–96, 1977.

23 Validation of a Multisegment Foot and Ankle Kinematic Model for Pediatric Gait*

Kelly A. Myers, Mei Wang, Richard M. Marks, and Gerald F. Harris

CONTENTS

* © 2004 IEEE. Reprinted, with permission, from *IEEE Trans Rehab Eng.,* 12:1, 122–130, 2004.

23.1 INTRODUCTION

The foot and ankle is a complex structural system. Motions at joints during gait are a function of bony repositioning. The foot serves to support and propel the body, transfer forces from the ground, and provide rotation for adaptations on uneven terrain. Dysfunctions of the foot have numerous origins, which are broadly categorized as either injury or pathology. It is crucial to properly treat foot and ankle anomalies, as they may lead to pain, further dysfunction, and erosion of proximal ability.

A currently accepted approach to quantifying foot and ankle kinematics during gait is to represent the entire foot as a single rigid body with a revolute ankle joint.[1] Although useful for overall sagittal plane studies, this method is inadequate for portraying true three-dimensional (3D) motion. More sophisticated models that segment the foot further and provide multiplanar rotation offer valuable insight into the segmental foot kinematics.

Few models include multisegmental kinematics for both the stance and the swing periods of gait. More typically, the biomechanical foot model is constrained to a limited number of segments and includes rotational limitations that restrict joint motion to a single axis of rotation.[2-5] Such rotational limitations lead to the inability to track well-documented, multiaxis joint rotations.[3,5-8]

There are many noteworthy, recently developed, biomechanical models that include multiple segments (three or more) to describe foot and ankle kinematics. Carson et al. document a four-segment foot model with rigorously defined segments using surface markers. However, no data are presented with regard to the accuracy, reliability, or validity of the biomechanical model.[10] Udupa et al. introduced a novel approach to kinematic foot analysis with the use of magnetic resonance (MR) imaging for 3D reconstruction of the foot and ankle segments.[11] Accurate and reproducible results were obtained. This MR method is particularly advantageous over the classical marker stereophotogrammetry methods, because the actual bone movements can be tracked as opposed to external landmarks. Unfortunately, this practice cannot be applied directly to gait. Rattanaprasert et al. provided a four-segment foot and ankle model. Each segment was assumed to have three degrees-of-freedom motion between the adjacent segments, with the exception of the hallux segment, which was limited to two degrees of freedom.[12] The developed model was tested for static accuracy and subject repeatability, and reported satisfactory results. The subjects included adults, and gait analysis was limited to the stance phase. Another model that was limited to the stance phase of gait was that of Leardini et al. This study segmented the foot and ankle into five parts: tibia/fibula, calcaneus, midfoot, first metatarsal, and hallux.[7] Repeatability measures were assessed, but a validation protocol was absent. Cornwall and McPoil used an electromagnetic system to develop a four-segment model to analyze the stance phase of gait.[13] All angular displacements were expressed relative to the leg segment, which does not correspond with the traditional method of graphical presentations, where segments are measured relative to the proximal segment. Additionally, there is no mention of model validation or accuracy testing. A study by Simon et al. complements the conventional segments by also defining functional segments that give insight into the combined motions of the foot.[14] The talus is defined as an individual segment in this model, although it cannot be defined with the use of surface markers alone.[15] In this case, a mathematical minimization problem has been deduced based on the positioning of adjacent segments. Thus assumptions are made assuming the joint's center location and its ability to be accurately traced during the gait cycle.[14,15] Many studies that present foot and ankle models include detailed development of the 3D segment but do not elaborate on validation procedures, including reliability and accuracy testing.[15,16]

With regard to the pediatric population, there are only limited biomechanical models to assess foot and ankle motion.[18,19] As with the adult populations, pediatric models of the foot and ankle strive to accurately describe the complex kinematics of foot motion in order to better understand kinematics and pathology and to improve treatment. Challenges in developing appropriate pediatric foot models include small foot sizes and close marker spacing, which frequently exceed the technical capabilities of the motion analysis system. Although reliability tests show good results for pediatric models, validation protocols are lacking in biomechanical model development.[18]

To date, there is no biomechanical model with pediatric applications that has demonstrated validity, accuracy, and reliability. The objective of this study was to develop an accurate biomechanical foot and ankle model to describe the kinematics of pediatric gait during both stance and swing. It was hypothesized that this pediatric system could function with equivalent or greater resolution, accuracy, and reliability when compared to existing adult foot and ankle model systems.

23.2 METHODOLOGY

23.2.1 Foot and Ankle Model

The pediatric biomechanical model defines the foot and ankle as four distinct segments: (1) tibia and fibula, (2) talus and calcaneus, (3) distal tarsals and metatarsals, and (4) hallux (Figure 23.1). An unrestricted 3D joint to the next distal segment couples each rigid body segment.

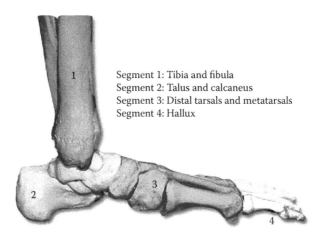

Segment 1: Tibia and fibula
Segment 2: Talus and calcaneus
Segment 3: Distal tarsals and metatarsals
Segment 4: Hallux

FIGURE 23.1 Bones of the foot and ankle with their associated model segment. (© 2004 IEEE)

The biomechanical model used a series of Euler rotations to determine the angle of the distal segment rotating with respect to the proximal segment. The order of rotations is sagittal, coronal, and then transverse planes of motion. This particular order was chosen with clinical applications in mind and realizing that as consecutive rotations are made, the accuracy of the model decreases.[6] Taking into account camera electronics, arrangements, and geometry, as well as planar motion of each of the segments, the derotation order was established as mentioned above. Each segment was assigned its own axis system. For instance, the left tibia segment is defined as:

$$t_{origin} = \begin{bmatrix} (M2_x + M3_x)/2 \\ (M2_y + M3_y)/2 \\ (M2_z + M3_z)/2 \end{bmatrix} \qquad (23.1)$$

$$t_2' = \begin{bmatrix} M3_x - t_{origin\,x} \\ M3_y - t_{origin\,y} \\ M3_z - t_{origin\,z} \end{bmatrix} \qquad (23.2)$$

$$t_1' = t_2 \times \begin{bmatrix} M1_x - t_{origin\,x} \\ M1_y - t_{origin\,y} \\ M1_z - t_{origin\,z} \end{bmatrix} \qquad (23.3)$$

$$t_3' = t_1' \times t_2' \qquad (23.4)$$

$$T = [t_1'\ t_2'\ t_3'] \qquad (23.5)$$

T is the 3×3 rotation matrix for the left tibia segment comprising the three unit vectors, t_1', t_2', and t_3'. One segment is expressed relative to the adjacent segment by multiplying the transposed 3×3 rotation matrix of the proximal segment by that of the distal segment. Therefore, the tibia segment is expressed relative to the global or lab coordinate system. The hindfoot is measured relative to the tibia, the forefoot to the hindfoot, and the hallux to the forefoot.

23.2.2 INSTRUMENTATION

A 15 camera VICON 524 (Oxford Metrics, Oxford, England) motion analysis system was used to acquire 3D marker data at 120 frames/sec (fps). The capture volume was defined with dimensions of 1.3 m (height) by 1.0 m (width) by 4.9 m (length). This volume ensured collection of complete stance and swing phase gait data. Three markers

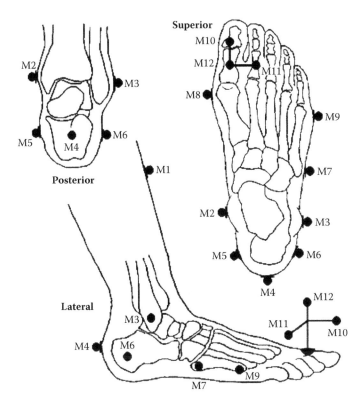

FIGURE 23.2 Marker locations of the pediatric foot and ankle model. (© 2004 IEEE)

were placed on bony landmarks (Figure 23.2) to define each segment of the model (Table 23.1). At a minimum, three noncollinear markers define a segment in space. The markers are small ($d =14.5$ mm), lightweight, and covered with reflective tape. To compensate for the small size of the hallux segment, which does not allow room for the placement of three markers, a hallux triad was used (Figure 23.2). A rotation matrix was developed for the hallux segment based on the geometry of the triad, so that the segment axis could be oriented more closely with the anatomical axes.

For the dynamic testing procedures, a Biodex System 3 (Biodex Medical Systems, Inc., New York, New York) was used to generate defined angular rotations. A Biodex machine uses a programmable rotational shaft in conjunction with a dynamometer. It can be positioned in multiple orientations to move through various ranges of motions. Biodex outputs that are of interest in this study include time, angular position (range = 330° and accuracy = ±1° of rotation), and angular velocity (range = 1 to 500°/sec and accuracy = ±1°/sec).

23.2.3 SUBJECT POPULATION

Three normal children, between the ages of 6 and 11, made up the subject population of this study. They had no history of gait abnormalities or any previous orthopedic

TABLE 23.1
Marker Locations of the Pediatric Foot and Ankle Model

Segments	Marker Number	Marker Name	Anatomical Location
1	M1	(R/L)MSAT	Medial surface of the anterior tibia
1	M2	(R/L)MMAL	Medial malleolus
1	M3	(R/L)LMAL	Lateral malleolus
2	M4	(R/L)TCAL	Calcaneal tuberosity
2	M5	(R/L)MCAL	Medial calcaneus
2	M6	(R/L)LCAL	Lateral calcaneus
3	M7	(R/L)T5ML	Tuberosity of the 5th metatarsal laterally
3	M8	(R/L)MH1M	Medial head of the 1st metatarsal
3	M9	(R/L)LH5M	Lateral head of the 5th metatarsal
4	M10	(R/L)XHAL	Anteriorly directed hallux marker
4	M11	(R/L)YHAL	Laterally directed hallux marker
4	M12	(R/L)ZHAL	Superiorly directed hallux marker

surgeries. Upon completion of instrumentation, each subject was asked to walk at a self-selected pace (approximately 1.10 m/sec) a distance of 5 m. No less than nine trials were collected for each subject, according to standard clinical protocol. This ensured enough trials to provide for more reliable estimates of gait patterns.

23.2.4 VALIDATION PROTOCOL

23.2.4.1 Linear Testing

Resolution and accuracy of the foot and ankle system were determined both statically and dynamically.[6,21,22] For static linear testing, four markers were placed on a dummy segment representing the approximate shortest and longest intermarker distances of the pediatric foot and ankle model (Figure 23.3). The short and long distances measured 39.9 and 140.7 mm, respectively. A midpoint distance was also explored (70.5 mm). The marker positions were measured with a vernier caliper (±0.02 mm tolerance). The dummy segment was placed in the capture volume and oriented along the x, y, or z global reference system axis. Data were collected for six trials of 3-sec duration for each orientation. To assess reliability, the testing procedures were repeated 2d later. Taking the same dummy segment and moving it through the capture volume at the average pediatric gait speed fulfilled dynamic linear testing.

23.2.4.2 Angular Testing

Dynamic angular testing used the Biodex System 3 to rotate through a known range of 305°. A dummy segment with three markers, representative of a proximal foot segment, was mounted onto the stationary Biodex, representing the distal segment (Figure 23.4). The Biodex was programmed to rotate through 305° at 180°/sec.

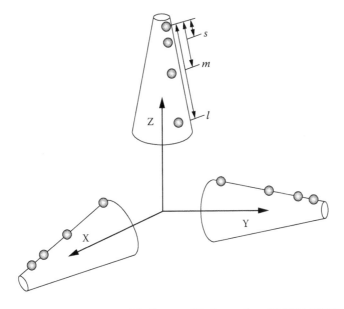

FIGURE 23.3 Dummy segment used in linear validation testing. (© 2004 IEEE)

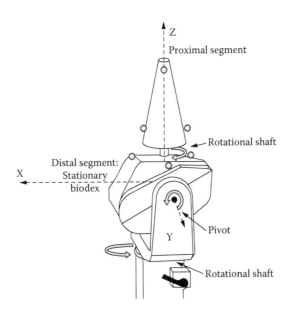

FIGURE 23.4 Biodex orientation for angular validation testing. (© 2004 IEEE)

The system provided the required angular output over time and was compared to the biomechanical model's output at various positions in the range. This procedure was repeated for x, y, and z orientations.

23.2.4.3 Accuracy and Resolution Equations

System resolution was calculated from the following equation[6]:

$$R = \left| D - \frac{1}{n} \sum_{i-0}^{n=1} d_i \right| + t\left(\frac{s}{\sqrt{n}} + \varepsilon_r + \varepsilon_m \right)$$

(23.6)

D = measured distance
n = total number of samples
d_i = computed distance
t = t-test coefficient (from statistical tables[23])
s = sample standard deviation
ε_r = round-off error = $(5/10^m)$
ε_m = measurement error, based on micrometer resolution (-0.02 mm)
m = number of significant digits.

System accuracy was computed as[6]:

$$A = \left(1 - \frac{\left| x_w - \frac{1}{n} \sum_{i=0}^{n=1} d_i \right|}{\frac{1}{n} \sum_{i=0}^{n=1} d_i} \right) \times 100\%$$

(23.7)

A = percentage system accuracy
x_w = "worst" data point.

23.2.5 KINEMATIC DATA ANALYSIS

3D marker data were run through two separate biomechanical foot and ankle models. The first was the pediatric model developed in this study. Secondly, the same trial data set was processed with the Milwaukee adult foot and ankle system. Marker data were labeled in VICON motion capture software, and gait events such as foot contact and toe-off were identified. The marker coordinates were processed with a Woltring filter, with a mean square error value of 20. Data were then processed with the VICON Body Builder for Biomechanics software. The marker data were also processed with the Milwaukee adult foot and ankle model.[6] Each model output was 12 joint rotation angles, one for each foot segment in each of the three anatomical planes.

The data were exported to MATLAB for graphical processing. Data sets were interpolated to 150 data points and normalized to percentage of gait cycle (0 to 100%)

for comparison. A cross-correlation function was used to compare the two models. The cross-correlation was calculated with the following equation[24]:

$$R_{xy}(\tau) = \lim_{T \to \infty} \frac{1}{T} \int_0^T x(t)y(t+\tau)\, dt \tag{23.8}$$

$x(t)$ = adult Milwaukee model kinematic output
$y(t)$ = pediatric model output
τ = frame lag.

Each cross-correlation curve was normalized, so that perfect correlation would equal 1. The point of maximal correlation was labeled and recorded for statistical purposes.

23.3 RESULTS

23.3.1 VALIDATION PROTOCOL

23.3.1.1 Linear Testing Results

The results of the static linear testing are shown in Table 23.2. Markers placed at 140.7 mm represent the long distance, at 70.5 mm the mid-distance, and at 39.9 mm the shortest distance. For comparative statistical purposes, t-test coefficients were selected at the 0.05 and 0.01 levels of significance. Accuracy was exceptional in all

TABLE 23.2
Linear Static Resolution and Accuracy Testing Results (© 2004 IEEE)

Orientation	Marker Position	Accuracy (%)	Resolution (mm)	p-Value
	Short-	100	0.30 – 0.14	0.05
			0.30 – 0.23	0.01
x-axis	Mid-	100	0.50 – 0.14	0.05
			0.50 – 0.23	0.01
	Long-	99.98	0.41 – 0.17	0.05
			0.41 – 0.29	0.01
	Short-	100	0.60 – 0.14	0.05
			0.60 – 0.23	0.01
y-axis	Mid-	99.90	0.53 – 0.18	0.05
			0.53 – 0.30	0.01
	Long-	100	0.10 – 0.14	0.05
			0.10 – 0.23	0.01
	Short-	99.95	0.18 – 0.17	0.05
			0.18 – 0.29	0.01
z-axis	Mid-	99.88	0.31 – 0.17	0.05
			0.31 – 0.29	0.01
	Long-	99.94	0.48 – 0.17	0.05
			0.48 – 0.29	0.01

TABLE 23.3
Linear Dynamic Resolution and Accuracy Testing Results
(© 2004 IEEE)

Marker Position	Accuracy	Resolution (mm)	P-Value
Short-	99.84%	0.53 – 0.18	0.05
		0.53 – 0.31	0.01
Mid-	99.81%	0.43 – 0.23	0.05
		0.43 – 0.39	0.01
Long-	99.91%	0.23 – 0.23	0.05
		0.23 – 0.39	0.01

three orientations, with the highest percentage of accuracy in the x-axis orientation followed by the y- and z-axes. The mean average accuracies of the short-, mid-, and long-distances (s, m, and l, respectively) were 99.99%, 99.96%, and 99.92% for the x-, y-, and z-orientations, correspondingly. The greatest resolution was documented in the s-, l-, and s-distances in the x-, y-, and z-orientations, respectively. The poorest resolution was seen at the m-, s-, and l-distances in the x-, y-, and z-orientations, respectively. The worst resolution was $0.53 - 0.18$ mm at 0.05 level of significance, m-distance, and 99.90% accuracy. The greatest resolution was seen in the y-orientation with the l-distance at $0.10 - 0.14$ mm and 0.05 level of significance.

Table 23.3 summarizes the results of the dynamic linear testing. The markers were oriented along the z-axis for the trials. The markers that represent distance l demonstrate both the highest percentage of accuracy (99.91%) and the greatest resolution ($0.23 - 0.23$ mm at 0.05 level of significance). The resolution is second greatest at distance m ($0.43 - 0.23$ mm at 0.05 level of significance) followed by the poorest resolution at s-distance ($0.53 - 0.14$ at 0.05 level of significance).

23.3.1.2 Angular Testing Results

Table 23.4 shows the computations of resolution and accuracy for the angular testing. The Biodex was programmed to rotate at a rate of 180°/sec. The x-, y-, or z-axis given is the axis in which the Biodex arm rotates around (i.e., the z-axis is analogous to transverse plane motion). The range of motion was set from 0° to 305°; however, the positions of rotation were measured with a constant angular velocity of 180°/sec. Consequently, there is a window of 200° at the center of the range of motion where the velocity of the arm is 180°/sec. The five positions where measurements were taken are equally distributed throughout this window. The mean accuracy of the dynamic angular test results was the highest with rotation about the x-axis (99.69%), followed by the y-axis (99.57%), and then the z-axis (99.51%). The resolution was the greatest with rotation about the z-axis ($0.78 - 1.23$ mm), then the x-axis ($0.86 - 0.34$ mm), and then the y-axis ($0.89 - 0.83$ mm).

TABLE 23.4
Dynamic Angular Test Results (© 2004 IEEE)

Position	x-Axis		y-Axis		z-Axis	
	Resolution (mm)	Accuracy (%)	Resolution (mm)	Accuracy (%)	Resolution (mm)	Accuracy (%)
1	0.82 – 3.56	99.39	0.41 – 3.50	99.19	0.22 – 3.57	99.18
2	0.28 – 3.42	99.66	0.24 – 3.58	99.56	0.09 – 3.90	98.92
3	1.0 – 3.35	99.77	0.55 – 3.54	99.64	0.51 – 3.36	99.75
4	1.1 – 3.81	99.81	0.93 – 3.43	99.81	0.10 – 3.35	99.87
5	0.99 – 3.50	99.82	2.32 – 3.62	99.67	2.96 – 3.53	99.83
Average	0.8612	99.69	0.8936	99.57	0.7794	99.51
Standard deviation	0.342	0.001	0.836	0.002	1.23	0.004

Note: Biodex velocity = 180°/sec and $p = 0.01$ level of significance.

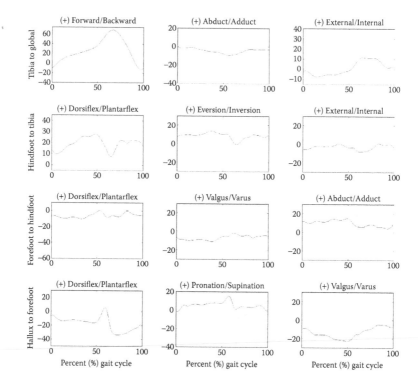

FIGURE 23.5 Kinematic data from one trial of representative subject. (© 2004 IEEE)

23.3.2 KINEMATIC DATA ANALYSIS

The kinematic output data of the foot and ankle model are shown in Figure 23.5. The trial presented is best representative of the pediatric walking trials. The motion of the tibia segment is expressed relative to the global lab coordinate system. The hindfoot, forefoot, and hallux segments are calculated relative to the adjacent proximal segment. The columns denote the sagittal, coronal, and transverse planes of motion, while the rows signify the relative angles between the lab and the tibia, tibia and hindfoot, hindfoot and forefoot, and forefoot and hallux. The axis labels on each of the graphs are identical. The y-axis is the intersegment rotation angle in degrees and the x-axis is the percentage gait cycle. The gait cycle is defined from heelstrike to the next consecutive heelstrike of the same foot and therefore includes both stance and swing phases.

Figure 23.6 shows the results of the pediatric foot model and then the Milwaukee foot model as reported by Kidder et al.[6] The solid line represents the pediatric model results, and the dotted line denotes the same data processed with the Milwaukee foot and ankle software. The cross-correlation graphs in Figure 23.7 show the

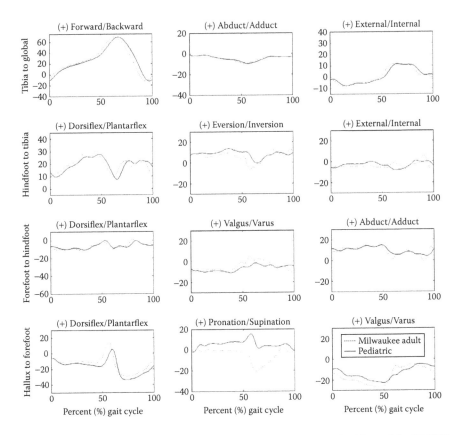

FIGURE 23.6 Kinematic results of pediatric and Milwaukee foot and ankle models. (© 2004 IEEE)

relationship between the two sets of kinematic data. The x-axis of the cross-correlation graphs is the lag in frame number. Normalized correlation coefficients are located on the y-axis. For positive correlation, the range is from 0 to 1, with 1 equaling perfect correlation. Table 23.5 summarizes the statistical analyses of the cross-correlation graphs. The table presents the mean and standard deviation of each trial for the three subjects involved in the study. The frame lag was equated to lag expressed as a percentage of the gait cycle. Correlation coefficients range from 0.988 ± 0.001 to 0.749 ± 0.200 (this range excludes the negatively correlated coronal plane hallux segment). Highest correlation was found between the sagittal plane tibia segments and the lowest correlation within the transverse plane hindfoot segments. The lag at which the correlation coefficients occur lie between a maximum of 3.55% gait cycle (coronal plane hallux segment) and 0.44% gait cycle (coronal plane hindfoot segment).

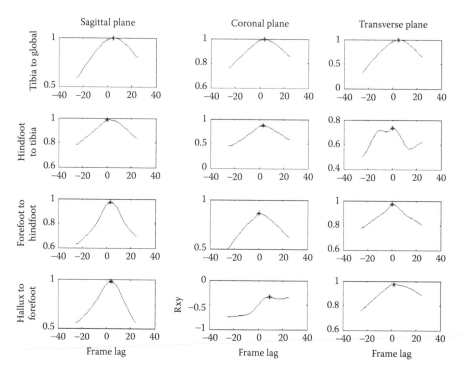

FIGURE 23.7 Cross-correlation graphs between pediatric and Milwaukee models. (© 2004 IEEE)

TABLE 23.5
Statistics of Cross-Correlation Graphs (© 2004 IEEE)

Segment	Plane	Mean Lag Percentage Gait Cycle	Standard Deviation	Mean Correlation Coefficient	Standard Deviation
Tibia	Sagittal	3.00	0.36	0.998	0.001
Tibia	Coronal	0.77	1.22	0.985	0.009
Tibia	Transverse	1.89	1.71	0.991	0.010
Hindfoot	Sagittal	0.89	1.38	0.994	0.004
Hindfoot	Coronal	0.44	0.81	0.948	0.047
Hindfoot	Transverse	0.77	1.71	0.749	0.200
Forefoot	Sagittal	0.67	1.03	0.969	0.016
Forefoot	Coronal	1.11	1.77	0.883	0.092
Forefoot	Transverse	0.67	1.12	0.957	0.038
Hallux	Sagittal	1.89	0.98	0.965	0.016
Hallux	Coronal	3.55	2.33	-0.096	0.299
Hallux	Transverse	1.67	1.51	0.934	0.066

23.4 DISCUSSION

23.4.1 Validation Protocol

For the results of the linear static testing, the resolution was slightly greater when the segment was oriented along the z-axis. Accuracy values are acceptable regardless of orientation or testing procedure. The comparable adult foot and ankle system reported static resolution as 0.01 ± 1.2 mm, with an accuracy at 99.4% (assuming a 0.01 level of significance) in the sagittal plane.[6] The coronal resolution for the adult model was 0.6 ± 1.1 mm with 99.5% accuracy. Transverse plane information was not provided. For the dynamic testing, resolution increased with decreasing marker distance. This result is typical of most imaging systems. However, the resolution for the short marker separation is still in a satisfactory range. Kidder et al. documented average resolution along the x-axis as 0.65 ± 0.07 mm and average accuracy as 98.9%.[6] y- and z-axes resolutions and accuracies are 0.94 ± 0.08 at 98.8% and 0.97 ± 0.13 at 99.04%, respectively, at a 0.05 level of significance.[6]

23.4.2 Kinematic Analysis

Comparisons between the adult Milwaukee foot and ankle kinematic analysis and the pediatric biomechanical model are presented. Figure 23.6 shows the two model outputs plotted on the same graphs. From these plots, it is evident that the tibia motion in the sagittal, coronal, and transverse planes matches closely with that of the adult Milwaukee foot and ankle model. The segment ranges of motion in each of the planes are also quite similar. It is difficult to make additional comparisons of these graphs to femur-referred gait data, as the current study refers the tibia to the lab-based global coordinate system. However, there are studies that make a global-based reference with similar curve patterns and ranges of motion in all three anatomical planes.[6,26]

The hindfoot segment in the sagittal plane shows ranges of motion similar to that in the adult Milwaukee foot model. The pediatric foot model also demonstrates a slight inversion shift from the Milwaukee foot model during midstance. Similar patterns are documented in other studies, which show good correlation between curve contour and ranges of motion.[1,3,5,6,26,28] Leardini et al. reported a diminished range of motion in a two-camera adult foot study.[7] Hindfoot motion in the coronal and transverse planes demonstrated a somewhat decreased range of motion compared to the Milwaukee model. These patterns and ranges are similar to normal reported adult data in the coronal plane [1,5–7,26,29] and also in the transverse plane.[1,6,7,26]

Hallux kinematics in the sagittal plane demonstrate similar ranges of motion. There is good correlation with the normal data published by Leardini et al.,[7] D'Andrea et al.,[29] and DeLozier et al.[28] In the coronal plane, the pediatric model demonstrates a pronation shift from about 5° at initial contact to a maximum of 10° in midstance. The hallux motion in the transverse plane is similar in the two models, with a slight valgus shift in the pediatric model. Forefoot motions in the sagittal and coronal planes are comparable in overall range of motion in the pediatric and adult models. The motions of the forefoot in the transverse plane are nearly identical. Recent publications report similar ranges of motion and curve morphology, although D'Andrea, while citing larger ranges of motion, reports similar patterns in the sagittal plane.[7,26,29]

23.4.3 CROSS-CORRELATION ANALYSIS: MILWAUKEE FOOT MODEL

MATLAB V.6 R-12 was used to perform cross-correlation analyses of the two model outputs (Figure 23.7). When comparing the subject trials, it is important to investigate the overall correlation as well as phase shift. Of the 12 graphs, 11 graphs have positive correlations. The hallux segment in the coronal plane exhibits negative correlation. This may be due to the initial curve divergence and offset that is present through the majority of the gait cycle. In the case of negative correlation, ranging from −1 to 0, 0 is the point of perfect correlation. The representative trial presented shows very good correlation between the Milwaukee and pediatric models. The point of maximum correlation is not less than 0.8421 (transverse plane hindfoot). The mean correlation coefficient of the 11 graphs of the representative trial is 0.961 ± 0.044 (this measurement excludes the coronal plane hallux segment). Table 23.5 reports the mean and standard deviation of the lag and correlation coefficients over all trials. The highest correlation is demonstrated in the sagittal plane tibia segment (0.998 ± 0.001). Examining each segment individually shows that the highest correlation is always in the sagittal plane. Also, when looking at each plane, the order of correlation (high to low) is the tibia, hindfoot, forefoot, and hallux. These trends are likely due to the order of rotations (sagittal, coronal, and transverse). The first rotation yields the highest accuracy. Consecutive rotations have diminished accuracy and the same is true when moving toward distal segments.

The lag at which maximum correlation occurs varies between graphs. The lag value other than 0 is indicative of a phase shift. The representative trial shows a mean lag of $1.4 \pm 1.6\%$ gait cycle. The maximum lag is 4.6% gait cycle (coronal plane hallux) and the minimum is 0 (coronal and transverse tibia, all planes of the hindfoot, and the transverse plane hallux). The phase shift may be attributed to the filtering devices used in the Milwaukee foot and ankle model. (It is unknown which filter the data are run through in the proprietary Milwaukee software.)

23.4.4 CLINICAL APPLICATION

Both the adult and pediatric Milwaukee foot models will accept radiographic input data. While it remains a goal to keep radiation exposure to a minimum, especially in pediatric subjects, there may be an advantage in referencing detailed foot motion to the underlying bony anatomy.[30] Use of these methods requires control of variation in radiograph measurement techniques, which easily add sources of error into the kinematic modeling program. Influences of radiographic variability on the foot and ankle model output have not been thoroughly examined. Future applications of this model may incorporate optional radiographic inputs if strongly desired. This may be beneficial in the case of a severely deformed foot, where the marker placement may not truly reflect the anatomy of the foot. Also, further use of the static foot position may be used to offset some errors not yet quantified to more closely align the foot segments to the true anatomical orientation.

23.5 CONCLUSION

The static and dynamic test results confirm the system accuracy and ability to track 3D motion during pediatric gait. The resolution and accuracy computations are comparable and even surpass similar measurements for the existing Milwaukee adult foot and ankle model. The dynamic angular test results also verify the ability of the biomechanical model to track rotations accurately. In the light of the current study results, the model is considered sufficient for further clinical application. The small number of clinical patients included in this study ($n = 3$) does not allow for detailed clinical descriptions of pediatric gait. Further work should include normal pediatric subjects and subjects with pathologies. It is hoped that quantification of normal and pathological pediatric gaits will ultimately lead to improved characterization, rehabilitation, and surgical treatment.

ACKNOWLEDGMENTS

The authors would like to thank the Marquette University Department of Engineering, Medical College of Wisconsin Department of Orthopaedic Surgery, Shriners Hospital for Children (Chicago, IL), and the Orthopaedic Research and Engineering Center for providing resources to complete this project. Much gratitude also goes to Lyon, Ropella, Van Bogart, and Tulchin, for consulting.

REFERENCES

1. J. Apkarian, S. Naumann, and B. Cairns, "A three-dimensional kinematic and dynamic model of the lower limb," *J Biomech,* vol. 22, no. 2, pp. 143–155, 1989.
2. T.M. Kepple, S.J. Stanhope, K.N. Lohmann, and N.L. Roman, "A video based technique for measuring ankle-subtalar motion during stance," *J Biomech Eng,* vol. 105, pp. 136–144, 1983.
3. S.H. Scott and D.A. Winter, "Talocural and talocalcaneal joint kinematics and kinetics during the stance phase of walking," *J Biomech,* vol. 24, pp. 743–752, 1991.
4. S.H. Scott and D.A. Winter, "Biomechanical model of the human foot: kinematics and kinetics during the stance phase of walking," *J Biomech,* vol. 26, pp. 1091–1104, 1993.
5. K.L. Seigal, T.M. Kepple, P.G. O'Connell, L.H. Gerber, and S.J. Stanhope, "A technique to evaluate foot function during the stance phase of gait," *Foot Ankle,* vol. 16, pp. 764–770, 1995.
6. S.M. Kidder, F.S. Abuzzahab, G.F. Harris, and J.E. Johnson, "A system for the analysis of foot and ankle kinematics during gait," *IEEE Trans Rehab Eng,* vol. 4, pp. 25–32, 1996.
7. A. Leardini, M.G. Benedetti, F. Catani, L. Simoncini, and S. Giannini, "An anatomically based protocol for the description of foot segments during gait," *Clin Biomech,* vol. 14, pp. 528–536, 1999.

8. T. Stahelin, B.M. Nigg, D.J. Stafanyshyn, A.J. van den Bogart, and S.J. Kim, "A method to determine bone movement in the ankle joint complex in vitro," *J Biomech*, vol. 30, pp. 513–516, 1997.

9. M. Carson, M. Harrington, N. Thompson, and T. Theologis, "A four segment in vivo foot model for clinical gait analysis," *Gait Posture*, vol. 8, p. 73, 1998.

10. J.K. Udupa, B.E. Hirsch, H.J. Hillstrom, G.R. Bauer, and J.B. Kneeland, "Analysis of in vivo 3-D internal kinematics of the joints of the foot," *IEEE Trans Biomed Eng*, vol. 45, no. 11, pp. 1387–1396, 1998.

11. U. Rattanaprasert, R. Smith, M. Sullivan, and W. Gilleard, "Three dimensional kinematics of the forefoot, rearfoot, and leg without the function of tibialis posterior in comparison with normals during stance phase of walking," *Clin Biomech*, vol. 14, pp. 14–23, 1999.

12. M.W. Cornwall and T.G. McPoil, "Three-dimensional movement of the foot during the stance phase of walking," *J Am Podiatr Med Assoc*, vol. 89, no. 2, pp. 56–66, 1999.

13. J. Simon, D. Meaxiotis, A. Siebel, H.G. Bock, and L. Döderlein, "A multi-segmented foot model," *Gait and Clinical Movement Analysis Society Abstracts*, 6th Annual Meeting, Sacramento, CA, 2001.

14. J. Simon, D. Metaxiotis, A. Siebal, H.G. Bock, and L. Döderlein, "A model of the human foot with seven segments," *Gait Posture*, vol. 12, pp.63–64, 2000.

15. M. Carson, M. Harrington, N. Thompson, J.J. O'Connor, and T.N. Theologis, "Assessment of a multi-segment foot model for gait analysis," *Gait Posture*, vol. 12, pp.76–77, 2000.

16. J. Henley, K. Wesdock, G. Masiello, and J. Nogi, "A new three-segment foot model for gait analysis in children and adults," *Gait and Clinical Movement Analysis Society Abstracts*, 6th Annual Meeting, Sacramento, CA, 2001.

17. P. Smith, J. Humm, S. Hassani, and G. Harris, "3-D Motion analysis of the pediatric foot and ankle," In *Pediatric Gait*, G.F. Harris and P.A. Smith, eds., pp. 183–188. Piscataway, NJ: IEEE Press Inc., 2000.

18. M.P. Kadaba, M.E. Wooten, H.K. Ramakrishnan, D. Hurwitz, and G.V.B. Cochran, "Assessment of human motion with VICON," *ASME Biomechan Symp*, vol. 84, pp. 335–338, 1989.

19. A.J. van den Bogart, G.D. Smith, and B.M. Nigg, "In vivo determination of the anatomical axes of the ankle joint complex: an optimization approach," *J Biomech*, vol. 27, no. 12, pp. 1477–1488, 1994.

20. L. Ott, *An Introduction to Statistical Methods and Data Analysis*. Boston, MA: PWS-Kent, 1988, p. A5.

21. J.S. Bendat and A.G. Piersol, *Random Data Analysis and Measurement Procedures*. New York: John Wiley & Sons, Inc., 2000.

22. J.E. Johnson, S.M. Kidder, F.S. Abuzzahab, and G.F. Harris, "Three-dimensional motion analysis of the adult foot and ankle," In *Human Motion Analysis*, G.F. Harris and P.A. Smith, eds., pp. 351–369. Piscataway, NJ: IEEE Press Inc., 1996.

23. G.S. DeLozier, I.J. Alexander, and R. Narayanaswamy, "A method for measurement of integrated foot mechanics," in *Proc 1st Int Symp Three-Dimensional Anal. Human Motion*, Montreal, PQ, Canada, July 1991.

24. S. D'Andrea, C. Tylkowski, J. Losito, W. Arguedas, T. Bushman, and V. Howell, "Three-dimensional kinematics of the foot," in *Proc 8th Annu East Coast Clin Gait Lab Conf,* Rochester, MN, pp. 109–110, May 5–8, 1993.

25. J.E. Johnson, R. Lamdan, W.F. Granberry, G.F. Harris, and G. F. Carrera, "Hindfoot coronal alignment: a modified radiographic method," *Foot Ankle Int,* vol. 20, no.12, pp. 818–825, 1999.

24 Measurement of Foot Kinematics and Plantar Pressure in Children Using the Oxford Foot Model

Julie Stebbins, Marian Harrington, Tim Theologis, Nicky Thompson, Claudia Giacomozzi, and Velio Macellari

CONTENTS

24.1 INTRODUCTION

The foot is a complex entity, composed of over 100 ligaments, 30 muscles, and 26 bones.[1] It has intricate movement patterns, which, at present, are not well understood. The foot provides a crucial mechanical role during locomotion, which may be summarized by the following four functions:[2]

It provides a stable base of support to minimize muscular effort.

It accommodates rotation of more proximal limb segments during the weight-bearing phase of the gait cycle.

Flexibility of the structures within the foot allows shock absorption and accommodation of the terrain.

Rigidity of structures within the foot allows leverage during push-off.

Normal patterns of motion within the foot during gait have been described by various authors using a variety of measurement techniques.[2–9] Impact at initial contact is partially absorbed through ankle plantarflexion, which proceeds from slight dorsiflexion to approximately 20° of plantarflexion during the initial stage of the gait cycle.[6] During this load acceptance phase, the body's entire weight is gradually transferred to the supporting limb,[9] as the lower leg internally rotates. Early experimental results by Hicks[10] suggested that the hindfoot tended to invert during this period. However, more recent studies using three-dimensional (3D) gait analysis appear to contradict this finding. Eversion of the hindfoot during early stance has been demonstrated by a number of authors, using both surface markers and bone pins.[4,6,8] Since these studies measured dynamic, *in vivo* motion, rather than relying on cadaveric analysis, it is probable that this reflects, more accurately, true motion of the hindfoot. The hindfoot also initially abducts during the first 20% of the gait cycle.[6] The general position of the hindfoot during the initial phase of stance allows flexibility for shock absorption and conformity to irregular surfaces.[2]

Between 15 and 50% of the gait cycle, the lower leg dorsiflexes over the foot,[9] the tibia rotates externally,[2,9] and the hindfoot tends to invert.[4,6,8] Toward terminal stance, the hindfoot again progresses to plantarflexion as the heel is raised off the ground.[2]

The hindfoot rapidly dorsiflexes during the initial swing phase to promote clearance of the foot. During terminal swing, the foot begins to plantarflex once again, which prepositions the foot for initial contact.

Very little information is available regarding forefoot motion during gait. Improvements in camera sensitivity have only recently begun to allow distinction between different segments of the foot during 3D motion analysis. However, this type of research is still in its infancy; thus, a degree of caution is warranted when interpreting results.

Interestingly, there is very little cadaveric research investigating forefoot motion. Much of the attention over recent years has focussed on the ankle and hindfoot, particularly the subtalar joint. The few studies available which address forefoot motion[5,11] have all employed 3D motion analysis. Results suggest that the forefoot tends to be slightly plantarflexed and supinated relative to the hindfoot at initial contact, progressing to slight dorsiflexion throughout the first half of stance, while maintaining a neutral position in the frontal plane.

During terminal stance, the forefoot rapidly plantarflexes, supinates, and adducts until toe-off occurs. During swing phase, it remains slightly plantarflexed and supinated.

Soft tissue and bony deformities within the foot compromise its role during gait. Altered bony alignment restricts the available range of motion, which inhibits shock absorption and accommodation functions of the foot. Poor biomechanical alignment also limits the generation of propulsive power, increasing the amount of muscular work required to propel the body forward.

Current methods of 3D motion analysis are inadequate for measuring and describing these patterns of movement within the foot. This is particularly apparent when considering measurement of the forefoot, or when deformity is present. A new system of measuring motion and loading of the foot, which is clinically relevant and able to be practically implemented, is required. The purpose of the current study was to develop a multisegment foot model, appropriate for use in children over the entire gait cycle. Five variations of this model were then tested to determine the most appropriate method for measuring intersegment motion within the foot for both healthy and pathological conditions, such as cerebral palsy. A second aim of this study was to provide a reliable and automated method for measuring plantar pressure in children, which may also be applied in the presence of foot deformity.

24.2 METHODOLOGY

24.2.1 Testing Protocol

Fifteen healthy children aged 6 to 14 yr (average age 9.5 yr, five male and ten female) were tested at the Oxford Gait Laboratory on three separate occasions. Visits were spaced between 2 weeks and 6 months apart. Each child had reflective markers placed on his or her dominant foot[12] and a conventional marker set on the lower body.[13] A 12-camera VICON 612 system (Vicon Motion Systems Ltd., Oxford, U.K.) was used to collect 3D kinematics of one foot and both lower limbs for each subject at 100 Hz. Data were also collected from a piezoresistive pressure platform (Istituto Superiore di Sanita, Rome, Italy) with a spatial resolution of 5 mm, sampling at 100 Hz.[14] This was rigidly mounted to and time synchronized with an AMTI force plate, with a minimum sampling frequency of 500 Hz (OR6 platform, Advance Mechanical Technology Inc., Massachusetts, U.S.). Results were validated by comparing center of pressure and total force output from the AMTI force plate with that of the pressure mat. Subjects were asked to walk at their usual walking speed along a 10-m walkway. Three representative trials for each visit were used in the analysis. These trials were identified visually by looking at all traces from the session (average 20 trials). A static standing trial was also performed to define the segment axes prior to four markers being removed, as shown in Table 24.1, for the walking trials.

24.2.1.1 Foot and Ankle Model

The Oxford Foot Model defined by Carson et al.[12] was modified for children and for application to deformity, such as that seen in cerebral palsy. The original model

TABLE 24.1

Names and Positions of Markers Used in the Foot Model

Marker Name	Position	Segment
KNE	Femoral condyle	Femur
TTUB	Tibial tuberosity	Tibia
HFIB	Head of fibular	Tibia
LMAL	Lateral malleolus	Tibia
MMAL[a]	Medial malleolus[a]	Tibia[a]
SHN1	Anterior aspect of shin	Tibia
CAL1	Posterior distal aspect of heel	Hindfoot
CAL2[a]	Posterior medial aspect of heel[a]	Hindfoot[a]
CPEG	Wand marker on posterior calcaneus aligned with transverse orientation	Hindfoot
LCAL	Lateral calcaneus	Hindfoot
STAL	Sustentaculum tali	Hindfoot
P1MT	Base of first metatarsal	Forefoot
P5MT	Base of fifth metatarsal	Forefoot
D1MT[a]	Head of first metatarsal[a]	Forefoot[a]
D5MT	Head of fifth metatarsal	Forefoot
TOE	Between second and third metatarsal heads	Forefoot
HLX	Base of hallux	Hallux

[a]Names are used in the static trial only and are removed for dynamic trials.

comprised a rigid tibial segment (tibia and fibula), a rigid hindfoot (calcaneus), a forefoot (five metatarsals), and a hallux (proximal phalanx of the hallux). The tibia was redefined using the knee joint center for compatibility with the lower body model. The hindfoot segment was altered to be independent of neighboring segments, which is particularly important in cases where foot deformity is present. For the forefoot, the position of the proximal marker on the first metatarsal (P1MT) was changed to be medial to the extensor hallucis longus tendon, in order to provide greater consistency in placement; the forefoot anterior/posterior axis was adjusted accordingly. The hallux segment was replaced by a single vector. This gave the following foot segment definitions for what was considered to be the *default model,* with markers listed in Table 24.1, and shown in Figure 24.1(a and b)

24.2.1.1.1   Tibia

24.2.1.1.1.1   Anatomical Definition

It is composed of the tibia and fibula and assumed to move as a single rigid body. Segment is based on the plane defined by the line from the knee joint center to the ankle joint center and the transmalleolar axis. Longitudinal axis is from the ankle joint center to the knee joint center. Anterior axis is perpendicular to the plane defined by the longitudinal axis and the transmalleolar axis. Transverse axis is mutually perpendicular.

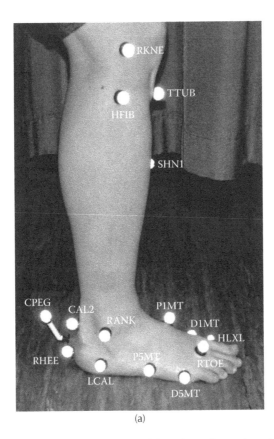

(a)

FIGURE 24.1   (a) Markers on the lower leg and foot shown from a lateral view. (b) Markers on the foot and ankle shown from a dorsal view.

24.2.1.1.1.2   Static Calibration

Vertical axis is from the mid-point between the MMAL and LMAL to the KJC (defined by the lower body model[13]). Anterior axis is perpendicular to the plane defined by the vertical axis and the vector from the MMAL to the LMAL. Transverse axis is mutually perpendicular.

24.2.1.1.2   Hindfoot

24.2.1.1.2.1   Anatomical Definition

The calcaneus defines the hindfoot. Motion at the talocrural and subtalar joints are considered to contribute jointly to motion of the hindfoot relative to the tibia. Segment is based on orientation of the mid-sagittal plane of the calcaneus in standing posture (defined by the line that passes along posterior surface of the calcaneus, which is equidistant from both the lateral and medial borders of this surface, and the point midway between the sustentaculum tali and the lateral border of the calcaneus). Anterior axis is from the most posterior aspect of the calcaneal tuberosity, in the plane defined above, and parallel to the plantar surface of the hindfoot. Lateral axis is perpendicular to this plane.

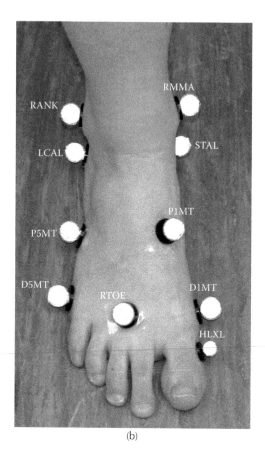

(b)

FIGURE 24.1 (Continued).

24.2.1.1.2.2   Static Calibration

Anterior axis is parallel to the floor and in the plane of CAL1, CAL2, and CPEG. Transverse axis is perpendicular to this plane. Vertical axis is mutually perpendicular.

24.2.1.1.3   Forefoot

24.2.1.1.3.1   Anatomical Definition

Comprises the five metatarsals and assumed to move as a single rigid body. Segment is based on the plane defined by the center of distal heads of the first and fifth metatarsals and the proximal head of the fifth metatarsal. Superior axis is perpendicular to this plane. Longitudinal axis is the projection of the line from the mid-point of the proximal heads of the first and fifth metatarsals to the mid-point of the distal heads of the second and third metatarsals into this plane.

24.2.1.1.3.2   Static Calibration

Vertical axis perpendicular to plane containing D1MT, D5MT, and P5MT. Longitudinal axis is the projection onto this plane of the line from the mid-point of P1MT and P5MT to TOE. Transverse axis is mutually perpendicular.

24.2.1.1.4   Hallux

24.2.1.1.4.1   Anatomical Definition

Comprises the proximal phalanx of the hallux. Based on a longitudinal line along the proximal phalanx.

24.2.1.1.4.2   Static Calibration

Mediolateral axis aligned with lateral axis of forefoot. Anterior axis from D1MT (at height of HLX) to HLX. Angles of rotation for each segment were calculated according to the joint coordinate system of Grood and Suntay.[15]

This model was implemented using BodyBuilder software (Vicon Motion Systems Ltd., Oxford, U.K.). The four markers on each segment (except the hallux) give redundancy in case of marker loss. This information was also exploited to calculate intersegment angles in different ways. Five variations of the default model were tested for anatomical feasibility and repeatability:

> Using a scaled virtual point between D1MT and D5MT to define the distal point of the longitudinal axis of the foot (DistFF). The point was chosen as the scaled distance that produced the same angle of forefoot abduction as using the TOE marker. It was thought that this would prove more reliable than placing the TOE marker on the foot.

> Tracking the forefoot segment with markers on the lateral part only — anatomically defined as comprising metatarsals 2 to 4 (eliminating the use of P1MT for dynamic trials). To quantify the sensitivity of the measurements to movement of P1MT relative to the forefoot (i.e., flexibility of the forefoot segment in the default model), P1MT was moved up and down by 5 mm within the forefoot coordinate system of one representative subject, using BodyBuilder software (Vicon Motion Systems Ltd, Oxford, U.K.). The resulting changes on forefoot pronation and supination were calculated. A value for forefoot "arch height" of the foot was also calculated. This was defined as the absolute distance between the marker on the dorsal surface of the base of the first metatarsal (P1MT) and the same point projected on the plantar surface of the forefoot as defined by the model in the static trial. This was then normalized to foot length by dividing by the distance from CAL1 to TOE, which gave the arch height as a percentage of foot length. The maximum and range of this distance were recorded.

> Tracking the hindfoot segment in walking trials without the use of the wand marker on the rear of the calcaneus (CPEG). This was performed since it appeared that the wand marker was prone to being knocked, and therefore a potential source of variability.

> Using markers on the tibia itself to define the longitudinal axis of the tibia (as in the original version of the model[4]), rather than the knee joint center from the conventional lower body model. This was also believed to potentially improve repeatability, since the assumption of a fixed knee joint center may be a source of variability.

> Static calibration of hindfoot and dynamic tracking of hindfoot without reference to CPEG. It was thought that this would prove to be more accurate and repeatable than visually lining up the CPEG with the orientation of the hallux.

Parameters that were analyzed included clinically significant maximums, minimums, and ranges of intersegment angles. These were determined after an initial visual analysis of the data, as well as consideration of routine clinical practice. Data from three trials for each visit were averaged and then one-way analysis of variance (ANOVA) tables were used to determine within-subject standard deviations (SDs) to give a measure of repeatability. Each variation of the model was compared to the default model. Changes in within-subject SDs greater than 1° were considered significant. Mean values for each variable were also calculated and differences were assessed with paired t-tests ($p < .01$).

24.2.2 PLANTAR PRESSURE

The pressure footprint was divided into five subsections. These were medial heel, lateral heel, midfoot, medial forefoot, and lateral forefoot. The positions of the markers on the foot were superimposed onto the pressure footprint at a time corresponding to mid-stance, defined by the instant when the summed vertical distance between all the markers on the foot and the floor was at a minimum. The medial/lateral and anterior/posterior coordinate of each marker was then projected vertically onto the footprint (Figure 24.2). This provided the means to automatically divide the foot on the basis of anatomical landmarks (Table 24.1). Peak force values (normalized to body mass) were obtained for each subarea, for each gait cycle, and repeatability of these measurements was assessed using SPSS software (SPSS Inc, version 11.0). ANOVA tables were used to define within-subject SDs for the healthy children. A normal range with 95% confidence intervals was established from the data from all the healthy children.

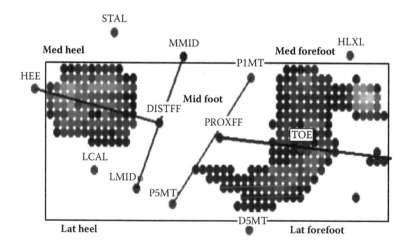

FIGURE 24.2 Pressure footprint showing five sub-areas: medial heel, lateral heel, midfoot, medial forefoot, and lateral forefoot. The labeled circles represent the projected positions of markers on the foot.

24.3 RESULTS

24.3.1 MULTISEGMENT FOOT KINEMATICS*

Measured variables from foot kinematics for each subject were compared between days. For the default model, the patterns of movement were found to be consistent but some offsets between days were observed (Figure 24.3). Within-subject SDs were lowest in the sagittal plane (between 2 and 4°). The highest variability was in the transverse plane at the hindfoot and forefoot, with SDs of 8 and 7°, respectively.

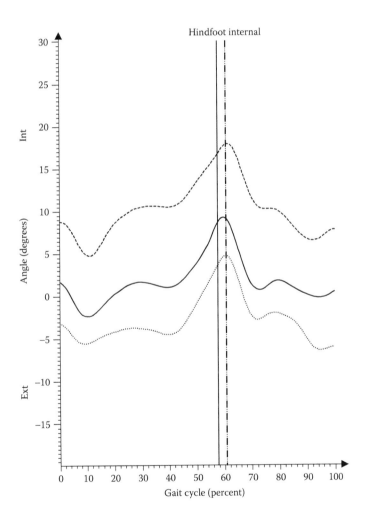

FIGURE 24.3 Example of inter-day variability in foot motion. Patterns consistent but offset apparent. Solid line from visit 1, dashed line from visit 2, dotted line from visit 3. Vertical lines divide stance and swing phase.

---

* The results of this section have been previously published.[16]

TABLE 24.2

Comparison of Means and Within-Subject SDs for the Default Model and Variations (1) and (2), Which Affect the Position of the Forefoot Relative to the Hindfoot and Tibia

	Default		DistFF Point (1)		Lateral Markers Only (2)	
	Mean	SD	Mean	SD	Mean	SD
Maximum forefoot dorsiflexion	9.8	3.4	9.8	3.3	10.1	3.3
Maximum forefoot supination	6.5	5.3	6.4	5.9	6.5	5.4
Minimum forefoot abduction	5.0	7.4	4.1	7.1	0.6[a]	7.1
Range forefoot dorsiflexion	20.8	2.7	20.8	2.7	19.2[a]	2.5
Range forefoot supination	8.8	1.6	8.6	1.6	7.8[a]	2.0
Range Forefoot Adduction	9.9	2.4	9.9	2.6	8.8[a]	2.3
Maximum FF/Tib dorsiflexion	19.9	3.7	19.9	3.5	NA	NA
Maximum FF/Tib supination	11.8	4.2	12.8	3.4	NA	NA
Maximum FF/Tib adduction	16.8	8.4	19.6	7.8	NA	NA
Range FF/Tib dorsiflexion	44.0	4.5	44.1	4.5	NA	NA
Range FF/Tib supination	15.2	3.1	16.4	3.3	NA	NA
Range FF/Tib adduction	17.3	3.7	18.4	3.4	NA	NA

NA = Not Available
[a]Significant difference in the mean value.

All five variations of the model were compared for repeatability to the default model. Changes in definitions of the model produced only minimal changes in repeatability. The only variation producing change in the repeatability was variation 5, which reduced variation of the hindfoot in the transverse plane between days from 8 to 6° (Table 24.2 and Table 24.3).

24.3.1.1 Variation 1

Using a scaled point, 53% of the distance between the heads of the first and fifth metatarsals produced no significant change in the measured angle of maximum forefoot adduction relative to the hindfoot, when compared to using the TOE marker (Table 24.2). It was therefore accepted that this scaled distance produced similar results to the TOE marker and was used for further comparison. No difference was noted in repeatability in using this point instead of the TOE marker.

24.3.1.2 Variation 2

Using markers on the lateral part of the forefoot only to track the forefoot had the effect of making the forefoot appear less adducted in swing than if markers on the entire forefoot were used (mean change from 5 to 1° adduction, $p < .01$) (Figure 24.4). It also reduced the range of forefoot motion (dorsi/plantar flexion: 21 to 19°; abduction/adduction: 9 to 8°; and pronation/supination: 10 to 9°, $p < .01$) (Table 24.2).

TABLE 24.3

Comparison of Means and Within-Subject SDs for the Default Model and Variations 3, 4, and 5, Which Affect the Hindfoot

	Default		No CPEG (3)		Tibia Markers (4)		No CPEG Static (5)	
	Mean	SD	Mean	SD	Mean	SD	Mean	SD
Maximum knee flexion	59.2	2.5	NA	NA	64.5[a]	3.1	NA	NA
Maximum hindfoot dorsiflexion	11.2	3.0	10.9	2.9	12.2	3.5	10.7	2.8
Maximum hindfoot inversion	9.0	5.2	8.8	5.4	9.3	5.6	7.6	4.6
Maximum hindfoot rotation	13.8	8.4	15.6	8.3	15.3	8.1	13.9	6.6[b]
Range knee flexion	56.9	3.0	NA	NA	61.2[a]	3.2	NA	NA
Range hindfoot dorsiflexion	24.2	2.7	23.7[a]	2.8	20.4[a]	2.6	23.8	2.8
Range hindfoot inversion	10.8	2.2	11.5	2.1	10.2	1.9	11.4	2.0
Range hindfoot rotation	12.3	2.7	12.4	2.0	11.1	2.0	12.1	2.1

NA = Not Available

[a]Significant difference in mean value.

[b]Significant difference in repeatability.

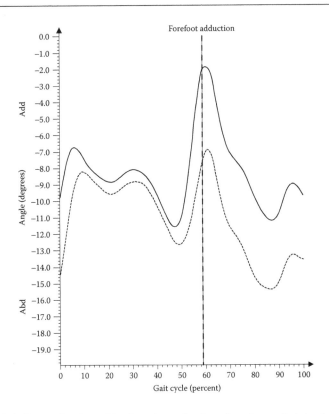

FIGURE 24.4 Change forefoot adduction when using lateral markers only to track the forefoot (dashed line). Solid line represents tracking all four markers on the forefoot (default model).

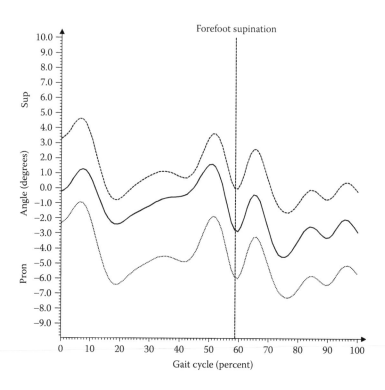

FIGURE 24.5 Change in forefoot angles as a result of shifting P1MT up (dashed line) by 5mm and down (dotted line) by 5mm. Solid line is neutral position of P1MT as in default model. Vertical dashed line divides stance and swing phase. Trace is from one representative subject.

The calculated forefoot "arch height" had a mean value of 23% (SD 4%). This changed within the gait cycle by 7% (SD 2%). Sensitivity analysis on the position of the proximal marker on the first metatarsal revealed that a movement of 10 mm in the vertical direction produced a maximum change of 9° in supination of the forefoot (Figure 24.5).

24.3.1.3 Variation 3

When the wand marker on the rear of the calcaneus was eliminated from use in calculating hindfoot angles in dynamic trials, repeatability was unchanged. However, it tended to reduce the range of hindfoot dorsiflexion (from 24.2 to 23.7°, $p < .01$) (Table 24.3).

24.3.1.4 Variation 4

Using anatomical markers on the tibia itself, rather than on the knee joint center, produced a significant increase in the mean maximum knee flexion angle (from 59 to 65°, $p < .01$)

and range of knee flexion (from 57 to 61°, $p < .01$). It also reduced the range of measured hindfoot dorsiflexion (from 24 to 20°, $p < .01$) (Table 24.2).

24.3.1.5 Variation 5

Elimination of the CPEG wand marker during static calibration was the only variation to significantly improve repeatability, which reduced the SD for hindfoot rotation from 8 to 6°. There were no significant changes in mean values.

Table 24.2 and Table 24.3 show a summary of the comparison of within-subject SDs for each of the methods described above, as well as comparisons of mean values. Figure 24.6 shows the average foot kinematics from 14 healthy children on the basis of the default version of the model. One subject was excluded from this average due to obvious toe walking.

24.3.2 Plantar Pressure*

Normalized peak force showed the highest values in the medial heel and medial forefoot, with the lowest value at the midfoot. Peak force repeatability varied from 0.2 to 1.8 N/kg for the different subareas, for intrasubject SD. Peak force showed the most variability in the medial heel (Figure 24.7).

24.4 DISCUSSION

24.4.1 Multisegment Foot Kinematics

A comprehensive study has been carried out on the repeatability of foot kinematics in healthy children of a model adapted to the assessment of foot deformity in children with cerebral palsy. This provided objective data on which to base a final version of the model.

For the default model, good consistency between patterns of foot motion was observed but some offsets in the curves between days were noted. This was quantified by comparing intrasubject SDs in peak and range values for the intersegment angles where the peak values between adjacent segments showed greater variability (2 to 8°) than the ranges (2 to 3°). The sagittal plane (dorsi/plantarflexion) was found to be the most repeatable and the highest variability was found in the transverse plane (internal/external rotation of the hindfoot and forefoot abduction/adduction). This variability is generally greater than previously reported values based on tests in adult subjects, as might be expected due to the smaller surface area of children's feet and the greater variability in their gait.[14] The trend in variability between planes (between 1 and 5°) is consistent with the results previously found when validating the Oxford Foot Model on two healthy adults.[4] Other investigators who have studied adult foot kinematics have found similar trends. Siegel et al.[18] reported similar SDs, with the sagittal plane having the least variability, followed by the coronal plane, and the transverse plane with the most variability. Moseley et al.[6] found 1 to 2° SDs, again with the greatest repeatability appearing in the sagittal plane, and the least in the

---

* The results of this section have been previously published.[17]

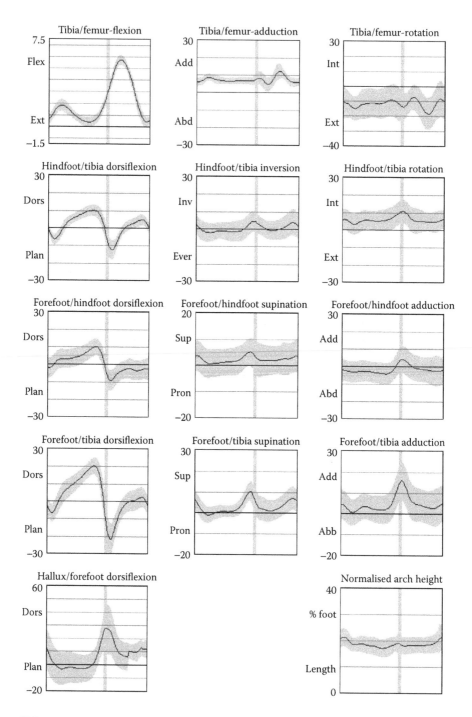

FIGURE 24.6 Inter-segment foot angles from 14 healthy children of final version of Oxford foot model normalized to 100% of the gait cycle. Shade band shows mean ±SD across all subjects.

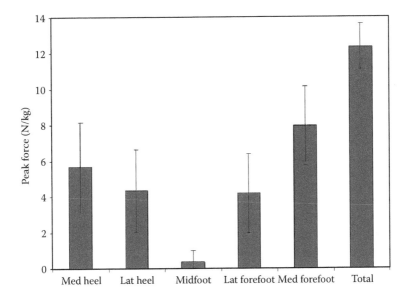

FIGURE 24.7 Normalized peak force among the five footprint sub-areas.

transverse plane. Kepple et al.[19] tested five healthy adults and found intrasubject SDs ranging up to 1.2°. They found the most variability in the transverse plane and the least in the coronal plane. Leardini et al.[11] reported acceptable levels of repeatability in the sagittal and coronal planes, but not in the transverse, for all intersegment pairings. They further stated that clinical conclusions on altered joint function in the transverse plane should therefore be handled more carefully. There have been some studies that found the most variability in the coronal plane.[20,21] The three studies of pathological feet[21–23] all found greater variability in the clinical cases when compared to the healthy controls.

It is difficult to directly compare results with other studies since there are differences between the definitions of axes and testing protocols. Most models[6,11] reference their dynamic angles to a standard neutral position, where all joint angles are defined to be zero. This would artificially reduce variation between sessions, as any error due to marker placement is reduced by shifting the reference position each time. The Oxford Foot Model does not reference to a measured neutral posture, but instead allows nonzero joint angle in the static reference position. This would account for some of the increased variability, but allows for measurement of foot deformity where achieving "neutral position" in a static standing posture is not always possible. Repeatability testing was also carried out on the same day by several researchers,[5,11,18,20,21,24] whereas the study described here was repeated on three separate days, which would also be likely to reduce repeatability. Furthermore, the method of quantifying repeatability differs between authors. In the current study, the variability in peak and range values are reported since these were considered to have clinical significance, whereas most previous studies report averaged values across a gait cycle or stance phase.[4,11]

The resulting differences in the repeatability from changes to the model tested within the current study were generally small. When the mid-point between the heads of the first and fifth metatarsals was used to define the longitudinal axis of the forefoot (instead of an actual "TOE" marker), repeatability was unchanged in all measured variables. Virtual markers have been reported to have greater reliability than physical markers,[25] and it was thought that identification of points on either side of the foot, rather than one on the top of the foot, would prove to be more accurate. This may still be the case in feet with significant deformity, where the metatarsals are no longer parallel and identification of a point between the second and third metatarsal heads may not represent the long axis of the forefoot. It may therefore be useful to maintain this as an option to calculate forefoot angles (since there is no significant difference in mean angles produced by this method and by using the TOE marker). Leardini et al.'s model[11] suggests a maximum forefoot adduction of around 10° as do Rattanaprasert et al.[21]. Hunt et al.[20] suggest a maximum of 2° in their model of forefoot motion, which is similar to the suggestions of Kidder et al.,[24] Wu et al.,[23] and MacWilliams et al.[5] Although these studies concerned adult feet, the results are similar to those found in the current study.

It was decided to attempt to track the forefoot with markers on the lateral part only in order to assess the relative movement of the P1MT marker and determine the validity of assuming this segment to be rigid. It was found that tracking with lateral markers only did not significantly improve repeatability. However, the measurement of arch height relative to the lateral forefoot was found to vary by an average of 7% of foot length within the gait cycle across all subjects. With the default definition of the forefoot, which considers the five metatarsals as a rigid body, this arch height measure would be constant. The variability in this measure is therefore due to flexibility between the medial and lateral forefoot. On this basis, a sensitivity analysis was conducted on one representative subject. Since this subject had a foot length of 180 mm, a change in arch height of 7% foot length would be equal to 12.6 mm. It was therefore concluded that P1MT was likely to move by at least this amount during the gait cycle. The effect on pronation and supination of the forefoot was assessed by shifting the position of P1MT up and down by 5 mm. It was discovered that the maximum effect of moving the marker up by 5 mm produced an increase in supination of 5°, while moving the marker down by 5 mm produced a reduction in supination of 4°, making a range of 9°. This suggests that the error induced in forefoot supination, by assuming the rigidity of the segment, may be as high as 9°, when the variation in forefoot arch height is around 7% of foot length. As a result of this analysis, it was decided to routinely record this measure of arch height and to assume that the value of range in arch height across the gait cycle (% foot length) roughly corresponds to the error in supination of the forefoot (°) when measuring it as one rigid segment.

The anterior axis of the hindfoot was assumed to be parallel to the floor for this study, since it involved only healthy children, all of whom were able to stand with feet flat on the floor. Where this is not achievable, a rotational offset in the sagittal plane may be input (on the basis of x-ray or additional marker position).

It was initially thought that using a wand marker on the rear of the calcaneus was the source of variability in hindfoot angles, since it was likely to be knocked out of place. When the repeatability of measuring hindfoot motion without this wand marker was examined, it was found that there was no significant change in repeatability when this marker was eliminated. When not using the wand, a lower range of measured dorsiflexion of the hindfoot was apparent. However, this value was very small (less than a degree) and not considered clinically relevant. It was decided to maintain the use of the wand marker, but to keep the option of tracking without it, in cases of obvious marker loss or knock, which can be assessed by comparing results from pre- and postassessment static trials.

Using physical markers on the tibia itself, rather than the calculated knee joint center from the conventional lower body model,[13] was expected to improve repeatability of measurements, but no significant change was noted. However, it significantly altered the absolute values of three of the eight kinematic variables. Primarily, it changed the apparent amount of knee flexion and also affected the range of hindfoot dorsiflexion. Maximum knee flexion was increased from 59 to 65° when markers on the tibia were used. The change in knee flexion angle when the knee joint center is not used may reflect translational error in the tibia and this effect may warrant further investigation. However, for consistency with conventional kinematics, it was decided to continue to use the knee joint center to align the long axis of the tibia, in order to be compatible with conventional lower body kinematic models.

When the CPEG marker was eliminated from the static calibration, an improvement of 2° in the within-subject SD was noted. It was thought that variability in aligning the CPEG marker with the transverse orientation of the hindfoot was the source of some variability in measuring of hindfoot rotation. The hypothetic line from CAL1 through the middle of the calcaneus is used to visually align the CPEG marker; so it was thought that directly using the line from CAL1 to the mid-point between STAL and LCAL (placed on either side of the calcaneus) would be a more repeatable estimate of the anterior axis of the hindfoot. While it is possible that this may reduce the sensitivity of the model to identifying deviation in the transverse plane, it is believed this is outweighed by the improvement in repeatability gained by using the mid-point between STAL and LCAL instead of the CPEG marker. This assumption will require further validation on feet with deformity of the hindfoot in the transverse plane.

The terminology for this model was adopted on the basis of clinical convenience and clarity. It is recognized that axes of rotation defined by the model do not always exactly replicate true anatomical axes. For example, Leardini et al.[26] confirmed *in vitro* that true inversion/eversion takes place at the subtalar or talocalcaneal joint about an axis whose position is load dependant. The present foot model combines the calcaneus and talus into a single segment (the hindfoot) and hence is unable to separate true inversion from overall relative motion between the tibia and hindfoot. However, the term "inversion/eversion" is meaningful to clinicians using this model, but it needs to be taken in the context of the definition described.

Taking into account repeatability and compatibility issues with the existing lower body model, it was decided to continue using the physical TOE marker to calculate the long axis of the forefoot, to eliminate use of the CPEG wand marker on the calcaneus, to use the conventional knee joint center to calculate the long axis of the tibia, and to measure forefoot arch height relative to the plantar surface defined by lateral markers on the forefoot to allow estimation of error produced in forefoot supination as a result of rigid body assumptions. Mean angles of this version of the model from the 14 healthy children are shown in Figure 24.6.

An awareness of the variability in the measurement of intersegment foot motion in children is vital for correct interpretation of results and should not be ignored when planning treatment and assessing outcomes. While a number of different variations of the model were assessed to achieve the optimal model for measuring foot motion, up to 7° variability was still apparent in the transverse plane. It was recognized that this may be in part due to inherent variability in children's gait. However, a significant factor is the consistency of marker placement between days on small feet. Therefore, clear protocols and practice in marker placement are crucial and improvements to fixation of the reflective markers should be considered.

24.4.2 PLANTAR PRESSURE

This study assessed the feasibility and repeatability of plantar pressure measurement of 15 healthy children using an automated subarea selection based on 3D marker positions.

There are many methods to achieve subdivision of the foot for detailed analysis. Since the ultimate aim of this study was to assess patients with foot deformity, it was considered important to define subdivisions of the foot, appropriate for these patients. The introduction of the current methodology was aimed at overcoming the difficulties that foot deformity in general poses when measuring plantar pressure. This is achieved by using anatomical markers projected on the footprint to determine subareas, and not relying on a "normal" alignment of the foot. Determination of transverse sections was in agreement with those defined previously, including hind-foot, midfoot, and forefoot (with the toes included with the forefoot).[27–32] However, the position of the dividing line between the segments was based on the position of markers on the foot, and therefore differed in principle to other methods. As the foot deformity associated with this population usually involves deviation in the coronal plane, it was decided to include further division of the transverse sections into medial and lateral components, apart from the midfoot, which was maintained as one area.

Automatic subarea definition based on marker placement was found to be reliable in healthy children. Since the protocol is not reliant on "normal" alignment of the foot, it allows assessment of feet where deformity is present. This is a further step to the method proposed by Giacomozzi et al.[14] and allows greater flexibility of application. Vertical projection of the position of markers onto the footprint was considered to be a valid assumption for healthy feet, since the entire foot is in contact with the pressure mat at mid-stance. In the presence of foot deformity when the plantar surface is not parallel to the floor at the time of mid-stance, the vertical projection of the markers may be slightly skewed on the footprint. However, the subarea selection method was chosen to have minimal effect on the selection of the areas that remain in contact with the floor and any discrepancy is likely to be within the spatial resolution of the mat. Further testing of subjects with foot deformity is required to validate this assumption.

Reporting of plantar pressure results in the literature is widely varied. There is little standardization in reporting units, definition of subdivisions, or normalization of results. However, where results are reported in kilopascals and subdivisions are similar to those used in this study, average peak pressure results are also similar to those reported in the literature. Average peak pressure from all healthy subjects varied from 80 kPa (at the midfoot) to 330 kPa (at the medial forefoot). This is similar to results reported by Meyring et al.[30] and Zhu et al.[33] Duckworth et al.[34] suggested that a range of 0 to 1000 kPa was evident during walking. Other researchers have reported results within similar ranges.[28,30]

24.5 CONCLUSION

The aim of this study was to provide a method for detailed assessment of foot motion and loading, capable of being applied to children with foot deformity. A multisegment foot model was validated for use with children — this was previously unavailable. The model proposed here produced results consistent with previous studies of foot kinematics in adults[5,12,20,21,24] and expected foot motion during normal gait.[7] The results in kinematic patterns were found to be more consistent than the absolute values. Absolute measurements in the transverse plane were found to be the least consistent, but repeatability was improved when the wand marker was eliminated from use on the hindfoot. The difference between measuring angles in slightly different ways gave only negligible differences in results, allowing for some flexibility in implementation in the presence of severe deformity.

The second aim of this study was to address the lack of consistency in plantar pressure measurement and reporting of results and provide a means to reliably measure plantar pressure in the presence of foot deformity. It was thought that the best way to achieve this was to automate the process as much as possible, while still maintaining clinical relevance and accuracy. Synchronization of plantar pressure, ground reaction force, and 3D position of markers on the foot was found to be a reliable method for providing information on localized forces under the sole of the foot.

This validation allows clinical implementation of the model, integrated with plantar pressure measurement, with an understanding of its reliability, enabling objective outcome studies in children with foot deformity.

ACKNOWLEDGMENT

We acknowledge the generous support of Action Medical Research in funding this project. We would also like to thank Maria Seniorou and the rest of the team at the Oxford Gait Laboratory for their assistance and the Centre for Statistics in Medicine, Oxford University, for statistical support.

REFERENCES

1. Allard, P. et al., Kinematics of the foot, *Can J Neurol Sci*, 9, 119, 1982.
2. Morris, J.M., Biomechanics of the foot and ankle, *Clin Orthop Relat Res*, 122, 10–17, 1977.

3. Bently, G. and Shearer, J., *The Foot and Ankle*. Mercer, 1996.

4. Liu, W. et al., Three-dimensional, six-degrees-of-freedom kinematics of the human hindfoot during stance phase of level walking, *Hum Mov Sci*, 16, 283, 1997.

5. MacWilliams, B.A., Cowley, M., and Nicholson, D.E., Foot kinematics and kinetics during adolescent gait, *Gait Posture*, 17, 214, 2003.

6. Moseley, L. et al., Three-dimensional kinematics of the rearfoot during the stance phase of walking in normal young adult males, *Clin Biomech (Bristol, Avon)*, 11, 39, 1996.

7. Perry, J., *Gait analysis: normal and pathological function*. Slack International, New Jersey, 1992.

8. Reinschmidt, C. et al., Tibiofemoral and tibiocalcaneal motion during walking: external vs. skeletal markers, *Gait Posture*, 6, 98, 1997.

9. Wright, D.G., Desai, M.E., and Henderson, W.H. Action of the subtalar and ankle-joint complex during stance phase of walking, *J Bone Joint Surg Am*, 46-A, 361, 1964.

10. Hicks, J.H., The mechanics of the foot, *J Anat*, 87, 345, 1953.

11. Leardini, A. et al., An anatomically based protocol for the description of foot segment kinematics during gait, *Clin Biomech (Bristol, Avon)*, 14, 528, 1999.

12. Carson, M.C. et al., Kinematic analysis of a multi-segment foot model for research and clinical applications: a repeatability analysis, *J Biomech*, 34, 1299, 2001.

13. Davis, R.B. and Deluca, P.A. Clinical Gait Analysis, in *Human Motion Analysis*, G.F. Harris, P. Smith, IEEE Press, New Jersey, 14, 1996.

14. Giacomozzi, C. et al., Integrated pressure-force-kinematics measuring system for the characterisation of plantar foot loading during locomotion, *Med Biol Eng Comput*, 38, 156, 2000.

15. Grood, E.S. and Suntay, W.J., A joint coordinate system for the clinical description of three-dimensional motions: application to the knee, *J Biomech Eng*, 105, 136, 1983.

16. Stebbins, J., Harrington, M., Thompson, N., Zavatsky, A., Theologis, T., Repeatability of a model for measuring foot kinematics in children, *Gait Posture*, 23(4): 401–10, 2006 Jun.

17. Stebbins, J. et al., Assessment of sub-division of plantar pressure measurement in children, *Gait Posture*, 22(4): 372–6, 2005 Dec.

18. Siegel, K.L. et al., A technique to evaluate foot function during the stance phase of gait, *Foot Ankle Int*, 16, 764, 1995.

19. Kepple, T.M. et al., A video-based technique for measuring ankle-subtalar motion during stance, *J Biomed Eng*, 12, 273, 1990.

20. Hunt, A.E. et al., Inter-segment foot motion and ground reaction forces over the stance phase of walking, *Clin Biomech (Bristol, Avon)*, 16, 592, 2001.

21. Rattanaprasert, U. et al., Three-dimensional kinematics of the forefoot, rearfoot, and leg without the function of tibialis posterior in comparison with normals during stance phase of walking, *Clin Biomech (Bristol, Avon)*, 14, 14, 1999.

22. Woodburn, J., Helliwell, P.S., and Barker, S., Three-dimensional kinematics at the ankle joint complex in rheumatoid arthritis patients with painful valgus deformity of the rearfoot, *Rheumatology (Oxford)*, 41, 1406, 2002.

23. Wu, W.L. et al., Gait analysis after ankle arthrodesis, *Gait Posture*, 11, 54, 2000.

24. Kidder, S.M. et al., A system for the analysis of foot and ankle kinematics during gait, *IEEE Trans Rehabil Eng*, 4, 25, 1996.

25. Soutas-Little, R.W., The use of "virtual markers" in human movement analysis, *Gait Posture*, 4, 176, 1996.

26. Leardini, A., Stagni, R., and O'Connor, J.J. Mobility of the subtalar joint in the intact ankle complex, *J Biomech*, 34, 805, 2001.

27. Oeffinger, D.J., Pectol, R.W., Jr., and Tylkowski, C.M. Foot pressure and radiographic outcome measures of lateral column lengthening for pes planovalgus deformity, *Gait Posture*, 12, 189, 2000.

28. Morag, E. and Cavanagh, P.R., Structural and functional predictors of regional peak pressures under the foot during walking, *J Biomech*, 32, 359, 1999.

29. Wearing, S.C., Urry, S.R., and Smeathers, J.E., Ground reaction forces at discrete sites of the foot derived from pressure plate measurements, *Foot Ankle Int*, 22, 653, 2001.

30. Meyring, S. et al., Dynamic plantar pressure distribution measurements in hemiparetic patients, *Clin Biomech (Bristol, Avon)*, 12, 60, 1997.

31. Nyska, M. et al., Effect of the shoe on plantar foot pressures, *Acta Orthop Scand*, 66, 53, 1995.

32. Chang, C.H., Miller, F., and Schuyler, J., Dynamic pedobarograph in evaluation of varus and valgus foot deformities, *J Pediatr Orthop*, 22, 813, 2002.

33. Zhu, H. et al., Walking cadence effect on plantar pressures, *Arch Phys Med Rehabil*, 76, 1000, 1995.

34. Duckworth, T. et al., The measurement of pressures under the foot, *Foot Ankle*, 3, 130, 1982.

25 The Design, Development, and Initial Evaluation of a Multisegment Foot Model for Routine Clinical Gait Analysis

Roy B. Davis, III, Eugene G. Jameson, Jon R. Davids, Lisa M. Christopher, Benjamin M. Rogozinski, Jason P. Anderson

CONTENTS

25.1 INTRODUCTION

In the late 1970s and early 1980s, a commonly used foot model[1] in clinical gait analysis was developed at the Newington Children's Hospital (Newington, CT), extending the theoretical work of Shoemaker.[2] As shown in Figure 25.1, this single-segment foot model is based on a vector that passes from the calcaneus to the space between the second and third metatarsals. The plantar surface of the foot provides a reference for the sagittal plane alignment of this vector. The ankle center (AC) and toe marker are

425

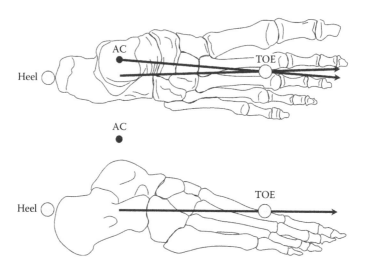

FIGURE 25.1 The most commonly used foot model at present consists of a single segment referenced to the plantar surface of the foot to define sagittal plane position/motion. The ankle center (AC) and the space between the second and third metatarsals (TOE) define transverse plane position/motion.

intended to provide references for transverse plane alignment, although sometimes the heel marker and toe marker are used instead.

This foot model offers limited and sometimes ambiguous or misleading information depending upon the shape and structural integrity of the patient's foot. It is assumed that the foot segment is relatively "rigid" between the heel and toe markers, and that the motion of this foot vector about the ankle flexion/extension axis represents ankle plantar flexion and dorsiflexion. Clearly, however, talocrural joint displacement, mid-foot (navicular and cuboid) movement relative to the hindfoot (talus and calcaneus), and forefoot (cuneiforms, metatarsals, and phalanges) motion relative to the mid-foot are all captured by this single-segment model with the toe marker placed on the dorsum of the forefoot (Figure 25.1 and Figure 25.2a). The potential for measurement artifact is exacerbated when the integrity of the mid-foot is compromised or "broken down." As illustrated in Figure 25.2b, toe marker placement on the forefoot captures this mid-foot displacement relative to the hindfoot and exaggerates the apparent ankle dorsiflexion. If this potential for artifact is recognized by the clinical team, then the toe marker can be placed more proximally (Figure 25.2c) to minimize the effect of the mid-foot movement artifact.

Transverse plane foot deformity also challenges the utility of this single-segment foot model. For example, an adducted forefoot presents a measurement quandary (Figure 25.3). If the toe marker is placed distally over the forefoot (Figure 25.3a, b), then the adducted position of the forefoot is included in the transverse plane kinematic results. If, however, the clinical team elects to document the transverse orientation of the hindfoot relative to the tibia, then the toe marker is placed proximally to the forefoot (Figure 25.3c). This proximal placement may be more consistent with

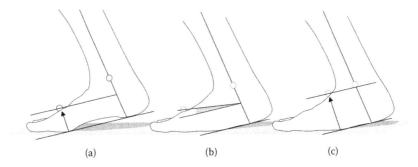

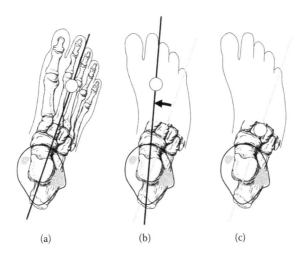

FIGURE 25.2 (a) The most commonly used current foot model relies on a retroreflective marker placed on the dorsum of the foot between the second and third metatarsals. (b) When the patient presents with mid-foot deformity or instability, this standard placement can result in a measure that indicates excessive ankle (talocrural) dorsiflexion. (c) If the deformity is appreciated by the clinical team, the reference marker can be placed proximal to the deformity to avoid or reduce measurement artifact.

FIGURE 25.3   (a) The most commonly used current foot model relies on a retroreflective marker placed on the dorsum of the foot between the second and third metatarsals. (b) When the patient presents with forefoot deformity (such as the excessive adduction illustrated here), this standard placement can result in a measure that indicates excessive internal foot progression, which may be consistent with the clinical impression of the examiner(s). (c) If, however, foot progression is defined consistent with the other foot/ankle kinematic measures associated with this model, then the reference marker must be placed proximal to the deformity. There exists no standard protocol in this area, leading to ambiguity with respect to the quantitative measure of "foot progression."

the sagittal plane goal of capturing talocrural motion, but it may produce quantitative results that conflict with visual assessments of foot position in the transverse plane during gait. Another fundamental challenge is that different clinical groups may instrument the foot with forefoot deformity differently, but refer to the kinematic results in the same way, e.g., transverse plane foot progression.

Given these limitations, why was this foot model ever adopted for clinical use? This single-vector foot model is linked to the technology that was available for motion data capture in the early 1980s. The original motion analysis laboratory at Newington Children's Hospital incorporated only three motion measurement cameras (one on either side and one at the end of the straight walkway). The limited optical and electronic resolutions of those cameras (relative to current technology) meant that the camera images of the markers (2.5 cm diameter) would readily "merge" in the camera view if placed too closely together on the segment of interest. When used for the computation (or reconstruction) of the three-dimensional (3D) marker trajectories, merged marker images may significantly reduce the quality of the 3D marker coordinate data. Consequently, only one marker was tolerated on the dorsum of the foot, and the heel marker (used only during a static subject calibration) was removed during the walking trials to avoid its image merging with that of the marker placed on the lateral malleolus. In fact, the original toe markers were placed over the head of the fifth metatarsal and equipped with nonreflective shields to allow only two cameras at a time to track the marker (as required by the Newington 3D data reconstruction algorithm). This primitive foot model was developed and adopted for clinical use in the early 1980s, because it was the best that the measurement technology would allow at the time. The foot model and its associated clinical protocol were intimately tied to the capability and limitations of the technology available at that time.

Contemporary technology, however, offers greater spatial measurement resolution, thereby potentially allowing more markers to be used to underpin a multisegment foot model, which better reflects the anatomical functional complexity of the foot. More sophisticated foot models can now be investigated to better meet the clinical needs of patients with foot deformity.

25.2 FOOT MODEL/ANALYSIS — CLINICAL REQUIREMENTS

The measurement goals associated with a foot model vary depending on the clinical population to be served, e.g., degree of anticipated foot deformity, specific clinical questions to be addressed. The adult patient with little or no significant foot deformity offers opportunities for the use of more markers or at least more widely spaced markers on the foot, as well as the potential for the routine palpation of a number of anatomical landmarks. By contrast, the pediatric patient with significant deformity of the hindfoot, mid-foot, and forefoot may offer a much more limited measurement opportunity, i.e., intermarker distances are reduced, and, normally, superficial anatomical landmarks may be obscured by the foot deformity.

Children with cerebral palsy are the primary clinical population served by the Motion Analysis Laboratory at the Shriners Hospitals for Children (Greenville, SC).

They commonly present with some degree of foot deformity[3] as well as a variety of other soft tissue and bony abnormalities. Of interest to the clinical team, with respect to quantitative foot assessments during gait, are the triplanar motions of the forefoot relative to the hindfoot (plantar flexion/dorsiflexion, inversion/eversion, and adduction/abduction) and of the hindfoot relative to the shank or tibia (plantar flexion/dorsiflexion, inversion/eversion, and internal/external rotation). Foot progression (the angles formed between the longitudinal axes of the foot segments and the direction of progression) during gait is also useful because of the association between foot segmental alignment and biomechanical support of the lower extremity. For this particular population, a multisegment foot model that is useful in routine, clinical gait analysis must:

1. Quantify the absolute and relative position and motion of two foot segments: hindfoot (including the talus and calcaneus) and forefoot (including the cuneiforms and metatarsals, but not the phalanges)

2. Be appropriate for pediatric patients: This is the focus of efforts at the Motion Analysis Laboratory at Shriners Hospitals for Children Greenville (SHCG) as well as many other clinical gait analysis facilities. While many foot models are developed with adult test subjects, pediatric application requires that the models remain sufficiently reliable and robust with the reduced intermarker distances associated with smaller-than-adult feet.

3. Be appropriate for patients with significant foot deformity: The main clinical population served by the Motion Analysis Laboratory at SHCG is children with cerebral palsy who commonly present with some degree of foot deformity.[3] An appropriate foot model must be sufficiently flexible to accommodate a wide variety of foot shapes.

4. Not require foot radiographs for the alignment of the anatomical coordinate systems: This requirement speaks to the practicality of the multisegment foot protocol for routine gait analysis, which is typically performed in laboratories that do not have direct access to radiography.

5. Allow for simultaneous whole-body gait data collection over an entire gait cycle (i.e., both stance and swing) without requiring a reconfiguration of the motion cameras: Simultaneous whole-body data capture and analysis provides an opportunity to correlate foot kinematics and kinetics with whole-body gait biomechanics. A comprehensive patient evaluation in the motion analysis laboratory can require 2 to 3 h of time. The practicality of a multisegment foot model is reduced substantially if additional time for reconfiguration and recalibration of the motion cameras is required for its use.

6. Build upon the current single-segment foot protocol with respect to the identification of key anatomical landmarks by the clinical evaluator: The current single-segment foot model requires the palpation and identification of two particular anatomical landmarks, the posterior aspect of the calcaneus and the space between the second and third metatarsals. These landmarks are readily available on children with foot deformity, as demonstrated by more than 20 yr of experience with the single-segment foot model.

7. Remain consistent with the current single-segment foot model to the degree possible with respect to the alignment of the anatomical coordinate

system associated with each foot segment: This facilitates a case-by-case comparison of the kinematic results provided by a new multisegment foot model with the current single-segment model, so that measurement and clinical differences can be appreciated.

25.3 CURRENTLY AVAILABLE MULTISEGMENT FOOT MODELS

A good deal of work has already been done with respect to the development of multisegment foot models[4-20] Most of these models, however, have been developed in the context of healthy adult feet.[4,7-10,12,13,15,17,18,20] Many are associated with protocols that would require motion camera repositioning and would not allow simultaneous whole-body gait data collection.[4,12,16]

More recently, two groups of investigators (in the Department of Biomedical Engineering, Marquette University, Marquette, Wisconsin and at the Oxford Gait Laboratory, Nuffield Orthopaedic Centre, Oxford, England) have adapted their respective adult multisegment foot models[4,9] for use in children.[14,19] In both cases, the model and/or associated measurement protocol have been simplified, e.g., number of instrumented foot segments and reflective markers reduced, for pediatric application. Both groups have examined aspects associated with the reliability of their models. The Marquette group describes a systematic evaluation of the reliability of the motion data-capture system.[14] The Oxford group has investigated tester reliability with respect to marker placement.[19] Simultaneous whole-body data collection appears to be possible with both the Marquette and the Oxford multisegment foot models. Neither of the models produces results that are readily compared with the measurements provided by the current single-segment model because of differences in the anatomical alignment of the segmental coordinate systems. The Marquette model utilizes radiographic data when available to align the segment anatomical coordinate systems, although radiographic data are not strictly required. It is not clear how the anatomical coordinate systems are approximated, if radiographic data are not available.

Both the Marquette and the Oxford pediatric foot models require the placement of markers on significantly more anatomical landmarks on the foot than the current single-segment model, such as markers on the head of the first metatarsal, the head and base of the fifth metatarsal, and the medial/lateral/posterior aspect of the calcaneus. In a study designed to explicitly investigate the reliability of the placement of markers at these same locations in both healthy adults and children, Henley et al.[5] carefully controlled (and validated) the repeatability of foot placement between days with individualized plaster molds. The study findings demonstrated good marker placement reliability between days and with the same clinician evaluator. However, marker placement reliability was found to be unacceptably poor between testers. These findings are consistent with the significant between-day variability reported by the Oxford group.[19] Both of these studies that focused on marker placement repeatability raise significant concerns about the feasibility of utilizing multisegment foot models that require the precise placement of a significant number of anatomical markers.

25.4 SHCG FOOT MODEL

25.4.1 Basis and Protocol

The Shriners Hospital for Children (SHCG) Foot Model is a two-segment foot model (forefoot and hindfoot) that reflects a straightforward extension of the current single-segment model. Principle references for the alignment of the anatomical coordinate systems for the forefoot and hindfoot are similar to the current single-segment model. Also shared between the two approaches is the palpation and identification of the required anatomical landmarks.

Based on its configuration of reflective markers (Table 25.1, Figure 25.4), the SHCG foot model appears quite similar to both the Marquette and the Oxford foot models. A key distinction between the SHCG approach and the other two models is that the three reflective markers on forefoot (MT1H, MT1B, and MT5H) and two of the three markers on the hindfoot (MCAL and LCAL) are "technical" markers and consequently do not require precise anatomical positioning on the foot. The foot model utilizes data provided by the medial and lateral ankle malleoli markers (MANK and LANK) that are placed for simultaneous full-body gait analysis. The only additional "anatomical" marker, PCAL, needed for the SHCG foot model

TABLE 25.1

Physical (Anatomical and Technical) and Virtual Marker Configuration: Shriners Hospitals for Children Greenville Multisegment Foot Model

	Anatomical Markers	
PCAL	Posterior calcaneus; medial/lateral placement strict; vertical placement approximate	Hindfoot
LANK	Lateral malleolus; placement approximate for foot model	Hindfoot
MANK	Medial malleolus; placement approximate for foot model	Hindfoot
	Technical Markers	
MCAL	Medial calcaneus; placement approximate	Hindfoot
LCAL	Lateral calcaneus; placement approximate	Hindfoot
MT1B	Base of first metatarsal; placement approximate	Forefoot
MT1H	Head of first metatarsal; placement approximate	Forefoot
MT5H	Head of fifth metatarsal; placement approximate	Forefoot
	Virtual Markers	
HFV1	Midpoint between MCAL and LCAL markers	Hindfoot
AC	Midpoint between MANK and LANK markers	Hindfoot
MT23B	Space between bases of the second and third metatarsals; medial/lateral identification with dynamic pointer strict; longitudinal identification approximate	Forefoot
MT23H	Space between heads of the second and third metatarsals; medial/lateral identification with dynamic pointer strict; longitudinal identification approximate	Forefoot

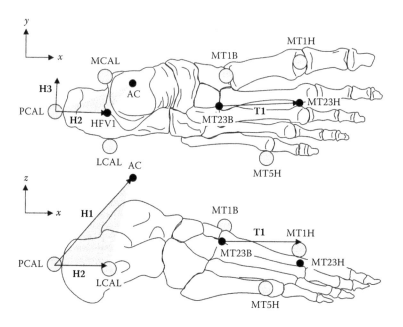

FIGURE 25.4 The anatomical references for the SHCG Foot Model are the anatomical marker PCAL and virtual markers AC and HFV1 for the hindfoot and virtual markers MT23B and MT23H for the forefoot. The plantar surface of the foot is a primary reference for both the hindfoot and the forefoot segment. Consequently, the hindfoot anatomical x-axis (the unit vector of **H2**) and the forefoot anatomical x-axis (the unit vector of **T1**) would be parallel to the floor/ground in the plantigrade patient. MCAL, LCAL, MT1B, MT1H, and MT5H are technical markers that allow the hindfoot and forefoot segments to be tracked during gait and that allow the hindfoot and forefoot anatomical coordinate systems to be constructed with the gait data.

requires repeatable positioning only with respect to its medial/lateral placement on the posterior calcaneus (i.e., its precise vertical placement is not critical). The only other alignment task by the clinical tester is the identification of virtual points (MT23H and MT23B) on the forefoot, using a dynamic pointer technique (Figure 25.5).[21] The longitudinal location of these two points over the metatarsals is not critical to the model, only their medial/lateral location between the second and third metatarsals. The three fundamental strengths of the SHCG approach with respect to its clinical practicality are that

- The flexibility provided by the approximate (as opposed to precise) positioning of the technical markers allows the clinician to readily respond to the foot shape variations that arise with foot deformity
- The anatomical marker placement and alignment requirements are consistent with more than 20 yr of experience with the current single-segment foot model
- The anatomical marker placement and alignment responsibilities of the clinician are minimized, thereby streamlining the clinical protocol while reducing the number of sources of marker placement variability.

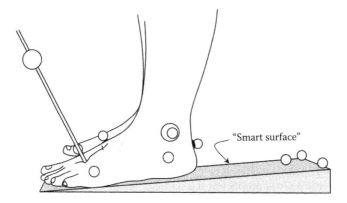

FIGURE 25.5 For the SHCG foot model, the plantar surface of the foot is a primary reference for both the hindfoot and the forefoot segment. A "smart surface" is used for patients who cannot stand plantigrade during the static subject calibration trial. The smart surface is instrumented with three reflective markers, so that the surface can be placed as needed by the clinician and its attitude determined by the motion measurement system. For particularly complex foot deformity, more than one smart surface can be used simultaneously. Illustrated here also is the tip of the dynamic pointer[21] that is used to identify key anatomical landmarks MT23B and MT23H on the forefoot (refer to Figure 25.4).

Both the hindfoot and the forefoot anatomical coordinate systems are based on data collected during a static subject calibration. The attitude of these anatomical coordinate systems relative to hindfoot and forefoot technical coordinate systems (based on the three technical markers on each respective segment) is also computed using the static data. These coordinate system transformation relationships are then used to determine the spatial position and alignment of the hindfoot and forefoot anatomical coordinate systems during the motion trials. The latter two steps are consistent with techniques used in whole-body gait analysis.[1] The remainder of this section describes the determination of the hindfoot and forefoot anatomical coordinate systems based on the static subject calibration.

25.4.2 HINDFOOT ANATOMICAL COORDINATE SYSTEM ALGORITHM

The primary anatomical reference for the hindfoot anatomical coordinate system is the plane formed by **PCAL**, **AC**, and **HFV1** (Figure 25.4). The secondary reference is the plantar surface of the hindfoot. The coordinate system is computed as follows:

1. An intermediate computational vector **H1** is computed from **PCAL** to the virtual **AC** (located midway between markers placed on the lateral and medial malleoli, consistent with whole-body gait analysis), **H1** = **AC** − **PCAL**.
2. An intermediate computational vector **H2** is computed from **PCAL** to the virtual point **HFV1**, **H2** = **HFV1** − **PCAL**, where virtual point **HFV1** is

determined midway between **LCAL** and **MCAL**, **HFV1** = (**LCAL** + **MCAL**)/2.

3. For a plantigrade subject, **H2** is set parallel to the floor. For a nonplantigrade subject, a "smart surface" is used to identify the plantar surface of the hindfoot, and **H2** is set parallel to the smart surface (Figure 25.5)

4. The vector cross product of **H1** and **H2** yields the intermediate computational vector **H3**. $H3 = H1 \times H2$.

5. The unit vector of **H2** becomes the anterior–posterior coordinate axis for the hindfoot e_{hfx}.

6. The unit vector of **H3** becomes the medial–lateral coordinate axis for the hindfoot e_{hfy}.

7. The vector cross product of e_{hfx} and e_{hfy} yields the superior–inferior axis for the hindfoot e_{hfz}.

25.4.3 FOREFOOT ANATOMICAL COORDINATE SYSTEM ALGORITHM

The primary anatomical reference for the forefoot anatomical coordinate system is the vector from virtual point **MT23B** to virtual point **MT23H** (Figure 25.4). The secondary reference is the plantar surface of the forefoot. The coordinate system is computed as follows.

1. An intermediate computational vector **T1** is computed from **MT23B** to **MT23H**, $T1 = MT23H - MT23B$.

2. For a plantigrade forefoot, **T1** is set parallel to the floor. For a nonplantigrade forefoot, a "smart surface" is used to identify the plantar surface of the forefoot and **T1** is set parallel to the smart surface (Figure 25.5).

3. The unit vector of **T1** becomes the anterior–posterior coordinate axis for the forefoot e_{ffx}.

4. For a plantigrade forefoot, the vertical axis of the laboratory (global) coordinate system becomes the superior–inferior axis for the forefoot e_{ffz}. For a nonplantigrade forefoot, the unit vector perpendicular to the smart surface becomes the superior–inferior axis for the forefoot e_{ffz}.

5. The vector cross product of e_{ffz} and e_{ffx} yields the medial–lateral axis for the forefoot e_{ffy}, $e_{ffy} = e_{ffz} \times e_{ffx}$.

25.4.4 INITIAL EVALUATION

Note: All quantitative tests described below were conducted in the Motion Analysis Laboratory at Shriners Hospitals for Children Greenville. For motion data capture, the laboratory is equipped with a Vicon 512 system with 12 M-1 motion cameras (Oxford Metrics Group, Oxford, England). The cameras are arrayed to provide a $6.7 \times 2.3 \times 2.0$ m measurement volume. 14.5 mm diameter retroreflective markers were used in all tests.

The evaluation of any new model and associated protocol must consider two key questions: Can the motion data-capture system provide 3D marker trajectory data of sufficient quality to support the new model? Can the data collection protocol, e.g., placement of anatomical markers, associated with the new model be performed with sufficient reliability and repeatability?

25.4.4.1 Measurement of System Reliability

To evaluate motion measurement system performance, it is not uncommon for investigators to move a pair of reflective markers, rigidly attached together at some fixed distance apart, through the measurement volume of the motion capture system. For example, a rod with two 50 mm diameter markers attached was held vertically and translated through the measurement volume of the SHCG motion capture system. The test yielded a mean intermarker distance of 500.0 (±0.2) mm, with an associated mean measurement error of 0.01 (±0.01) mm or 0.003%. Based on these results, one might conclude that the SHCG measurement system offers more than sufficient accuracy and precision for a variety of applications. This simple test, however, merely "demonstrates" that the measurement system is functional and that it can measure the distance between two markers with submillimeter precision under these circumstances. The same rod was moved randomly through the measurement volume, resulting in a mean intermarker distance of 500.2 (±0.8) mm with a mean measurement error of 0.02 (±0.8) mm or 0.05%. The same rod and markers were used, but the results differed significantly between the two tests. Different camera contributions in the 3D data reconstruction process give rise to marker trajectory variability. Also, the random movement of the rod increases the probability that the quality of the two-dimensional camera image data is reduced (e.g., merged marker images). The two test results differ because the second test is more challenging for the motion capture system than the first. Neither test, however, demonstrates that the motion capture system can deliver sufficient measurement quality for a new foot model for gait analysis.

To evaluate the capability of the measurement system relative to a new gait model, tests must be devised that determine whether the marker configuration associated with the new gait model can be adequately monitored while moving through the measurement volume in a manner consistent with gait. Similar to the marker configuration associated with the proposed multisegment foot model, a rigid marker triad of known geometry was fixed to the dorsum of the forefoot (Figure 25.6). The marker triad was then "walked" through the measurement volume a number of times with the subject equipped with the triad alone on the foot as well as with the other shank and foot markers associated with this foot model (Table 25.1). In this way, a rigid marker configuration that approximated the forefoot model was moved through the measurement volume in a manner consistent with routine patient evaluation. By varying the spacing of the markers on the triad, it was possible to investigate the impact of the reduced intermarker distances associated with pediatric patients. The data shown in Figure 25.7 suggest that the lower limit with respect to the spacing between the MT1H (or MT1B) and MT5H markers on the forefoot is approximately 50 mm with appropriate marker trajectory filtering (a Woltring filter with a mean square error value of 20 was used for this exercise). These results also illustrate the negative impact of the juxtaposition of the other nontriad markers

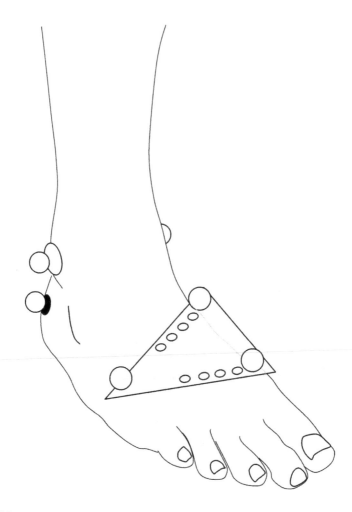

FIGURE 25.6 To evaluate the capability of the motion measurement system with respect to marker trajectory data accuracy and precision, a rigid triad of markers was placed on the test subject's forefoot. Intermarker spacing on the device was varied and the data for multiple walks were collected. The results of this testing are provided in Figure 25.7.

on the triad marker data. That is, the triad marker results were degraded by inappropriate ray contributions from the other markers and merged marker image data during 3D reconstruction.

25.4.4.2 Marker Placement Reliability

The system reliability testing has shown that the measurement system can (with identified limits) deliver 3D marker trajectory data of sufficient quality for the proposed foot model. However, can the foot markers be placed by the clinician with sufficient reliability and repeatability? To begin to investigate this question, a single subject (adult male, age: 50 yr, height: 1.9 m, mass: 86 kg) was evaluated by two

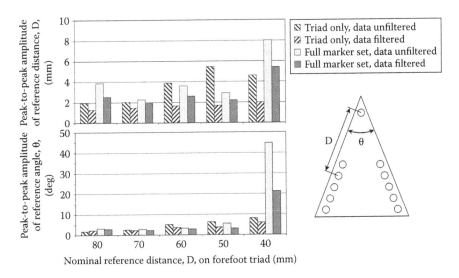

FIGURE 25.7 The accuracy and precision of the motion measurement system were evaluated with a rigid triad of markers that was placed on the test subject's forefoot (Figure 25.6). With the substantial increase in reference distance and angle noise between the nominal reference distances of 50 and 40 mm, the lower acceptable limit with respect to the intermarker spacing in the clinical utilization of the SHCG Foot Model (with the current motion measurement configuration) would be 50 mm with the use of a Woltring filter (mean square error of 20).

clinicians on each of five different days for a total of ten test sessions. Both testers were well experienced with anatomical palpation and marker placement for routine clinical gait analysis. The spatial position of the subject's foot during the standing subject calibration trials was controlled using a wooden platform equipped with blocks abutting the bony processes of the test foot. After static subject calibration, five walking trials per session were collected as the subject walked at a self-selected speed along a level, straight 10 m walkway. Euler angles (plantar/dorsiflexion, in/eversion, int/external rotation) were used to represent both standing posture and walking kinematics.[22]

As one might anticipate, marker placement variability increased from "within session" to "between day, same tester" to "between day, between tester" as reflected in the mean and maximum differences in marker coordinate values as well as the associated coefficients of variation (Table 25.2). These findings are consistent with those described by Henley et al.[5] Generally, within-session repeatability of the subject's foot placement within the test apparatus was satisfactory with a mean difference in coordinate values of 0.7 ± 0.6 mm. The greatest within-session variability was seen with the mediolateral positioning of PCAL (3.7 mm maximum marker coordinate difference). The maximum between-day, between-tester variation in marker coordinate values (29 mm) was associated with the anterior–posterior positioning of the MT23B landmark (Table 25.2 and Table 25.3). The marker coordinate range over the ten test sessions (Table 25.3) was greatest in the vertical (z) direction (mean of 11 ± 5 mm) and least for the mediolateral (y) direction (mean of

TABLE 25.2

Test–Retest Differences in Marker Coordinate and Segment Angle Values during Standing, Static Subject Calibrations over Ten Test Sessions with Two Evaluators

	Mean Difference		Maximum Difference		Mean COV[a]
	Markers (mm)	Angles (°)	Markers (mm)	Angles (°)	Markers
Within-session	0.7 (±0.6)	0.8 (±1)	3.7	5.4	0.4%
Between-Day, tester 1	4.6 (±2.5)	9 (±5)	14	14	1.5%
Between-Day, tester 2	5.5 (±2.9)	9 (±7)	14	19	1.9%
Between-Day, between tester	8.4 (±5.5)	5 (±12)	29	31	2.4%

[a]Coefficient of variation.

TABLE 25.3

Range of Test–Retest in Marker Coordinate and Segment Angle Values during Standing, Static Subject Calibrations Over Ten Test Sessions with Two Evaluators

	Marker Coordinates[a] (mm)			Segment Angles (°)			
	x	y	z		x	y	z
LANK	9	2	12	Shank (absolute position)	0	0	6
MANK	5	2	6	Hindfoot (absolute position)	31	5	13
MCAL	7	6	16	Forefoot (absolute position)	0	0	8
PCAL	4	7	16	Hindfoot-relative-to-Shank	30	5	16
LCAL	9	5	11	Forefoot-relative-to-Hindfoot	31	0	13
MT1B	10	7	9				
MT1H	5	7	4				
MT5H	6	6	6				
MT23B	29	8	18				
MT23H	8	5	10				
Mean	9 ± 7	5 ± 2	11 ± 5				

[a]x, y, z coordinate system axes are consistent with those depicted in Figure 25.4.

5 ± 2 mm). The range over the ten test sessions associated with standing hindfoot inversion/eversion was 31°.

The magnitude of the range associated with standing hindfoot inversion/eversion merits further examination. The maximum deviation of the hindfoot from neutral measured by tester 1 was 19° of inversion and by tester 2 was 12° of eversion. Consequently, the range between these two tests was 31°. It is noted, however, that without these two trials, the range over the other eight trials is reduced to 8°, with a mean inverted hindfoot position of 6° (±2°). In the trial associated with tester 1, it appears that poor within-session foot placement repeatability on the part of the subject was the primary reason for the elevation in hindfoot inversion. The measurement of 12° of eversion resulted from the medial misplacement (4 mm) of the PCAL marker by tester 2 along with a simultaneous medial deviation in the AC location (2 mm) due to subject foot placement variability.

This significant hindfoot eversion measurement outlier prompted a perturbation analysis to catalog the sensitivities of the angular measures relative to marker misplacement artifact. The results in Table 25.4 are specific to this particular model and the average marker coordinates associated with the ten trials by the two clinicians. Generally, the model is not sensitive to perturbations in marker placement artifact in the vertical (z) direction, consistent with the use of the plantar surface as a reference for anatomical coordinate system alignment. Moreover, sensitivity to marker placement artifact in the anterior–posterior (x) direction is relatively low as well. The sensitivity of the model to marker perturbation in the mediolateral (y) direction is more significant. The probability of mediolateral misplacement of the medial and lateral ankle markers (MANK and LANK) is low as demonstrated by the data presented in Table 25.3. As already illustrated by tester 2, hindfoot inversion/eversion and internal/external rotation measurements are quite sensitive to the mediolateral placement of the posterior calcaneus marker (PCAL). Hindfoot inversion/eversion as predicted by this model with these marker data is most sensitive to mediolateral placement of the medial (MCAL) and lateral (LCAL) calcaneus markers (approximately 2°/mm).

The average kinematic results of the walking trials collected over the ten test sessions for this single adult are presented in Figure 25.8 and Figure 25.9. The patterns associated with this single subject are consistent to a degree with other reported models and results after noting the approximately 5 to 10° of hindfoot inversion demonstrated in his gait data.[14,19] The variability of the walking data (as reflected by the standard deviations associated with each plot) is consistent with the standing data variability, e.g., standard deviation in sagittal plane motion of the foot segments is small by comparison to coronal and transverse plane motions. The impact of the one errant PCAL placement is illustrated in Figure 25.10, as the variability associated with the coronal plane hindfoot motion is substantially reduced when this one trial is removed.

A fundamental challenge in foot modeling is the reduced distance between markers (as compared with intermarker distances utilized for larger body segments). Consequently, one must maximize the distances where possible. The experimental data presented in this single-subject study illustrate this point. For example, for the errant "12° of eversion" trial described above, if the MCAL and LCAL markers had

TABLE 25.4
Mean Angular Sensitivity to ±5 mm Perturbations in Marker Coordinate Values Expressed as degree/mm

| | Hindfoot Angles | | | | | | | | | | | | | | | Forefoot Angles | | | | | |
| | LANK | | | MANK | | | MCAL | | | PCAL | | | LCAL | | | MT23B | | | MT23H | | |
	x^a	y	z	x	y	z	x	y	z	x	y	z	x	y	z	x	y	z	x	y	z
In/Eversion	0.2	1.2	0.1	0.2	1.2	0.1	-0.3	-2.0	0.0	0.3	1.7	-0.3	-0.3	-2.0	0.0	0.0	0.0	0.0	0.0	0.0	0.0
Pl/Dorsiflexion	0.0	0.2	0.0	0.0	0.2	0.0	0.0	-0.3	0.0	0.0	0.1	0.0	0.0	-0.3	0.0	0.0	0.0	0.0	0.0	0.0	0.0
In/External Rot	0.0	0.0	0.0	0.0	0.0	0.0	0.1	0.7	0.0	-0.2	-1.5	0.0	0.1	0.7	0.0	-0.2	-1.7	0.0	0.2	1.7	0.0

[a] x, y, z coordinate system axes are consistent with those depicted in Figure 25.4.

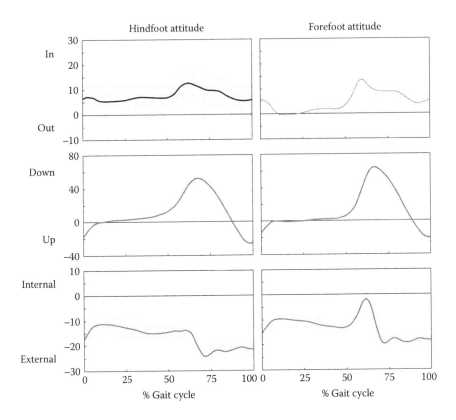

FIGURE 25.8 Shown are average (with one standard deviation, gray band) hindfoot and forefoot attitude (absolute angles relative to the inertially fixed laboratory coordinate system) during straight, level walking for a single adult subject evaluated on five separate days by two clinicians working independently (for a total of ten trials).

each been placed 15 mm further forward (in the x direction), then the standing hindfoot measurement would have been 8° of inversion instead of 12° of eversion. That is, the H2 vector, oriented principally in the anterior–posterior direction, would have increased in magnitude, thereby making it less susceptible to medial–lateral marker placement variability. More generally, if these same changes were introduced in the average marker coordinate data that provided the basis for the marker perturbation analysis, then the marker placement sensitivities would have been substantially lower, e.g., the LCAL sensitivity of 2°/mm is reduced to 1.1°/mm. Arguably, then, more explicit guidance to the clinicians in the placement of the markers (specifically, PCAL, MCAL, LCAL, and the identification of virtual points MT23B and MT23H), to maximize the associated intermarker distances, will improve the reliability of the model.

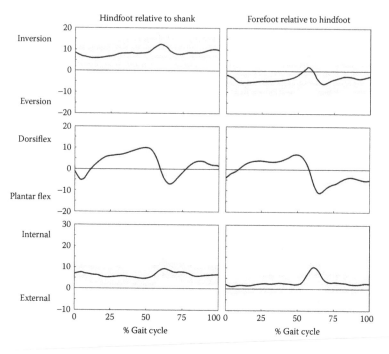

FIGURE 25.9 Shown are average (with one standard deviation, gray band) hindfoot relative to shank and forefoot relative to hindfoot kinematics during straight, level walking for a single adult subject evaluated on five separate days by two clinicians working independently (for a total of ten trials).

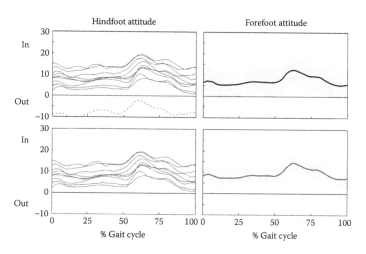

FIGURE 25.10 Shown in the top two hindfoot attitude graphs are the individual and average results of ten walking trials (single adult subject evaluated on five separate days by two clinicians). The bottom two graphs illustrate the reduction in the variability of the average results (i.e., the standard deviation, gray band) achieved by removing the one outlier trial (dashed curve in the upper left graph) from the average results.

25.5 SUMMARY

Relative to other models described in the literature, the SHCG multisegment foot model described in this chapter significantly reduces the marker alignment responsibilities of the clinician during data collection. With only one physical anatomical marker (PCAL) to place and two virtual points (MT23B and MT23H) to identify precisely, it is anticipated that the model can be readily adapted to a wide variety of foot anatomical deformities. Moreover, these anatomical points are consistent with the current single-segment foot model. Consequently, the clinical application of the new model draws upon two decades of experience in the palpation and identification of these landmarks in a variety of patient populations. The model also shows good potential for routine clinical use, in that it allows for simultaneous whole-body gait data collection over an entire gait cycle (i.e., both stance and swing) and does not require a reconfiguration of the motion cameras.

While the testing results presented here are promising, they reveal that additional clinician instruction and further evaluation are needed before the model is acceptable for clinical utilization. Future investigation must also include the examination of the reliability of the model with pediatric subjects with foot deformity (who are seldom included in model validation exercises).

These empirical results, particularly as related to reliability of the placement of markers MT1B, MT1H and MT5H, reiterate the concerns posed by Henley et al.[5] regarding the use of these markers in the anatomical alignment of the foot segmental coordinate systems. Based on the insights provided by the perturbation analysis described here, it is appropriate that such numerical analyses be repeated for the models already described in the literature and developed in the future.

REFERENCES

1. Davis R.B. et al., A gait analysis data collection and reduction technique, *Hum Mov Sci*, 10, 575, 1991.
2. Shoemaker P.A., Measurements of relative lower body segment positions in gait analysis, M.S. thesis, University of California, San Diego, 1978.
3. O'Connell P.A. et al., Foot deformities in children with cerebral palsy, *J Pediatr Orthop*, 18, 743, 1998.
4. Carson M.C. et al., Kinematic analysis of a multi-segment foot model for research and clinical applications: a repeatability analysis, *J Biomech*, 34, 1299, 2001.
5. Henley J. et al., Reliability of a clinically practical multi-segment foot marker set/model, In: *Proc. Gait and Clinical Movement Analysis Soc. Meeting*, Lexington, KY, 2004, 62.
6. Humm J.R. et al., Kinematic morphology of segmental foot motion in normal pediatric subjects, *Gait Posture*, 9, 115, 1999.
7. Hunt A.E. et al., Inter-segment foot motion and ground reaction forces over the stance phase of walking, *Clin Biomech*, 16, 592, 2001.
8. Kepple T.M. et al., A video-based technique for measuring ankle-subtalar motion during stance, *J Biomed Eng*, 12, 273, 1990.
9. Kidder S.M. et al., A system for the analysis of foot and ankle kinematics during gait, *IEEE Trans Rehabil Eng*, 4, 25, 1996.

10. Leardini A. et al., An anatomically based protocol for the description of foot segment kinematics during gait, *Clin Biomech*, 14, 528, 1999.
11. Liu W. et al., Three-dimensional, six-degrees-of-freedom kinematics of the human hindfoot during stance phase of level walking, *Hum Mov Sci*, 16, 283, 1997.
12. MacWilliams B.A., Cowley M., and Nicholson D.E., Foot kinematics and kinetics during adolescent gait, *Gait Posture*, 17, 214, 2003.
13. Moseley L. et al., Three-dimensional kinematics of the rearfoot during the stance phase of walking in normal young adult males, *Clin Biomech*, 11, 39, 1996.
14. Myers K.A. et al., Validation of a multisegment foot and ankle kinematic model for pediatric gait, *IEEE Trans Neural Syst Rehabil Eng*, 12, 122, 2004.
15. Rattanaprasert U. et al., Three-dimensional kinematics of the forefoot, rearfoot, and leg without the function of tibialis posterior in comparison with normals during stance phase of walking, *Clin Biomech*, 14, 14, 1999.
16. Scott S.H. and Winter D.A., Biomechanical model of the human foot: kinematics and kinetics during the stance phase of walking, *J Biomech*, 26, 1091, 1993.
17. Siegel K.L. et al., A technique to evaluate foot function during the stance phase of gait, *Foot Ankle Int*, 16, 764, 1995.
18. Simon J. et al., The Heidelberg foot measurement method: development, description and assessment, *Gait Posture*, 23, 401, 2006. available online.
19. Stebbins J. et al., Repeatability of a model for measuring multi-segment foot kinematics in children, *Gait Posture*, 23, 411, 2006. available online.
20. Woodburn J. et al., A preliminary study determining the feasibility of electromagnetic tracking for kinematics at the ankle joint complex, *Rheumatology*, 38, 1260, 1999.
21. Davis R.B., Jameson G.G., Davids J.R., A simple tool for the identification of virtual anatomical landmarks during a static subject calibration, 12th Annual Meeting of the European Society for Movement Analysis in Adults and Children, Marseille, France, Sep, 2003.
22. Greenwood D.T., *Principles of Dynamics,* Prentice-Hall, Edgewood Cliffs, NJ, 1965, 333.

26 Reliability of a Clinically Practical Multisegment Foot Marker Set/Model

John Henley, James Richards, David Hudson, Chris Church, Scott Coleman, Lauren Kersetter, and Freeman Miller

CONTENTS

26.1 INTRODUCTION

Improvements in image resolution within the digital camera industry have dramatically increased our ability to accurately track small markers and small marker clusters. These abilities have generated substantial interest in improving aspects of gait analysis associated with measuring the kinematics and kinetics of foot motion. As a result of this interest, numerous multisegment foot marker sets have been proposed for use in clinics and research.[1–28] In theory, these models represent a substantial improvement over traditional single-segment models that treat the foot as a single rigid body.

The traditional foot model utilizes two actual markers (one on the dorsum of the forefoot traditionally between the second and third metatarsals just proximal to the metatarsophalangeal joint and one on the back of the calcaneus) and one virtual marker (the ankle joint center). Because the three markers often become collinear on patients with small or low-arched feet, this marker set cannot be used to determine varus–valgus or pronation–supination orientations of the foot. Another popular traditional marker set utilizes three markers on the forefoot, either by rigid marker-triad plate or as individual markers on the heads of the first and fifth metatarsal bones and near the base of the second and third metatarsals. This marker set does have the ability to measure all three angular rotations; however, it still treats the foot as a single rigid segment and integrates forefoot motion with motion from the talocural and the subtalar joints (referred to here as ankle motion).

While the ideal foot model would consider the function of all the bones in the foot, it is obviously impossible to account for every aspect of the foot's skeletal anatomy by monitoring markers placed on the skin. Consequently, concessions have to be made regarding how the foot is modeled and how marker locations are defined to enable measurement of the model's components. Because of the complexity of the foot, the substantial number of models that can be imagined to represent the foot and the number of laboratories working independently on this problem, many different multiple segment foot models have been proposed.[1–28] These models differ in the number of segments used to define the foot, the anatomical structures used to define the segments, and the manner in which segments are represented mathematically. Specifically, there are differences in the definitions of local anatomical coordinate systems that define these subsegments and joints. These issues represent problems of choice, in that clinicians will eventually have to choose a model with defined structural and mathematical properties that best suits their needs. Despite the diversity of models that are currently proposed, it is likely that the gait community will settle on a model that a vast majority of clinicians find acceptable. However, there is another, more general problem that needs to be addressed prior to the implementation of any of the proposed multimarker foot models — the ability of clinicians to accurately implement the model.

As markers are placed in proximity to other markers, the precision of marker placement becomes more critical to the validity of the results. More to the point, as markers are placed closer together, small errors in placement have a larger effect on the orientation of segments defined by the markers. For example, if two markers were placed on the shank with a center-to-center distance of 300 mm, and one marker had a lateral displacement error (displacement orthogonal to the vector formed by the two markers) of 1 mm, the resulting error in orientation of the vector formed by the two markers would be 0.19°. Likewise, a lateral displacement error of 2 mm would result in 0.38° of orientation error, and a lateral displacement error of 3 mm would result in 0.57° of orientation error. Now, consider two markers placed on the back of the calcaneus with a center-to-center distance of 18 mm. In this situation, a 1-mm lateral displacement error for one marker will yield a 3.18-degree error in the vector orientation. Likewise, a 2-mm lateral displacement error would yield 6.34°

of orientation error, and a 3-mm lateral displacement error would yield 9.46° of orientation error. Laterally misplacing both markers in different directions would amplify the orientation error. In the case of calcaneus markers used in this example, the errors would primarily affect the amount of rearfoot inversion/eversion — a critical component of pronation/supination.

Errors in marker placement can occur for a number of reasons, most of which are associated with our abilities to visualize or palpate anatomical landmarks and to place the markers on the exact points of identification. The ability to visualize or palpate anatomical landmarks is complicated by the fact that most landmarks are covered by skin, fat tissue, muscle, and/or tendon. It would be convenient if all subjects had freckles or birthmarks at the precise locations where we desire to place the markers. Instead, landmarks consist of flat surfaces, depressions, or points (such as an epicondyle or a tubercle), and each of these has its own unique issues. The flat surface identifies an area for marker placement but provides no precise point. Consequently, the clinician is faced with the decision of determining the exact location for placement of the marker center within the area, and this is open to interpretation on the part of the clinician. Pointed surfaces present both a palpation/visualization problem and a marker attachment problem. For example, the shape of the medial malleolus resembles a ridge more than a point, and the clinician is again faced with determining the location on the ridge where the marker should be placed. The lateral malleolus, on the other hand, resembles more of a point and provides a more precise landmark. However, attachment of the marker over the lateral malleolus is more difficult because of the fact that it resembles a point, and because of the peroneal tendons, which can move beneath the marker and result in unwanted marker motion. More subtle landmarks that are found in the foot (i.e., the navicular or cuboid surfaces) are difficult to palpate and almost impossible to visualize in many subjects. Given that anatomical structures are not clean simple geometric shapes and they exhibit variability even bilaterally within an individual (i.e., the left and right feet of an individual are not mirror images of one another), precise marker placement is not an easy accomplishment. Tendons, fat pads, veins, and interference from other structures such as the opposing limb may alter the appropriateness of specific landmarks and require that markers be placed in other locations. Additionally, the presentation of these structures may be altered as a result of therapeutic interventions such as surgery.

In summary, since current camera systems are able to detect smaller markers placed in proximity, the problem shifts from limitations of technology to clinical practicalities and the limiting factor becomes the ability to accurately and reliably place markers on the foot.

26.2 PURPOSE

To better understand these limitations, we conducted a study to determine the reliability associated with placing markers on specific anatomical landmarks about the foot and ankle. The experiment took place in three different clinical gait analysis laboratories configured to capture multiple strides in a single trial.

26.3 METHODS

26.3.1 DATA COLLECTION PROTOCOL

Marker reliability measures were obtained using 14 adult feet (mean = 30 ± 7.8 yr, average foot length = 246 mm ± 22 mm) and 8 pediatric feet (mean = 6.5 ± 2.6 yr, mean foot length=196 mm ± 28 mm). Three clinicians with extensive experience in gait analysis identified anatomical landmarks on the foot necessary to produce the desired four-segment foot model. The landmarks identified were center of the proximal posterior calcaneus, center of the distal posterior calcaneus, medial and lateral malleoli, navicular, base of the fifth metatarsal, heads of the first and fifth metatarsals, between the heads of second and third metatarsals, and hallux nail bed (Figure 26.1).

Data collection consisted of two parts. First, a method to ensure that the subjects' feet could be positioned in the exact location and orientation within the camera volume was tested. The method consisted of creating plaster of Paris molds that formed a cast around the sole of each subject's feet (Figure 26.2).

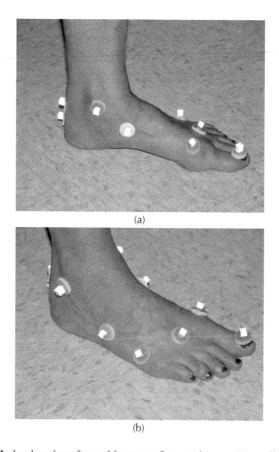

(a)

(b)

FIGURE 26.1 Marker locations for multisegment foot marker set, (a) medial and (b) lateral.

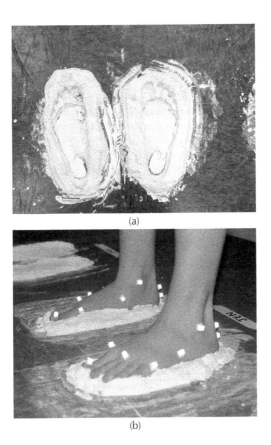

FIGURE 26.2 (a) Plaster of Paris mold. (b) Multisegment foot marker set in plaster of Paris mold.

The molds were formed directly on the laboratory floor and were immovable. The ability of subjects to place their feet in the exact same position and orientation in the calibrated volume was tested by having one clinician place the markers previously described on the feet of each subject.

The subjects then placed their feet in their molds, and the positions of the markers were recorded using an eight-camera motion analysis system for 0.5 sec at 60 Hz in a 3 m × 7 m volume. The subjects removed their feet from their molds, walked around the perimeter of the laboratory, and then repositioned their feet in the molds without disturbing the original marker placement. A second measurement was taken with the motion analysis system. The positions of each marker on each subject's feet were then compared between trials.

The second part of data collection had two goals:

To measure the ability of a single clinician to repeatedly place markers on the same landmarks on each subject's feet

To determine the agreement between different clinicians placing markers on the same landmarks on each subject's feet

Three clinicians placed the marker set on each subject's feet twice. Clinicians and trials were randomized for each subject. Following marker placement by an individual clinician, the subject stepped into the plaster casts and the marker positions were recorded. The subject then stepped out of the casts, and the markers were removed. A second clinician would then apply the markers and the measurement process was repeated. This continued until each clinician applied the markers to each subject twice.

26.3.2 DATA ANALYSIS

The reliability and objectivity of foot marker placements were analyzed in two manners. The first part of the analysis examined the absolute marker positions within marker application, between marker applications, and between clinicians.

26.3.2.1 Within Marker Application (Reliability)

The three-dimensional positions of the markers were analyzed between trials when the subjects stepped in and out of the molds without removing the markers. Deviation ranges and intraclass correlation coefficients (ICCs) were calculated for each marker along each axis.

26.3.2.2 Between Marker Application (Reliability)

The three-dimensional positions of the markers were analyzed between each marker application for each of the three clinicians. Deviation ranges and intraclass correlation coefficients (ICCs) were calculated for each marker along each axis, and statistical values were pooled across clinicians.

26.3.2.3 Between Clinicians (Objectivity)

The three-dimensional positions of the markers were analyzed between marker applications from each of the three clinicians. Deviation ranges and intraclass correlation coefficients (ICCs) were calculated for each marker along each axis, and statistical values were pooled across trials.

The second part of the analysis examined the effects of marker variability on foot kinematics using the same three comparisons defined above. Kinematics were defined as follows.

The foot model consisted of the hindfoot, forefoot, first ray, fifth ray, and hallux. The hindfoot anatomical coordinate system was created from the two posterior calcaneal markers and the ankle joint center, which was simply defined as the bisection of the medial and lateral malleolus markers. The z-axis of the hindfoot anatomical system was the unit cross product of the vector from the bottom calcaneus marker to the ankle joint center (vector 2; Figure 26.3) with the vector from the bottom calcaneus marker to the top calcaneus marker (vector 1; Figure 26.3). The anatomical y-axis of the hindfoot was the unit vector parallel to the cross product of the global z-axis (vertical, vector 3, Figure 26.3) and the z hindfoot anatomical axis. This was determined with the foot settled into the mold. The anatomical x-axis

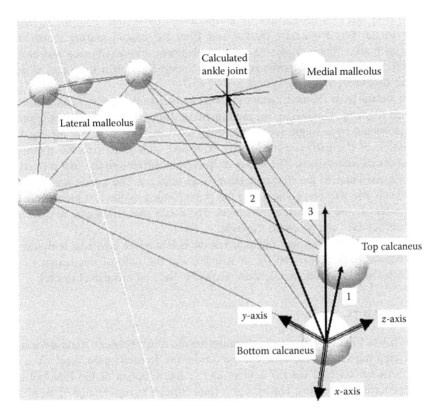

FIGURE 26.3 Hindfoot local coordinate system: where 1 — vector from bottom calcaneus to top calcaneus, 2 — vector from bottom calcaneus to ankle joint, and 3 — global vertical.

of the hindfoot was formed from the unit cross product of the y and the z hindfoot anatomical axes. Thus the z-axis points to the right of both feet, the y-axis points anteriorly, and the x-axis points toward the plantar surface. By utilizing the global vertical when the foot was flat on the ground, the calcaneal markers defined the eversion/inversion attitude of the hindfoot. The plantar/dorsiflexion attitude of the hindfoot was defined as parallel to the floor when the foot was settled into the mold. The internal/external rotation attitude of the hindfoot was defined by the plane formed by the calcaneal markers and the ankle joint center.

Applying an zyx Euler rotation sequence to define the orientation between the shank (defined as the room's coordinate system with the global x-axis pointing vertically down, the y-axis pointing anteriorly, and the z-axis pointing laterally to the right) and the hindfoot anatomical coordinate systems, plantar flexion was positive about the global z-axis, eversion for the left foot and inversion for the right foot were positive about the intermediate y-axis, and in-toeing for the left foot and out-toeing for the right foot were positive about the x-axis of the hindfoot. We need to pick a convention for the xyz axes.

The first and fifth metatarsals were represented by vectors from the navicular marker to the first metatarsal marker and from the cuboid marker to the fifth metatarsal marker, respectively. As vectors, plantarflexion/dorsiflexion and abduction/adduction could be determined, but not rotation about their long axes as seen from the hindfoot coordinate system.

The vector from the first metatarsal head marker to the hallux marker defined the hallux segment. As with the first and fifth metatarsal segments, the hallux segment was represented by a single vector, and long axis rotations were not measurable. The motion of the hallux segment was expressed with respect to the following forefoot coordinate system: The y-axis of the forefoot followed the first metatarsal (from the navicular to the first metatarsal head marker). The x-axis was oriented dorsoplantar and was perpendicular to the plane formed by the first metatarsal, the fifth metatarsal, and the navicular markers. The z-axis was orthogonal to the x and the y forefoot axes and points to the right.

The height of the arch was calculated as the height of the navicular with respect to the bottom of the foot, and the arch index was the ratio of this height to the distance between the bottom calcaneus marker to the first metatarsal marker.

26.4 RESULTS

Figure 26.4 to Figure 26.6 visually demonstrate the errors between trials associated with placing markers for the different test conditions. In each figure, black lines are drawn between selected marker centers and in the direction of the hindfoot and forefoot coordinate systems. The light gray lines indicate the orientation of the global coordinate system. Figure 26.4 demonstrates the ability of a single subject to repeatedly place the foot in the same location on the plaster molds. Comparison of Figure 26.4 and Figure 26.5 demonstrates the variability introduced when the markers are removed and replaced by a single individual. Comparison of Figure 26.5 and Figure 26.6 provides

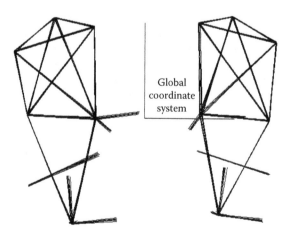

Global coordinate system

FIGURE 26.4 Overlay of ten trials of a single subject after stepping in and out of the mold without having markers removed and replaced between trials.

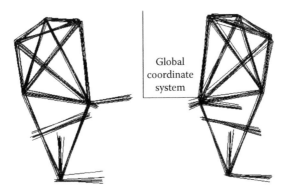

FIGURE 26.5 Overlay of ten trials of a single subject after having markers removed and replaced between trials by a single clinician.

a sense of the additional variability when multiple clinicians place the markers. Note that each series of figures was performed on the same individual ten times.

ICCs for the within-application test indicated that the subjects were reliable in placing their feet in the same location (Table 26.1). The average intraclass correlation (ICC) for each marker in each direction was 0.965, with a low of 0.826 for the fifth metatarsal marker in the vertical direction.

The ICC for each marker in the between-application comparison averaged 0.856, with a low of 0.487 for the fifth metatarsal in the vertical direction (Table 26.2).

ICCs for the clinician comparison were below 0.500, with the marker position average at 0.429 and a low of −0.098 for the cuboid in the vertical direction (Table 26.3). All the ICCs are significant at $p = .05$.

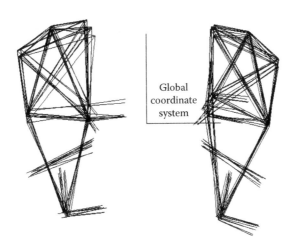

FIGURE 26.6 Overlay of ten trials of a single subject after having markers removed and replaced between trials by three clinicians.

TABLE 26.1
Within-Application Marker Position Reliability ICCs

	Inferior/Superior	Medial/Lateral	Anterior/Posterior
Lower calcaneus	0.949[a]	0.984[a]	0.987[a]
Upper calcaneus	0.961[a]	0.989[a]	0.991[a]
Navicular	0.986[a]	0.992[a]	0.993[a]
Cuboid	0.932[a]	0.973[a]	0.997[a]
First metatarsal head	0.959[a]	0.984[a]	0.986[a]
Second and third metatarsal spaces	0.969[a]	0.987[a]	0.989[a]
Fifth metatarsal head	0.826[a]	0.936[a]	0.946[a]
Hallux	0.902[a]	0.965[a]	0.970[a]

[a]Significant F, $p = .05$.

In summary, the average within-application ICC was 0.965, between-application ICC 0.856, and between-clinician ICC 0.429 (Figure 26.7). Only the between-clinician ICCs were significant.

These ICCs were produced by differences in marker position. For the within-application condition, the average of marker position errors had a range of 1.33 mm with a maximum range of 1.87 mm for the navicular marker in the anterior posterior direction and a minimum of 0.59 mm for the marker between the second and third metatarsal spaces in the inferior superior direction (Table 26.4).

For the between-application condition, the marker position had an average range of 2.39 mm, with a maximum range of 3.57 mm for the navicular marker in the inferior-superior direction and a minimum of 0.81 mm for the hallux marker in the inferior-superior direction (Table 26.5).

TABLE 26.2
Between-Application Marker Position Reliability ICCs

	Inferior/Superior	Medial/Lateral	Anterior/Posterior
Lower calcaneus	0.684[a]	0.875[a]	0.839[a]
Upper calcaneus	0.800[a]	0.873[a]	0.879[a]
Navicular	0.887[a]	0.920[a]	0.923[a]
Cuboid	0.664[a]	0.866[a]	0.881[a]
First metatarsal head	0.918[a]	0.955[a]	0.958[a]
Second and third metatarsal spaces	0.863[a]	0.940[a]	0.946[a]
Fifth metatarsal head	0.487[a]	0.795[a]	0.822[a]
Hallux	0.877[a]	0.945[a]	0.950[a]

[a]Significant F, $p = .05$.

TABLE 26.3
Between-Clinician Marker Position Objectivity ICCs

	Inferior/Superior	Medial/Lateral	Anterior/Posterior
Lower calcaneus	0.371[a]	0.457[a]	0.475[a]
Upper calcaneus	0.370[a]	0.460[a]	0.475[a]
Navicular	0.474[a]	0.476[a]	0.487[a]
Cuboid	−0.098[a]	0.481[a]	0.480[a]
First metatarsal head	0.462[a]	0.488[a]	0.487[a]
Second and third metatarsal space	0.420[a]	0.493[a]	0.487[a]
Fifth metatarsal head	0.131[a]	0.492[a]	0.487[a]
Hallux	0.440[a]	0.497[a]	0.492[a]

[a]Significant F, $p = .05$.

For the between-clinician condition, the marker position had an average range of 5.10 mm, with a maximum range of 8.97 mm for the marker between the second and third metatarsal space in the anterior–posterior direction and a minimum of 1.29 mm for the hallux marker in the inferior–superior direction (Table 26.6).

In summary, there was an increase in marker movement from a low of 1.33 mm in repositioning the feet to 2.39 mm when the markers are replaced to 5.10 mm when the markers were replaced by different individuals (Figure 26.8).

The variability in marker placement, in turn, produced variability in the orientation of the foot model segments. Flexion/extension of the hindfoot was the least

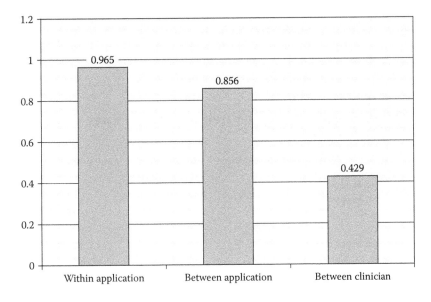

FIGURE 26.7 Summary of ICCs.

TABLE 26.4
Within-Application Marker Position Variability Range of Position (mm)

	Inferior/Superior	Medial/Lateral	Anterior/Posterior
Lower calcaneus	1.12	1.81	1.72
Upper calcaneus	1.03	1.60	1.57
Navicular	1.53	1.81	1.87
Cuboid	1.12	1.05	1.86
First metatarsal head	1.15	1.08	1.30
Second and third metatarsal spaces	0.59	1.12	1.38
Fifth metatarsal head	1.32	1.00	1.75
Hallux	0.60	0.99	1.45

affected and insensitive to condition (Figure 26.9). Orientation differences in internal/external rotation and inversion/eversion increased when the markers were replaced by the clinician and then more so when different clinicians replaced the markers. The inversion/eversion orientation of the hindfoot was affected the greatest.

In the first ray, the internal/external (abduction/adduction) orientation with respect to the hindfoot was affected to a greater extent than the flexion/extension orientation regardless of condition (Figure 26.10). Similar to the hindfoot, the effect increased from within applications to between applications to between clinician conditions.

The results for the fifth ray orientation (Figure 26.11) and for the hallux (Figure 26.12) were similar to that of the first ray, with the exception that the hallux orientation was almost equally affected in each direction.

TABLE 26.5
Between-Application Marker Position Variability Range of Position (mm)

	Inferior/Superior	Medial/Lateral	Anterior/Posterior
Lower calcaneus	3.02	2.71	1.85
Upper calcaneus	3.03	2.48	1.85
Navicular	3.57	2.05	3.30
Cuboid	2.93	1.57	3.20
First metatarsal head	1.83	2.07	3.27
Second and third metatarsal spaces	1.48	2.45	2.93
Fifth metatarsal head	2.09	2.10	3.36
Hallux	0.81	1.53	1.89

TABLE 26.6
Between-Clinician Marker Position Variability Range of Position (mm)

	Inferior/Superior	Medial/Lateral	Anterior/Posterior
Lower calcaneus	7.39	4.93	3.14
Upper calcaneus	6.60	4.27	3.20
Navicular	7.96	4.01	6.60
Cuboid	7.25	3.10	7.06
First metatarsal head	3.46	3.79	8.03
Second and third metatarsal space	4.41	4.45	8.97
Fifth metatarsal head	4.83	3.98	7.51
Hallux	1.29	2.60	2.81s

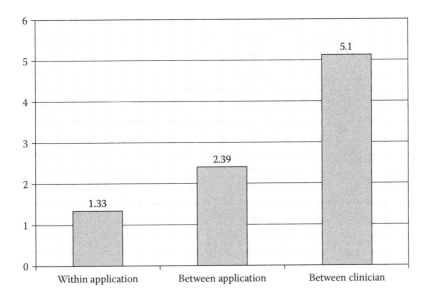

FIGURE 26.8 Summary of marker placement variability (mm).

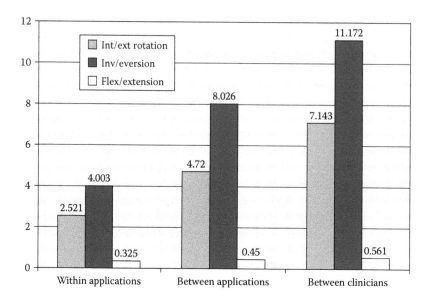

FIGURE 26.9 Errors in hindfoot orientation (expressed relative to room), in degrees.

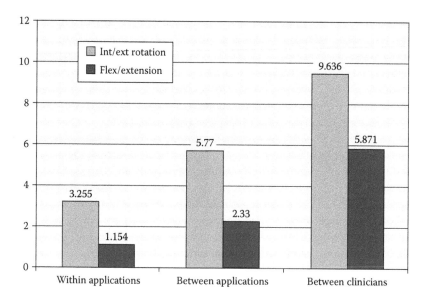

FIGURE 26.10 Errors in first ray orientation (relative to hindfoot), in degrees.

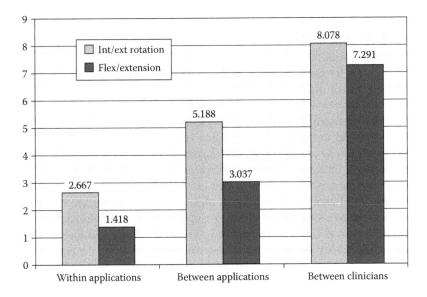

FIGURE 26.11 Errors in fifth ray orientation (relative to hindfoot), in degrees.

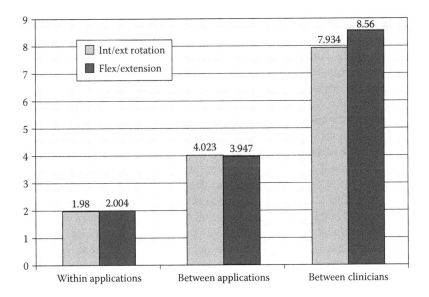

FIGURE 26.12 Errors in hallux orientation (relative to forefoot), in degrees.

26.5 DISCUSSION

Our analyses indicate that the precision of marker placement at these specific anatomical locations on the foot is limited. The motion capture system produced less than 1 mm error for markers placed at least 1 cm apart, indicating that this was not a substantial source of error.

The small deviations in marker position and large ICCs for the within-application condition demonstrated that the subjects were able to reliably place their feet in the same location and that the stepping motion did not cause substantial movement. Repeated trials by one or more clinicians resulted in larger errors — an issue that must be considered in utilizing multisegment foot marker sets. The between-application errors indicate the range of variability that can be expected due to limits in human motor control and limits in the ability: to identify the same unmarked location. The first refers to the precision capabilities: how well an object can be placed on a targeted location. The second refers to variability in visualizing unmarked locations. As an example, imagine locating the center of a square without drawing the diagonals. One would be close but not exact. The difficulty of this task increases with finding the center of irregular shapes. The surface structure of the foot makes placement difficult; flat surfaces lack the landmarks needed to reference marker placement, while angular surfaces provide good reference but magnify marker misplacement through added angular deflection. Unfortunately, in the foot, small misplacements result in large angular deviations due to the proximity of the markers.

Some segment orientation directions were more susceptible to marker misplacement than others. In general, the flexion/extension was the least susceptible, except for the hallux, where each direction seemed to be equally affected. The long axis orientations of the hallux and the first and fifth rays were not measured due to modeling these segments as vectors.

A change in orientation between marker placement trials could be a possible source of variability. Since the cubes are covered with a retroreflective tape, light is reflected back to the camera from each side of the cube that is visible to the camera, not just the face of the cube that is most orthogonal to the line of sight of the camera. With a spherical marker, a constant circle is presented to each camera and the center remains fixed, even if the marker is rotated. With a cubic marker, the presentation shape slightly varies with the orientation; thus the centroid will vary slightly, but the variation will be less than if only the surface facing the camera reflected light. The markers used in this experiment measured 6 mm on each side and were captured in a very large volume, which would minimize errors from this source. By spinning markers about a fixed position within the defined volume, the centroid movement averaged approximately 0.2 mm, or about the same as that associated with spherical markers. Therefore, it is possible that nonuniformity in the retroreflective tape, and dirt or skin oils that accumulate on the surface with use, will alter the amount of light reflected back from various areas of the marker, thereby changing the observed centroid just as much as the actual shape of the marker (Figure 26.13).

Two factors helped to decrease the variability associated with marker placement. First, markers can only be placed on a surface, not above or below. Therefore deviations perpendicular to the skin surface are minimized. Second, not all deviations

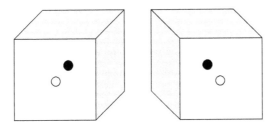

FIGURE 26.13 Position of true marker centroid (black circle) relative to the reflecting centroid (white circle).

in marker placement create deviations in segment orientation. Some marker placement deviations are bound to occur parallel to the vector that the markers are defining, which would have no effect on segmental orientation.

In this study, we looked at how small changes in marker relationships could alter the determination of segmental orientation. We assumed that the relationship between the coordinate systems calculated from marker positions (technical coordinate system) and the local anatomical coordinate systems for each segment was known. There are two limitations associated with this assumption. First, an offset exists between the marker centroid and the anatomical point that the marker is trying to represent. This creates a fixed rotational and translational offset between the anatomical and the technical coordinate systems. One can compensate for the difference between the two coordinate systems if the magnitude and direction of the marker centroid-anatomical point offset can be measured in the technical coordinate system. This is difficult to do in a clinical setting. Second, the anatomical coordinate systems of the foot segments are not well defined. This is especially true for foot segments that are composed of multiple bones such as the forefoot. Even in the hindfoot segment, which may be modeled by just the calcaneus (some models include the talus), it is difficult to define an anatomical coordinate system due to the irregularity and lack of symmetry of the bone. Therefore, because there is some fixed but undefined offset between a coordinate system defined by skin markers and the true segmental anatomical coordinate system, there must be some fixed offset in our measurements. This situation makes it difficult to determine zero or neutral points in calculated motion curves. However, the range of motion will not be affected.

The range of motion will be affected if the relationship between the technical coordinate system and the anatomical coordinate system is not fixed. When the foot moves, the skin and other soft tissues move relative to the underlying bone, undermining the assumption of a fixed relationship between the anatomical and technical coordinate systems. The amount and direction of soft tissue movement depend on the suppleness of the tissue, the amount of motion, the direction of motion, and the speed and acceleration in the motion, to name a few. Many research studies have been devoted to quantifying and devising methods to minimize this issue either by mechanical or mathematical means. At present, this problem has not been resolved.

26.6 CONCLUSION

As current camera systems are able to detect smaller markers placed in proximity, the problem shifts from limitations of technology to clinical practicalities, and the limiting factor becomes the ability to accurately and reliably place markers on the foot. We found good reliability of repeatedly placing markers on the foot by a single clinician, but poor reliability when multiple clinicians were involved. Although the specific numerical results are applicable only to our model, we feel that it is safe to generalize these trends to all multisegment foot models. That is, the high within-clinician reliability and lower between-clinician reliability suggest that measures of multisegment foot kinematics are related to the clinicians' sense of the foot anatomy and their preferences in placing markers on irregular surfaces. In light of the work by Gorton et al.,[29] in looking at a laboratory's ability to utilize full body marker sets, foot marker sets are not unique. However, due to the proximity of the markers utilized in multisegment marker sets, the variability associated with placing markers has a more detrimental effect. Researchers need to be aware of this issue and not rely on reports of motion analysis system accuracy and marker tracking ability as the sole limitations in the accuracy of data. At this juncture, the accuracy of marker placement is likely to have a more profound effect. More work is needed to determine if practice improves the agreement between clinicians.

REFERENCES

1. Abuzzahab, F.S. et al., Foot and ankle motion analysis system instrumentation calibration and validation, in *Human Motion Analysis*, Harris, G.F. and Smith, P.A. Eds., Piscataway, NJ, IEEE Press, 1996, 152.
2. Abuzzahab, F.S. et al., A system for foot and ankle motion analysis during gait, in *Proceedings of the 8th Annual West Coast Gait Conference*, 1993, 137.
3. Carson, M.C. et al., A four segment in vivo foot model for clinical gait analysis, *Gait Posture* 8, 73, 1998.
4. Carson, M.C. et al., Assessment of a multi-segment foot model for gait analysis, *Gait Posture* 12, 76, 2000.
5. Carson, M.C. et al., Kinematic analysis of a multi-segment foot model for research and clinical applications: a repeatability analysis, *J Biomech* 34, 1299, 2001.
6. Catani, F. et al., An anatomical protocol for 3D kinematics assessment of five-segment foot and ankle complex, in *Abstracts of the 9th Meeting of the European Society of Biomechanics and II World Congress of Biomechanics*, Amsterdam, 1994, 151.
7. Catani, F. et al., 3D kinematic assessment of foot-ankle complex, *Rehabilitation R&D Progress* 33, 36, 1995.
8. Cowley, M., MacWilliams, B.A., and Meek, S., A multi-segment kinematic and kinetic foot model for clinical decision making, *Gait Posture* 13, 297, 2001.
9. DeLozier, G.S., Alexander, I., Narayanaswamy, R., A method for measurement of integrated foot kinematics in *Proceedings of International Symposium on 3D Analysis of Human Movement*, Montreal, Canada, 1991
10. Henley, J. et al., Reliability of a clinically practical multi-segment foot marker set/model, in *Abstracts of Ninth Annual Gait and Clinical Movement Analysis Society*, Lexington, KY, 2004.

11. Henley, J. et al, A new three-segment foot model for gait analysis in children and adults, *Gait Posture*, 13, 284, 2001.

12. Humm, J.R. et al., Kinematic morphology of segmental foot motion in normal pediatric subjects, *Gait Posture* 9, 115, 1999.

13. Johnson, J.E. et al., (1996) Three dimensional motion analysis of the adult foot and ankle, in *Human Motion Analysis,* Harris, G.F. and Smith, P.A. Eds., Piscataway, NJ, IEEE Press, 1996, 351.

14. Kidder, S.M. et al., A system for the analysis of foot and ankle kinematics during gait, *IEEE Trans Rehabil Eng*, 4, 25, 1996.

15. Kidder, S.M. et al., A biomechanical model for foot and ankle motion analysis, in *Human Motion Analysis,* Harris, G.F. and Smith, P.A. Eds., Piscataway, NJ, IEEE Press, 1996, 133.

16. Kotajarvi, B.R. et al., Dynamic foot biomechanics of children with clubfoot, *Gait Posture*, 13, 257, 2001.

17. Leardini, A. et al., An anatomically based protocol for the description of foot segment kinematics during gait, *Clin Biomech*, 14, 528, 1999.

18. MacWilliams, B.A., Cowley, M., and Nicholson, D.E., Foot kinematics and kinetics during adolescent gait. *Gait Posture,* 17, 214, 2003.

19. Morlock, M. and Nigg, B.M., Theoretical considerations and practical results in the influence of the representation of the foot for the estimation of internal forces with models, *Clin Biomech,* 6, 3, 1991.

20. Rattanaprasert, U. et al., Three dimensional kinematics of the forefoot, rearfoot, and the leg without the function of the tibialis posterior in comparison with normals during stance phase of walking, *Clin Biomech,* 14, 14, 1999.

21. Scott, S. and Winter, D.A., Talocural and taolcalcaneal joint kinematics and kinetics during the stance phase of walking, *J. Biomech,* 24, 743, 1991.

22. Scott, S. and Winter, D.A., Biomechanical model of the human foot: kinematics and kinetics during the stance phase of walking, *J. Biomech,* 26, 1091, 1993.

23. Simon, J. Wolf, S., and Doderlein, L., Gait analysis of the growing foot, *Gait Posture,* 16, s110, 2002.

24. Simon, J. et al., A model of the human foot with seven segments, *Gait Posture*, 12, 63, 2000.

25. Simon, J. et al., A multisegmented foot model, *Gait Posture* 13, 269, 2001.

26. Smith, P. et al., Three dimensional motion analyses of the pediatric foot and ankle, in *Pediatric Gait: A New Millennium in Clinical Care and Motion Analysis Technology,* Harris, G.F. and Smith, P.A. Eds., Piscataway, NJ, IEEE Press, 183, 2000.

27. Stroud, C. et al., Foot/Ankle motion analysis in patients with posterior tibial tendon dysfunction, in *Pediatric Gait: A New Millennium in Clinical Care and Motion Analysis Technology,* Harris, G.F. and Smith, P.A. Eds., Piscataway, NJ, IEEE Press, 173, 2000.

28. Theologis, T. et al., Dynamic foot movement in children treated for congenital talipes equinovarus, *J. Bone Joint Surg*, 85, 572, 2003.

29. Gorton, G. et al., in *Proceedings of the 6th Annual GCMAS Meeting,* Sacramento, CA, 2001.

27 A Multisegment, 3D Kinematic Model of the Foot and Ankle

Kenton R. Kaufman, Harold P. Kitaoka, Diana K. Hansen, Duane A. Morrow, and Brian R. Kotajarvi

CONTENTS

27.1 INTRODUCTION

The foot and ankle joint complex (FAC) consists of several joints with different characteristics, which are involved in motion occurring between the foot and the lower leg. There is an interdependence of the FAC with the more proximal joints of the lower extremity. The great weight-bearing stresses to which these joints are subjected can result in a wide range of alignment and contribute to the diversity of difficulties in the joints of the FAC. The frequency of ankle and foot problems can be traced readily to the foot's complex structure, the need to sustain large weight-bearing stresses, and the multiple and somewhat competing functions that the foot must perform. Acting as both a shock attenuator and a power transmitter, the FAC meets its diverse requirements through its 28 bones that form 25 complex joints. These joints include the proximal and distal tibiofibular joints, the talocrural or ankle joint, the talocalcaneal or subtalar joint, the talonavicular and the calcaneal cuboid joints, the five tarsometatarsal joints, five metatarsophalangeal joints, and the interphalangeal joints.

Clinical motion analysis involves the comparison of a person's gait to that of normal individuals. A person's gait is classified as abnormal when their gait parameters deviate excessively from normal. Currently, a number of methods have been suggested for measurement of lower extremity kinematics.[1-5] In these models, the human body is modeled as a system of articulated, rigid links, which represent the lower limb segments and the upper body. By modeling the body as an ensemble of rigid-body segments, it is possible to calculate the kinematics at any articulation. However, these models describe the foot as one rigid segment. Little attention has been given to the development of models to describe the foot and ankle. This has been due, historically, to hardware limitations of motion analysis systems and the relatively small size of the foot in relation to the other lower extremity segments analyzed in a standard gait assessment. Recently, following advances in digital camera resolution, efforts have begun to develop specific techniques and marker segments for use in foot and ankle motion analysis.[6-8] The purpose of this chapter is to describe a multisegment model of the foot and ankle complex.

27.2 METHODS

The foot and ankle complex was divided into three functional segments: the lower leg, the hindfoot, and the forefoot. A three-segment rigid-body model was used to describe the kinematics of the foot and ankle during ambulation. The three rigid-body segments were defined by markers attached to each of these segments (Figure 27.1). The lower leg segment includes the tibia and fibula. The hindfoot is defined by markers on the calcaneus. The forefoot is defined by markers on the first and fifth metatarsals. To describe the foot and ankle segment kinematics, a minimum of three noncollinear markers are needed on each segment. A total of 11 markers were used to define the three-segment foot and ankle model (Table 27.1). The markers were 1.0 cm in diameter. Double-sided adhesive tape was used to fix the marker bases to the subject's skin.

Video-based methods from motion analysis were used for data collection. A ten-camera real-time system (Motion Analysis Corporation, Santa Rosa, CA) was used

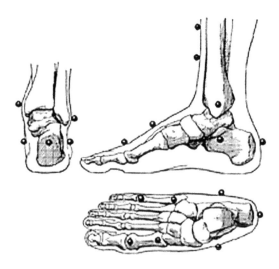

FIGURE 27.1 Position of retroreflective markers used to define foot model segments.

TABLE 27.1
Anatomical Marker Positions

Markers	Anatomical Location
1	Anterior surface of the tibia 6 cm above the malleoli
2	Anterior surface of the tibia 2 cm above the malleoli
3	Medial malleolus
4	Lateral malleolus
5	Tuberosity of the calcaneus
6	Medial calcaneus
7	Lateral calcaneus
8	Base of the first metatarsal
9	Head of the first metatarsal
10	Base of the fifth metatarsal
11	Head of the fifth metatarsal

at a sampling rate of 60 frames/sec to collect the two-dimensional trajectory data of the reflective markers placed on the subject. Each camera was fit with a near infrared light emitting diode (LED) ring light and an optical filter specific to that frequency of light, enhancing the image of reflective targets in the view space while allowing reasonable ambient lighting conditions. A calibrated view volume measuring 5 m long × 3 m wide × 3 m high was used for data collection. The EVaRT (EVa Real-Time, Motion Analysis, Santa Rosa, CA) software package was used for creating the three-dimensional (3D) marker trajectories from two or more camera views of a marker within the calibrated view volume. Recorded marker trajectories were processed to reconstruct the absolute positions and orientation of the body segments, as well as the relative positions of the segments to describe joint motions.

Local coordinate systems were constructed for the lower leg, rearfoot, and forefoot rigid-body segments. Local coordinate axes were developed for each model segment based upon the global, laboratory-referenced, 3D marker coordinates. The construction of each segment coordinate axes was unique to that segment. Once the local coordinate axes were defined, the relative orientations of segment axes could be used to express the relative motion between the body segments. The anatomical description of the relative orientation of the two segments was conveniently obtained by relating the two coordinate systems embedded in the proximal and distal segments. Motion of the distal segment orientation was expressed relative to the next proximal segment using the unified definition of joint motion.[10,11] An Eulerian angle system was used for specification of the joint motions. This method allowed the joint rotations to be described about clinically meaningful axes, i.e., flexion/extension, abduction/adduction, and internal/external rotation. The 3D coordinate systems were constructed with an anteriorly directed x-axis, y-axis pointed to the body's left side, and a superiorly directed z-axis. With these embedded coordinate systems, the joint angles were determined using the following conventions: Flexion occurred about the mediolateral y-axis of the proximal body (the sign of this variable was reversed in order to correspond with other published reports), adduction occurred about the x-axis perpendicular to the first and third axes, and rotation occurred about the proximally directed z-axis of the distal body.

Data were collected from ten asymptomatic subjects (aged 31 ± 6 yr). An initial 1-second standing reference data collection was taken to define the orientation of the embedded coordinate systems in a neutral position. This static reference position was captured in a weight-bearing stance with the midline of the posterior aspect of the calcaneus and the second toe on a line parallel to the line of progression (global x-axis) of the laboratory. The leg was positioned such that the tibia was oriented vertically in both the frontal and sagittal planes. Ten walking trials were then collected. Joint angles from all dynamic data trials were calculated frame by frame with respect to the static reference position using the least squares position orientation algorithm.[12]

27.3 RESULTS

Sagittal plane hindfoot motion results (Figure 27.2a) indicate that the hindfoot moves into plantarflexion after foot contact and then reverses and begins to dorsiflex until late stance, when the hindfoot plantarflexes before toe-off. A plot of coronal-plane hindfoot motion (Figure 27.2b) demonstrates an initial eversion, with movement back into inversion. Data of transverse-plane hindfoot motion (Figure 27.2c) show internal rotation during first rocker, external rotation during second rocker, and internal rotation during third rocker. Examination of sagittal plane forefoot motion (Figure 27.3a) reveals dorsiflexion until opposite foot strike, when the forefoot again goes into plantarflexion. The dorsiflexion during mid-stance represents a flattening of the longitudinal arch as the body progresses over the stance foot. In the coronal plane, the forefoot motion (Figure 27.3b) shows a trend of progressive eversion. Motion of the forefoot in the transverse plane (Figure 27.3c) starts in abduction and then moves into adduction. The forefoot returns to abduction during terminal stance.

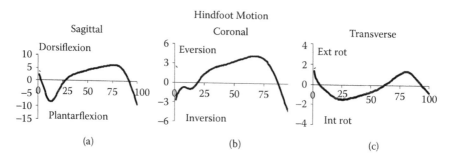

FIGURE 27.2 Hindfoot motion for (a) sagittal, (b) coronal, and (c) transverse planes. The mean and standard deviation for ten subjects are shown.

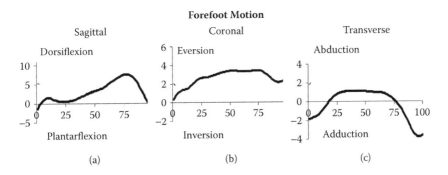

FIGURE 27.3 Forefoot motion for (a) sagittal, (b) coronal, and (c) transverse planes. The mean for ten subjects is shown.

27.4 DISCUSSION

A 3D model for measuring normal foot and ankle motion has been developed. The foot and ankle motion measured in this study has demonstrated good agreement with other studies in adults. The patterns of ankle motion in the sagittal plane agree very well with other investigators.[6–8,13–15] Hindfoot motion reported in this study also agrees with published results.[6–8,15] Comparison of the motion of the forefoot segment with respect to the hindfoot is more difficult due to the disparity of published reports. In general, the results of this study compared with those published by Kidder et al. [7]

One of the challenges of developing a clinically useful model for the foot and ankle complex is the difficulty of differentiating markers using a video-based motion analysis system. A compromise must be made between measurement volume, marker size, and marker location on the foot. Previous analog camera technology was limited in resolution and resulted in trials with missing data or marker "drop-out." In contrast, the current camera technology has improved to digital cameras with greater than 1 megapixel resolution. These imaging advances have made it possible to track foot markers while maintaining a large measurement volume used for full-body gait analysis. These advances now make it conceivable to use a multisegment foot model with standard lower extremity biomechanical models.

27.5 CONCLUSIONS

A useful technique for quantifying the foot and ankle kinematics has been described. This model divides the foot and ankle complex into lower leg, hindfoot, and forefoot segments. The 3D rotations of these segments are quantified. Objective measurement of foot and ankle motion will enable clinicians to more effectively treat foot and ankle disorders and is essential for the assessment of treatment outcome.

ACKNOWLEDGMENT

This work was supported by a grant from the National Institutes of Health-AR44513 and also by the Mayo Clinic/Mayo Foundation.

REFERENCES

1. Davis, RB, Ounpuu, S, Tyberski, D, and Gage, JR. A gait analysis data collection and reduction technique. *Hum Mov Sci* 1991; 10:575–587.
2. Kadaba, MP, Ramakrishnan, HK, and Wootten, ME. Measurement of lower extremity kinematics during level walking. *J Orthop Res* 1990; 8:383–392.
3. Apkarian, J, Naumann, S, and Cairns, B. A three-dimensional kinematic and dynamic model of the lower limb. *J Biomech* 1989; 22:143–155.
4. Cappozzo, A, Leo, T, and Pedotti, A. A general computational method for the analysis of human locomotion. *J Biomech* 1975; 8:307–320.
5. Kaufman, KR, An, KN, and Chao, EY. A comparison of intersegmental joint dynamics to isokinetic dynamometer measurements. *J Biomech* 1995; 28:1243–1256.
6. Delozier, G, Alexander, I, and Narayanaswamy, R. A method for measurement of integrated foot kinematics. In *7th Annual Summer Meeting, American Orthopedic Foot and Ankle Society.* 1991. Boston, MA.
7. Kidder, S, Abuzzahab, FS, Jr., Harris, GF, and Johnson, JE. A system for the analysis of foot and ankle kinematics during gait. *IEEE Trans Rehabil Eng* 1996; 4:25–32.
8. D'Andrea, SD, Tylkowski, C, Losito, J, Arquedas, W, Bushman, T and Howell, V. Three-dimensional kinematics of the foot. In *Proceedings of the 8th Annual East Coast Gait Conference.* 1993. Rochester, MN.
9. Chao, E. Justification of triaxial electrogoniometer for the measurement of joint rotation. *J Biomech* 1980; 13:987–1006.
10. Grood, E and Suntay, W. A joint coordinate system for the clinical description of three-dimensional motions: applications to the knee. *J Biomech Eng* 1983; 105:136–143.
11. Soderkvist, I and Wedin, P. Determining the movements of the skeleton using well-configured markers. *J Biomech* 1993; 26:1473–1477.
12. Sutherland, DH, Olshen, RA, Biden, EN and Wyatt, MP. The development of mature walking. In *The Development of Mature Walking.* Mac Keith Press, Oxford, England, 1988.
13. Scott, S and Winter, DA. Talocrural and talocalcaneal joint kinematics and kinetics during the stance phase of walking. *J Biomech* 1991; 28:743–752.
14. Kepple, T, Stanhope, SJ, Lohmann, KN, and Roman, NL. A video-based technique for measuring ankle-subtalar motion during stance. *J Biomech Eng* 1990; 12:273–280.
15. Padilla, J. Foot and ankle motion in cadaveric specimens; Validation of an optoelectronic motion detection system. M.S. thesis, Department of Orthopedics, Mayo Graduate School, Rochester, MN, 1995.

28 A Spatial Linkage Model of the Ankle Complex

Dragomir C. Marinkovich

CONTENTS

28.1 INTRODUCTION

Current motion analysis methods provide an acceptable tool to analyze motion of the pelvis, hip, knee, and ankle. These predominantly noninvasive systems utilize markers placed externally on known anatomical landmarks to track motion of the individual joints of the lower extremities. The marker motions are tracked by cameras or electromagnetic field sensors, depending on the type of markers, and typically provide feedback on pelvis, hip joint, knee joint, and ankle joint motions in the sagittal, coronal, and transverse planes. Lower extremity motion analysis has been established as a tool for evaluating gait patterns for both children and adults, and the results of these analyses are used in treatment planning for a variety of pathologies.

Classical lower extremity motion analysis focused on the foot as a single rigid segment and did not acknowledge its multiple degrees of freedom (DOF). Recent developments in motion analysis have focused on the kinematics of multiple segments of the foot.[1] However, a common limitation of these systems is their inability to capture the motion of the talus bone (the common component between the ankle and subtalar joints). Abnormalities in the foot can cause irregular loading and motion of the talus. Knowledge of talar motion would be beneficial to evaluation and treatment of these pathologies.

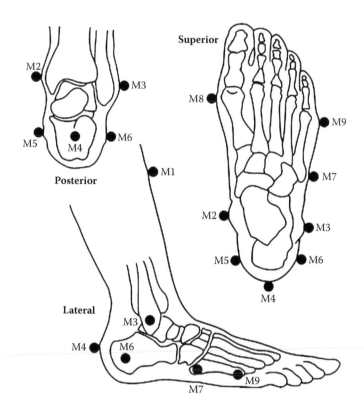

FIGURE 28.1 MFM marker placement.

Kidder et al.[1] developed the Milwaukee Foot Model (MFM) to describe the kinematics of the foot and ankle during locomotion using a passive marker motion analysis system. This rigid body model is composed of four segments made up of the following structures: (1) the tibia and fibula (tib/fib segment); (2) the calcaneus, talus, and navicular (hindfoot segment); (3) the cuneiforms, metatarsals, and cuboid (forefoot segment); and (4) the proximal phalanx of the hallux (hallux segment). Each segment is coupled using an unrestricted three-dimensional (3-D) joint. A total of 12 reflective markers are used to track the motions. Figure 28.1 shows the locations of the markers. The model utilizes an Euler method to describe the relative motion between the distal segments with respect to the adjacent proximal segments. The advantages of this system have been indicated previously.[1] Some limitations include the following: (1) errors induced by relative motion between the bones and markers attached to soft tissue; (2) the results of the Euler transformations are dependent on the sequence of rotations chosen to represent the movement; and (3) the system is not able to track subtalar joint motion, as the talus cannot be marked with a reliable external anatomical landmark.

A new geometric model of the ankle complex was developed to be used with video-based motion analysis systems in order to predict subtalar motion based on the motion of other segments of the foot. The proposed model is unique in that it closely represents the actual anatomical and kinematic aspects of the ankle joint complex. It incorporates a revolute joint for the ankle joint and a unique spatial mechanism for the subtalar joint that is based on key anatomical features and ligaments of the ankle complex. A cadaveric study was done to gather data to be used with this new model. The actual motions of the bone segments of the ankle and subtalar joints were compared with the marker-based motion of the model segments. It was hypothesized that mathematical modeling techniques could be used in conjunction with motion analysis information to predict subtalar motion during foot/ankle articulations.

28.1.1 Current Foot and Ankle Models

Current foot and ankle models fall into at least three categories: (1) both the talocrural and the subtalar joints are represented as revolute joints, (2) the ankle complex is represented by a spherical joint, or (3) the ankle joint is represented by a four-bar linkage (4BL) system.[2]

Dul et al.[3] developed a biaxial model of the ankle and subtalar joints using a rigid three-body system comprising a leg, talus, and foot segment. The segments are connected using two revolute joints, each with one DOF. The orientation of the ankle joint axis is defined by the line derived from a point on the lateral malleolus to a point on the medial malleolus. The subtalar axis is defined by the line derived from a point on the posterior lateral aspect of the calcaneus to a point on the superior midpoint of the navicular.

Van den Bogert et al.[4] also developed a biaxial, subject-specific model of the ankle comprising the tibia/fibula (or leg), calcaneus, and talus segments, which was based on the work done by Arebald et al.[5] The ankle and subtalar joints are each represented by revolute joints with the joint axes determined from motion data recorded from a total of six reflective markers placed on the leg and shoe. The axis orientations are determined using a least squares approach to solve for 12 model parameters. The resulting subtalar axis approximation is constant throughout the motion of the foot. However, Lundberg et al.[6], Leardini et al.,[7] and Lewis and Piazza[8] most recently discussed that the axis orientation of the subtalar joint *in vivo* is not constant throughout the cycle. This approximation of the subtalar axis may not be sufficient when used clinically.

Smith et al.[9] used a similar optimization approach to van den Bogert et al.[4] in determining the orientations of the talocrural and subtalar joints, assuming that the two joints were pure hinge joints. The methodology was sound when used with a mechanical device simulating the two axes. However, the results for *in vitro* testing showed a significant difference between predicted and measured axes orientations. This again suggests that the subtalar joint cannot be accurately modeled simply as a pure hinge.

Leardini et al.[2,10] formulated a model of the ankle joint based on a 4BL concept rather than the predominantly used revolute joint concept. This approach is a departure from the traditional approaches in that it uses actual representations of anatomical features and components of the ankle in their model. The advantage of this

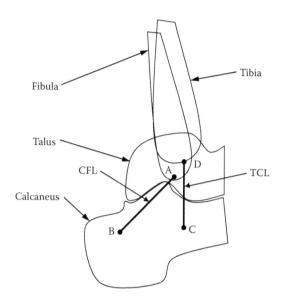

FIGURE 28.2 4BL model of ankle complex. (With permission from Leardini, A., O'Connor, J.J., Catani, F., Giannini, S., *J Biomech*, 32(6), 1999, 585–591.)

model over others is that it simulates rolling and sliding between the articular surfaces of the tibia and talus, which is not possible with a hinge joint. This model is unique for this application and uses representations of the ligaments that control mobility and the tibiocalcaneal (TCL) and calcaneofibular (CFL) ligaments, as two of the links of the system and the tibia/fibula segment as the coupler link. Figure 28.2 shows a schematic of the model.

The pin joint locations of the system (A, B, C, and D) were determined through dissection and are the attachment points of the TCL and CFL ligaments. This presents a disparity when compared to the classical method of determining the ankle joint axis. Traditionally, the axis is located anatomically using the tips of the lateral and medial malleoli. This creates an axis that is obliquely oriented to the sagittal plane. Leardini et al.'s[2] method also uses the tips of the lateral and medial malleoli but projects those points onto the sagittal plane, as two joints of the 4BL. In doing so, this limits the motion of the ankle joint strictly to the sagittal plane. Because points A and D are collinear in the traditional approach, a 3° rotation is applied with respect to the tibia/fibula anatomical frame to orient the mechanism more closely to the traditional approach.

Additional models of the foot and ankle have been proposed, which were not specifically used for gait analysis. Some of these foot and ankle models have modeled the foot and ankle joints as combinations of hinge and ball joints.[3] Dubbledam et al.[11] used a foot and leg model developed at the University of Virginia for the Mathematical Dynamic Modeling (MADYMO) body simulation program that included the major ligaments of the foot and ankle. That model was used to study injuries of the lower extremities due to impacts and was not specifically designed for gait analysis.

28.2 METHODS

28.2.1 SPATIAL LINKAGE MODEL

The proposed model expands upon the work done by Leardini et al.[2] and the biaxial approaches. The ankle joint is defined in most literature as a one DOF joint. Lundberg et al.[6] found the relative rotation between the talus and the tibia/fibula mortise joint in the coronal and transverse planes during weight-bearing to be between −1 and 1°. The new model continues to model the ankle joint as a revolute joint, but approximates the ankle complex including the subtalar joint as a spatial linkage.

The linkage system is based on the premise that as the subtalar joint is articulated, the positions of the TCL and CFL ligaments are either determined by the motion of the subtalar joint or that they determine the position of the subtalar joint. Additionally, the main feature that holds the talus and calcaneus together is the interosseous ligament. Using these assumptions, a spatial linkage system can be derived to approximate the subtalar joint.

Leardini et al.[2] identified that the TCL and CFL ligaments remain isometric during plantar and dorsiflexion, and surmised that they control and guide ankle joint motion. Renstrom et al.[12] studied the strains in the CFL and the anterior talofibular ligament (ATFL), and found that the CFL was essentially isometric during flexion and that the CFL's strain increased during supination and external rotation. Colville et al.[13] also found that both the CFL and the ATFL strains increased during ankle inversion. Additionally, the interosseous talocalcaneal ligament and ligamentum cervicis guide and limit the extremes of motion in the subtalar joint.[14,15] The interosseous ligament also provides the strongest connective tissue bond between the talus and calcaneus and is an extremely strong and relatively inelastic ligament. These ligaments, as well as the articular surfaces between the talus and calcaneus, dictate the motion between the talus and calcaneus. The proposed model approximates the articular surfaces of the subtalar joint and the interosseous ligament as a single spherical joint, and uses representations of the TFL and CFL as links in a mechanism that more closely mimics the actual motion of the ankle and subtalar joints vs. a biaxial model. The attachment points of the TCL and CFL are represented as spherical joints. Figure 28.3 shows a schematic diagram of the spatial linkage model (SLM).

The SLM is composed of five links, five spherical joints, and one revolute joint. It maintains the current thinking that the ankle complex has two DOFs: one DOF for the ankle joint and one DOF for the subtalar joint. The locations of the spherical joints are determined from anatomical features of the ankle complex and are coincident with the MFM skin-marker locations. The CFL ligament (Link 1) is attached to the apex of the lateral malleolus (Joint 5) and extends downward and posteriorly to a tubercle on the lateral surface of the calcaneus (Joint 4). The former attachment point corresponds to the lateral malleolus marker of the MFM, and the latter attachment point is very close to the lateral calcaneal marker. The TCL ligament (Link 2) is attached to the apex of medial malleolus (Joint 2) and extends downward to the sustentaculum tali of the calcaneus (Joint 3). The malleolar attachment point corresponds directly to a marker on the MFM. The latter point location can either be calculated as a phantom point using the medial malleolus, medial calcaneus, and medial head of the first metatarsal marker locations or by an addition of a marker attached to the skin over the

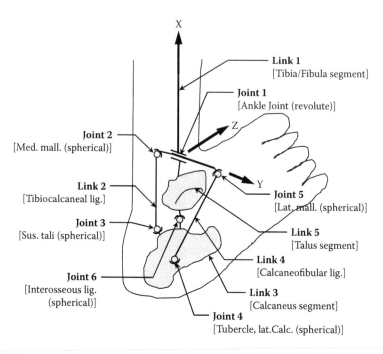

FIGURE 28.3 Schematic diagram of SLM.

sustentaculum tali. The ankle joint axis is defined by the lateral and medial malleoli markers (Joints 2 and 5). Additionally, those two markers and a marker on the medial surface of the anterior tibia define the reference frame for the system.

In the current adaptation of the model, joint positions 2, 4, and 5 are given from marker data. The Joint 1 location is the midpoint between Joints 2 and 5. The Joint 3 location is calculated as the point where a perpendicular line from joint location 2 intersects a line formed by markers on the medial calcaneus and the medial head of the first metatarsal. Alternatively, a marker can be placed over the sustentaculum tali to locate this joint.

The key variable of the model is Joint 6, representing the interosseous ligament and articular surfaces between the calcaneus and talus. It is the common point between those two segments. The initial location was determined with the foot in the neutral position. It is a point directly below Joint 1 located within the sinus tarsus. Referring to the Figure 28.3 coordinate system, Joint 6 has the same y- and z-coordinates as Joint 1 and the same x-coordinate as Joint 3. The sensitivity of the Joint 6 location was analyzed and is presented later in the chapter. Once the location of Joint 6 is established, the calcaneus and talus segments can be calculated. The calcaneus segment is determined from the points represented by Joints 3, 4, and 6. The talus segment is determined from the points representing Joints 1, 2, and 6. When the foot is motioned, three equations can be solved at each time step to determine the three unknown x-, y-, and z-coordinates of Joint 6. The calcaneus and talus segments are then defined. MatLab (The Mathworks Company, Natick, MA)

TABLE 28.1
Specimen Physical Characteristics

Specimen	Test Date	Sex	Age	Height (in.)	Weight (lbs)
1	14-May-04	F	84	67	200+

was used for the calculations and analysis. The end result of this model is that the relative motion between the talus and calcaneus (subtalar motion) can be predicted.

28.2.2 SPECIMEN TESTING PROCEDURE

A cadaveric study was designed to gather data to be used to test the new proposed model. A cadaver specimen with intact foot and ankle was motioned through plantarflexion/dorsiflexion and inversion/eversion using a controlled dynamometer while reflective skin and implanted bone markers were tracked. The cadaveric specimen was amputated below the knee with the tibial and fibular heads intact. The physical characteristics of the amputee are shown in Table 28.1.

A two-piece fixture (leg and foot) was designed to separately hold the leg portion and the foot portion of the specimen in place while allowing free movement of the foot and ankle. The leg fixture was constructed to hold the specimen distally from the knee and proximal to the ankle joint. The leg was placed horizontally in a modified ankle fixation orthotic (AFO) that was fastened to a nylon plate. The leg was held in place using two hook and loop straps, one of which was fixed to the AFO. The straps were adjusted to prevent transverse plane (with respect to the lab coordinate system, Figure 28.4) movement of the leg. The nylon plate of the leg fixture was

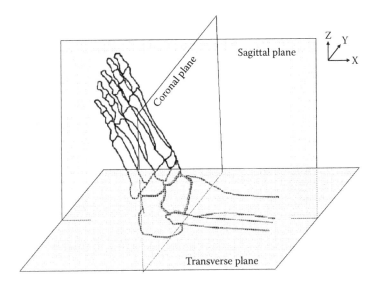

FIGURE 28.4 Description of planes of motion.

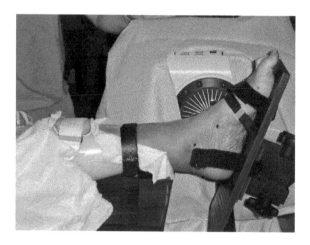

FIGURE 28.5 Leg and foot fixture setup for plantarflexion/dorsiflexion testing.

attached to a wooden platform that was secured to the seat/platform portion of a Biodex System 3 (Biodex Medical Systems, Shirley, NY) computer-controlled dynamometer. The Biodex allows computer control of movement through a specified range of motions and rates. The primary motions of interest were plantarflexion/ dorsiflexion and inversion/eversion.

The foot fixture was constructed to attach to the dynamometer component of the Biodex and to secure the foot. This fixture was designed to allow the foot to plantarflex and dorsiflex in one configuration, and to allow the foot to invert and evert in another configuration. The foot was secured to the foot fixture using two hook and loop straps. Both straps secured the forefoot between the midfoot and distal heads of the metatarsals so as to not interfere with marker or triad placements. A heel cup was used to secure the heel. The heel cup was adjusted to hold the foot in place such that the ankle joint axis and the Biodex dynamometer axis were nearly coincident to each other when the fixture was attached to the dynamometer. Figure 28.5 shows the specimen testing setup for plantarflexion/dorsiflexion, and Figure 28.6 shows the setup for inversion/eversion.

Anterior/posterior and lateral radiographic images were taken of the specimen prior to its placement in the leg and foot fixtures using a GE OEC Stenoscope 9 in. C-arm fluoroscope (GE OEC Medical Systems, Milwaukee, WI). The images revealed no underlying conditions or evidence of orthosis.

The order of testing was chosen so that there would be a minimal amount of disturbance to the marker and triad placements and was as follows:

1. Plantar/dorsiflexion with skin markers
2. Inversion/eversion with skin markers
3. Inversion/eversion with triads inserted and no skin markers
4. Plantar/dorsiflexion with triads inserted and no skin markers

After the specimen was secured in the foot and leg fixtures, the Biodex chair, dynamometer locations, and the foot fixture were adjusted so that the ankle joint

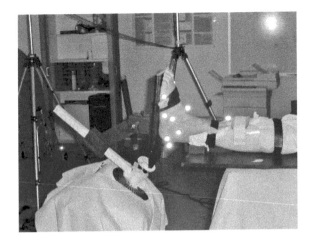

FIGURE 28.6 Leg and foot fixture setup for inversion/eversion testing.

axis and dynamometer axis were nearly coincident in the sagittal plane. The point where the ankle axis bisects the midplane of the ankle was used to approximate the alignment axis. The range of motion of the specimen was determined by physically moving the foot through plantarflexion and dorsiflexion until moderate resistance was felt at the extremes. The Biodex dynamometer motion range was recorded and then adjusted to 75% of the measured range in both plantar and dorsiflexion in order to prevent any distortion caused by the Biodex at the extremes. Table 28.2 shows the measured and tested ranges of motion and the rates of testing.

Twelve reflective markers were placed on the leg as shown in Figure 28.7. Markers 1 through 6 and 10 through 12 correspond to marker locations from the MFM. Markers 7 to 9 were added as redundant markers and were not used in the analysis. The anatomical locations of the markers are listed below and in Figure 28.7:

1. Anterior on the tibia and distal to the tibial tuberosity
2. Lateral malleolus
3. Medial malleolus
4. Calcaneal tuberosity

TABLE 28.2
Measured and Tested Ranges of Motion

Plantarflexion		Dorsiflexion		Inversion		Eversion			
Maximum Range	Tested Range	Maximum Range	Tested Range	Maximum Range	Tested Range	Maximum Range	Tested Range	Rate (degrees/sec)	Pause at ends (sec)
0	30	10	8	25	25	25	25	20	1

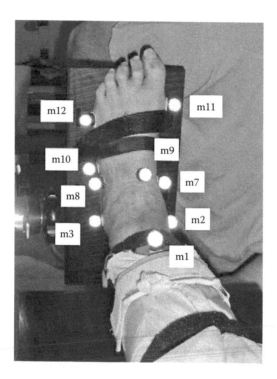

FIGURE 28.7 Reflective marker placement.

  5. Medial calcaneus
  6. Lateral calcaneus
  7. Navicular tuberosity
  8. Lateral aspect of the cuboid
  9. Dorsal aspect of the intermediate cuneiform
 10. Tuberosity of the fifth metatarsal
 11. Head of the fifth metatarsal
 12. Head of the first metatarsal

A 15-camera Vicon 524 Motion Analysis System (Vicon Motion Systems, Lake Forest, CA) tracked and recorded the 3D positional information from the markers. Figure 28.8 shows the placement and height of the 15 cameras.

Static marker location data were recorded with the leg and foot in the neutral position, defined as the foot being at a 90° angle with respect to the leg. The specimen was ranged through five trials, each containing seven cycles. One cycle consisted of starting in the neutral position, plantarflexing 25°, returning to the neutral position, dorsiflexing 8°, and then returning to the neutral position.

Upon completion of the plantarflexion/dorsiflexion (P/D) trials, the dynamometer and foot fixture were reconfigured for inversion/eversion testing. The foot fixture was designed to allow the foot to remain fastened while the conversion was made.

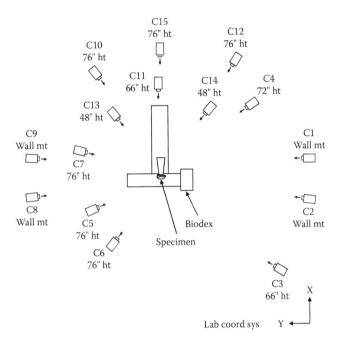

FIGURE 28.8 Camera positions and heights.

Figure 28.6 shows the configuration of the fixture and Biodex for internal/external rotation (I/E) testing. The fixture was adjusted so that the Biodex axis was approximately in line with the subtalar axis of the specimen. The specimen was again ranged through five trials, each containing seven cycles.

Upon completion of the I/E trials, the specimen's position on the fixture and strap locations were marked prior to removal from the fixture. The skin was carefully dissected in four locations on the foot in order to drill and place marker triads into the calcaneus, talus, cuboid, and navicular. The tissue was dissected in such a way as to not affect the stabilizing components of the foot and ankle or to affect the movement of the triads during the trials. A drill was used to insert the triads directly into the respective bones. Additionally, a triad was inserted into an exposed section of the tibia just distal to the tibial head. The specimen was placed again in the fixture and testing continued with I/E first followed by P/D using the same number of trials and cycles. Figure 28.9 shows the locations of the triads.

28.3 RESULTS

Four cases were analyzed and compared from the test data:

1. The relative motion between the calcaneus and talus (subtalar motion) during inversion/eversion
2. The relative motion between the talus and tibia/fibula segment during inversion/eversion

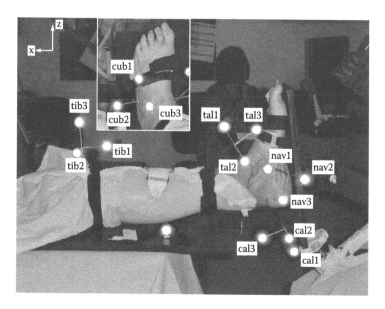

FIGURE 28.9 Bone marker triad placements and marker names.

3. The relative motion between the calcaneus and talus (subtalar motion) during plantarflexion/dorsiflexion
4. The relative motion between the talus and tibia/fibula segment during plantarflexion/dorsiflexion

In each of these cases, the data from the bone marker implants were compared to the skin-marker data. A similar method to that used with the MFM[13] was utilized to calculate the relative motions between the segments. The data are presented as relative rotations between the segments of interest using Euler rotations. The data are presented as rotations with respect to the lab coordinate planes (sagittal, coronal, and transverse) as shown in Figure 28.4.

Figure 28.10 shows the subtalar motion during inversion/eversion testing of the specimen. The left graph is derived from motion data taken from bone marker data and shows the rotations of the implanted calcaneus marker relative to the implanted talus marker. The right graph shows subtalar motion defined as the motion of the skin-marker–based hindfoot with respect to the talus segment derived from the SLM.

Figure 28.11 shows the talar motion within the ankle joint mortise during the inversion/eversion testing. The left graph shows the relative rotations of the talus bone marker with respect to the tibia bone marker. The right graph shows the rotations of the talus segment with respect to the tibia/fibula segment, both derived from skin-marker data.

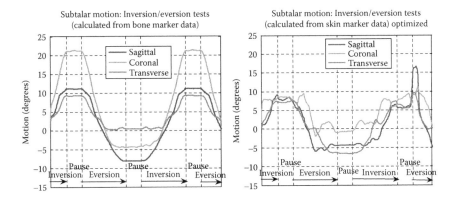

FIGURE 28.10 Subtalar motion during inversion/eversion testing.

Figure 28.12 shows the subtalar motion during plantarflexion/dorsiflexion testing of the specimen. The left graph is derived from motion data taken from bone marker data and shows the rotations of the implanted calcaneus marker relative to the implanted talus marker. The right graph shows subtalar motion defined as the motion of the skin-marker–based hindfoot with respect to the talus segment derived from the SLM.

Figure 28.13 shows the talar motion within the ankle joint mortise during the plantarflexion/dorsiflexion testing. The left graph shows the relative rotations of the talus bone marker with respect to the tibia bone marker. The right graph shows the rotations of the talus segment with respect to the tibia/fibula segment, both derived from skin-marker data.

A sensitivity study was done to determine the "optimal" initial location of Joint 6 of the SLM. As indicated previously, the initial position was based on the y- and z-coordinates of Joint 1 (the ankle joint) and the x-coordinate of Joint 3 (the distal

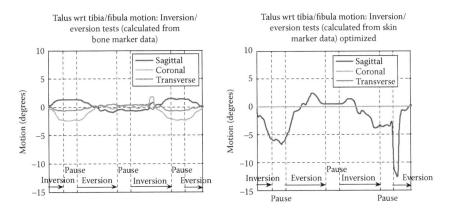

FIGURE 28.11 Talus with respect to tibia/fibula motion during inversion/eversion testing.

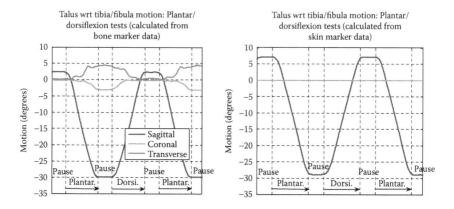

FIGURE 28.12 Talus with respect to tibia/fibula motion during plantarflexion/dorsiflexion testing.

attachment point of the TCL ligament). The initial coordinates of Joint 6 were each varied in five iterative steps from –20 mm to +20 mm of the original assumed location. Table 28.3 shows the sensitivity (low, medium, and high) that each change in the x-, y-, and z-coordinates had to the rotations. An optimal value was also determined from the iterations that most closely matched the bone-marker motions. The shaded blocks in Table 28.3 indicate the optimal values with medium-to-high sensitivity that most closely matches their respective bone marker motion counterparts. That corresponded to a Æx of + 10 mm, a Æy of 0 mm, and a Æz of + 10 mm. The table also shows the respective corresponding range of motions for each variable and the comparative values from the bone-marker motion data. The rightside graphs of Figure 28.10 to Figure 28.13 were calculated using these delta values for Joint 6.

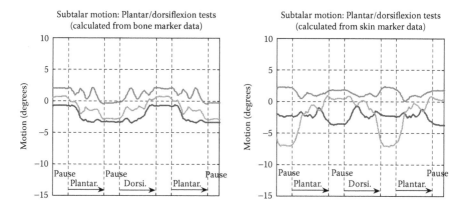

FIGURE 28.13 Subtalar motion during plantarflexion/dorsiflexion testing.

TABLE 28.3
Sensitivity Study of Joint 6 of the Spatial Linkage Model

	Inversion/Eversion		Plantarflexion/Dorsiflexion		Plantarflexion/Dorsiflexion	
	Calcaneus wrt Talus (Skin Markers)		Calcaneus wrt Talus (Skin Markers)		Talus wrt Tibia (Skin Markers)	
	Sensitivity	Optimal Value (Corr. Range)	Sensitivity	Optimal Value (Corr. Range)	Sensitivity	Optimal Value (Corr. Range)
x-variable						
Sagittal	Medium	$x = +15...(-7.5 + 12.5)$ᵃ	High	$x = +10...(-4...-2)$ᵃ	High	$x = +10...(-7.5...+29)$ᵃ
Coronal	Low	$x = -20...(-2...+7)$	Low	$x = -20...(-6...+1)$	n/a	n/a
Transverse	Low	$x = +15...(-8...+8)$	High	$x = +10...(0...+1)$ᵃ	n/a	n/a
y-variable						
Sagittal	Medium	$y = -20...(-9...+11)$ᵃ	Medium	$y = +20...(-3...+3)$	Medium	No optimal value
Coronal	Low	$y = -10...(-2...+8)$	Low	$y = +20...(0...-5)$	n/a	n/a
Transverse	Low	$y = +20...(-7...+8)$	Low	$y = +20...(0...+2)$	n/a	n/a
z-variable						
Sagittal	High	$z = +10...(-7...+11)$ᵃ	Low	$z = +20...(-2.5...-1)$ᵃ	Low	$z = +20...(-8...+28)$
Coronal	Low	$z = -10...(-3...+6)$	Low	$z = -20...(+1...-5)$	n/a	n/a
Transverse	Low	$z = 0...(-7.5...+8)$	Low	$z = -10...(+1...+1)$	n/a	n/a
Comparative Values			**Comparative Values**		**Comparative Values**	
Bone marker data (calculated wrt talus)	Sagittal	$(-8...+11)$	Bone marker data (talus wrt tibia)	Sagittal $(-3...-1)$	Bone marker data (talus wrt tibia)	Sagittal $(-2.5...+30)$
	Coronal	$(-4...+7)$		Coronal $(-3...+1/2)$		Coronal —
	Transverse	$(-9...+9)$		Transverse $(0...+2)$		Transverse —

ᵃ Indicates optimal values.

28.4 DISCUSSION

The leg specimen was ranged from 25° inversion to 25° eversion during the inversion/eversion testing. Figure 28.10 shows the results with respect to the lab coordinate planes in a triplanar manner. The SLM shows similar trends as the bone-marker derived data. It is apparent looking at Figure 28.11 that there is little movement within the ankle joint during the bone-marker testing. However, there was about 5° of motion in the ankle joint during the skin-marker testing. This would lower the peak values of Figure 28.10 (right). This difference in Figure 28.11 is quite possibly caused by a slight change in the leg position during the changeover from skin markers to bone markers. The specimen was removed from the fixture after the skin-marker testing to insert the bone-marker triads. Figure 28.11 (right) shows no rotations in the coronal and transverse planes. The model defines that the rotation in the ankle joint (Joint 1) is only in the sagittal plane.

   Figure 28.12 (left) shows that there is slight rotation in the coronal and transverse planes during plantarflexion/dorsiflexion with the bone markers. The tested range of motion was from 8° dorsiflexion to 30° plantarflexion. The measured range was from about 3 to 30°. The SLM-based motion was from about 7 to 29°. This is very close to the tested range. The differences again may be attributed to specimen trial placement errors. The comparison between bone marker and SLM motion is very good.

28.5 CONCLUSION

The SLM is an intriguing concept to implement for modeling the ankle and subtalar joints. It mimics the actual motion of the subtalar joint and agrees with other observations that the subtalar axis is not fixed during motion. Further study is needed to better develop the location of skin markers and to determine the sensitivity of marker location. The model holds promise for improving the diagnostic capabilities of gait analysis.

ACKNOWLEDGMENTS

The author thanks Marquette University and the Orthopaedic Rehabilitation and Engineering Center (OREC) for providing resources for this project. The author also thanks G. Harris, Ph.D.; G.E.O. Widera, Ph.D.; R. Marks, M.D.; M. Wang, Ph.D.; N. Nigro, Ph.D.; and J. Long, M.S. for their assistance.

REFERENCES

1. Kidder, S.M., Abuzzahab, F.S., Harris, G.F., Johnson, J.E., "A system for the analysis of foot and ankle kinematics during gait," *IEEE Trans of Rehab Eng*, 4(1), 1996, 25–32.
2. Leardini, A., O'Connor, J.J., Catani, F., Giannini, S., "A geometric model of the human ankle joint," *J Biomech*, 32(6), 1999, 585–591.

3. Dul, J., Shiavi, R., Green, N.E., "Simulation of tendon transfer surgery," *Eng Med,* 14, 1985, 31–38.

4. van den Bogert, A.J., Smith, G.D., Nigg, B.M., "In vivo determination of the anatomical axes of the ankle joint complex: an optimization approach," *J Biomech,* 27(12), 1994, 1477–1488.

5. Arebald, M., Nigg, B.M., Ekstrand, J., Olsson, K.O., Ekstrom, H., "Three-dimensional measurement of rearfoot motion during running," *J Biomech,* 23, 1990, 933–940.

6. Lundberg, A., Svensson, O.K., Nemeth, G., Selvik, G., "The axis of rotation of the ankle joint," *J Bone Joint Surgery,* 71B, 1989, 94–99.

7. Leardini, A., Stagni, R., O'Connor, J.J., "Mobility of the subtalar joint in the intact ankle complex," *J Biomech,* 34, 2001, 805–809.

8. Lewis, G.S., Piazza, S.J., "Functional location of subject-specific joint axes of the human ankle complex," *Intl Mech Engr Cong Expo,* 2004, 379–380.

9. Smith, R., Hunt, A., Buchen, P., Poon, S., "Finding the talocrural and subtalar joint axis orientations," IX Intl Symp on Comp Simul in Biomech, July 2–4, 2003.

10. Leardini, A., O'Connor, J.J., Catani, F., Giannini, S., "Kinematics of the human ankle complex in passive flexion; a single degree of freedom system," *J Biomech,* 32, 1999, 111–118.

11. Dubbledam, R., Nilson, G., Pal, B., Eriksson, N., Owen, C., Roberts, A., Crandall, J., Hall, G., Manning, P., Wallace, A., "A MADYMO Model of the Foot and Leg for Local Impacts," *43rd Stapp Car Crash Conference Proceedings,* vP-350, 1999, 185–202.

12. Renstrom, P., Wertz, M., Incavo, S., Pope, M., Ostgaard, C. Arms, S., Haugh, L., "Strain on the lateral ligaments in the ankle" [Abstract], Orth Res Soc Annual Meeting, Atlanta, Feb 1998.

13. Colville, M.R., Marder, R., Boyle, J., Zarins, B., "Strain measurement in the human ankle ligaments" [Abstract], Orth Res Soc Annual Meeting, Atlanta, Feb 1988.

14. Neumann, D.A., *Kinesiology of the Muscoskeletal System: Foundations for Physical Rehabilitation,* 1st ed., Mosby Inc., St. Louis, 2002.

15. Norkin, C.C., Levangie, P.K., *Joint Structure and Function: A Comprehensive Analysis,* 2nd ed., F.A. Davis Co., Philadelphia, 1992.

29 Multisegment Foot Biomechanics in Dynamic Hindfoot Varus

Matthew R. Walker, Frank L. Buczek, Kevin M. Cooney, Neil A. Sharkey, and James O. Sanders

CONTENTS

29.1   INTRODUCTION

Dynamic hindfoot varus (DHV) is a common presentation among children with hemiplegic cerebral palsy (Figure 29.1) and among patients of any age with stroke or traumatic brain injury, yet methods to accurately determine the source of the deformity remain unsatisfactory. Overactive or out-of-phase tibialis anterior (TA) and tibialis posterior (TP) muscles are most often cited as the cause, and surgical corrections are typically focused on these muscles (Table 29.1). TA originates on the anterior, proximal tibia and interosseus membrane, and inserts on the medial side of the medial cuneiform and on the base of the first metatarsal. It primarily serves to dorsiflex the foot while secondarily serving as an invertor of the hindfoot and supinator of the forefoot. This muscle normally acts eccentrically at initial contact to control the heel rocker prior to foot-flat, and it acts concentrically during the swing phase to dorsiflex the foot and promote ground clearance. Continuous or out-of-phase activity of TA, often seen subsequent to stroke or traumatic brain injury, is typically treated with a

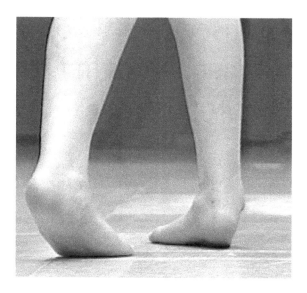

FIGURE 29.1 Photograph of a subject with DHV (right foot).

split anterior tibialis tendon procedure (SPLATT), which balances the coronal plane action on the foot while preserving sagittal plane dorsiflexion.

TP is a deep muscle that originates on the posterior, proximal tibia, fibula, and interosseus membrane and inserts on the tuberosity of the navicular, the underside of the cuneiforms, and the base of the second, third, and fourth metatarsals, after its tendon passes posterior to the medial malleolus. It is a weak plantarflexor and a strong invertor. Although normally active only during stance phase to assist the triceps surae with plantarflexion during push-off, in some cases it may be active only during swing phase to assist with ground clearance through inversion.[1] Continuous activity of TP, often seen in cerebral palsy, may be treated by lengthening

TABLE 29.1
Typical Surgical Decision Criteria for Treating DHV

EMG Activity	Tibialis Anterior	Tibialis Posterior
Continuous	Split tendon	Lengthen tendon Release tendon Split tendon
Out-of-phase	Split tendon	Transfer tendon

From Vaughan, C.L., Nashman, J.H., and Murr, M.S., What is the normal function of tibialis posterior in human gait?, in *The Diplegic Child: Evaluation and Management*, Sussman, M.D., Ed., American Academy of Orthopaedic Surgeons, Rosemont IL, USA, 1992, Chapter 31. With permission.

or releasing its tendon, or by a split posterior tibialis tendon procedure (SPOTT). The latter balances coronal plane action on the foot while preserving sagittal plane plantarflexion. Out-of-phase activity of TP is most often treated with a tendon transfer to eliminate unwanted plantarflexion.

It is clear that the activity of TA and TP plays an important role in treatment selection, yet difficulties arise when these muscles are active simultaneously. Here, it is especially difficult to determine the primary deforming force. Over an 18-month period, we evaluated 12 patients referred to our Motion Analysis Laboratory for DHV (Table 29.2). All of these patients demonstrated varus hindfoot (HF) during stance phase, simultaneous with both TA and TP activity, each with varying intensities. However, 11 of these same patients also demonstrated varus HF during swing phase; TA was active for all 11 of these patients, while TP was active for only 8. Surgical recommendations based upon instrumented gait analysis included five SPLATTs, six SPOTTs, one TA tendon lengthening, and six TP tendon lengthenings. Perhaps most telling, for six patients, instrumented gait analysis remained ambiguous enough to require subsequent referral to clinical judgment, and in 5 out of the 12 cases, the actual surgeries performed differed from those we recommended. This was quite disappointing, as each child endured fine-wire electromyography (EMG) to determine TP activity, yet this information proved inconclusive.

Detailed knowledge of foot motion is critical not only to understand clinical foot deformities, but also to understand lower extremity mechanics during locomotion. The human foot has traditionally been modeled as a single rigid segment, and in some cases as a simple vector lacking a valgus/varus degree of freedom (DoF) at the ankle.[2] Other models allow measurement in all three planes of movement, but still consider the foot as a single segment with motion occurring only at the ankle. Single-segment foot models, originally developed and since utilized because of the technical constraints inherent in traditional methodologies, have recently been described as overly simplified[3] and inadequate[4] for the clinical analysis of foot mechanics. It has been known for some time that the foot deforms during movement, as it is composed of 26 bones and over 30 joints that each have six DoF movement capacity.[5] Treating separate segments as a single rigid body adversely affects inverse dynamics results,[3] as these calculations require detailed understanding of force transfer from the ground, across adjoining segments, to the shank (SH). A more detailed foot model not only increases our understanding of foot kinematics and deformities,[6-9] but would also allow increased fidelity in kinetics calculations.

Biomechanists have begun to adopt enhanced foot models. Advances in motion capture technology have improved the ability to track an increased number of small markers, thus reducing movement artifact from larger markers and allowing reliable modeling of the foot as more than a single segment.[5] Rigid body mechanics require a minimum of three noncollinear markers to reconstruct three-dimensional motion; least squares techniques use at least one additional marker to control for measurement error. For multisegment foot modeling, practical and technical challenges include the placement of several markers on small foot segments, and the effects of skin movement artifact on relatively small motions. In light of these challenges, we believe foot models should be developed specifically to answer the questions being addressed.

TABLE 29.2
Clinical Experiences at Shriners Hospitals for Children — Erie, PA

PT	Stance			Swing			Recommendation						Surgery Performed				
	VH	TA	TP	VH	TA	TP	SPLATT	SPOTT	TA tdn	TP tdn	HCL	CLIN	SPLATT	SPOTT	TA tdn	TP tdn	HCL
1*	2	1	2	1	2	1		X		X	X	X		X			X
2	2	1	2	0	2	1	X			X	X	X	X			X	
3*	2	1	2	2	2	1	X		X					X			X
4	2	2	2	1	2	1					X	X		X			X
5*	2	1	2	2	2	1		X			X						
6*	2	1	2	2	2	1		X			X			X			X
7	2	2	1	2	2	1						X					
8	2	2	2	2	2	0		X			X	X		X			X
9	1	2	2	1	2	0	X			X			X			X	
10	2	2	2	2	2	0	X			X			X			X	
11	2	2	2	2	1	1	X	X		X		X		X			
12*	2	2	2	1	2	1		X		X							
Totals							5	6	1	6	6	6	3	6	0	3	5

PT: patients (* used in feasibility study), VH: varus hindfoot observed, TA: tibialis anterior surface EMG present,

TP: tibialis posterior fine-wire EMG present; tdn: tendon lengthening; HCL: heel-cord (teno-Achilles) lengthening; 2: greater intensity or duration; 1: lesser intensity or duration; 0: nonexistent; CLIN: clinical judgment.

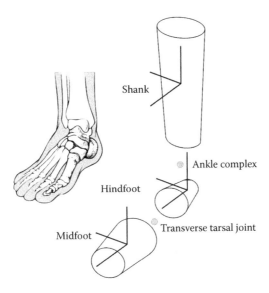

FIGURE 29.2 Schematic of body segments and joints modeled in this feasibility study (right foot).

To better serve our patients, we wished to develop a multisegment foot model of sufficient accuracy to determine individual contributions to the varus deformity made by TA and TP. Our ideal kinetic model would include SH, HF, midfoot (MF), and forefoot (FF) segments, accurately defined without medical imaging while accounting for important muscles crossing these segments. Ultimately, we envisioned the use of optimization techniques to identify muscle contributions to the varus deformities without the need for fine-wire EMG. As a first step in this difficult process, we conducted a feasibility study of multisegment foot kinematics. We hypothesized that an anatomically based, nonradiographic kinematic model (Figure 29.2) of the SH, HF, and MF could differentiate between normal subjects and patients with DHV.

29.2 METHODS

29.2.1 HUMAN SUBJECT TESTING

The patients seen in this study underwent a full clinical examination and conventional gait analysis, often lasting a minimum of 2h, prior to multisegment foot data collection. After much instrumentation and a needle stick for the fine-wire EMG placement, these children became intolerant of additional procedures. Thus, we avoided the collection of medical imaging and motion capture calibration trials by using a single kinematic frame at mid-stance for anatomical calibration of the multisegment foot model. (Consequences of this choice are explained in the Discussion.) For this feasibility study, we examined five children diagnosed with neurological involvement and DHV (patients, Table 29.3), and six children with no neurological

TABLE 29.3
Subject Characteristics

Variable	Normals	DHV Patients
Number of subjects	6	5
Sex (male, female)	2 M / 4 F	4 M / 1 F
Age (yr)[a]	8.8 (2.9)	8.5 (3.6)
Mass (kg)[a]	26.7 (11.1)	40.3 (23.2)
Height(cm)[a]	126.6 (15.9)	132.6 (20.2)
Side tested (L/R)	2 L / 4 R	2 L / 3 R
Strides used per subject[b]	6.0 (6, 6)	4.8 (3, 6)

[a]Data are means and (standard deviations).

[b]Data are means and (minimum, maximum).

impairments and no known or apparent foot or ankle pathology (normals). Independent ambulation, with or without an assistive device, was required for subject inclusion in the patients group.

Prior to testing, subjects and/or their guardians signed informed consent documents approved by our human subjects committee. Surface EMG electrodes (Motion Lab Systems, MA-300, Baton Rouge, LA, U.S.) were placed bilaterally over the rectus femoris, vastus medialis, semitendinosis, TA, and gastrocnemius muscles. For the involved side of patients, a fine-wire EMG electrode was inserted into the belly of TP, in place of the vastus medialis surface electrode. All of the fine-wire procedures were performed using sterile techniques by the same investigator certified in these methods. The wire placements were confirmed by eliciting an expected movement using a functional electrical stimulator (Focus NMES, Empi Inc., St. Paul, MN, U.S.). Motion capture markers were fixed to the skin based on palpable bony landmarks (Figure 29.3). Subjects were then instructed to perform multiple walking trials at their self-selected speed. Sagittal and coronal views of the subjects were recorded using Super-VHS (S-VHS) observational video. Two different Vicon motion capture systems were used (Oxford, Metrics Group, Oxford, England, U.K.) as a laboratory upgrade occurred between the collections for patients and normals. Kinematic data for patients were collected at 60 Hz using a six-camera Vicon 370 system, but due to equipment limitations, gaps occurred in some marker trajectories. Gaps of less than ten samples were considered acceptable and were filled using a cubic spline interpolation; trials with larger gaps were eliminated from the study. Kinematic data for normals were collected at 120 Hz using an upgraded ten-camera Vicon 612 system, without the need for interpolation. All marker trajectories were low-pass filtered using a dual-pass, second order, recursive Butterworth filter and a cutoff frequency of 6 Hz.[10]

Though not used for this kinematics study, ground reaction forces and plantar pressures were also collected to help prepare for future work. EMG and ground reaction forces from three strain-gauge force plates (OR6-7, Advanced Mechanical Technology Inc., Watertown, MA, U.S.) were collected at 1200 Hz and 1560 Hz for

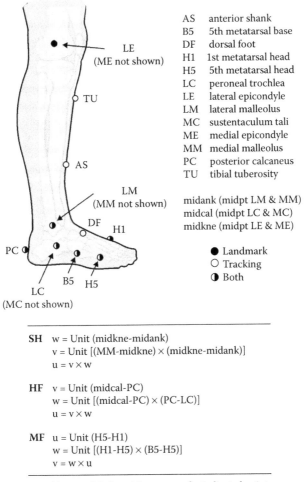

AS	anterior shank
B5	5th metatarsal base
DF	dorsal foot
H1	1st metatarsal head
H5	5th metatarsal head
LC	peroneal trochlea
LE	lateral epicondyle
LM	lateral malleolus
MC	sustentaculum tali
ME	medial epicondyle
MM	medial malleolus
PC	posterior calcaneus
TU	tibial tuberosity

midank (midpt LM & MM)
midcal (midpt LC & MC)
midkne (midpt LE & ME)

● Landmark
○ Tracking
◑ Both

SH w = Unit (midkne-midank)
       v = Unit [(MM-midkne) × (midkne-midank)]
       u = v × w

HF v = Unit (midcal-PC)
       w = Unit [(midcal-PC) × (PC-LC)]
       u = v × w

MF u = Unit (H5-H1)
       w = Unit [(H1-H5) × (B5-H5)]
       v = w × u

Variables are global position vectors for indicated points.
"Unit" = Unit vector parallel to calculated vector.

FIGURE 29.3 Schematic detailing the locations and descriptions of external motion capture markers (right foot). Right local reference frame derivations are described below the illustration. (Adapted from Walker, M.R., Cooney, K.M., Sharkey, N.A., Sanders, J.O., and Buczek, F.L., Multi-segment foot kinematics of dynamic hindfoot varus, *J. Orthop. Sports Phys. Ther.*, 34, A11–12, 2004. With permission from the Orthopaedic and Sports Physical Therapy Sections of the American Physical Therapy Association.)

patients and normals, respectively. EMG data were analog band-pass filtered to retain frequencies between 25 and 500 Hz. Plantar pressure data were collected at 1200 Hz from patients (but not normals) using an EMED 2016/2 platform (Novel, Munich, Germany).

29.2.2 Multisegment Foot Model

Our kinematic model (Figure 29.2) consisted of an SH (tibia and fibula), HF (calcaneus and talus), and "MF" (remaining tarsals and metatarsals). In each segment of the model, right-handed local reference frames included three unit direction vectors: "u" pointed laterally for right segments and medially for left segments, "v" pointed anteriorly, and "w" pointed superiorly. Local reference frames were derived using the anatomical "landmark" markers (Figure 29.3) from a single mid-stance frame in one of the walking trials. The singular value decomposition method[11] was used to obtain optimal rigid body rotation matrices in the walking trials.

Intersegmental motion was then expressed in terms of Cardan angles (distal relative to proximal segment) by Euler decomposition of the transformation matrix describing the movement from the pose of the distal segment to that of the proximal segment. Angular outputs were made anatomically consistent between the left and right legs, normalized to gait cycles, and ensemble averaged (mean ± 1 standard deviation) for both subject groups.

29.2.3 Terminology

The first rotation, termed dorsi/plantar flexion, is about the mediolaterally directed "u" axis of the distal segment. The second rotation, termed sustentaculum-tali (ST) valgus/varus, is about an anteriorly directed floating axis. (The more superior position of marker MC relative to LC results in a varus offset when HF is in subtalar neutral. Consequently, we refer to these rotations as ST valgus/varus to distinguish them from more conventional definitions for this DoF.) The final rotation, termed external/internal rotation, is about the superiorly directed "w" axis of the proximal segment.

29.3 RESULTS

29.3.1 Angular Results

We first present sagittal plane motion of HF with respect to (wrt) SH, followed by MF wrt HF; we then repeat this sequence for coronal and transverse plane motions. Finally, we present transverse plane motion of MF wrt SH. Here, ensemble averages are used to illustrate general findings.

For normals, HF was plantarflexed wrt SH at initial contact, but quickly moved into dorsiflexion for much of stance phase (Figure 29.4, top left); push-off, initial swing, and terminal swing were all characterized by plantarflexion. Although the corresponding curve for patients had the same general shape, it demonstrated greater variability and remained in plantarflexion throughout the gait cycle (compared to normals, average root-mean-square (RMS) difference: 16.4°). For normals, MF was slightly plantarflexed wrt HF from early to mid-stance, at push-off, and throughout swing, with mild dorsiflexion occurring only in late stance (Figure 29.4, top right). In contrast, patients have increased MF dorsiflexion wrt HF throughout the gait cycle (average RMS difference: 21.7°).

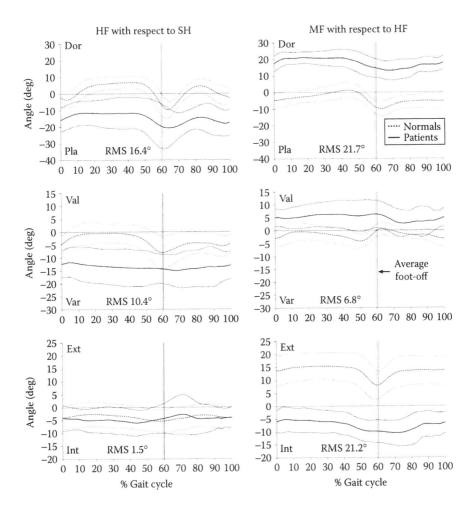

FIGURE 29.4 Ensemble average angular kinematics (mean ± 1 standard deviation) of HF wrt SH (first column) and MF wrt HF (second column) highlight differences between normals (dotted) and patients (solid). From top to bottom row: dorsi/plantar flexion (dor/pla), ST valgus/varus (val/var), and external/internal rotation (ext/int). Average foot-off events are indicated by vertical lines, and average RMS differences are noted in degrees.

In the coronal plane, (Figure 29.4, middle left), motion of HF wrt SH for normals revealed slight ST varus at initial contact, nearly neutral alignment at mid-stance, and maximum ST varus at push-off. Patients demonstrated increased amounts of ST varus at a near constant 12 to 13° (average RMS difference: 10.4°). Motion of MF wrt HF for normals also exhibited mild amounts of ST varus at initial contact (Figure 29.4, middle right), a brief period of neutral alignment, and a return to ST varus in late stance. Patients demonstrated a near constant 5° of ST valgus for MF wrt HF (average RMS difference: 6.8°).

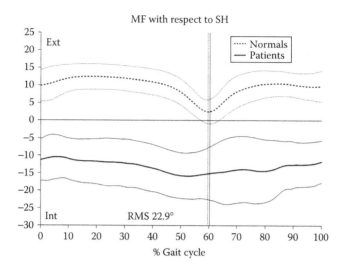

FIGURE 29.5 Ensemble average transverse plane kinematics (mean ± 1 standard deviation for external/internal rotation) of MF wrt SH highlight differences between normals (dotted) and patients (solid). Average foot-off events are indicated by vertical lines, and the average RMS difference is noted in degrees.

In the transverse plane, there was little difference between patients and normals for HF wrt SH (Figure 29.4, bottom left), with both groups averaging near 5° of internal rotation (average RMS difference: 1.5°). Motion of MF wrt HF for normals demonstrated approximately 14° of external rotation throughout the gait cycle, with decreased external rotation occurring at push-off (Figure 29.4, bottom right), whereas patients exhibited internal rotation throughout the gait cycle (average RMS difference: 21.2°).

Motion of MF wrt SH (Figure 29.5) closely followed that of MF wrt HF (Figure 29.4, bottom right) for both patients and normals, but was biased by approximately 5° of additional internal rotation. This was about the same amount of internal rotation as seen for HF wrt SH (Figure 29.4, bottom left).

29.3.2 CASE PRESENTATIONS

In a single patient trial (Figure 29.6), increased ST varus for HF wrt SH, from late swing through late stance, coincided with remarkable TP EMG activity; more neutral ST varus motion was observed at the stance/swing transition when TP EMG activity was nearly absent. There was near constant amplitude of TA EMG activity throughout the gait cycle, which suggested that TP was the likely source for the varus deformity. Such a persuasive result was not seen in most patients. In another single DHV patient trial (Figure 29.7), substantially increased ST varus of the HF relative to the SH was exhibited with TA and TP EMG activity continuous throughout the gait cycle, with few discernable "on" and "off" states. There was increased TA EMG amplitude in

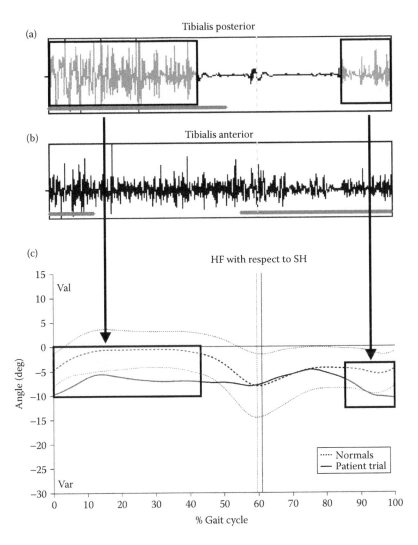

FIGURE 29.6 Graphs from one patient trial showing TP EMG activity (graph a) and increased ST varus rotation of HF wrt SH (graph c) occurring at the same times in the gait cycle (boxed areas). Low amplitudes of TP EMG activity (graph a) are consistent with more normal amounts of ST varus rotation. TA EMG activity (graph b) is nearly constant throughout the gait cycle. The graphs suggest that TP is the primary contributor to the varus deformity.

early swing, but the muscle was still active throughout stance phase. The EMG data were not normalized, and thus TA and TP EMG magnitudes could not be compared. In this patient, the muscular contributions to the varus deformity were not definitive.

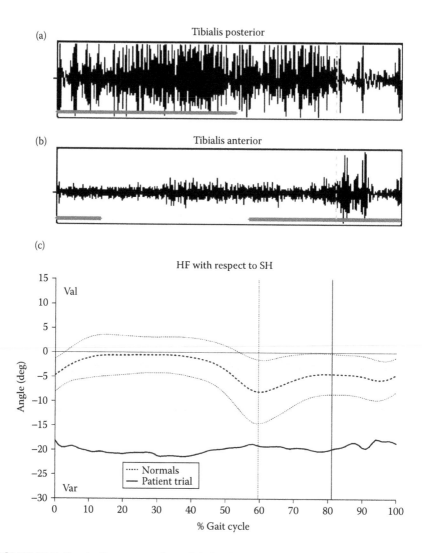

FIGURE 29.7 Graphs from one patient trial showing TA (graph a) and TP (graph b) EMG activity with markedly increased ST varus rotation of HF wrt SH (graph c). Both muscles are active continuously. Because the EMG data are not normalized, we cannot make EMG amplitude comparisons between the muscles. In this case, alternative diagnostic measures are necessary to discern individual muscle contributions to the varus deformity.

29.4 DISCUSSION

Normal kinematics (Figure 29.4) obtained using our model compared well to those reported by others,[6,12–14] accounting for differences in nomenclature and alignment of local reference frames. Although the general curve shapes were similar across patients and normals, in almost all cases intersegmental rotations were less extreme or dampened in the patients, with nearly constant malalignments throughout gait.

These findings are consistent with chronic tissue deformation resulting in aberrant foot positions. In four of the six intersegmental motions examined (Figure 29.4), patients displayed large and consistent shifts in rotation over the entire gait cycle when compared to normals. These four distinct motion differences were increased plantarflexion of HF wrt SH, increased dorsiflexion of MF wrt HF, increased internal rotation of MF wrt HF, and increased ST varus of HF wrt SH. These results are consistent with the clinical interpretation of supination resulting in HF plantarflexion and inversion, and forefoot/MF internal rotation (adduction).

Increased HF plantarflexion wrt SH in patients is likely a consequence of tight or overactive triceps surae or TP muscles, resulting in an equinus pattern also typical in children with cerebral palsy. Increased MF dorsiflexion wrt HF in patients is suggestive of MF break (i.e., rocker bottom deformity) due to chronic tissue stress as the MF accepts an abnormally high proportion of the ground reaction forces. The ability of this model to distinguish MF break is a definitive advantage over single-segment foot models.

Excessive MF internal rotation wrt HF in patients is also likely a consequence of tissue stress due to aberrant application of ground reaction forces in the HF equinovarus posture. For patient trials, the point of application of the ground reaction force vector was typically near the lateral aspect of the MF. In the latter half of stance, an antero-medially directed ground reaction force applied to the lateral aspect of the MF would tend to internally rotate MF wrt HF. Overactivity of either TA or TP may exacerbate these effects. Over time, this pattern of walking would stretch the ligaments at the calcaneocuboid, talonavicular, and midtarsal joints, resulting in the observed malalignment. In our model, HF was tracked with markers applied only to the calcaneus, and from this we inferred motion of the calcaneus and talus. Because of this, we were concerned that increased MF internal rotation wrt HF could cause the talonavicular joint to reach its end range-of-motion, allowing the MF and talus to rotate as one unit, separate from the calcaneus. If this were true, the SH would follow the motion of the MF and talus, resulting in decreased MF internal rotation wrt SH, compared to MF wrt HF. However, our data do not support this conclusion. Examination of the transverse plane motion for MF wrt SH (Figure 29.5) instead reveals increased MF internal rotation wrt SH, compared to MF wrt HF. This increase was approximately equal to the amount of internal rotation for HF wrt SH. These data suggest that the MF reached its end range-of-motion wrt HF, and pulled the HF into internal rotation wrt SH.

ST valgus/varus kinematics for normals suggest that, at initial contact, ground reaction forces drive the HF into decreased ST varus wrt SH. The MF follows until foot-flat, at which time it begins a shift into ST varus wrt HF to remain flat on the ground. As the heel leaves the ground, the Achilles tendon pulls the HF into ST varus due to its medial insertion on the calcaneus. The MF remains firmly positioned on the ground, resulting in a brief period of ST valgus wrt HF at terminal stance. Patients are continually in maximum ST varus for HF wrt SH, presumably due to spastic invertors (e.g., TA or TP). Motion of MF wrt HF is more difficult to explain in patients; MF is on the ground in stance resulting in ST valgus relative to the inverted HF, and after the heel leaves the ground, MF seems to be pulled into less ST valgus. This pattern may be due to deformities associated with chronic stress as the MF lies flat on the ground in the presence of HF varus.

A single frame at mid-stance was used for anatomical calibration of our multi-segment foot model rather than separate medical imaging and calibration trials. Consequently, a varus offset resulted from the placement of HF markers, and we used the term ST valgus/varus for coronal plane rotations. Other studies have used calibration jigs[6] and routines to align local reference frames with radiographs,[12] yet these techniques have limitations of their own. The use of a jig to maintain a neutral posture for a calibration trial appears reasonable; however, even this procedure would have been difficult for our patients, likely resulting in either atypical walking patterns or refusal to walk entirely. Kidder et al.[12] noted radiograph measurement difficulties, and there is an assumption that bones are in the same positions for both radiographs and motion capture calibration trials.

In a separate motion capture analysis, we determined that the varus offset induced by our model averaged approximately 5.5° when nine adult subjects (with no foot or ankle pathology) were held in subtalar neutral for one trial each. Root et al.[15] explained that subtalar neutral is expected just after initial contact. The mean ST varus for HF wrt SH in normals was approximately 5° immediately after initial contact (Figure 29.4), thus providing good agreement with our 5.5° offset. Although a more conventional, anatomically oriented axis would be more meaningful to clinicians, the use of an offset axis did not hinder the ability of our model to differentiate patients from normals.

This feasibility study attempted to use EMG and kinematics to discern contributions to the varus deformity from TA and TP. Despite the use of a multisegment foot model and fine-wire EMG, we had a mix of successful outcomes (Figure 29.6) and ambiguous outcomes (Figure 29.7). The latter results may have been more conclusive had we been able to normalize EMG for patients to a maximum voluntary contraction, as this would have allowed us to compare EMG amplitudes across muscles. However, with compromised selective motor control associated with cerebral palsy, particularly cocontraction of antagonist muscles, such normalization techniques are not typically considered possible. Furthermore, to infer musculotendinous forces from normalized EMG, we would have needed an additional patient calibration (e.g., joint torque vs. EMG amplitude), and all such calibrations were specifically avoided in our protocol. For these reasons, we believe muscle modeling that employs optimization techniques will be worth exploring for these patients.

Several biomechanical modeling issues are relevant for this feasibility study. As a convenience, we combined the metatarsals (typically considered part of the forefoot) with bones commonly defined in the MF, in what we called our "MF" segment. However, a recent study using a 14-segment cadaveric foot model, with wires inserted directly into bones, found considerable motion during the stance phase between the metatarsals and MF bones with which they articulated.[16] Although our model successfully differentiated MF motion between patients and normals, findings by Liu et al.[16] argue for the modeling of separate MF and forefoot segments. Increased accuracy in our model may also be attained by tracking the SH with a cluster of markers proximal to the ankle joint (i.e., near-marker AS), rather than tracking with markers on the malleoli. Such a marker cluster would avoid the marker slippage that occurs near bony prominences[17] and the majority of muscular movement that occurs at the proximal end of the SH. We must also consider alternative methods to calibrate for subtalar neutral to improve the anatomical relevance of the varus measurement. The next iteration of our multisegment foot model will address these kinematic limitations, add muscle modeling and kinetics, and include a repeatability analysis.

29.5 FUTURE DIRECTIONS

As our ultimate goal is to identify muscle contributions to the varus deformities without the need for fine-wire EMG, we require a kinetic, musculoskeletal, multisegment foot model. New challenges for developing such a model include locating the three-dimensional position of joint centers, calculating ground reaction forces on individual foot segments, and developing a muscle model likely to be different for normals and patients.

The use of palpable bony landmarks and anthropometry to define virtual points within the body is not new, but this technique does require validation often through medical imaging. We have derived preliminary methods to estimate the location of joint centers at the junction of the MF and HF segments (i.e., along the transverse tarsal joint, Figure 29.8), and the HF and SH segments (i.e., at the center of the ankle complex). We

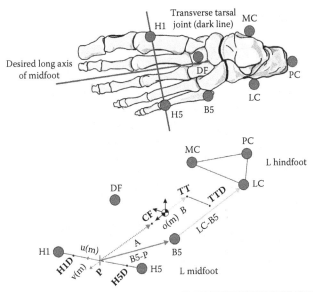

Key (see Figure 29.3 for marker locations)	**Vector Algebra**

Key (see Figure 29.3 for marker locations)

o(m) = origin of LRF, at center-of-mass of midfoot
u, v(m) = unit direction vectors of midfoot Figure 29.3
P = midpoint of H1-H5
H1D = derived point based upon distal midfoot radius
H5D = derived point based upon distal midfoot radius
TTD = derived point based upon proximal midfoot radius
CF = intermediate calculation point (near cuneiforms)
TT = approximation to transverse tarsal joint

Vector Algebra

A $= v(m)*\{v(m) \cdot [B5 - P]\}$
B $= v(m)*0.5*\{v(m) \cdot [LC - B5]\}$
CF $= P + A$
TT $= CF + B$
H5D $= P - u(m)*[\text{distal radius}(mf)]$
H1D $= P + u(m)*[\text{distal radius}(mf)]$
TTD $= TT - u(m)*[\text{proximal radius}(mf)]$
· = vector dot product

FIGURE 29.8 Derivation of the center of the transverse tarsal joint for the left foot (needed for inverse dynamics) based upon external marker positions and anthropometry measures alone. Algorithms such as these need to be validated through comparison with medical imaging.

need to derive similar methods for the junction of the new forefront segment (FF) and the MF (i.e., along the metatarsal/metacarpal joint line), and to validate all of these methods, with medical imaging for samples of normals and patients with DHV.

In the general case, more than one segment in a multisegment foot model will be in contact with the ground, complicating force plate–based inverse dynamics. For some time now, devices to measure plantar pressures have been combined with force plates to estimate equivalent force systems on separate segments of the foot.[4,18–20] In essence, a force plate provides a single force system (normal force, shear forces, and free moment) that when applied to the rigidly modeled foot at the center-of-pressure (COP) (also output from the force plate) causes the foot to move mechanically in the same way it moves under the influence of the actual pressure distribution. Pressure data can be subdivided into areas beneath separate segments of the foot, and mathematically integrating the pressure over these individual areas provides both a resultant normal force and its COP. Because pressure-measuring devices do not simultaneously measure shear, an assumption is typically made that the net shear forces and free moment measured by the force plate are distributed across the segments contacting the force plate in the same proportions as the normal forces, as guided by pressure data.[4,18–20] This assumption has been validated analytically[19] but not experimentally. We plan to validate this proportionality assumption experimentally, and then calculate multisegment kinetics using traditional inverse dynamics

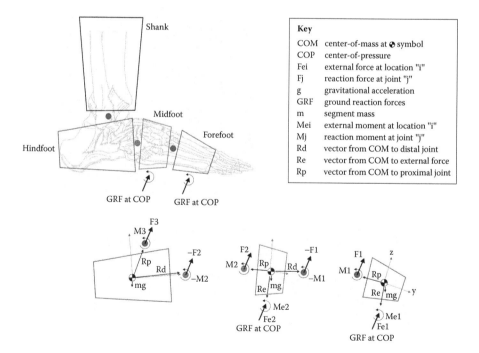

FIGURE 29.9 Free-body diagram of a kinetic, multisegment, foot model. GRFs are calculated and applied at the COP based upon simultaneous plantar pressure and force plate data. In this example of heel rise, no contact occurs between the heel and the ground.

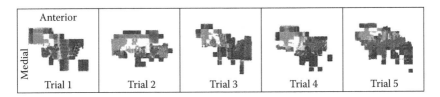

FIGURE 29.10 Sample plantar pressure plots from one patient. Large trial-to-trial variability necessitates simultaneous collection of plantar pressure and force plate data for kinetic modeling.

with separate ground reaction force systems (GRFs) applied to each segment (Figure 29.9). Note that until methods are developed to reliably provide force systems between mediolaterally adjacent segments, our multisegment foot model will use only distal/proximal segmentation.[21] There also exist practical difficulties in masking plantar pressures to the foot model. A recent study by MacWilliams et al.[4] collected pressure and force plate data during separate walking trials in normals, and later combined these to create separate force systems applied to individual foot segments. Pressure measurements from patients in our study were highly variable between strides (Figure 29.10), suggesting that the approach used by MacWilliams et al. for normals would be impractical for children with DHV. Consequently, we plan to identify the pressure subareas based upon simultaneously collected foot kinematics, plantar pressures, and force plate data. This technique, as suggested by MacWilliams,[22] has the advantage of assuring that the pressure subareas are in agreement with the anatomically based kinematic model.

Finally, with multisegment foot kinetics available, we plan to use muscle modeling to identify contributions to the varus deformity associated with TA, TP, and any other structures found to be relevant (e.g., tight triceps surae). Such a model will allow calculation of musculotendinous forces, the line-of-action of these forces, and their associated varus moments about joints of interest, thereby guiding treatment selection. An obvious and nontrivial difficulty will be the modeling of spastic muscles in children with cerebral palsy. However, validation of this muscle model may be accomplished with *in vitro* tests using a dynamic gait simulator,[23] capable of reproducing foot kinematics, ground reaction forces, and plantar pressure patterns, through control of individual musculotendinous forces.

29.6 CONCLUSIONS

This feasibility study has increased our knowledge of foot biomechanics in patients with DHV, and of multisegment foot modeling. The nonradiographic kinematic model was able to successfully differentiate kinematics between normals and patients. However, EMG and multisegment foot kinematics were not definitive indicators of the relative muscle contributions to the varus deformity. Improved treatment selection for DHV relies on a quantitative understanding of the dynamic contributions of TA and TP to the inversion moment. A validated kinetic and musculoskeletal multisegment foot model will allow quantification of the deformity, and of the respective muscular forces causing the deformity.

REFERENCES

1. Vaughan, C.L., Nashman, J.H., and Murr, M.S., What is the normal function of tibialis posterior in human gait?, In *The Diplegic Child: Evaluation and Management,* Sussman, M.D., Ed., American Academy of Orthopaedic Surgeons: Rosemont IL, 1992, Chapter 31.
2. Sutherland, D.H., Olshen, R., Cooper, L., and Woo, S.L., The development of mature gait, *J. Bone Joing Surg. Am.,* 62-A, 336, 1980.
3. Lundberg, A., The foot: block, gearbox or cushion? Some concepts in foot kinematics, *J. Orthop. Sports Phys. Ther.,* 34, A6, 2004.
4. MacWilliams, B.A., Cowley, M., and Nicholson, D.E., Foot kinematics and kinetics during adolescent gait, *Gait Posture,* 17, 214, 2003.
5. Davis, I. (Ed.), Foot and ankle research retreat: consensus statement, *J. Orthop. Sports Phys. Ther.,* 34, A2, 2004.
6. Carson, M.C., Harrington, M.E., Thompson, N., O'Connor, J.J., and Theologis, T.N., Kinematic analysis of a multi-segment foot model for research and clinical applications: a repeatability analysis, *J. Biomech.,* 34, 1299, 2001.
7. Stebbins, J.A., Harrington, M.E., Thompson, N., and Theologis, T.N., Advances in the measurement of foot kinematics in children, *J. Orthop. Sports Phys. Ther.,* 34, A11, 2004.
8. Walker, M.R., Cooney, K.M., Sharkey, N.A., Sanders, J.O., and Buczek, F.L., Multi-segment foot kinematics of dynamic hindfoot varus, *J. Orthop. Sports Phys. Ther.,* 34, A11, 2004.
9. Woodburn, J., Nelson, K.M., Lohmann Siegel, K., Kepple, T.M., and Gerber, L.H., Multisegment foot motion during gait: proof of concept in rheumatoid arthritis, *J. Orthop. Sports Phys. Ther.,* 34, A10, 2004.
10. Winter, D.A., *Biomechanics and Motor Control of Human Gait,* 2nd Ed, University of Waterloo Press: Waterloo, Canada, 1991, p.18.
11. Söderkvist, I. and Wedin, P., Determining the movements of the skeleton using well-configured markers, *J. Biomech.,* 26, 1473, 1993.
12. Kidder, S.M., Abuzzahab, F.S., Harris, G.F., and Johnson, J.E., A system for the analysis of foot and ankle kinematics during gait, *IEEE Trans. Rehab. Eng.,* 4, 25, 1996.
13. Leardini, A., Benedetti, M.G., Catani, F., Simoncini, L., and Giannini, S., An anatomically based protocol for the description of foot segment kinematics during gait, *Clin. Biomech.,* 14, 528, 1999.
14. Rattanaprasert, U., Smith, R., Sullivan, M., and Gilleard, W., Three-dimensional kinematics of the forefoot, rearfoot, and leg without the function of tibialis posterior in comparison with normals during stance phase of walking, *Clin. Biomech.,* 14, 14, 1999.
15. Root, M.L., Orien, W.P., and Weed, J.H., *Clinical Biomechanics: Normal and Abnormal Functions of the Foot,* Vol. II, Clinical Biomechanics: Los Angeles, 1977.
16. Liu, A., Nester, C.J., Ward, E., Howard, D., Derrick, T., Cocheba, J., and Patterson, P., Development of an improved rigid body model of the foot, *J. Orthop. Sports Phys. Ther.,* 34, A15, 2004.

17. Cappozzo, A., Cappello, A., Della Croce, U., and Pensalfini, F., Surface-marker cluster design criteria for 3-D bone movement reconstruction, *IEEE Trans. Biomed. Eng.*, 44, 1165, 1997.
18. Abuzzahab, F.S. Jr., Harris, G.F., and Kidder, S.M., A kinetic model of the foot and ankle, *Gait Posture*, 5, 148, 1997.
19. Giacomozzi, C. and Macellari, V., Piezo-dynamometric platform for a more complete analysis of foot-to-floor interaction, *IEEE Trans. Biomed. Eng.*, 5, 322, 1997.
20. Giacomozzi, C., Macellari, V., Leardini, A., and Benedetti, M.G., Integrated pressure-force-kinematics measuring system for the characterisation of plantar foot loading during locomotion, *Med. Biol. Eng. Comput.*, 38, 156, 2000.
21. Buczek, F.L., Walker, M.R., Rainbow, M.J., Cooney, K.M., and Sanders, J.O., Impact of mediolateral segmentation on a multi-segment foot model, *Gait Posture*, 23(4), 519–22, 2006.
22. MacWilliams, B.A., Kinetic measures of the foot: overcoming current obstacles, presented at Foot and Ankle: New Horizons in Clinical Treatment and Innovative Technology: Bestheda, MD, 2003.
23. Sharkey, N.A. and Hamel, A.J., A dynamic cadaver model of the stance phase of gait: performance characteristics and kinetic validation, *Clin. Biomech.*, 13, 420, 1998.

Section D

Technical Advances in Foot
and Ankle Motion Analysis

30 The Accuracy and Utility of Virtual Markers

Michael H. Schwartz and Adam Rozumalski

CONTENTS

30.1 INTRODUCTION

Three-dimensional (3D) human movement analysis relies on detecting and tracking markers or orientation sensors mounted on the skin of subjects. This tracking is done by video cameras, electromagnetic sensors, or microphones. The focus of this chapter will be on systems that track individual markers, not orientation sensors. Similar principles apply to electromagnetic systems, with some subtle differences that are not particularly germane to this discussion.

Each point tracked by the motion system is referred to as a physical marker (PM). These PMs form the basis of coordinate systems that (ideally) move in harmony with the underlying body segment. Such a coordinate system is commonly referred to as a technical coordinate system (TCS). The positions and orientations of the TCSs provide the basis for determining segment and joint kinematics, from which numerous scientifically and clinically relevant data are derived.

It is frequently desirable to track points or landmarks that cannot accommodate PMs. Some examples include joint centers, medial bony landmarks, and the plantar

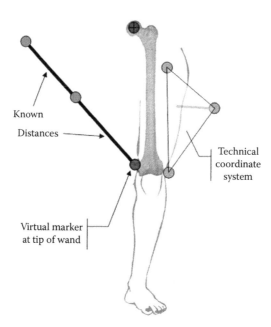

Known
Distances

Technical
coordinate
system

Virtual marker
at tip of wand

FIGURE 30.1 *IP:* A typical device used for acquiring VMs. The tip of the rod is at a known distance and orientation relative to the markers. By capturing a frame of data with the rod placed on a landmark of interest, the position of the landmark relative to the global (or local) coordinate system can be found.

surface of feet. While it may be impossible to directly track these landmarks with PMs, the locations can be tracked indirectly as long as the position and orientation of the location can be defined relative to a TCS. These indirectly tracked objects are referred to as *virtual*. A point tracked in this manner is referred to as a virtual marker (VM). There are many examples of the use of VMs in standard movement analysis methodology. For example, the standard models used in clinical gait analysis include VMs at the hip, knee, and ankle joint centers.[1] These joint center VMs are defined from anthropometric regression equations or joint geometry. The Calibrated Anatomical System Technique (CAST) protocol makes use of 22 VMs throughout the lower extremity.[2] An extension of the CAST protocol identifies 14 VMs on a five-segment shank-foot model.[3]

The markers in the CAST protocol, and the related shank-foot extension, are defined using an instrumented pointer (IP) rather than regression equations (Figure 30.1). In the IP method, a rod is equipped with two or more markers. The tip of the rod is at a precisely known distance and direction relative to the PMs on the rod. To obtain a VM, the tip of the rod is placed on the desired landmark. The motion system records the 3D positions of the rod's markers, which can then be used to determine the 3D position of the rod's tip relative to the laboratory coordinate system. The VM can then be expressed in any coordinate system the user desires, including a segmental PM-based coordinate system.

This chapter will deal with two aspects of VMs. First, the positional accuracy of VMs will be examined by means of a Monte-Carlo simulation. Results that are specifically appropriate for foot models will be included. Next the use of VMs to create a virtual shape (VS) will be described, including specific examples of virtual lines, circles, and planes derived.

30.2 ACCURACY

The precision and accuracy of PM reconstruction have been reasonably well characterized by both equipment manufacturers and independent tests conducted by movement analysis laboratories. Despite their extensive use in movement analysis, the same cannot be said for VMs. It is therefore of interest to examine the behavior of VMs vis-à-vis the better understood issue of PM accuracy.[4] A Monte-Carlo simulation was used to evaluate the accuracy of VMs. The model and simulation are as follows.

30.2.1 MODEL

The model from which error estimates are derived consists of three PMs and one VM (Figure 30.2). The three PMs form an angle, the vertex of which is considered to be the origin. The distance from the origin to each PM is the same, thus forming two legs of an isosceles triangle. This distance is called the PM spacing and is denoted L_{PM}. The angle formed by the legs is called the PM angle and is denoted

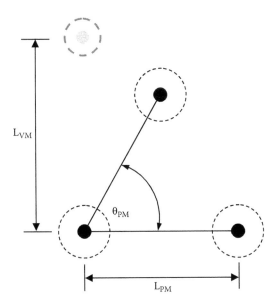

FIGURE 30.2 *Monte-Carlo simulation:* The parameters of the simulation are the PM spacing (L_{PM}), PM angle (Θ_{PM}), and the distance to the VM (L_{VM}). The errors in the PM locations are modeled as independent random variables. The relative error (ρ) is the resulting VM error divided by the PM error. Values of $\rho > 1$ indicate an amplification of reconstruction error, while $\rho < 1$ indicates an attenuation of error.

Θ_{PM}. A VM is located at a distance L_{VM} from the origin in an arbitrary direction. This is a prototype marker arrangement and is specifically constructed to reflect marker sets commonly used in clinical gait analysis. Application-specific marker sets could be easily introduced if desired.

Errors in the position of the PMs, denoted ε_{PM}, are assumed to be independent random variables. This is intended to model the reconstruction error in the marker positions — not the errors due to palpation, marker misplacement, or soft tissue artifact (especially those of the en masse variety), which are beyond the scope and intent of this analysis.

30.2.2 SIMULATION

The Monte-Carlo simulation consists of repeated estimations of the VM position. The first step in the simulation is to choose the PM spacing and PM angle — L_{PM} and Q_{PM}, respectively. Next, define a TCS, using a Gramm–Schmidt procedure, from the nominal (error free) PM positions. The Gramm–Schmidt method is not ideal, as has been shown by several authors including Veldpaus et al.[5] However, Gramm–Schmidt represents the most commonly used method in clinical gait analysis. Denote the TCS thus defined by the unit vectors $(\hat{e}_1, \hat{e}_2, \hat{e}_3)$. Next, assign random errors to each PM. For this study, the errors were assumed to be random and uncorrelated. This idealization could certainly be relaxed if a more realistic model of the PM errors were known. Denote this TCS by the unit vectors $(\hat{e}_1^*, \hat{e}_2^*, \hat{e}_3^*)$. Once the error-laden TCS has been created, compute nominal and error-laden VM positions, r_{VM}, r_{VM}^* respectively, for VMs located a distance $L_{VM} = |r_{VM}|$ away from the origin. At this point, both the nominal and error-laden VM positions are known, and thus the error in the VM position, $\varepsilon_{VM} = |r_{VM} - r_{VM}^*|$, can be calculated.

The *relative accuracy* of the VM is defined as the ratio of VM accuracy to PM accuracy, $\rho = \varepsilon_{VM}/\varepsilon_{PM}$. There is an unavoidable amount of error in the PMs. The question at hand is whether or not using VMs amplifies, maintains, or attenuates this error. It will be shown that the answer depends on the layout of the PMs and the distance of the VM from the PM origin. For this reason, the simulation is repeated numerous times (on the order of 1000 per configuration) for an array of L_{PM}, Θ_{PM}, and L_{VM} values. The results of the simulations can be arranged in graphical form to display the mean errors. Mean relative errors (ρ) < 1.0 indicate attenuation of PM error, while $\rho > 1.0$ indicates amplification of PM error. Other statistics (max, min, etc...) could also be computed, but were felt to be less instructive.

30.2.3 RESULTS

Results are displayed for two different simulations in Figure 30.3 and Figure 30.4. The difference between the simulations is the layout of the PMs (intermarker spacing L_{PM}). The abscissa of each graph shows different values of L_{VM}, while the ordinate shows different values of Θ_{PM}. It is clear that the ideal marker configuration consists of PMs at right angles to one another and as far apart as possible. This is logical and adheres to the conventional wisdom prevalent in the motion analysis community at large. What is more instructive is to be able to identify critical regions in the

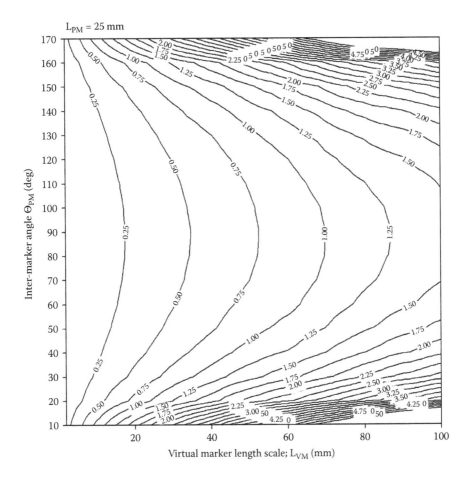

FIGURE 30.3 *Monte-Carlo results: 25 mm PM spacing:* Regions of error amplification and attenuation can clearly be seen. Amplification occurs primarily when PMs are nearly colinear, or when VMs are far from the PMs. This coincides with the conventional wisdom and logic. There are, however, advantages to knowing the precise amount of error, as well as the regions in which the error changes rapidly.

L_{PM}–Θ_{PM} space, where the accuracy deteriorates rapidly. This knowledge can be used to design marker sets (both physical and virtual) to produce data of a given level of accuracy. It can be seen, for example, that nearly colinear markers ($\Theta_{PM} <$ 30° or > 150°) cause rapid deterioration of accuracy for nearly all L_{VM}s. However, even PMs with internal angles of 30° result in rapid deterioration of VM accuracy for L_{VM} > 30 mm. Increasing PM spacing has a pronounced effect on the accuracy maintaining/enhancing region of the L_{VM}–Θ_{PM} space.

While this simulation focused specifically on VM positional accuracy, it would be a straightforward extension to examine the accuracy of VM-based coordinate systems (position and orientation) or of angles (segmental or intersegmental) defined by VMs. Further extensions/enhancements to this model and simulation would

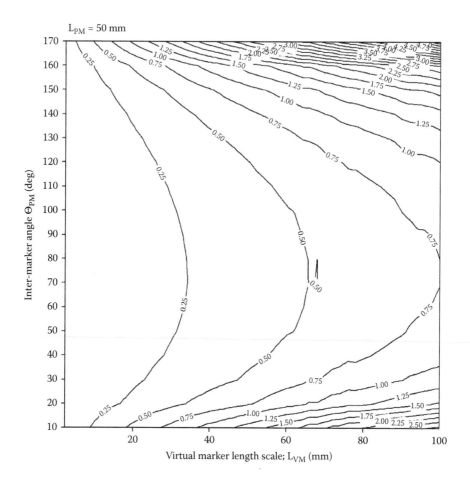

FIGURE 30.4 *Monte-Carlo results: 50 mm PM spacing:* The effect of increasing PM spacing is evident (compare with Figure 30.3). Larger regions of error attenuation appear, while the general pattern of attenuation/amplification regions is similar to the 25 mm model.

include more realistic PM errors, as well as possible models of soft tissue artifacts. Despite its simplicity, the model is able to provide valuable quantitative information that can be useful in the planning, conducting, and analysis of movement data that incorporate VMs.

30.3 VIRTUAL SHAPES

Traditionally an IP is used to define a specific point in space that becomes a VM as described earlier. However, not every anatomical landmark is aptly modeled as a single point. The malleoli, for example, are large enough and blunt enough that a single point is a poor representation. The circumference of the malleoli, on the other hand, provides both the point approximation (center of the circle) and more detailed information about the anatomy (position, orientation, and diameter of the landmark), which may be useful for other purposes.

The basic methods used to define VMs can be easily extended to create entities other than points. A VS is an object derived from a distribution of VMs. The object can be simple, such as a point, line, circle, or plane, or it can be complex, such as the condyles of the femur or the plantar surface of the calcaneous. Anatomical items of interest can be defined by VSs in a simple and flexible way using the IP to trace the different geometries. These VSs can, in turn, be used to define or align coordinate systems based on relevant anatomy. Creating a VS requires two steps: *collection* of a VM array and *fitting* of the array to a template.

30.3.1 Collection

The first step in defining a VS is to collect an array of VMs. This can be as simple as pointing to a specific landmark, or as complex as tracing out the contour of a bony landmark. The VM array is acquired by capturing data while the IP is moved over the region(s) of interest. When collecting the VM array, it is important to identify as much of the shape as possible. This will help minimize errors and uncertainties associated with irregularities in the surface to be identified. At each captured frame of a VS definition trial, a VM is defined at the end of the IP. For the purposes of this chapter, the array of VMs will be denoted $S = \{\mathbf{v}_k, k = 1, N\}$, where $\mathbf{v}$ is the VM in the global reference frame, k is the frame number, and N is the total number of frames captured.

30.3.2 Fitting

Once the VS definition trial has been completed, the next step is to fit the VM array to an underlying shape template (e.g., circle). The VM array (S) is fit to the template by minimizing a cost function, such as the sum of squared errors between the VM array and the template. The cost can be based on point-by-point matching between the VM and the template[6] or by using the entire array of VMs to derive the equation for a more general geometry such as a line or plane. In the procedure presented here, the cost functions are derived such that the difference between the VM array and the template shape is minimized in a least squares sense. The choice of a least squares minimizer is arbitrary but well documented.[7] The number of VSs that are possible is obviously limitless. For the sake of clarity and practicality, several common/useful shapes will be described in more detail. These are the *point, line, circle*, and *plane*.

30.3.2.1 Point

A point is the simplest VS possible. Some examples for virtual points are the tibial tubercles, metatarsal heads, and acromium processes. In fact, a point VS can be defined as a single frame capture of a VM. For the sake of introducing the VS fitting concept, however, the entire point VS method will be explicitly described.

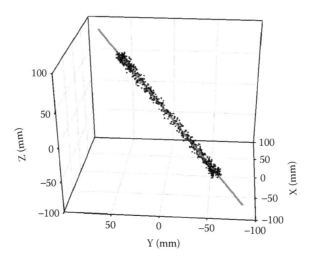

FIGURE 30.5 *Virtual line:* A virtual line fit to an array of VMs.

For this and subsequent examples, consider the task of locating the template shape relative to the global reference system. The problem of transforming between global and local reference systems is well understood and not the focus of this chapter.

The template for a point VS is a single point in space $t = (t_x, t_y, t_z)$. As noted earlier, the VM array is a set of points in space $S = \{v^k, k = 1, N\}$. The procedure is to minimize the distance between the template point and the array of points in a least squares sense. Of course, this is a trivial task for the case of a point VS. If the error associated with identifying the point (IP instability, reconstruction error, etc.) is assumed to be symmetric, the least squares answer is the mean of the array of points, so $t = (v^k = \bar{v})$.

30.3.2.2 Line (Figure 30.5)

A virtual line is defined using the IP to trace a portion of line on a body segment. For example, the tibial ridge is used to define the superior/inferior direction of the tibial coordinate system. The template line consists of a point on the line $p = (p_x, p_y, p_z)$ and an unknown unit direction vector parallel to the line $\hat{e} = (e_x, e_y, e_z)$. The VM array consists of a set of points along a line traced by the IP. Alternatively, two VMs or point VSs could be used. The advantage to the traced line is that it provides a richer set of information, such as the precise shape of the landmark and how closely the landmark fits the template (the cost).

The first step is to translate the array so that its centroid ($\bar{v}$) is at the origin. This is not necessary, but simplifies the computations since it allows p to be chosen as the origin. Let the translated VM array be $\bar{S} = \{\tilde{v}^k = (v^k - \bar{v}), k = 1, N\}$. The distance from each $\tilde{v}_k$ to the line of best fit is then $d_k = d(\tilde{v}^k) = \sqrt{|\tilde{v}^k|^2 - (e\tilde{v}^k)^2}$. Choose an objective function to be the sum of the squared distances $\Phi = \sum_{i=1}^{n} d_k^2$. The goal is then to find

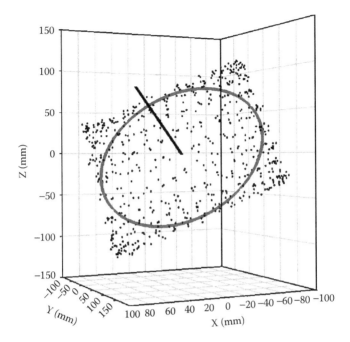

FIGURE 30.6 *Virtual plane:* A virtual plane fit to an array of VMs. The method is generalizable to any surface, no matter how nonplanar.

ê that minimizes Φ, subject to the constraint that $|\hat{e}| = 1$. This is a standard minimization problem that can be solved in a number of different ways, most conveniently using the normal equations, as described in multiple places including Ref. 8. Once the unit direction vector is found, the line is translated from the origin back to its original location in space.

30.3.2.3 Plane (Figure 30.6)

Defining a plane is done in much the same way as defining a line. Instead of moving the pointer along a line, it is moved along a surface. An example is the plantar surface of the calcaneous (or entire foot). The template plane consists of a point on the plane $p = (p_x, p_y, p_z)$ and an unknown unit direction vector normal to the plane $\hat{e} = (e_x, e_y, e_z)$.

As with the line, the array is translated so that its centroid is at the origin. Again, let the translated VM array be $\overline{S} = \{\tilde{v}^k = (v^k - \overline{v}), k = 1, N\}$. It can be shown that the centroid of the original distribution lies on the plane of best fit. Thus the distance from each $\tilde{v}$ to the plane of best fit is then $d_k = d(\tilde{v}^k) = (\hat{e}\tilde{v}^k)$. The objective function $\Phi = \sum_{i=1}^n d_k^2$ is once again minimized relative to the unit normal vector constraint $|\hat{e}| = 1$, and the resulting plane is translated back to the original centroid.

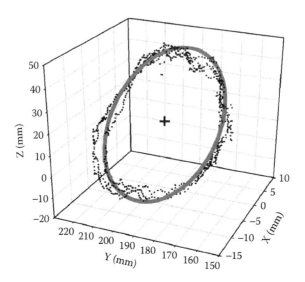

FIGURE 30.7 *Virtual circle.* A virtual circle fit to an array of VMs. The markers were traced along the perimeter of the first author's medial malleolus.

30.3.2.4 Circle (Figure 30.7)

More complex geometries can also be used as templates for VSs. A circle, for example, can be defined around the malleoli or the condyles of the femur. Several revolutions are traced around the anatomical landmark using the IP. Finding the best-fit circle consists of several steps:

A plane of best fit is found as described above. Once the plane is found, all points in the distribution are projected onto this plane. Next, the data are rotated so that the least squares plane is the x–y plane (this step is for algebraic simplicity). Denote the projected and transformed VM array by $\bar{S} = \{\tilde{v}^k \ projected \ \& \ rotated, k = 1, N\}$. A circle is fit to the projected and rotated points using a least squares approach. The template circle consists of the unknown center coordinates (x_c, y_c) and the radius of the circle (r). It is straightforward to show that the distance function becomes $d_k = d(\bar{v}^k) = \sqrt{(\tilde{v}_x^k - x_c)^2 - (\tilde{v}_y^k - y_c)^2} - r$. Choose an objective function to be the sum of the squared distances $\Phi = \sum_{i=1}^{n} d_k^2$. The unconstrained minimum of Φ can be found to yield the center and radius of the circle. Once the circle is found, it can be transformed back to the original coordinate system.

30.4 DISCUSSION

Both VMs and VSs can be valuable tools for defining anatomical coordinate systems or identifying anatomical landmarks. A whole host of anatomical landmarks can be identified, which would otherwise require PMs. In addition, landmarks/regions not well modeled by individual markers can be mapped using VSs. This technique has the potential to improve the flexibility of model design and data acquisition. VSs represent a novel extension of the VM paradigm. A uniform approach to defining VSs using least squares estimates should make the development of processing software simple. More elaborate applications of VSs, such as template bone matching algorithms, offer exciting possibilities for the application of VM and VS methods to subject-specific musculoskeletal modeling tasks.[6]

VMs are as accurate as their physical counterparts as long as care is taken to place PMs appropriately. Even in cases where accuracy must be sacrificed due to geometric constraints, the results of the study presented here give guidelines as to how deleterious consequences can be minimized. In practice, adding VSs (and VMs) to standard collection protocols adds only a few minutes of testing time and processing time. Given these facts, VMs should be exploited in clinical gait analysis and advanced modeling of the foot and ankle.

REFERENCES

1. Davis, R.B., Ounpuu, S., Tyburski, D., and Gage, J., A gait collection and reduction technique, *Hum Mov Sci* 10, 575–587, 1991.
2. Capozzo, A., Catani, F., Della Croce, U., and Leardini, A., Position and orientation in space of bones during movement: anatomical frame definition and determination, *Clin Biomech* 10 (4), 171–178, 1995.
3. Leardini, A., O'Connor, J. J., Catani, F., and Giannini, S., A geometric model of the human ankle joint, *J Biomech* 32 (6), 585–591, 1999.
4. Morrow, D., Hansen, D., and Kaufman, K., Assessing the accuracy of virtual markers for tracking ankle location in gait, in *GCMAS Annual Meeting*, Rochester, MN, 2001.
5. Veldpaus, F., Woltring, H., and Dortmans, L., A least squares algorithm for the equiform transformation from spatial marker co-ordinates, *J Biomech* 21, 45–54, 1988.
6. Donati, M., Camomilla, V., and Cappozzo, A., Automatic virtual palpitation of bone landmarks, in *GCMAS Annual Meeting*, Portland, OR, 2005, pp. 28.
7. Shakarji, C., Least-Squares Fitting Algorithms of the NIST Algorithm Testing System, *J Res Natl Inst Stand Technol* 103, 633–641, 1998.
8. Press, W., Teukolsky, S., Vetterling, W., and Flannery, B., General Linear Least Squares, in *Numerical Recipes in Fortran: The Art of Scientific Computing*, 2nd ed. Cambridge University Press, Cambridge, 1986, pp. 665–675.

31 Determination of Subject-Specific Ankle Joint Axes from Measured Foot Motion

Stephen J. Piazza and Gregory S. Lewis

CONTENTS

31.1 INTRODUCTION

Joint kinematics can vary substantially between individual subjects, and errors in joint definitions can have pronounced effects on the results of clinical gait analyses.[1-3] This variation in joint mechanics has motivated the development of "functional" methods, in which the locations of joint centers and joint axes are determined from the measured joint rotations rather than being defined relative to bony landmarks. Functional methods for location of the flexion axis of the knee[1,4,5] and the center of rotation of the hip[1,6-10] have been widely studied in research settings, and these methods are gaining acceptance in clinical laboratories. Evaluations of functional methods under controlled conditions suggest that they are more accurate, robust, and reproducible than methods that rely upon anatomical landmark location.[1,4,8]

The development and implementation of functional methods for the location of ankle joint axes, however, have lagged behind those proposed for the hip and knee. The ankle complex has received less attention for two reasons: First, the mechanical analog commonly used to represent the joints of the ankle is more complex than those in use at the other joints. The knee is usually modeled as a simple uniaxial hinge joint, and the hip is modeled as a ball-and-socket joint, while the combined talocrural (TC) (tibiotalar) and subtalar (ST) (talocalcaneal) joints are often described as functioning like a universal joint consisting of two successive, nonparallel hinge joints.[11] Second, to characterize hip and knee motions, one must record the motions of large, easily identifiable body segments, the pelvis and thigh for the hip and the thigh and shank for the knee. At the ankle, one of the body segments, the talus, is inaccessible and cannot be tracked with skin-mounted markers.

It is possible, however, to use numerical optimization to compute the locations of two joint axes from the motions of the proximal and distal segments, even when the motion of the intermediate segment cannot be measured. Sommer and Miller[12] described such an algorithm and its implementation for the location of wrist joint axes, and van den Bogert[13] used a similar approach to locate the TC and ST joint axes. Aside from the joints upon which the algorithms were tested, the primary difference between the two studies is that the algorithm used by Sommer and Miller minimized differences between experiment and model as represented by translations and Euler rotations, while the algorithm of van den Bogert minimized differences between experimental and model-reconstructed marker positions. In both studies, the repeatability of the optimization methods, rather than their accuracy, was the primary criterion for their evaluation. Promising repeatability results were reported by van den Bogert for the ankle complex, but aside from the optimized axes being generally consistent with previous *in vitro* studies, there was no indication that those axes properly represented the true anatomical joint axes. Siston et al.,[14] however, recently used two-axis optimization to define a point ankle joint center that did correspond well to the center of the distal tibial articulating surface.

The purpose of the present study was to assess the accuracy of two functional methods for ankle joint axis location. One of these methods is a two-axis optimization, similar to those proposed by previous authors;[12,13] the other is a motion-based technique for location of the ST joint axis alone. Both methods were evaluated using a cadaver model in which the motions of the tibia, talus, and calcaneus could be measured directly using bone-mounted markers.

31.2 OPTIMIZATION-BASED LOCATION OF TWO AXES

31.2.1 OPTIMIZATION ALGORITHM

A technique similar to that described by Sommer and Miller[12] was implemented for fitting a kinematic model to measured tibia–calcaneus motion. The kinematic model consisted of two fixed revolute (hinge) joints. Twelve parameters described the placement of the TC joint axis relative to the tibia, of the ST joint axis relative to the calcaneus, and of the two axes relative to one another. These parameters were adjusted by the optimization algorithm until the motion of the model best fit the experimentally measured motion. The fit of the model kinematics to the experimental kinematics was assessed by decomposing tibia-to-calcaneus transformation matrices into three translations $(r_1, r_2, r_3,$ in units of cm) and three Euler angles $(\psi_1, \psi_2, \psi_3,$ in units of radians). The differences between model and experimental values were computed, and the sum of the squares of these residuals over all frames was computed:

$$f = \sum_{k=1}^{m} \left[\sum_{i=1}^{3} \left(r_i' - r_i \right)_k^2 + \left(\psi_i' - \psi_i \right)_k^2 \right] \tag{31.1}$$

where m is the number of frames, the primed terms denote the experimental values, and unprimed terms denote the model values. The above objective function f was minimized using a Levenberg–Marquardt algorithm that was implemented in MatLab (ver. 6.5, Mathworks, Natick, MA). A Gauss–Newton algorithm was used for an "inner" optimization executed for each frame to estimate the TC and ST joint angles in the model.

31.2.2 EXPERIMENTS

31.2.2.1 Mechanical Linkage

Initial experimental tests were performed on an anthropomorphic mechanical linkage that incorporated both TC and ST joints (Figure 31.1). These mechanical joints produced idealized hinge motions that were affected by stereophotogrammetric error. The orientations of the revolute joints were adjustable, so that different axis configurations could be tested. The testing protocol for the linkage was similar to that described below for cadaver specimens.

31.2.2.2 Cadaver Specimens

Three fresh-frozen lower right leg specimens were tested (80 yr. F, 69 yr. M, and 68 yr. M). The specimens were thawed and sectioned 35 cm above the plantar surface. Soft tissues were removed from the proximal 10 cm to accommodate attachment of coupling hardware and a steel rod to the proximal tibia. A single

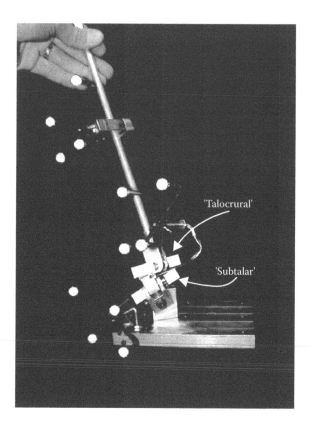

FIGURE 31.1 Mechanical linkage used for initial experimental assessment of the two-axis optimization algorithm. Marker clusters are mounted on tibia, talus, and calcaneus segments. Two hinges represent the TC and ST joints.

screw was used to fix the fibula to the tibia in its physiological position at the proximal end of the specimen.

31.2.2.3 Cadaver Testing Apparatus

A custom-designed apparatus (Figure 31.2) was used to apply a constant load along the long axis of the tibia during continuous movements of the ankle complex. The foot rested on a nonskid base plate and was otherwise unconstrained during the tests. The proximal tibia was moved in plantarflexion/dorsiflexion and inversion/eversion, and combinations of these motions while the foot remained nearly stationary. A square plate was attached proximal to the tibia rod, and a thin nylon cord was attached to each corner of this plate. These cords were passed through holes in the base plate, and weights were attached to each cord, resulting in a constant compressive force directed along the tibial shaft. Each cord remained nearly parallel to the tibial long axis during the ankle motions, with the cords sliding slightly in the holes of the base plate during motion.

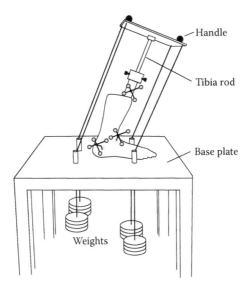

FIGURE 31.2 Schematic diagram of apparatus used for *in vitro* testing of the two-axis optimization method. A constant axial load is applied to the tibia while it is manually moved in dorsiflexion/plantarflexion and inversion/eversion. Marker clusters are attached to the bones for tracking of the tibia, talus, and calcaneus.

An Eagle video-based motion analysis system (Motion Analysis Corp., Santa Rosa, CA) was used to track bone motions. Rigid marker clusters, each consisting of four 10 mm in diameter spherical markers with inter-marker distances of 4 to 8 cm, were fixed on a pin rigidly fastened to the proximal tibia, superior neck of the talus, and medial calcaneus. The soft tissues in the vicinity of the mounting points were dissected away, and screws were used to attach the clusters. Three cameras operating at 100 Hz were positioned so that they surrounded the lateral and posterior aspects of the foot. The calibrated volume was approximately $60 \times 60 \times 60$ cm, and the average residual from the manufacturer's dynamic calibration was approximately 0.15 mm.

31.2.2.4 Testing Protocols

To facilitate the creation of anatomical coordinate systems fixed to the bone segments, a series of static trials were performed with the foot and shank in an anatomically neutral position. A two-marker pointer[15] was used to locate the following anatomical landmarks: lateral malleolus, medial malleolus, two points on opposite sides of the tibia rod, the most posterior point on the heel, the dorsum of the second metatarsal head, and three non-collinear points on the base plate. The coordinates of the markers attached to the bones were also recorded during these trials.

During dynamic trials, the proximal tibia was moved manually while the motions of the tibia, talus, and calcaneus markers were recorded. The proximal tibia was moved in a cross-pattern (dorsiflexion/plantarflexion followed by inversion/eversion) followed by a box pattern (dorsiflexion–eversion, dorsiflexion–inversion, plantar-flexion–inversion, and plantarflexion–eversion). An axial load of 225 N was applied to the tibia. Five trials, each approximately 30 sec in duration, were performed for each specimen. The first specimen was a pilot specimen for which a 300 N load was applied and three trials were performed. For mechanical linkage testing, ranges of motion similar to those applied to the specimens were applied. Five trials were collected for each of three axis configurations.

31.2.2.5 Kinematic Data Processing and Axis Fitting

The static trial data were used to establish bone-fixed anatomical coordinate systems for each of the three segments. For the tibia coordinate system: (1) the origin was positioned midway between the malleoli; (2) the Z-axis pointed along the transmalleolar line laterally; (3) the X-axis pointed anteriorly and perpendicular to a plane made by the malleoli and the midpoint of the two tibia rod points; and (4) the Y-axis pointed superiorly and was orthogonal to the X- and Z-axes. The calcaneus-fixed coordinate system had a roughly similar orientation: (1) The origin was positioned at the head of the second metatarsal; (2) the Y-axis pointed superiorly and perpendicular to the plane containing the three base plate points; (3) the X-axis pointed anteriorly along the projection on the base plate plane of the vector from the heel point to the head of the second metatarsal; and (4) the Z-axis pointed laterally and was orthogonal to the X- and Y-axes. The talus coordinate system was located with the same position and orientation as the tibia coordinate system at the neutral position.

The dynamic data were first filtered using a low-pass, fourth order, Butterworth filter with a 10-Hz cutoff frequency implemented in MatLab. The data were then resampled to reduce the number of data frames using a method based on distance moved by tibia markers, resulting in retained frames that were not equally spaced in time but rather were more evenly distributed in space.[13] A frame was retained only if at least one tibia marker had moved greater than a given distance (typically 4 to 7 mm) from its position at the last previously retained frame. The number of retained frames was between 225 and 275 for each trial.

The resampled marker trajectories were then used along with the known coordinates of the segment markers relative to their respective anatomical coordinate systems to compute the global rigid body kinematics of each bone for each frame. Homogeneous transformation matrices were computed using a least-squares method[16] in order to take advantage of the redundant fourth marker in each segment cluster.

Finite helical axes were computed in order to locate the "true" joint axes. Relative motions of the tibia and talus were used to locate the TC axis, and the ST axis was determined from relative motions of the calcaneus and talus. For every possible pair of retained data frames, the position and orientation of the helical axis were computed along with the rotation about and translation along that axis.[17] Helical axis decompositions with rotations smaller than 7.5° were discarded due to the potentially greater influence of measurement noise. A single "mean" helical axis was computed for each joint using a least-squares method that minimized the sum of the perpendicular

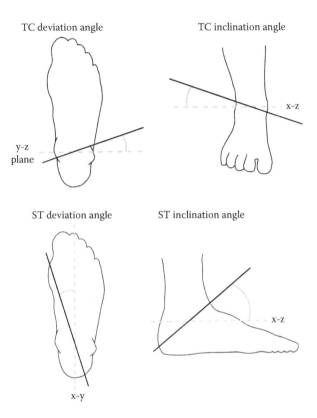

FIGURE 31.3 Definitions of inclination and deviation angles for both the TC and the ST joints. Positive angles are shown. The angles are measured from anatomically aligned planes of the calcaneus coordinate system (indicated by the dashed lines).

distances from all individual axes to the mean axis. Inclination and deviation angles were computed, which described the orientations of the joint axes relative to the planes of the calcaneus coordinate system with the foot in the neutral position (Figure 31.3).

The optimization method was used to determine TC and ST axis locations from the relative motions of the tibia and calcaneus. Ten optimizations with ten different sets of initial parameter estimates were executed for each trial. The final 12 parameters and associated axis locations were almost always insensitive to the starting guess, suggesting that global minima of the objective function (Equation 31.1) were achieved. Inclination and deviation angles of the axes resulting from optimization were computed relative to the calcaneus coordinate system in the anatomically neutral position (Figure 31.3).

The TC and ST axis locations resulting from optimization were compared to the corresponding mean helical axis in order to assess the accuracy of the optimization. For both joints, the angle between the optimization axis and the helical axis was computed. The shortest distance between the axes occurring within an anatomically relevant region was also determined. For the TC joint, this region was bounded

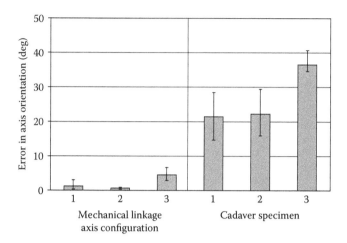

FIGURE 31.4 Angular errors for the two-axis optimization method for both the mechanical linkage and the cadaver tests. Similar results were obtained for the TC axis, although those results are not shown.

by the two malleoli, and for the ST joint, the region was bounded by the posterior aspect of the heel and a point 10 cm anterior to the heel.

31.2.3 RESULTS

Mechanical linkage axes located using the two-axis optimization were quite close to their counterparts found using helical axis decomposition, but this was not true for joint axes found in the cadaver specimens (Figure 31.4). Axis location errors were typically 5° or smaller for the linkage but were 20° or larger for the cadaver tests. The distances between optimized and true axes were also larger for the cadaver tests (range across specimens: 1.3 to 14.5 mm) than for the linkage (range across configurations: 0.6 to 1.2 mm).

31.3 "SUBTALAR ISOLATION" METHOD FOR SUBTALAR JOINT LOCATION

31.3.1 RATIONALE

If the talus did not move with respect to the tibia, then the motion of the calcaneus with respect to the tibia would be identical to the motion of the ST (talocalcaneal) joint. Location of the ST joint could then be accomplished using helical axis decomposition of the tibia–calcaneus motion. This immobilization of the talus may occur when the foot is placed in a slightly dorsiflexed position, because the dome of the talus, which is wider anteriorly than posteriorly,[18,19] becomes wedged in the mortise formed by the distal tibia and fibula. The potential for dorsiflexion to reduce talar motion is the reason that dorsiflexion is often applied during clinical examinations of the ST joint[20] and in part forms the basis for the palpation-based method for ST joint location proposed by Kirby.[21] We sought to examine the possibility that talar immobilization could be achieved and thus permit location of the ST joint from measured foot motion.

31.3.2 CADAVER EXPERIMENTS

31.3.2.1 Cadaver Specimens

Six fresh-frozen, unpaired lower leg specimens (from donors aged 56 to 79 yr; 5 M, 1 F; 3 R, 3 L) were tested. The specimens were prepared as described previously for the two-axis optimization testing, with the exception that the Achilles tendon was left intact proximally.

31.3.2.2 Cadaver Testing Apparatus

A custom-designed apparatus (Figure 31.5) was used to apply motion to the foot. The specimen was attached to the apparatus with the foot hanging down. A horizontal bar was secured to the plantar surface of the forefoot using a nylon cable tie, and

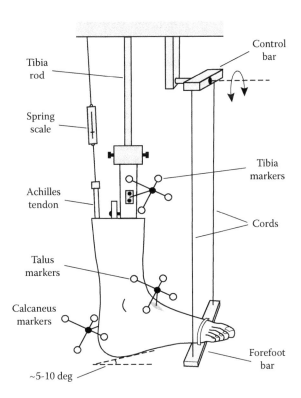

FIGURE 31.5 Apparatus used to apply foot motions in the "ST isolation" tests. The upper horizontal bar is manually rotated to induce motion in the forefoot and at the ST joint.

this bar was connected to a second, parallel bar above the specimen using two thin nylon cords. The upper horizontal bar could then be manually rotated about a fixed hinge to produce foot motion. The position of the specimen was adjusted prior to the motion trials such that the foot was in 5 to 10° of dorsiflexion. The Achilles tendon was clamped in series with a spring scale, and a tension of 25 N was applied to it.

31.3.2.3 Testing Protocol

The motion analysis system setup; attachment of reflective marker clusters to the tibia, talus, and calcaneus; and static trial protocol were similar to that described above for cadaver tests of the two-axis optimization method. The dynamic trials consisted of applying foot motions and measuring the motions of the tibia, talus, and calcaneus segment markers. In each trial, the upper horizontal bar was rotated until resistance to the motion was felt by the tester. Approximately six cycles of motion were completed during the trial in 30 sec. Ten trials were performed for each specimen. Specimen 1 was a pilot specimen for which only five trials were performed, and this specimen was previously dissected of all soft tissues except ligaments proximal to the midfoot.

31.3.2.4 Kinematic Data Processing and Helical Axis Decomposition

The bone-fixed anatomical coordinate systems for each segment were established from the static trials as described previously, except that the calcaneus coordinate system origin was positioned at the heel. The dynamic trial data were filtered using a low-pass, fourth order, Butterworth filter with a 10-Hz cutoff. The data were resampled to change the sampling frequency from 100 to 10 Hz (with equal temporal spacing). The global rigid body kinematics of the tibia, talus, and calcaneus anatomical coordinate systems were then computed as in the previous set of experiments.

Finite helical axes were computed from calcaneus–talus motion to locate the "true" ST joint axis. Finite helical axes were also computed for calcaneus–tibia motion. For both sets of helical axes, a single "mean" helical axis was computed, and these two axes were compared in order to assess the accuracy of the ST isolation technique.

Motions at the TC joint were also quantified by decomposing the transformations associated with the relative motion of the tibia and talus. Three angles, α, β, and γ, were extracted from the rotation submatrix for each frame using a Z–X–Y fixed (with respect to tibia) angles convention. In the anatomically neutral position, α, β, and γ were all zero, because the talus coordinate system was aligned with the tibia coordinate system.

31.3.3 Results

Errors in locating the true ST joint axis using the ST isolation method were variable across the specimens tested (Figure 31.6). For four of the six specimens (1, 2, 4,

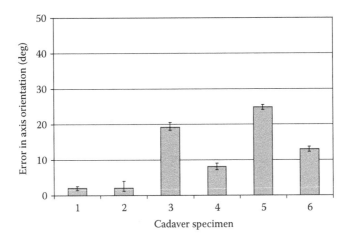

FIGURE 31.6 Angular errors for the "ST isolation" method in cadaver tests. The angle between the calcaneus–tibia mean helical axis and the calcaneus–talus (ST) mean helical axis, averaged across trials with error bars indicating the range, is shown.

and 6), the errors in axis orientation were approximately 10° or smaller, but for two specimens (3 and 5), these errors were 20° or larger. Similar results were obtained for the minimum distances between the fit and true axes, with errors of 3 and 4 mm for specimens 3 and 5, and errors approximately 1 mm or less for the other four specimens. Examination of the TC joint rotations (Figure 31.7) explained the differences among specimens in the measured errors: Specimens for which small TC rotations were measured (e.g., specimen 2) had small-axis location errors and specimens with larger TC rotations (e.g., specimen 5) generally had larger-axis location errors.

31.4 DISCUSSION

31.4.1 EVALUATION OF EXPERIMENTAL AXIS LOCATION ACCURACY

Previous studies using cadaver models have indicated that intersubject differences in the orientations of ankle joint complex axes are as high as 40°.[22,23] Estimates of ST joint kinetics during walking have suggested that the ground reaction force vector passes close to the joint axis, perhaps between 0 and 5 cm away. Given this degree of variability and the required precision for inverse dynamic computations, a reasonable expectation is that methods for locating these axes should be accurate to within 5° and 2 mm. Neither of the methods tested in this study consistently met this standard, but results for the ST isolation method were promising. Errors in two of six specimens were sufficiently small to indicate that clinically useful axes were determined, and the accuracy threshold was nearly met in two additional specimens.

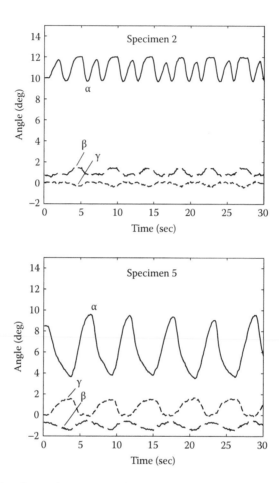

FIGURE 31.7 Angular motions at the TC joint during cadaver tests of the "ST isolation" method. Angles α, β, and γ, which describe orientations of the talus with respect to the sagittal, frontal, and transverse planes, respectively, of the tibial anatomical coordinate system, are plotted for single trials for two specimens. The range of α (amount of dorsiflexion/plantarflexion movement of the talus) is considerably larger for specimen 5; this specimen also had the worst ST axis location errors.

31.4.2 Limitations

The primary limitations of this study were that testing was performed on cadaver specimens rather than on living subjects, and that a small number of specimens were tested for each method. Cadaver testing permits invasive tracking of bone motions but leaves open the question of whether accurate axis locations could be repeated in patients under conditions of realistic joint loading. There are many different ways to formulate and solve the two-axis optimization problem,[12–14,24] and it is difficult to know if the poor results discovered for it here could be overcome by different choices for the objective function, optimization algorithm, and the locations of the marker clusters relative to the bones. Work is currently underway in our laboratory to address these questions.

31.4.3 INHERENT DIFFICULTIES WITH TWO-AXIS OPTIMIZATION

There is strong evidence suggesting that the simultaneous identification of fixed TC and ST joints from measured tibia–calcaneus motion is an ill-posed problem. Previous studies of *in vivo* ankle joint kinematics using three-dimensional location of radio-opaque markers implanted in the tibia, talus, and calcaneus[25] have shown that neither of these joints is fixed as movement occurs, and that the TC joint, in particular, undergoes substantial changes in orientation with dorsiflexion and plantarflexion. It may not be possible, simultaneously, to characterize these joints using fixed-axis models. In the present study, the optimization performed well on the mechanical linkage but poorly on the cadaver specimens. The primary difference between the two tests was that the mechanical linkage had fixed axes while the specimens did not.

When two hinge axes are fit to tibia–calcaneus motion, it is possible that errors in locating one axis will compensate for errors in locating the second axis. In such cases, the motion reconstructed from the optimized model is essentially the same as the measured motion, but both axis locations will be wrong. A model of an idealized universal joint (Figure 31.8) was analyzed to illustrate this point. Two segments, A and B, are connected by two intersecting, orthogonal joint axes about which rotations α and β occur.

The angle ϕ describes the rotation of the universal joint with respect to A below the joint, and a rotation of $-\phi$ is applied above the joint. When $\phi = 0°$, the transformation $^B_A T^{(1)}$ describing the pose of B relative to A is

$$
^B_A T^{(1)} =
\begin{bmatrix}
c\beta_1 & -s\beta_1 & 0 & -s\beta_1\, l_B \\
c\alpha_1\, s\beta_1 & c\alpha_1\, c\beta_1 & -s\alpha_1 & c\alpha_1\, c\beta_1\, l_B + l_A \\
s\alpha_1\, s\beta_1 & s\alpha_1\, c\beta_1 & c\alpha_1 & s\alpha_1\, c\beta_1\, l_B \\
0 & 0 & 0 & 1
\end{bmatrix}
\tag{31.2}
$$

where α_1 and β_1 are the two joint angles for this configuration, and l_A and l_B are the distances from the intersection point of the two joint axes to o_A and o_B, respectively.

For $\phi \neq 0°$, the universal joint is rotated in the horizontal plane while the segments A and B are held in place; such a configuration can be taken to represent an axis location that is erroneous compared to the true axis location given by $\phi = 0°$. The components of the transformation $^B_A T^{(2)}$ describing the pose of B relative to A are given by

$$_A^B T^{(2)}{}_{11} = c^2\phi\, c\beta_2 + c\phi\, s\phi\, s\alpha_2\, s\beta_2 + s^2\phi\, c\alpha_2$$

$$_A^B T^{(2)}{}_{12} = -c\phi\, s\beta_2 + s\phi\, s\alpha_2\, c\beta_2$$

$$_A^B T^{(2)}{}_{13} = -c\phi\, s\phi\, c\beta_2 - s^2\phi\, s\alpha_2\, s\beta_2 + c\phi\, s\phi\, c\alpha_2$$

$$_A^B T^{(2)}{}_{14} = (-c\phi\, s\beta_2 + s\phi\, s\alpha_2\, c\beta_2)\, l_B$$

$$_A^B T^{(2)}{}_{21} = c\phi\, c\alpha_2\, s\beta_2 - s\phi\, s\alpha_2$$

$$_A^B T^{(2)}{}_{22} = c\alpha_2\, c\beta_2$$

$$_A^B T^{(2)}{}_{23} = -s\phi\, c\alpha_2\, s\beta_2 - c\phi\, s\alpha_2$$

$$_A^B T^{(2)}{}_{24} = c\alpha_2\, c\beta_2\, l_B + l_A$$

$$_A^B T^{(2)}{}_{31} = -c\phi\, s\phi\, c\beta_2 + c^2\phi\, s\alpha_2\, s\beta_2 + c\phi\, s\phi\, c\alpha_2$$

$$_A^B T^{(2)}{}_{32} = s\phi\, s\beta_2 + c\phi\, s\alpha_2\, c\beta_2$$

$$_A^B T^{(2)}{}_{33} = s^2\phi\, c\beta_2 - c\phi\, s\phi\, s\alpha_2\, s\beta_2 + c^2\phi\, c\alpha_2$$

$$_A^B T^{(2)}{}_{34} = (s\phi\, s\beta_2 + c\phi\, s\alpha_2\, c\beta_2)\, l_B$$

$$_A^B T^{(2)}{}_{41} = 0$$

$$_A^B T^{(2)}{}_{42} = 0$$

$$_A^B T^{(2)}{}_{43} = 0$$

$$_A^B T^{(2)}{}_{44} = 1$$

$$(31.3)$$

The point o_B can be made to trace the same path in an A-fixed coordinate system for $\phi = 0°$ and for some arbitrary nonzero value of ϕ. Equating the translation vector of $_A^B T^{(1)}$ and $_A^B T^{(2)}$, we can determine the relationship between the joint angles for the two configurations such that o_B has the same position for both configurations:

$$\beta_1 = -\sin^{-1}(-c\phi\, s\beta_2 + s\phi\, s\alpha_2\, c\beta_2) \tag{31.4}$$

$$\alpha_1 = \sin^{-1}\left(\frac{s\phi\, s\beta_2 + c\phi\, s\alpha_2\, c\beta_2}{c\beta_1}\right) \tag{31.5}$$

If we now attach a marker P to B (as shown in Figure 31.8) and move the mechanism such that o_B traces the same path for both configurations, we find that

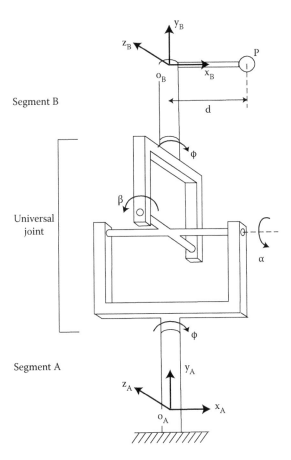

FIGURE 31.8 Simplified kinematic model used to demonstrate difficulties in applying the two-axis optimization method. Segment B is connected to segment A by a universal joint with intersecting, orthogonal axes.

the differences in the paths traced by marker P can be quite small. For example, consider P attached to B at a distance $d = 100$ mm from o_B along axis x_B. For $\phi = 30°$ (representing a 30° displacement of both joint axes), we compute the position of P in space using Equation 31.3 for a series of poses of the mechanism with joint angles α_2 and β_2 both ranging between $-30°$ and $30°$. For $\phi = 30°$, Equation 31.4 and Equation 31.5 are used to determine α_1 and β_1, such that the path of o_B is the same for both configurations. We then compute the position of P for $\phi = 0°$, using the calculated joint angles α_1 and β_1 and Equation 31.2. Finally, we compute the distance between the position of P for $\phi = 0°$ and the position of P for $\phi = 30°$ for all pairs of α_2 and β_2 (Figure 31.9).

We see from this analysis that when the relative segment motions are small, those motions are nearly identical for two very different joint axis orientations. Over much of the approximate ranges of motion of the TC and ST joints ($-10° < \alpha_2 < 10°$ and $-10° < \beta_2 < 30°$; indicated by the dashed box in Figure 31.9), the marker

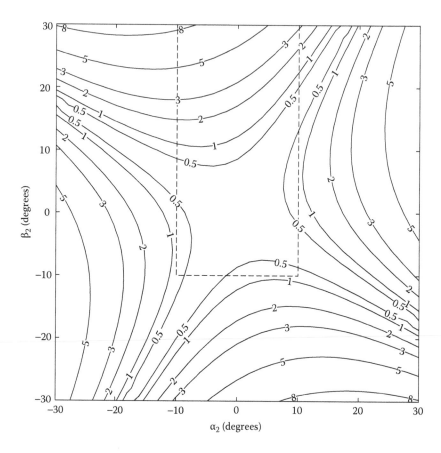

FIGURE 31.9 Contour plot showing errors in marker location in mm for mislocated axes computed using the model shown in Figure 31.8. Errors are distances between the positions of marker P obtained with $\phi = 0°$ and positions obtained with $\phi = 30°$ and are plotted vs. joint angles α_2 and β_2 (see text). The dashed box indicates the approximate expected range of ST and TC joint motion.

errors resulting from $\phi = 30°$ errors in axis location are less than 1 mm. With the added complications of moving joint axes, stereophotogrammetric error, and skin movement, the optimization algorithm likely has difficulty in "choosing" between different joint configurations, because the resulting differences in model kinematics (e.g., marker errors) may be small. Even when small marker errors are computed, it is possible that there are underlying large errors in axis location; optimization performed on a second anthropomorphic computer model with intentionally displaced joint axes underscores this point (Table 31.1).

TABLE 31.1

Marker Location Errors and Angular Axis Location Errors for Various Models Used to Locate Axes in the Ankle Complex

Model Investigated	Primary Source(s) of Marker Fit Error	Marker Fit Error (mm)[a]	Angular Errors In Locating True Axis			
			TC Deviation Error (°)	TC Inclination Error (°)	ST Deviation Error (°)	ST Inclination Error (°)
Mechanical linkage[b]	Marker tracking	0.3	2	1	2	1
Cadaver with bone-mounted markers[b]	Marker tracking + moving hinge axes	1.6	26	2	26	12
Human subject (van den Bogert et al., 1994)[13]	Marker tracking + moving hinge axes + skin, shoe movement	2.3	—	—	—	—
Human subject (Reinbolt et al., 2005)[c 24]	Marker tracking + moving hinge axes + skin movement	2.3	—	—	—	—
Computer simulation[d]	Forced error in joint axis orientation	0.9	28	19	28	5

[a] Marker-fit error as defined by van den Bogert et al. (1994).[13]

[b] Method similar to Sommer and Miller (1980)[12] used for optimization, which did not explicitly minimize marker-fit errors.

[c] Marker-fit error determined by dividing reported root-mean-squared (RMS) error by $\sqrt{3}$.

[d] An anthropomorphic kinematic model was used to generate marker data, then optimization (van den Bogert et al., 1994)[13] was executed but with one of the 12 optimization variables fixed with an error (specifically an Euler angle specifying the talocrural axis was fixed with an error of 30°).

31.5 CONCLUSION

It is important to have subject-specific determinations of ankle joint axes because these axes vary substantially from subject to subject, making generic joint models of limited use in patient evaluations. Isman and Inman[23] characterized the orientation of the ankle complex joint axes and found that the range of inclination and deviation angles formed by these axes with the cardinal planes (Figure 31.3) was greater than 40° in some cases. Knowledge of these axes together with marker sets that allow differential tracking of foot segment motions (such as those described elsewhere in this book) would facilitate more clinically meaningful gait analysis of movement disorders of the foot and ankle.

Although the "Subtalar isolation" method yielded inconsistent results across specimens in this study, we believe that it is worthy of further investigation. It may be possible to modify the application of loads to the foot, such that the dorsiflexion load applied to the forefoot is kept constant, and variations in the moments applied about the TC joint are minimized as ST joint motions are applied. Also unclear is the degree to which the TC joint is immobilized by dorsiflexion alone. These possibilities are currently being investigated using *in vitro* and *in vivo* models in our laboratory.

ACKNOWLEDGMENTS

The authors would like to thank Kevin Kirby and Andrea Cereatti for valuable discussions and H. Joseph Sommer III for contributing the algorithm for least-squares determination of the mean helical axis. This work was funded by grant number BES-0134217 from the National Science Foundation.

REFERENCES

1. Schwartz, M.H. and Rozumalski, A., A new method for estimating joint parameters from motion data, *J Biomech*, 38, 107–116, 2005.
2. Stagni, R. et al., Effects of hip joint centre mislocation on gait analysis results, *J Biomech*, 33, 1479–1487, 2000.
3. della Croce, U., Cappozzo, A. and Kerrigan, D.C., Pelvis and lower limb anatomical landmark calibration precision and its propagation to bone geometry and joint angles, *Med Biol Eng Comput*, 37, 155–161, 1999.
4. Hagemeister, N. et al., A reproducible method for studying three-dimensional knee kinematics, *J Biomech*, 38, 1926–1931, 2005.
5. Lewis, J.L. and Lew, W.D., A method for locating and optimal "fixed" axis of rotation for the human knee joint, *J Biomech Eng*, 100, 187–193, 1978.
6. Cappozzo, A., Gait analysis methodology, *Hum Mov Sci*, 3, 27–50, 1984.
7. Cereatti, A., Camomilla, V. and Cappozzo, A., Estimation of the centre of rotation: a methodological contribution, *J Biomech*, 37, 413–416, 2004.
8. Leardini, A. et al., Validation of a functional method for the estimation of hip joint centre location, *J Biomech*, 32, 99–103, 1999.

9. Piazza, S.J., Okita, N. and Cavanagh, P.R., Accuracy of the functional method of hip joint center location: effects of limited motion and varied implementation, *J Biomech,* 34, 967–973, 2001.
10. Piazza, S.J. et al., Assessment of the functional method of hip joint center location subject to reduced range of hip motion, *J Biomech,* 37, 349–356, 2004.
11. Wright, D.G., Desai, S.M. and Henderson, W.H., Action of the subtalar and ankle-joint complex during the stance phase of walking, *J Bone Joint Surg Am,* 46–A, 361–382, 1964.
12. Sommer, H.J. and Miller, N.R., A technique for kinematic modeling of anatomical joints, *J Biomech Eng,* 102, 311–317, 1980.
13. van den Bogert, A.J., Smith, G.D. and Nigg, B.M., *In vivo* determination of the anatomical axes of the ankle joint complex: an optimization approach, *J Biomech,* 27, 1477–1488, 1994.
14. Siston, R.A. et al., Evaluation of methods that locate the center of the ankle for computer-assisted total knee arthroplasty, *Clin Orthop Relat Res,* 439, 129–135, 2005.
15. Cappozzo, A. et al., Position and orientation in space of bones during movement: anatomical frame definition and determination, *Clin Biomech,* 10, 171–178, 1995.
16. Challis, J.H., A procedure for determining rigid body transformation parameters, *J Biomech,* 28, 733–737, 1995.
17. Spoor, C.W. and Veldpaus, F.E., Rigid body motion calculated from spatial co-ordinates of markers, *J Biomech,* 13, 391–393, 1980.
18. Barnett, C.H. and Napier, J.R., The axis of rotation at the ankle joint in man. Its influence upon the form of the talus and the mobility of the fibula, *J Anatomy,* 86, 1–9, 1952.
19. Inman, V.T., *The Joints of the Ankle,* Williams & Wilkins, Baltimore, 1976.
20. Greene, W.B., *Essentials of Musculoskeletal Care,* Amercian Academy of Ortho-paedic Surgeons, Rosemont, IL, 2001.
21. Kirby, K.A., Methods for determination of positional variations in the subtalar joint axis, *J Am Podiatr Med Assoc,* 77, 228–234, 1987.
22. Piazza, S.J., Mechanics of the subtalar joint and its function during walking, *Foot Ankle Clin,* 10, 425–442, 2005.
23. Isman, R.E. and Inman, V.T., Anthropometric studies of the human foot and ankle, *Bull Prosthet Res,* 97–129, 1969.
24. Reinbolt, J.A. et al., Determination of patient-specific multi-joint kinematic models through two-level optimization, *J Biomech,* 38, 621–626, 2005.
25. Lundberg, A., Kinematics of the ankle and foot, *In vivo* roentgen stereophotogram-metry, *Acta Orthop Scand Suppl,* 233, 1–24, 1989.

32 Dynamic Radiographic Measurement of Three-Dimensional Skeletal Motion

J. D. Yamokoski and Scott A. Banks

CONTENTS

32.1 INTRODUCTION

Measurement of three-dimensional (3D) human motion has been practiced in the clinic for almost 50 yr. These measurements have provided critical information for understanding and treating abnormalities of human gait, posture, balance, and sports performance. Over the past 10 to 15 yr, there has been a growing capability for more accurate and precise measurements of the moving human skeleton using dynamic radiographic imaging techniques. These observations permit novel analyses such as wear modeling of total knee replacement components[1] and assessing impingement and dislocation of total hip replacements.[2] To date, radiographic kinematic studies primarily have been carried out on the major weight-bearing joints of the body, determining the relative kinematics of large bones in the hip and knee.

Measuring the dynamic motions of joints in the foot and wrist, which involve numerous small bones interacting in complex motions, has proven challenging. Computed tomography (CT)/magnetic resonance (MR) imaging,[3] radiostereometric analysis (RSA),[4,5] *in vitro* tests,[6–8] mechanical devices,[9] and skin and bone-pin

543

mounted markers (both electromagnetic[10,11] and optical[12–17]) have contributed to our understanding of the kinematics of the foot/ankle complex. RSA and CT/MR methods provide excellent resolution but limited dynamic capability. *In vitro* methods suffer from uncertainty of muscle loads. Marker-based motion capture (MoCap), the standard for gross skeletal kinematic studies, suffers inaccuracy from skin movement relative to the underlying bones.[5,17,18] The ideal tool, then, permits accurate, noninvasive measurement of skeletal kinematics under normal loading conditions. Furthermore, it should allow the study of natural bones and artificial implants with equal facility.

In what follows, we will present a tool we believe addresses all these requirements — dynamic radiographic measurements. Our lab, along with colleagues across the globe, have used this measurement technique to characterize the motions in hundreds of knees, including healthy knees, knees with anterior cruciate ligament (ACL) injury and/or reconstruction, and knees with over 25 different types of arthroplasty. Figure 32.1 is an example of this technique applied to the study of the motions of the natural knee. Activities such as treadmill gait, stair, sit-to-stand, lunge, and kneeling have also all been studied. Other researchers have used the same method to characterize the motions of the hip.[2,19,20] This method is also currently being applied to the shoulder and elbow joints as well as the spine.

The organization of this chapter is as follows: First, we will describe the current state-of-the-art in dynamic radiographic measurements. Most of this discussion will focus on application to the knee joint since it is the joint that has received

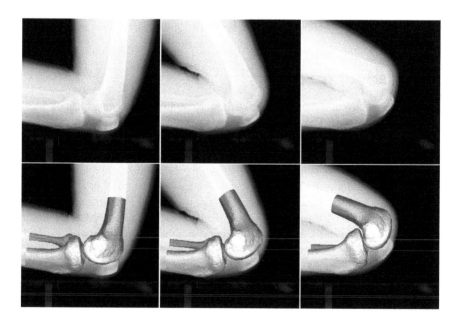

FIGURE 32.1 The top row is a series of x-ray images obtained from a dynamic movement trial, and the bottom row is their associated solutions found using single-plane shape registration methods. (Images contributed by Takaaki Morooka, M.D.)

the most attention to date. We will follow this with a discussion of how dynamic radiographic measurement methods might be applied to the foot/ankle complex. Finally, we will conclude with a discussion of new technologies we expect to be using within a few years.

32.2 STATE OF THE ART

32.2.1 OVERVIEW

The dynamic radiographic measurement approach is based on imaging the joint of interest as it moves, using x-ray fluoroscopy to obtain a sequence of images in which the bones or prostheses are projected as two-dimensional (2D) perspective silhouettes. These images are processed to remove any distortions created by the imaging hardware. From knowledge about the imaged objects (e.g., a computer-aided design (CAD) model or volumetric model from CT/MRI data) and the projection geometry, the image creation process can be recreated on a computer — essentially creating a virtual fluoroscope. With the only unknowns being the six pose variables of the imaged object (three translations and three rotations), an iterative generate and test process can be carried out on the virtual fluoroscope until some sort of match criterion is met between the output of the virtual fluoroscope and the real x-ray images. When the two projections match, the 3D pose of the model can be taken as an estimate of the real object's pose relative to the imaging reference frame.

32.2.1.1 Image Calibration

All methods of surface or volumetric registration to 2D images, whether a single- or biplane study, begin with a perspective model of the imaging hardware. Camera calibration is the process of determining the internal camera geometric and optical characteristics (intrinsic parameters) and/or the 3D position and orientation of the camera frame relative to a reference coordinate system (extrinsic parameters).[21] For dynamic radiograph measurements, all 3D position and orientation measurements are made relative to the fluoroscope. The reason for this will become clear when the shape-matching problem is formally defined. As a result, we can ignore the extrinsic parameters of the fluoroscope. Therefore, to recreate a perspective projection model of the fluoroscope, the intrinsic parameters of interest are the principal distance (C_{pd}) and principal point (u_0, v_0), as shown in Figure 32.2. Fluoroscopic images generally have significant geometric distortion due to the system of curved phosphors and lenses employed to form the image. Accurate comparisons between computer-synthesized and experimentally acquired images can only be made if there is no systematic geometric distortion in the experimentally measured views. There are other sources of distortion including those introduced by digitizing the fluoroscopic video as well as deviation from the perspective model due to x-ray scatter and beam-hardening phenomenon. These other sources, however, are generally negligible and not considered in most studies.

There are many approaches to single-camera calibration.[21–23] Zhang categorizes methods into those that observe a known 3D object (photogrammetric calibration)

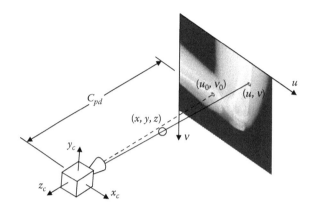

FIGURE 32.2 Pictorial representation of the camera intrinsic parameters. C_{pd} and (u_0, v_0) are the principal distance and principal point, respectively.

and those that film the same static scene from different viewpoints (self-calibration).[23] Most methods for fluoroscopic calibration fall in the photogrammetric category because it is relatively inexpensive and easy to construct a calibration object. Most published methods include extra parameters to account for the image distortion in addition to the geometric parameters. However, we separate the distortion removal and fluoroscope calibration into two steps. Doing so makes the forward projection model (simulating the fluoroscope) much simpler as we can ignore distortion in the model since it is removed from the original images. There are several methods that have been proposed for removing distortions from fluoroscope images.[24-29] Gronenschild reported a global dewarping method[27] with superior accuracy, noise sensitivity, and reproducibility compared to bilinear interpolation and two other local dewarping methods.[30]

Our method for determination of the other internal camera parameters is accomplished by imaging a star-shaped distribution of control points parallel to the fluoroscopic image intensifier. The relations between m Cartesian control points with spatial locations (x_i, y_i, z_i) for $1 \leq i \leq m$, the image coordinates (u_i, v_i) of the control points, and the internal orientation parameters can be derived from basic geometric principles

$$u_i = u_0 - \frac{C_{pd} * x_i}{z_i}$$
$$\qquad\qquad i = 1 \cdots m \qquad\qquad (32.1)$$
$$v_i = v_0 - \frac{C_{pd} * y_i}{z_i}$$

Equation 32.1 yields an overdetermined system of $2 * m$ equations and three unknowns. Solving Equation 32.1 to find the unknown intrinsic camera parameters can be posed as a least-squares–fitting problem: $\min_{w \in \mathfrak{R}^3}[\Phi(w, \eta_i) - \chi_i] \; \forall i,$

where $w = [u_0, v_0, C_{pd}]^T$ is a vector of the unknown intrinsic camera parameters. The control points in Cartesian space, $\eta_i = [x_i \ y_i \ z_i]^T$, are transformed by Φ (Equation 32.1) into image coordinates and compared to the measured image coordinates, $\chi_i = [u_i \ v_i]^T$.

32.2.1.2 Shape Registration

The problem of registering 3D models to 2D images is complex. We will restrict our discussion to rigid models of bone or implant surfaces or volumes. A general problem description for single-plane studies can be stated: Given a rigid body model, M, a target image, I, and a dissimilarity measure, E, find the best transformation, $_M^I T$, that associates any point of M to a corresponding point in I and minimizes the dissimilarity measure between the transformed model M' and the target image I. The problem statement for biplane studies is nearly identical. After calibration, we have knowledge of the transformation from image coordinates in I to an intermediate coordinate system, C, which we defined earlier in Equation 32.1 and can be manipulated into a transformation matrix we will call $_C^I T$. Therefore we can rewrite $_M^I T$ as

$$_M^I T = {_C^I T} * {_M^C T}$$
(32.1)

The unknown then becomes the transformation from the intermediate coordinate system to the model coordinate system, $_M^C T$. The pose of any object in space can be described with six independent variables, typically three Cartesian translations (x,y,z) and three Euler rotations (α, β, γ). In our studies, we typically use a 3-1-2 cardan sequence for body-fixed ordered rotations.[31] Finally, the unknown transformation, $_M^C T$, can be written as a function of these six independent variables,

$$_M^C T = \begin{bmatrix} c_\beta * c_\gamma + s_\alpha * s_\beta * s_\gamma & c_\alpha * s_\gamma & -s_\beta * c_\gamma + s_\alpha * c_\beta * s_\gamma & x \\ -c_\beta * s_\gamma + s_\alpha * s_\beta * c_\gamma & c_\alpha * c_\gamma & s_\beta * s_\gamma + s_\alpha * c_\beta * c_\gamma & y \\ c_\alpha * s_\beta & -s_\alpha & c_\alpha * c_\beta & z \\ 0 & 0 & 0 & 1 \end{bmatrix}$$
(32.2)

where c_k and s_k ($k = \alpha, \beta, \gamma$) are the cosine and sine of the respective angles.

The problem statement can then be more precisely stated as: find the best combination of $(x,y,z,\alpha,\beta,\gamma)$, which can be used along with camera calibration parameters to transform any point of M to a corresponding point in I and minimize the dissimilarity measure E between the transformed model M' and the target image I.

Typically we want to know the relative motions between multiple bones or implants (e.g., relative pose between a talus, M_1, and tibia, M_2). If $_{M_1}^C T$ and $_{M_2}^C T$ can be found by shape matching, then the transformation from M_1 to M_2 is given by

$$_{M_2}^{M_1} T = \left[{_{M_1}^C T}\right]^{-1} * {_{M_2}^C T}$$
(32.3)

With the problem defined, surface or volume registration reduces to a choice of similarity measure and optimization algorithm to iteratively determine the six independent pose variables.

32.2.1.2.1   Single-Plane Fluoroscopic Studies

Image registration techniques have been used for biomechanical measurements since 1991.[32] This involved a template matching technique based on computationally efficient Normalized Fourier Descriptors.[33] This technique worked well with limited computer power, but required the entire object boundary curve to be visible for accurate results. Techniques now employ numerical optimization and two classes of similarity measures: direct image-to-image and model-to-projection ray measures.

With the direct image-to-image similarity measure, You et al.[34] or Mahfouz et al.,[35] for example, took advantage of the increasing speed of the average personal computer. A projected image of the model and x-ray was compared directly in image space using a weighted average of the normalized cross-correlations between the intensity and edge images. Due to the large number of local minima (or false solutions) predicted by this similarity measure, Mahfouz utilized a global optimization method, simulated annealing. While a global optimizer generally takes much longer than a local optimization method to arrive at a solution, it decreased the solution's sensitivity to the initial pose guess. This aspect of their work is particularly appealing in a clinical setting, because it reduced the amount of work required by an operator to put a model into a good initial pose. From *in vitro* testing, they were able to report root-mean-square (RMS) errors of 0.68 mm, 1.7 mm, and 1.3°, in XY (in-plane) translation, Z (out-of-plane) translation, and rotation, respectively.

The second class of similarity measures was introduced for medical imaging by Lavallee and Szeliski.[36] They showed that the 3D pose of a model could be determined by projecting rays from contour points in an x-ray image back to the x-ray focus and noting that all of these rays are tangent to the model surface. Hence, an optimization method could be used to minimize the sum of Euclidean distances between all projected rays and the model surface. To reduce the time spent computing distances between projected rays and the model surface, a 3D distance map of the model was precomputed and used for these distance calculations. Lavallee and Szeliski developed their method for use with stereo images, and Zuffi et al. later applied it to single-plane fluoroscopy with total knee replacements.[37] Except for some problems with occlusion, they recorded relative pose errors between femoral and tibial components *in vitro* on the order of 1.5 mm and 1.5°, in position and orientation, respectively.

While both Mahfouz and Zuffi examined the application of single-plane fluoroscopy to knee arthroplasty kinematics, numerous factors prohibit direct comparison of the matching accuracy, including image quality and model geometry. To date, there has not been a thorough comparison of published methods to determine measurement accuracy as a function of image quality and model geometry.

All single-plane or monocular measurement techniques exhibit greater uncertainties for translations perpendicular to the image plane. One obvious solution is to add another, ideally orthogonal, perspective projection. Alternatively, the measurement technique can be augmented to better estimate out-of-plane translations. Yamazaki et al.[38] utilized Zuffi's 3D distance map technique to estimate the implant pose. They then used response-surface techniques[39] to refine the out-of-plane translations, reporting RMS errors improved from 3.2 to 1.4 mm for *in vitro* tests.

32.2.1.2.2   Biplane Fluoroscopic Studies

As mentioned above, the main shortcoming of single-plane studies are larger measurement errors for translations orthogonal to the image plane. The obvious solution is to add another simultaneous x-ray projection. If the two x-ray projections are made orthogonal, then out-of-plane translations in one image become the in-plane translations in the other. The addition of a second image complicates the similarity measure, but several groups have reported methods for matching CT/MRI-derived bone models or total knee replacement (TKR) models to biplane sequences.[34,40–44]

You et al.[34] used bone models derived from CT scans to create digitally reconstructed radiographs (DRRs). These DRRs were compared to x-ray images using a normalized cross-correlation, an approach similar to that of Mahfouz et al.[35] You et al. reported errors during *in vitro* testing on the order of 0.5 mm in translations and 1.4° for rotations. Other groups have reported similar results matching fluoroscopic images with implant components[42,43] and bones.[40,41] Finally, others have reported similar measurement results using manual alignment of a model's contours[41] or a point-cloud representation of the model[44] using commercial or custom software.

32.3 APPLICATION TO THE ANKLE JOINT SYSTEM

Fluoroscopic measurements have been applied to the foot/ankle complex.[45–48] These studies primarily have used fluoroscopy to gather 2D measurements of foot ground angle and ankle dorsi/plantar flexion angle. To date, no report applying shape matching techniques to determine the 3D kinematics of the bones of the foot has appeared in the English literature.

Measurements of the foot and ankle complex are possible, but present specific experimental challenges. The close apposition of bones in the foot results in overlapping or occluding of the bony outlines on radiographic projections. Lateral projections will show the talus and calcaneous clearly, while the navicular, cuboid, and cuneiforms will have overlapping projections. Transverse projections will reverse the situation. A sagittal oblique projection shows each of the hindfoot bones clearly and may prove useful for quantifying hindfoot bone kinematics during weight-bearing activities (Figure 32.3). Biplane imaging might also be used to provide better precision and more uniformly distributed errors.

The use of force platforms for simultaneous recording of ground reactions forces would seem an obvious and desirable adjunct to any dynamic radiographic study. Unfortunately, commercially available fluoroscopy units are quite difficult (or impossible) to use at ground level, necessitating a robust elevated walkway to support elevated force platforms. This inconvenience provides, in part, motivation for the development of a radiographic imaging platform with greater flexibility for dynamic studies of skeletal motions.

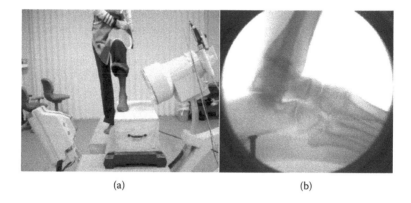

(a)   (b)

FIGURE 32.3 Current fluoroscopy systems have limited vertical travel, requiring patients to be elevated above the ground in order to obtain sagittal oblique projections of the foot/ ankle complex.

32.4 THE FUTURE OF DYNAMIC RADIOGRAPHIC MEASUREMENTS

Recovering 3D kinematic information from 2D x-ray or fluoroscopic images has proved to be a useful tool to clinicians and researchers. While several improvements and variations of single- and biplane fluoroscopy have been proposed since the method's introduction to the biomechanics community, much remains to be done.

Previous methods for analysis have focused on recovering the pose of an object one image at a time. This provides accurate data, but requires a trained operator to provide a good initial guess of the object's pose for each image in the sequence. Global optimizers have been introduced to make the pose estimation more robust to poor initial guesses,[35] but these still require the initial guess. If dynamic radiographic techniques for skeletal motion measurement are ever to find wide research or clinical utilization, then the algorithm should require minimal user supervision. Current shape-registration methods do not enforce continuity constraints on bone trajectories. Figure 32.4 shows a typical solution for the anterior and superior translations for a clinical image sequence obtained using traditional methods, showing numerous discontinuities. This issue typically is addressed by either filtering the time history data or fitting smooth functions to the discrete solutions. Because continuity was not enforced as a constraint during the initial optimization, the filtered or fitted data are no longer optimal. Furthermore, by optimizing on a per image basis, one cannot avoid the fact that the absolute best pose that can be achieved will be directly related to the noise in that particular image. Unfortunately in clinical x-ray studies, there are many sources of noise in an image, including image blur and edge erosion by soft tissue. We currently are addressing these problems with studies aimed at solving the sequence level optimization problem rather than the single-image optimization problem. Inspired by similar work done by Mazza and Cappozzo,[49] the unknown time history of the motion of the imaged object is parameterized by n equally spaced knots of a fifth order B-spline curve. The n knots are treated as the

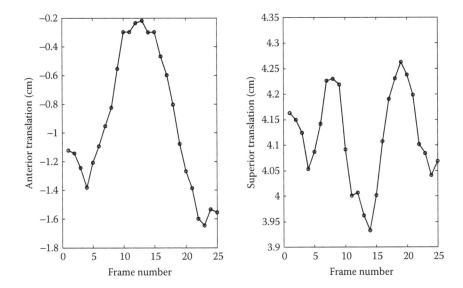

FIGURE 32.4 Typical solutions for the (a) anterior and (b) superior translations of the femur relative to the tibia from a single-plane fluoroscopic study. The data show the discrete and discontinuous nature of solutions determined one frame at a time with no continuity constraints imposed.

design variables of an optimization process. If an optimal set of B-spline knots can be found, which minimizes some similarity measure across the entire image sequence, then, by the properties of the B-spline parameterization, a continuous time-history solution can be found. Theoretically, we would expect this method to be more accurate and more robust than previous methods. Initial results have not yet proved this conjecture, but they have at least indicated that our early investigations are feasible and that they deserve further investigation.

Realizing that commercial fluoroscopic hardware is designed to image humans resting supine on an operating table, there is no surprise finding limitations when applying these devices to observe dynamic skeletal motion. We feel that the imaging hardware deserves attention equivalent to that given algorithms. Imaging hardware limitations directly influence the future impact of this measurement approach, and can be considered as follows: activity restrictions, anatomy limitations, exposure to ionizing radiation, and bone-model generation.

Patients can have quite different clinical outcomes depending upon how they recruit their muscles as dynamic joint stabilizers.[50] Similarly, the motions of joint replacements differ significantly depending upon the activity.[51] These findings underscore the need to observe motions during normal loading conditions when deciding on surgical interventions or assessing device design/performance relationships. The challenge is finding clinically important activities where the joint remains in a small volume of space suitable for fluoroscopic observation with a 23 to 30 cm field of view. This has been "solved" for the knee by using modified stairclimbing and gait activities where a combination of activity modification and multiple positions of the fluoroscope is used to obtain the required images. However, it has not been possible to observe knee joint motions during normal ground-level steady walking, stair descent, or chair sit/stand. As previously mentioned, available imaging systems do not permit observations centered less than ~100 cm from the ground, requiring platforms to elevate the subject into the field of view (Figure 32.3). This means more equipment is required, the subject is elevated into a visually uncomfortable position, and accessory sensors like floor-mounted force plates (for measuring ground reaction forces) are not easily used.

Current fluoroscopic imaging systems also impose restrictions on the anatomic locations, which can be observed during dynamic motion. "Lift with your legs" is a simple, sensible admonition to avoiding low back injury. However, it precludes fluoroscopic observation of the low back during relevant lifting activities due to a small field of view. Similarly, it is impossible to obtain a transverse view of the patella, a so-called skyline view, during a chair-rise or bicycle activity without an imaging system that can dynamically align the view to the anatomy of interest. Similar arguments apply to the shoulder, foot and ankle, and hip, where biomechanically interesting or clinically important observations are not possible because of the limited field of view or immobility of existing radiographic imaging systems.

Ionizing radiation of any level remains a critical concern for both research and clinical observations. Although radiation exposure often is justified by the clinical need or importance of the information so obtained, it must be minimized to the extent possible. Current fluoroscopic systems rely on human operators to initiate and terminate exposures. Because the operator has only qualitative feedback on the timing and alignment of the exposure, the patient receives greater than the minimum exposure required for the well-aligned and timed diagnostic image sequence. Thus, limiting radiographic exposures to only useful views by some automatic procedure has the potential to reduce exposure even during routine examinations.

Lastly, the model-based image measurement approach assumes a digital model of the implant, or bone surface is available for registration with the radiographic image sequence. Obtaining models for manufactured objects is not difficult. However, it is inconvenient, expensive, and time consuming to obtain separate tomographic scans of the patient or study subject to create the bone models required for dynamic radiographic motion analysis.

We now are attempting to address all of these hardware limitations by creating a novel imaging platform specifically intended for recording dynamic skeletal motion and cone-beam CT (Figure 32.5). This robot-based imaging platform will use real-time motion capture to measure the patient's movement and pass this information to the robotic system for automatic tracking and gated acquisition of the desired radiographic sequence. The same machine capabilities will permit cone-beam CT, so that dynamic imaging and bone-model creation can be performed using one imaging platform in a time- and space-efficient manner. These capabilities will remove or reduce the activity, anatomy, exposure, and bone-model generation limitations of standard fluoroscopy systems — permitting application of dynamic skeletal imaging and model-based analyses in a wide range of clinical and research contexts. We believe this technology has the potential to advance research and

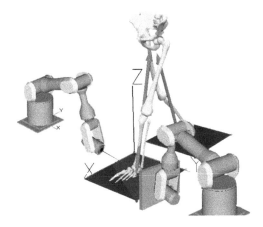

FIGURE 32.5 A robot-based x-ray imaging platform will permit dynamic imaging of all aspects of the moving skeleton and provide anatomic reconstructions using cone-beam CT techniques.

clinical diagnostic capabilities for conditions affecting hundreds of millions of people each year, and hope to demonstrate a working prototype of this system shortly after publication of this monograph.

32.5 CONCLUSIONS

Shape-matching based radiographic measurement techniques are currently used by many groups throughout the world to determine dynamic motion patterns in hips, knees, shoulders, and other joints, and to characterize joint function, surgical efficacy, implant performance, articular wear, and arthroplasty failure mechanisms. These techniques provide a valuable complement to traditional motion measurement capabilities, providing dynamic weight-bearing intra-articular motion measurements that are difficult to otherwise obtain. Current efforts focus on automating the analysis to provide skeletal kinematics from image sequences with little operator intervention, and to develop novel radiographic imaging platforms with specific capabilities for tomography and dynamic imaging of the skeleton in motion. In principle, and as a direct extension of existing capabilities, these same techniques could be used for evaluating dynamic 3D motion of the natural foot and ankle.

REFERENCES

1. B.J. Fregly, W.G. Sawyer, M.K. Harman, and S.A. Banks, "Computational wear prediction of a total knee replacement from *in vivo* kinematics," *J Biomech,* vol. 38, pp. 305–314, 2005.
2. H. Tanino, M.K. Harman, S.A. Banks, and W.A. Hodge, "Relationship between polyethylene liner design, impingement and dislocation on retrieved acetabular components," 51st Annual Meeting of the Orthopaedic Research Society, Washington, D.C., 2005.

3. J.J. Crisco, R.D. McGovern, and S.W. Wolfe, "Noninvasive technique for measuring *in vivo* three-dimensional carpal bone kinematics," *J Orthop Res*, vol. 17, pp. 96–100, 1999.

4. A. Lundberg, "Kinematics of the ankle and foot. *In vivo* roentgen stereophotogrammetry," *Acta Orthop Scand Suppl*, vol. 233, pp. 1–24, 1989.

5. R. Tranberg and D. Karlsson, "The relative skin movement of the foot: a 2D roentgen photogrammetry study," *Clin Biomech (Bristol, Avon)*, vol. 13, pp. 71–76, 1998.

6. C. Hurschler, J. Emmerich, and N. Wulker, "*In vitro* simulation of stance phase gait part I: Model verification," *Foot Ankle Int*, vol. 24, pp. 614–622, 2003.

7. T. Stahelin, B.M. Nigg, D.J. Stefanyshyn, A.J. van den Bogert, and S.J. Kim, "A method to determine bone movement in the ankle joint complex *in vitro*," *J Biomech*, vol. 30, pp. 513–516, 1997.

8. S. Siegler, J. Chen, and C.D. Schneck, "The three-dimensional kinematics and flexibility characteristics of the human ankle and subtalar joints — Part I: Kinematics," *J Biomech Eng*, vol. 110, pp. 364–373, 1988.

9. C. Giacomozzi, S. Cesinaro, F. Basile, et al., "Measurement device for ankle joint kinematic and dynamic characterisation," *Med Biol Eng Comput* vol. 41, pp. 486–493, 2003.

10. M.W. Cornwall and T.G. McPoil, "Three-dimensional movement of the foot during the stance phase of walking," *J Am Podiatr Med Assoc*, vol. 89, pp. 56–66, 1999.

11. M.W. Cornwall and T.G. McPoil, "Motion of the calcaneus, navicular, and first metatarsal during the stance phase of walking," *J Am Podiatr Med Assoc*, vol. 92, pp. 67–76, 2002.

12. T.M. Kepple, S.J. Stanhope, K.N. Lohmann, and N.L. Roman, "A video-based technique for measuring ankle-subtalar motion during stance," *J Biomed Eng*, vol. 12, pp. 273–280, 1990.

13. S.M. Kidder, F.S. Abuzzahab, Jr., G.F. Harris, and J.E. Johnson, "A system for the analysis of foot and ankle kinematics during gait," *IEEE Trans Rehabil Eng*, vol. 4, pp. 25–32, 1996.

14. W. Liu, S. Siegler, H. Hillstrom, and K. Whitney, "Three-dimensional, six-degrees-of-freedom kinematics of the human hindfoot during the stance phase of level walking," *Human Mov Sci*, vol. 16, pp. 283–298, 1997.

15. S.H. Scott and D.A. Winter, "Biomechanical model of the human foot: kinematics and kinetics during the stance phase of walking," *J Biomech*, vol. 26, pp. 1091–1104, 1993.

16. K.L. Siegel, T.M. Kepple, P.G. O'Connell, L.H. Gerber, and S.J. Stanhope, "A technique to evaluate foot function during the stance phase of gait," *Foot Ankle Int*, vol. 16, pp. 764–770, 1995.

17. J. Fuller, L.J. Liu, M.C. Murphy, and R.W. Mann, "A comparison of lower-extremity skeletal kinematics measured using skin- and pin-mounted markers," *Hum Mov Sci*, vol. 16, pp. 219–242, 1997.

18. A. Cappozzo, "Three-dimensional analysis of human walking: Experimental methods and associated artifacts," *Hum Mov Sci*, vol. 10, pp. 589–602, 1991.

19. A.V. Lombardi, Jr., T.H. Mallory, D.A. Dennis, R.D. Komistek, R.A. Fada, and E.J. Northcut, "An *in vivo* determination of total hip arthroplasty pistoning during activity," *J Arthroplasty*, vol. 15, pp. 702–709, 2000.

20. H. Inaoka, A. Ishidal, Y. Fukuoka, K. Suzuki, and M. Matsubara, "Pose estimation of artificial hip joint using a single radiographic projection," *Med Biol Eng Comput*, vol. 41, pp. 94–100, 2003.

21. R.Y. Tsai, "A versatile camera calibration technique for high-accuracy 3D machine vision metrology using off-the-shelf TV cameras and lenses," *IEEE J Robotics Automation*, vol. 3, pp. 323–344, 1987.
22. G.Q. Wei and S. Dema, "Implicit and explicit camera calibration — theory and experiments," *IEEE Trans Pattern Anal Mach Intell*, vol. 16, pp. 469–480, 1994.
23. Z.Y. Zhang, "A flexible new technique for camera calibration," *IEEE Trans Pattern Anal Mach Intell*, vol. 22, pp. 1330–1334, 2000.
24. V. Baltzopoulos, "A videofluoroscopy method for optical distortion correction and measurement of knee-joint kinematics," *Clin Biomech (Bristol, Avon)*, vol. 10, pp. 85–92, 1995.
25. J.M. Boone, J.A. Seibert, W.A. Barrett, and E.A. Blood, "Analysis and correction of imperfections in the image intensifier-TV-digitizer imaging chain," *Med Phys*, vol. 18, pp. 236–242, 1991.
26. D.P. Chakraborty, "Image intensifier distortion correction," *Med Phys*, vol. 14, pp. 249–252, 1987.
27. E. Gronenschild, "The accuracy and reproducibility of a global method to correct for geometric image distortion in the x-ray imaging chain," *Med Phys*, vol. 24, pp. 1875–1888, 1997.
28. H. Haneishi, Y. Yagihashi, and Y. Miyake, "A new method for distortion correction of electronic endoscope images," *IEEE Trans Med Imaging*, vol. 14, pp. 548–555, 1995.
29. W.A. Wallace and F. Johnson, "Detection and correction of geometrical distortion in x-ray fluoroscopic images," *J Biomech*, vol. 14, pp. 123–125, 1981.
30. E. Gronenschild, "Correction for geometric image distortion in the x-ray imaging chain: local technique versus global technique," *Med Phys*, vol. 26, pp. 2602–2616, 1999.
31. S.J. Tupling and M.R. Pierrynowski, "Use of cardan angles to locate rigid bodies in 3-dimensional space," *Med Biol Eng Comput*, vol. 25, pp. 527–532, 1987.
32. W.A. Hodge, S.A. Banks, P.O. Riley, and C. Spector, "*In Vivo* kinematics of a meniscal bearing TKR during constrained stair rising," *Annual Meeting of the Association of Bone and Joint Surgeons*, Florida, 1991.
33. S.A. Banks and W.A. Hodge, "Accurate measurement of three-dimensional knee replacement kinematics using single-plane fluoroscopy," *IEEE Trans Biomed Eng*, vol. 43, pp. 638–649, 1996.
34. B.M. You, P. Siy, W. Anderst, and S. Tashman, "*In vivo* measurement of 3D skeletal kinematics from sequences of biplane radiographs: application to knee kinematics," *IEEE Trans Med Imaging*, vol. 20, pp. 514–525, 2001.
35. M.R. Mahfouz, W.A. Hoff, R.D. Komistek, and D.A. Dennis, "A robust method for registration of three-dimensional knee implant models to two-dimensional fluoroscopy images," *IEEE Trans Med Imaging*, vol. 22, pp. 1561–1574, 2003.
36. S. Lavallee and R. Szeliski, "Recovering the position and orientation of free-form objects from image contours using 3D distance maps," *IEEE Trans Pattern Anal Mach Intell*, vol. 17, pp. 378–390, 1995.
37. S. Zuffi, A. Leardini, F. Catani, S. Fantozzi, and A. Cappello, "A model-based method for the reconstruction of total knee replacement kinematics," *IEEE Trans Med Imaging*, vol. 18, pp. 981–991, 1999.
38. T. Yamazaki, T. Watanabe, Y. Nakajima, et al., "Improvement of depth position in 2D/3D registration of knee implants using single-plane fluoroscopy," *IEEE Trans Med Imaging*, vol. 23, pp. 602–612, 2004.

39. R. Barton, "Metamodels for simulation input-output relations," Winter Simulation Conference, Arlington, Virginia, 1992.

40. S. Laporte, W. Skalli, J.A. de Guise, F. Lavaste, and D. Mitton, "A biplanar reconstruction method based on 2D and 3D contours: application to the distal femur," *Comput Methods Biomech Biomed Engin*, vol. 6, pp. 1–6, 2003.

41. G. Li, T.H. Wuerz, and L.E. DeFrate, "Feasibility of using orthogonal fluoroscopic images to measure *in vivo* joint kinematics," *J Biomech Eng*, vol. 126, pp. 314–318, 2004.

42. B.L. Kaptein, E.R. Valstar, B.C. Stoel, P.M. Rozing, and J.H. Reiber, "A new model-based RSA method validated using CAD models and models from reversed engineering," *J Biomech*, vol. 36, pp. 873–882, 2003.

43. A. Short, H.S. Gill, B. Marks, et al., "A novel method for *in vivo* knee prosthesis wear measurement," *J Biomech*, vol. 38, pp. 315–322, 2005.

44. T. Asano, M. Akagi, K. Tanaka, J. Tamura, and T. Nakamura, "*In vivo* three-dimensional knee kinematics using a biplanar image-matching technique," *Clin Orthop Relat Res*, pp. 157–66, 2001.

45. A. Gefen, M. Megido-Ravid, Y. Itzchak, and M. Arcan, "Biomechanical analysis of the three-dimensional foot structure during gait: a basic tool for clinical applications," *J Biomech Eng*, vol. 122, pp. 630–639, 2000.

46. V.L. Giddings, G.S. Beaupre, R.T. Whalen, and D.R. Carter, "Calcaneal loading during walking and running," *Med Sci Sports Exerc*, vol. 32, pp. 627–634, 2000.

47. D.R. Green, T.E. Sgarlato, and M. Wittenberg, "Clinical biomechanical evaluation of the foot: a preliminary radiocinematographic study," *J Am Podiatry Assoc*, vol. 65, pp. 732–755, 1975.

48. S.C. Wearing, S. Urry, P. Perlman, J. Smeathers, and P. Dubois, "Sagittal plane motion of the human arch during gait: a videofluoroscopic analysis," *Foot Ankle Int*, vol. 19, pp. 738–742, 1998.

49. C. Mazza and A. Cappozzo, "An optimization algorithm for human joint angle time-history generation using external force data," *Ann Biomed Eng*, vol. 32, pp. 764–772, 2004.

50. T. Alkjaer, E.B. Simonsen, S.P. Magnusson, H. Aagaard, and P. Dyhre-Poulsen, "Differences in the movement pattern of a forward lunge in two types of anterior cruciate ligament deficient patients: copers and non-copers," *Clin Biomech*, vol. 17, pp. 586–593, 2002.

51. S.A. Banks and W.A. Hodge, "2003 Hap Paul Award paper of the International Society for Technology in Arthroplasty: Design and activity dependence of kinematics in fixed and mobile-bearing knee arthroplasties," *J Arthroplasty*, vol. 19, pp. 809–816, 2004.

33 Exploring the Frontiers of *In Vivo* Multibody Ankle Dynamics Using Fast-Phase Contrast Magnetic Resonance Imaging

Frances T. Sheehan, Andrea R. Seisler, and Karen Lohmann Siegel

CONTENTS

33.1 INTRODUCTION

Movement of the rearfoot relative to the lower leg is influenced by the motion of two joints: the talocrural and subtalar joints. Fundamental understanding of how these two joints influence rearfoot movement is based on classic work that began in the 1940s and 1950s on anatomical specimens.[1–4] These early studies described talocrural joint rotation as occurring about a simple floating hinge joint, implying that the rotation direction was constant, but the axis of rotation could move during joint motion.[1,4] Rotation of the subtalar joint has been described as occurring about either a fixed hinge joint[1,3,5,6] or a fixed screw axis.[2] These earlier studies found that neither the talocrural joint nor the subtalar joint axes were oriented within one cardinal body plane so that rotations about these axes were triplanar. Thus the terms "supination" and "pronation" were coined,[2] terms that are still commonly, although not consistently, used today. Supination consists of plantar flexion (PF) in the sagittal plane, inversion in the frontal or coronal plane, and internal rotation or adduction in the transverse plane. Pronation consists of dorsiflexion (DF), eversion, and external rotation or abduction.[2] In total, these studies concluded that the talocrural joint axis was primarily a transverse axis, while the subtalar joint axis was directed anteriorly and superiorly. Thus, rearfoot PF was attributed almost purely to talocrural rotation, whereas inversion and internal rotation were attributed to subtalar rotation.[1,2,6,7]

Clinical measures of the foot and the treatment decisions on which they are based (e.g., adhesive strapping, footwear prescription, and orthotic device design) are still closely tied to the conclusions of these early studies, even though more recent work has thrown these original findings into question. The assumption that calcaneal inversion/eversion occurs predominantly at the subtalar joint was restated as recently as 2005.[8] However, in the late 1980s, investigators demonstrated that commonly held beliefs in regard to the rearfoot axes of rotation were true or partially true only under specific circumstances. In an *in vitro* study of 15 limbs, Siegler et al.[9] clarified that DF–PF was the dominant motion at the talocrural joint and inversion/eversion was the dominant motion at the subtalar joint at or near the neutral position, but less so toward the end of the range of motion. They also reported that less than 10% of the DF–PF range of motion was coupled with inversion/eversion or ab/adduction. In an *in vivo* study of eight subjects, Lundberg et al.[10] showed the association between inversion and PF was weak and even associated with DF in some subjects. For foot eversion, they found more total motion occurred at the talonavicular joint than at the subtalar joint.[10]

Therefore, while more recent literature has suggested that the partition of motion between the talocrural and subtalar joints and the coupling of motion across planes may be less distinct than once thought, these studies have been few in number. The paucity of data, possibly due to the lack of noninvasive or minimally invasive techniques available to measure talar motion, may explain why clinicians have been slow to incorporate these findings and continue to base clinical practice on the older classic anatomical papers.[1-4] For example, a recent gait study tracked calcaneal eversion relative to the tibia as a proxy measure of subtalar joint pronation, based on the assumption that the three-dimensional rotations could be distinctly divided between the two joints.[8] More contemporary studies of *in vivo* talocrural and subtalar joint motion are needed to provide additional evidence on which to base clinical practice. Therefore, the purpose of this study was to test the feasibility of applying a noninvasive *in vivo* technique for the study of three-dimensional joint motion, fast-phase contrast magnetic resonance imaging (fast-PC MRI) to the study of talocrural and subtalar joint kinematics. To this end, we addressed three specific questions: (1) Do the talus and calcaneus move independently of each other? (2) If they do, can the rotation observed at the calcaneal–tibial complex be separated between the two joints? (3) Are the motions in one plane coupled with motions in other planes of movement?

33.2 METHODS

Six healthy male subjects (age = 25.5 ± 3.4 yr; weight = 66.3 ± 11.0 kg; height = 175.6 ± 5.6 cm), free of any foot pathology or pain, participated in this Institutional Review Board–approved study. For one subject (A6 and A7) both feet were studied because time permitted. After obtaining informed consent, subjects were placed

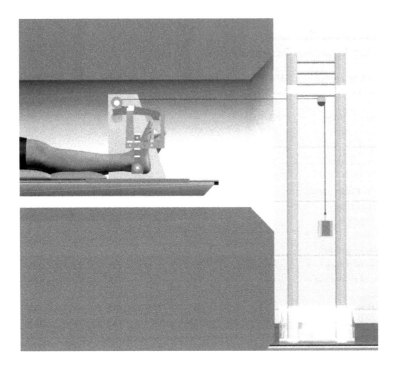

FIGURE 33.1 Subject placement within the MR imager. Each subject was placed in the MRI, such that the knee and hip were in full extension. The foot was then attached to the ALD using Coban® (3M, St. Paul, MN), so that the ball of the foot rested on the foot pedal of the ALD. A rope attached to the ALD passed over a pulley to a weight hanging outside the MRI, so that it provided resistance in PF. The ALD was designed so that the rope ran over a cam, creating a fixed moment arm for the tension in the rope.

supine in a 1.5 T MR scanner (LX; GE Medical Systems, Milwaukee, WI, U.S.), with the hip and knee maintained in full extension. A dual transmit–receive phased array MR coil was stabilized by a custom-built ankle loading device (ALD) medial and lateral to the ankle (Figure 33.1). The foot, covered only with a sock, was strapped to the freely moving foot pedal, with the heel resting in a heel groove located on the device base. A base plate extended from the pedal to the mid-calcaneus. This foot pedal allowed three degrees of rotational freedom at the ball of the foot. An optical trigger, which synchronized dynamic data collection to the motion cycle, was placed on the device, so that it would receive a signal at maximum DF.

After the subject was placed in the magnet and prior to the dynamic data collection, the ALD was locked into a position that allowed the subject to remain in the neutral position (tib–foot angle ≈ 0°– Figure 33.1) without muscle activation. The other two degrees of freedom were not locked. An axial gradient echo sequence (Table 33.1) was then acquired.

For the dynamic scans, the locking pins, used statically, were moved such that the subject's motion was limited to a comfortable, repeatable range. This range was

TABLE 33.1
Imaging Sequence Parameters

Imaging Sequences	3D GRE	Fastcard	Fast-PC	Fastcard
Plane	Axial	Sagittal oblique	Sagittal oblique	Axial
Number of slices	~ 80–100	1	1	2
Repetition time (msec)	12.2	5.0	9.0	5.0
Echo time (msec)	5.2	1.3	4.3	1.3
Field of view (cm)	24 × 24	24 × 24	30 × 30	24 × 24
Slice thickness (mm)	1.5	10.0	10.0	10.0
Flip angle (deg)	30	20	20	20
Max. velocity encoding	—	—	30	—
Number of averages	1	1	2	1
Number of views	—	16	2	16
Temporal resolution (msec)	—	54	72	54
Time frames	—	24	24	24
Imaging time	6:30	0:17	3:42	0:34

typically 1 to 5° less than the subject's maximum range of motion. The external weight system (Figure 33.1) was adjusted, so the cable was taut with a 2.3 kg (5 lb) weight, hanging freely outside of the bore. The weight system was specifically designed to apply a load to the ankle joint away from the subject, to ensure artifacts did not disrupt the MR images, and to provide resistance during PF. Subjects maintained a repeated DF–PF movement of the foot relative to the tibia at the rate of 35 cycles/min guided by an auditory metronome, for each dynamic sequence.

A dynamic exam involved three movement trials. A fastcard sequence (Table 33.1) in a sagittal–oblique imaging plane (Figure 33.2a) that bisected the Achilles tendon and passed through the tibia, talus, and calcaneus was acquired first. This dataset was used as a practice for the subject and also served to ensure that the fast-PC sequence was selected at the proper imaging location. Next, at a single sagittal or sagittal/oblique location, a full fast-PC dataset (Table 33.1 — anatomic and x, y, and z velocity images) was acquired (Figure 33.3). Finally, a fastcard sequence was acquired at two axial levels (Table 33.1). The axial planes were defined from the anatomic image representing neutral foot position, relative to the tibia, in the fast-PC image set (Figure 33.2b). The tib–foot angle (Figure 33.4) was defined as the angle between a vector perpendicular to the anterior edge of the tibia and a vector connecting the most inferior, posterior calcaneal point to the inferior metatarsal heads. The orientation and displacement of the calcaneus, talus, and tibia were individually quantified by integrating velocity data, obtained during the fast-PC acquisition, using Fourier integration.[11] The initial bone orientation was then calculated using anatomically based coordinate systems that were identified in a single

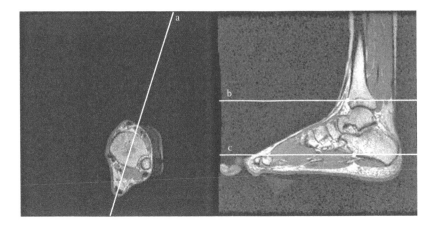

FIGURE 33.2 Dynamic imaging planes. *Line A:* Defined the sagittal–oblique imaging plane (seen on the right); bisected the Achilles tendon; and passed through the tibia, talus, and calcaneus. This imaging plane was used for acquisition of fast-PC data (anatomic and *x, y, and z* velocity images). *Line B:* Defined the tibial axial imaging plane (*left*) and was selected through the most anterior portion of the distal tibia in the sagittal view. *Line C:* Defined the calcaneal axial plane and was selected through the most anterior inferior point on the calcaneus. The latter two imaging planes were used for acquisition of fastcard data (anatomic images only).

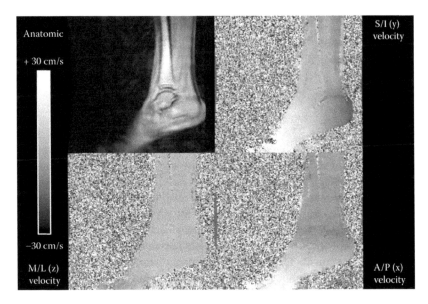

FIGURE 33.3 Fast-PC MRI images in the PF position. The above images represent a single time frame, out of 24, in the DF–PF cycle of ankle A4. Black and white pixels indicate the minimum (–30 cm/sec) and maximum (30 cm/sec) velocities, respectively. During this time frame, the foot is plantar flexing relative to the tibia. This results in an inferior movement of the toes and a superior movement of the calcaneus. These velocities are represented by the white pixels at the toes and the darker pixels at the calcaneus. Less velocity is seen in the other two directions.

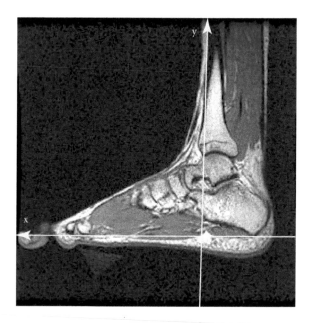

FIGURE 33.4 Determination of the tib-foot angle. The above figure is from the static series of A5. The tib-foot angle is the angle between y *and* $x - 90°$, where y is the line adjacent to the anterior tibia and x is the line connecting the most posterior, inferior point on the calcaneus and the inferior metatarsal heads. This calculation allows the neutral position to be defined as $0°$. The points defining x and y are defined once and tracked throughout the motion cycle based on the integrated fast-PC data. The point on the inferior metatarsal heads is assumed to be rigidly connected to the calcaneus. Note that this image was taken with a tib-foot angle slightly less than $0°$.

time frame only (Figure 33.5). Using matrix multiplication, the attitude of all three bones relative to the imaging coordinate system throughout the movement was defined using the anatomically based coordinate systems. Again, using matrix multiplication, the orientation matrices for each bone relative to the imager were converted into the orientation matrices of the talus relative to the tibia (talocrural joint), the calcaneus relative to the talus (subtalar joint), and the calcaneus relative to the tibia (calcaneal–tibial complex). The entire movement cycle was used for the integration process, but all further analysis and data presentation were limited to the PF portion of the movement. Then orientations for the talocrural, subtalar, and calcaneal–tibial joints were simplified to three cardan rotation angles using a zyx-body-fixed sequence. After the rotation angles were calculated, the rotations about the x- and y-axes and translations along the z-axis were negated for the right leg and the rotations about the z-axis were negated for both legs. Thus, the first rotation was about the z-axis, and PF was positive, the second rotation was about the y-axis and external rotation was positive, and the third rotation was about the x-axis and eversion was positive. Using the known time-dependent orientation and translations of the calcaneal–tibial complex, the tib–foot angle (Figure 33.4) was tracked by assuming

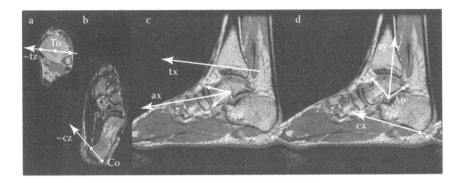

FIGURE 33.5 Anatomically based coordinate system. All axes were defined in the image representing the tib-foot angle as close to the neutral position as possible. The *x*-axis was defined first. The tibial **tx** (C) was defined as the line connecting the most anterior and posterior points on the distal tibia in the sagittal image. The calcaneal **cx** (D) was defined as the line connecting the most anterior inferior point and the most posterior inferior on the calcaneus in the sagittal image. The talar **ax** (C) was defined as the line that bisects the arc formed by the two lines connecting the talar sinus, with the most anterior superior and anterior inferior talar points in the sagittal image. A temporary *z*-axis (**tz**$_{temp}$, **cz**$_{temp}$) was formed for the tibia and calcaneus. The tibial **tz**$_{temp}$ (A) was defined as the line connecting the most lateral and medial points in the tibial axial image. The calcaneal **cz**$_{temp}$ (B) was defined as the line connecting the most convex point of the posterior medial curve and the most convex point of the posterior lateral curve of the calcaneus in the calcaneal axial image. A temporary *y*-axis (**ay**$_{temp}$) was formed for the talus. The talar **ay**$_{temp}$ (D) was defined as the line which bisected the arc formed by the lines from the talar origin, ao, to the anterior point at which the superior surface changes from concave to convex on the talar dome and the most posterior point on the talar dome in the sagittal image. The *y*-axis for the tibia and calcaneus was defined as the cross-product of the *x*-axis and its temporary *z*-axis. The *z*-axis for the talus was defined as the cross-product of the *x*-axis and its temporary *y*-axis. Then the tibial and calcaneal *z*-axis was defined as the cross-product between the *x*- and *y*-axes for each body. The talar *y*-axis was formed by the cross-product of the talar *z*-axis and the talar *x*-axis.

that the point on the inferior metatarsal heads was rigidly attached to the calcaneus. Since these data were taken with respect to time and not the tib–foot angle, interpolation was used to present the orientation angles with respect to tib–foot angle in 1° increments.

33.3 RESULTS

The rotations (Figure 33.6) and translations (Figure 33.7) of the talocrural and subtalar joints demonstrated that the two joints did not move as a single joint, as they are often modeled, nor did the joints rotate as typically described clinically. The majority of all rotations occurred at the talocrural joint, with minimal rotations occurring at the subtalar joint. At the talocrural joint, supination was observed for all subjects. The consistency across subjects varied based on the degree of freedom (three rotations

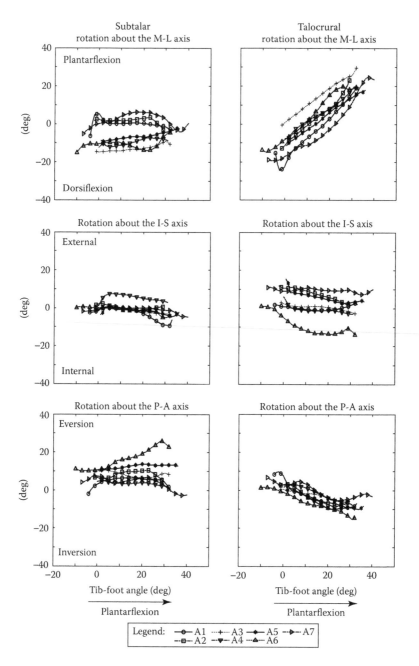

FIGURE 33.6 3D orientations of the calcaneus relative to the talus (*left column*) and talus relative to the tibia (*right column*). These angles are based on a *zyx*-body fixed cardan angle rotation sequence. To maintain anatomical directions, the rotations about the inferior–superior axis (*y*) and the posterior–anterior axis (*x*) are negated for the right leg, and rotations about the right–left axis are negated for both legs. Thus, PF, external rotation, and eversion are positive.

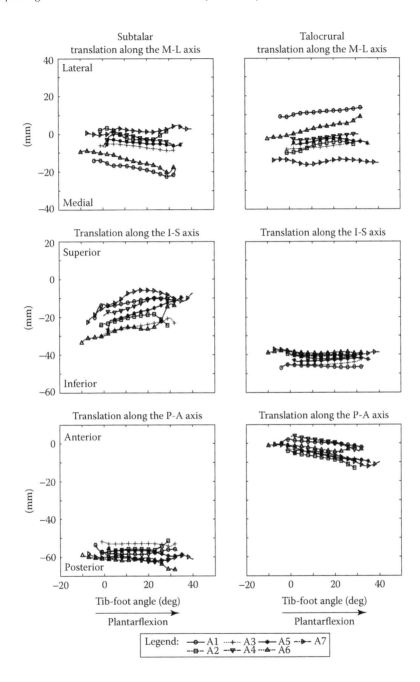

FIGURE 33.7 3D translations of the calcaneus origin relative to the talar coordinate system (*left column*) and the talus origin relative to the tibial coordinate system (*right column*). To maintain anatomical directions, the translation along the right–left axis are negated for the right leg. Thus, the anterior, superior, and lateral are positive.

TABLE 33.2
Change in Orientation for Each Joint during PF

	A1	A2	A3	A4	A5	A6	A7	Average
			Plantar Flexion (deg)					
Talocrural	44.1	36.1	30.0	27.5	29.2	34.5	44.2	35.1
Subtalar	11.8	−6.5	5.7	4.9	6.9	10.7	11.6	6.4
Cal-tib	37.6	31.4	33.5	31.5	35.5	42.8	47.7	37.1
			External Rotation (deg)					
Talocrural	3.8	−10.0	−5.6	−9.0	−12.6	−15.1	−3.8	−7.5
Subtalar	−9.6	−3.7	−3.4	6.4	4.5	−5.8	−5.8	−2.5
Cal-tib	−8.3	−10.4	−5.6	−5.8	−11.8	−18.0	−7.8	−9.7
			Eversion (deg)					
Talocrural	−18.8	−11.8	−10.1	−10.7	−11.2	−16.9	−12.1	−13.1
Subtalar	8.5	−5.2	−4.1	−3.7	3.8	15.6	−10.0	0.7
Cal-tib	−18.4	−10.0	−12.6	−14.3	−9.8	−6.0	−17.4	−12.6

Each entry represents the difference in value of rotational degree of freedom (PF — top, external rotation — middle, and Eversion — bottom) between maximum and minimum tib-foot angle. The sign associated with each entry defines if a positive or negative change in angle occurred between the maximum and minimum tib-foot angle. Due to the nonlinear nature of cardan rotation angles, the rotation at the talocrural and subtalar joints do not necessary need to sum to the rotation at the calcaneal–tibial complex.

and three translations), but for nearly all rotations, the variation became minimal in the range of maximum DF (~ −15°) to neutral ankle angle (0°).

PF occurred primarily at the talocrural joint, with little PF at the subtalar joint (Figure 33.6, top row). Talocrural PF was quite consistent across subjects, but the curves were offset from each other. On the other hand, subtalar PF demonstrated differences in both value and slope across subjects. One subject, A1, demonstrated a DF trend at the subtalar joint and a PF trend at the talocrural joint.

For the majority of subjects, there was only slight internal rotation, and this occurred primarily at the talocrural joint (Figure 33.6, middle row). Unlike the other two rotations, a small but consistent pattern of internal rotation was seen.

Inversion clearly occurred at the talocrural joint (Figure 33.6, bottom row), with an average internal rotation of 10.7° (Table 33.2). At the subtalar joint, there was typically minimal inversion, but interestingly, three subjects (A1, A5, and A6) demonstrated eversion at this joint. The strong eversion of A6 (15.6°) pulled the average rotation for all subjects up to 0.7° (Table 33.2). Internal rotation at the subtalar joint and inversion at the talocrural joint had the most consistent patterns and values, across subjects, out of all the angles reported.

All subjects followed consistent patterns of displacement for both joints (Figure 33.7). In general, the calcaneus shifted medially and superiorly with little anterior movement and the talus moved laterally, slightly inferiorly, and posteriorly during PF. While the patterns of rotation were consistent across subjects, there were larger offsets between subjects in lateral translation for both joints and superior translation of the subtalar joint.

33.4 DISCUSSION

In order to improve diagnostic accuracy, prevent injury, and reduce the impact of impairments on rearfoot function, an understanding of the *in vivo* kinematics of the talocrural and subtalar joints is critical. Previous studies have shown that fast-PC MRI[12] is an excellent tool for quantifying musculoskeletal dynamics and is both accurate[13] (system bias = 0.06 mm (SD, 0.35) and a measured average absolute error of 0.35 to 0.5 mm) and precise[14] (SD between two trials for six subjects was equal to 1.2, 1.5, and 0.7° for tibiofemoral extension, external rotation, and valgus, respectively). Such precision and accuracy are quite comparable to biplane radiographic imaging.[15] This study was able to build upon these earlier imaging studies and demonstrate that this noninvasive and nonionizing technique was a feasible and revealing tool for the *in vivo* study of talocrural and subtalar joint three-dimensional kinematics joints during volitional activity. The results from this and future fast-PC MRI studies will help advance clinical areas such as total ankle replacement development, orthosis design, and ankle pathology diagnostics.

The functional movement evaluated in the current study can be related to a subject standing with the balls of their feet on a beam under their own muscular control, raising and lowering partial body weight through a range of motion just shy of the maximum PF and DF. In general, intersubject variability was small and typically more variability occurred due to offsets between subjects than due to the pattern of movement. For nearly all rotations, the intersubject variability was lower from maximum DF to neutral tib–foot angle, and there was less nonsagittal plane rotation in this range than in later PF. These kinematic patterns are likely due to the talus "locking" into the mortise. Also, for the subtalar joint, the manner in which the current coordinate system was defined forced the external rotation angle to be zero at the neutral tib–foot angle. Alterations to the coordinate system are planned, which will eliminate any predefined relationships, with an ultimate goal of finding an easily defined coordinate system that produces minimal intersubject variability.

Classic clinical knowledge,[1,6,9,16] stating that the majority of the PF excursion observed at the calcaneal–tibial complex occurs at the talocrural joint, was confirmed in this study, with an average of 95% of total calcaneal–tibial motion occurring at the talocrural joint. However, these prior studies also predicted that motion in the frontal and transverse planes occurred at the subtalar, not the talocrural joint.[1,2,6,7,9,16] Total motion at the subtalar joint on average was less than 7° about any axis and much smaller than those reported in any prior study of this joint.[2,7,17] This study demonstrated that on average 77% of the total internal rotation of the calcaneus relative to the tibia occurred at the talocrural joint, not the subtalar joint. Even more surprisingly, total inversion excursion was slightly greater on average at the talocrural joint than at the calcaneal–tibial complex, with three subjects demonstrating eversion at the subtalar joint. It is important not to overstate this result; two (A1, A5) of the three subjects (A1, A5, A6) demonstrating eversion at the subtalar joint did so to only a small extent.

In total, these results call into question the assumptions of prior kinematic studies regarding, which joint motions calcaneal–tibial angles truly represent.[8]

Although direct comparison to previous studies is difficult due to the unique advancements of the current study, these past studies do provide excellent checks in terms of the observed ranges of motion. The current data do agree that calcaneal–tibial motion about a transverse axis showed the greatest excursion. On average 37.1° of PF was observed at the calcaneal–tibial complex with 35.1° occurring at the talocrural joint. Previous static evaluations of the talocrural joint have reported 43°,[18] 53°,[10] and 66°[09] of available DF–PF range of motion. As previously noted, subjects' volitional motion in this study typically occurred within 1 to 5° of their available maximum and Lundberg et al.[16] clearly stated that the 53° was not easily obtained in living subjects. The even greater amount of DF–PF seen in cadaver studies is likely outside a reasonable anatomical range due to the loss of soft-tissue forces. In these previous studies, total joint excursion was determined from the peak-to-peak motion during movement imposed in one plane of motion, while joint position in the other two planes was maintained near the neutral position. For these other axes of motion, 13.1° of talocrural inversion in this study is a bit higher than the reported 7.3°[10] and 9.8°[09] of total inversion/eversion excursion, and the average 7.5° of talocrural internal rotation appears more reasonable when compared to 11.8°[16] than 26.5°[09] of total internal/external rotation excursion reported in previous studies.

The likely reason for the discrepancies between the early cadaver studies and the current results is the fact that, in these cadaver studies, the talus was either forced against the tibia[6] or the talocrural joint was placed in a more dorsiflexed position, which would lock it into the mortise and limit its rotational freedom in inversion and internal rotation. Previous studies[1,6] distributed rotation among the talocrural and subtalar joints based on the joint axes of rotations, defined from statically positioning the joint in various poses. A later cadaver study[9] quantified the three-dimensional orientations of each joint, but proportionally assigned equal internal rotation to both joints. The feet were statically positioned through a range of postures by using a single-axis rotational displacement, while maintaining the orientation about the other axes near neutral position. Since the three-dimensional rotations of a joint are not independent from each other, single-axis rotation limits the ability to generalize these data. Also, when working with cadavers, the effect of volitional muscular control and postmortem changes cannot be easily quantified.

The work of Lundberg et al.[10,16] in living subjects clearly shows the limits of talus rotation when the calcaneal–tibia complex is put into a more dorsiflexed position. When subjects were statically positioned in varying degrees of tibial–calcaneal inversion/eversion,[10] with the joint maintained in a more dorsiflexed position, nearly all the rotation was isolated to the subtalar joint. Yet, when the foot was brought through a range of DF–PF in these same subjects,[16] nearly all the rotation occurred at the talocrural joint. Thus, it would appear that both the subtalar and the talocrural joints are able to invert and internally rotate, but these motions only occur at the talocrural joint if the talus is not locked into the mortise.

A recent invasive study[19] provided a methodology that was closer to the current study by evaluating *in vivo* rearfoot kinematics during gait, using bone screws, and found that PF occurred primarily at the talocrural joint. Note, that the range of PF was limited (average range was 13.5°) potentially by either the bone screws or the gait pattern studied. This gait study measured a three-dimensional orientation in terms of two-dimensional projection angles. Such projection angles could easily produce different results when compared to three-dimensional cardan rotation angles for the identical movement. Unlike previous cadaver studies, Arndt et al.[19] found that inversion and internal rotation was proportioned almost equally between the talocrural and subtalar joints, with high variability across subjects. Compared to this invasive study of rearfoot kinematics during gait, the current results showed greater excursions at both joints, with the exception of subtalar inversion and internal rotation.[13,14] The greater excursions are consistent with the greater DF–PF motion seen in the current data, and the exceptions at the subtalar joint are likely due to individual subjects who demonstrated a change in orientation that was opposite to the majority of subjects. For example, A4 demonstrated internal rotation except in the early portion of PF, creating an overall external rotation pattern. Thus, in general, this previous study[19] and the current study appear to support each other's results.

As noted above, PF clearly was associated with inversion and, to a lesser extent, internal rotation, the three components of supination. These results support the concept of coupled rotations across the three planes of movement first proposed in early studies,[2] but not the work of Siegler et al.,[9] who reported less than 10% of PF range of motion was coupled with inversion or adduction. Coupled rotations were clearly seen at the talocrural joint, but were more ambiguous at the subtalar joint. Paradoxically, three feet (A1, A5, and A6) demonstrated subtalar joint eversion during PF, while both the talocrural joint and the calcaneal–tibial complex showed inversion. Lundberg et al.[10] also reported some variability in the association between DF–PF and inversion/eversion in some of their subjects, but noted this at the subtalar, not the talocrural joint. In this study, internal rotation during PF was minimal at both the talocrural and the subtalar joints, suggesting this motion may occur at joints within the foot distal to the subtalar joint. While Lundberg[16] found comparable amounts of internal rotation at both the talocrural and the subtalar joints, they did note 10° more internal/external rotation at the talonavicular joint than at the two more proximal joints.

Joint translations were noted at both joints along all three directions of motion to varying extents. This is not consistent with early literature that described the talocrural and subtalar joints as simple fixed hinge joints.[1,3,5] The talus origin demonstrated posterior along with minimal superior displacement, indicating that the origin is likely close to the axis of rotation and that the whole bone translates posteriorly during PF. Similarly, the calcaneal origin translates superiorly with little anterior displacement, most likely indicating an overall anterior movement of the bone. Future analyses based on the finite helical axes are planned to better flush out the relationships between orientation and displacement, but from the current results, it is clear that neither joint is a fixed hinge joint.

33.5 CONCLUSIONS

This study accomplished its stated goal in demonstrating fast-PC MRI a feasible and useful tool to noninvasively study three-dimensional joint motion and provided new insight into the study of talocrural and subtalar joint kinematics. It revealed that the talocrural and subtalar joints do move independently of one another, but not in the manner described in classic anatomical studies. Talocrural motion accounted for greater than 77% of calcaneal–tibial motion in all three rotational directions, while subtalar joint motion was minimal. Results did confirm earlier reports of coupled motions, finding that PF was accompanied by inversion and, to a lesser extent, internal rotation, but these motions all occurred at the talocrural joint, not the subtalar joint. These findings call into question the earlier anatomical studies on which much of clinical practice on the foot and ankle is based. The two key sources for this discrepancy are the locking of the talus into the mortise during DF, and the realistic movements that are associated with noninvasive *in vivo* studies. Thus, future study is warranted.

ACKNOWLEDGMENTS

The authors would like to thank Tracy Rausch for her help with device design, device building, and data collection; Jeanine Graham for her support in patient data management; Jere McLucas for his assistance in figure preparation; and Steven Stanhope, Ph.D. for guidance throughout this project and his editorial comments. This material is based upon work supported by a Whitaker Young Investigator's Grant. Any opinions, findings, and conclusions or recommendations expressed in this material are those of the authors and do not necessarily reflect the views of the Whitaker Foundation, the National Institutes of Health, or the U.S. Public Health Service.

REFERENCES

1. Hicks, J.H., The mechanics of the foot. I. The joints, *J Anat*, 87, 345, 1953.
2. Manter, J.T., Movements of the subtalar and transverse tarsal joints, *Anat Rec*, 80, 397, 1941.
3. Root, M.L. et al., Axis of motion of the subtalar joint: an anatomical study, *J Am Podiatr Med Assoc*, 56, 149, 1966.
4. Barnett, C.H. and Napier, J.R., The axis of rotation at the ankle joint in man; its influence upon the form of the talus and the mobility of the fibula, *J Anat*, 86, 1, 1952.
5. Wright, D.G., Desai, S.M. and Henderson, W.H., Action of the subtalar and ankle-joint complex during the stance phase of walking, *J Bone Joint Surg*, 46-A, 361, 1964.
6. Isman, R.E. and Inman, V.T., Anthropometric studies of the human foot and ankle, *Bull Prosth Res*, 10–11, 97, 1969.
7. Close, J.R. et al., The function of the subtalar joint, *Clin Orthop Relat Res*, 50, 159, 1967.
8. Youberg, L.D. et al., The amount of rearfoot motion used during the stance phase of walking, *J Am Podiatr Med Assoc*, 95, 376, 2005.
9. Siegler, S., Chen, J. and Schneck, C.D., The three-dimensional kinematics and flexibility characteristics of the human ankle and subtalar joints—Part I: Kinematics, *J Biomech Eng*, 110, 364, 1988.
10. Lundberg, A. et al., Kinematics of the ankle/foot complex—Part 2: Pronation and supination, *Foot Ankle*, 9, 248, 1989.
11. Zhu, Y., Drangova, M. and Pelc, N.J., Fourier tracking of myocardial motion using cine-PC data, *Magn Reson Med*, 35, 471, 1996.

12. Foo, T.K. et al., Improved ejection fraction and flow velocity estimates with use of view sharing and uniform repetition time excitation with fast cardiac techniques, *Radiology*, 195, 471, 1995.

13. Sheehan, F.T., Zajac, F.E. and Drace, J.E., Using cine phase contrast magnetic resonance imaging to non-invasively study in vivo knee dynamics, *J Biomech*, 31, 21, 1998.

14. Rebmann, A.J. and Sheehan, F.T., Precise 3D skeletal kinematics using fast phase contrast magnetic resonance imaging, *J Magn Reson Imaging*, 17, 206, 2003.

15. Tashman, S. and Anderst, W., In-vivo measurement of dynamic joint motion using high speed biplane radiography and CT: application to canine ACL deficiency, *J Biomech Eng*, 125, 238, 2003.

16. Lundberg, A., Kinematics of the ankle and foot. In vivo roentgen stereophotogrammetry, *Acta Orthop Scand Suppl*, 233, 1, 1989.

17. Pearce, T.J. and Buckley, R.E., Subtalar joint movement: clinical and computed tomography scan correlation, *Foot Ankle Int*, 20, 428, 1999.

18. Sammarco, G.J., Burstein, A.H. and Frankel, V.H., Biomechanics of the ankle: a kinematic study, *Orthop Clin North Am*, 4, 75, 1973.

19. Arndt, A. et al., Ankle and subtalar kinematics measured with intracortical pins during the stance phase of walking, *Foot Ankle Int*, 25, 357, 2004.

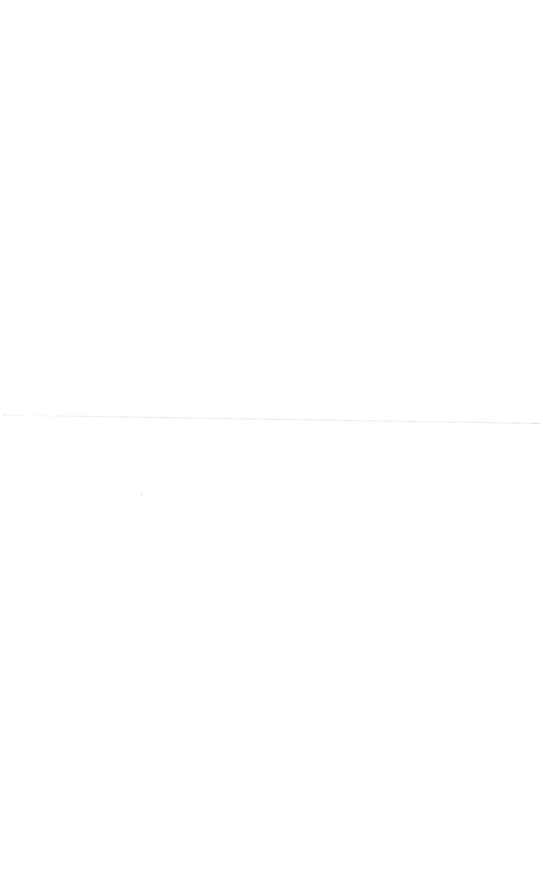

34 Kinetic Measures of the Foot: Overcoming Current Obstacles

Bruce A. MacWilliams

CONTENTS

34.1 INTRODUCTION

Analysis of net joint moments and powers is routinely used in gait analysis to assist with clinical decision making and in research to understand function and surgical outcomes. If a more detailed analysis of the motion of the foot was available, this could potentially lead to better clinical decision making and better understanding of both the normal and pathological functions of the foot. Unfortunately, standard gait models treat the foot as a single rigid segment and neither the motions nor the forces within the various joints in the foot are computed.

Recently, spurred by advancements in camera technology, there have been several publications concerning multisegment foot modeling.[1–9] These studies have all measured kinematics within various joints of the foot. Kinetic measures of these same joints are not computed due to a number of technological difficulties. This chapter will discuss these difficulties, how they may be overcome with current technology, and how future technological advancements may be applied to make this assessment a clinical reality. The methods described here have been used to report kinematics and kinetics of a normal pediatric population.[10] An expansion of the procedures used

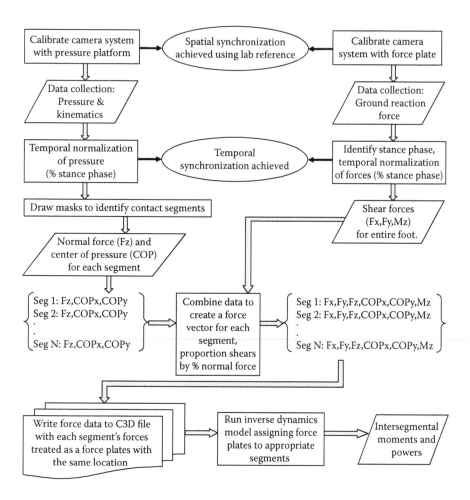

FIGURE 34.1 Flowchart depicting the sequence of methods used to derive kinetics in a multisegment foot model.

in this study is presented here along with additional suggestions, which may streamline and improve the process. The methodology is outlined in general terms and is not limited to a specific kinematic model. A flowchart of these methods is presented in Figure 34.1.

34.2 METHODS

34.2.1 DISTRIBUTED FORCE MEASURES

In clinical gait analysis, kinetic measurements are possible when a single force vector is measured acting on a single segment (typically the foot, treated as a single, rigid segment). As many movement lab practitioners are aware, when both feet contact the same force plate, kinetics are invalidated in the gait model. The problem is that a single force vector cannot be used to establish the relative forces and centers of pressure of multiple segments. When treating the foot as a multisegmental body, this situation of multiple segment contact on a force plate may be present throughout stance phase, depending on the location and definition of the individual segments.

Thus, to measure forces within multiple segments of the foot, some form of distributed force measure is required. This may be achieved through the use of either small force sensors placed in a shoe under the segments of interest or a contiguous grid of sensors to span multiple segments. Such grids are designed to either be placed in a shoe or as stationary mat or platform systems to walk over.

34.2.2 SHEAR FORCES

One drawback of these sensor grids is that they currently are only able to measure vertical force, equivalently expressed as pressure, giving rise to the term "pedobarograph." One potential solution to measure the full compliment of ground reaction forces is to integrate the pressure mat and forceplate technology. Normal forces and center of pressure may be determined by the sensor grid for each individual segment, and shear forces may be approximated by distributing the force vector among the various segments by a weighting scheme based on the percentage of normal force in each segment, such that the normal force Fn is the sum of each of its n components:

$$Fn = \sum_{i=1}^{N} Fn_i$$

The shear force Fs for any given segment i is given by

$$Fs_i = Fs\left(\frac{Fn_i}{Fn}\right)$$

This would be applied to each of the shear components, which include a medial/lateral shear force, anterior/posterior shear force, and moment in the plane normal to the plantar surface. If such a scheme is employed, it must be validated for any particular model, as it is possible to have high shears in some areas in the absence of significant normal force.

34.2.3 DATA COLLECTION AND SYNCHRONIZATION

Currently, collection of the full complement of data necessary to make kinetic computations of the foot is only achievable through separate systems of hardware and software. This requires postprocessing of the data to achieve both spatial and temporal synchronization. One possibility that solves or at least simplifies both the spatial and temporal issues is to physically integrate the hardware systems by attaching a mat system to a force plate; however, thickness of the pressure mat and the raised flooring necessary for some systems to accommodate this thickness may prove a deterrent. If data are collected in separate walking trials, identification of stance phase events (initial contact and final contact) and time normalization may be used to temporally synchronize the data. Spatial synchronization may be performed either by using reflective markers to identify pressure devices or through separate volume calibrations. If the latter approach is used, registration between the two devices may be achieved by aligning the reference frames with appropriate offsets. The local coordinate systems used during measurement in each system must also be appropriately accounted for with postprocessing. Ideally, force and pressure systems may be integrated such that data are collected simultaneously, with synchronized onsets of data collection and sampling at equal rates or multiples of rates (an example of the latter is video collected at 60 Hz and force plate data collected at 600 Hz or 1200 Hz).

In the cited publication, force and plantar pressure systems could not be integrated because of dimensional constraints, and data for each system had to be collected from separate trials.[10] Additionally, data from the plantar pressure system could only be collected at 50 Hz while data from the motion capture system could only be collected at multiples of 60 Hz. Thus, there were several obstacles to overcome regarding data synchronicity. First, it is recognized that although stance in healthy individuals is highly repeatable, there may be slight differences in stance time due to velocity or other changes, which may result in small differences between trials. To minimize these changes, the force plate trials were matched with plantar pressure trials according to stance time, which could be accurately determined by monitoring the forces and pressures to identify initial and final contact events. The single force plate trial, which most closely matched the average stance phase duration of the five pressure platform trials, was selected. To account for the differences in the data collection rates, each data set was time normalized and resampled at every 2% of the stance phase using a spline technique.[10] This procedure additionally allowed trials of varying stance times to be compared and averaged as data were interpolated to specific percentages of stance phase. While this procedure may be valid for highly repeatable stance phases, individuals with various pathologies may exhibit variations large enough that this process of trial matching would not yield accurate results.

34.2.4 PARTITIONING OF PRESSURE DATA

For kinetic computation, each segment of the foot, which contacts the ground, must have a specified six component ground reaction force vector consisting of a normal force (Fz), medial/lateral and anterior/posterior shear forces (Fx and Fy), normal moment (Mz), and a center of pressure location of the vector ($COPx$ and $COPy$). The measurements for each of these segments must somehow be derived from the force and/or pressure measurement technology used for data collection. How this is achieved is dependent upon the measurement technology used.

If in-shoe force sensors are used for measurement, the force locations relative to the foot may be known *a priori*; however, such force sensors may only cover small regions of the foot and some contact information may be lost. If a pressure

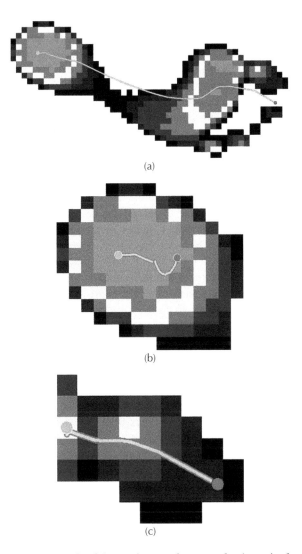

FIGURE 34.2 (a) Is an example of the continuum of pressure for the entire foot during stance with the center of pressure line indicated. Bottom images are examples of specific areas of the foot, which have been masked from the continuum. (b) Shows the entire heel as a segment; (c) Shows the hallux. The segmental center of pressure lines are shown for these segments.

sensor matrix is used, another set of problems arises. With this technology, the sensors span the various contact segments, resulting in a time-varying continuum of data representing the entire plantar surface. Some partitioning of the data must be undertaken to relate pressure regions to the segments of interest. In our own work, we resorted to hand drawing "masks" on pressure data to correlate with the contact segments defined in our kinematic model (Figure 34.2).[10] This process involves the qualitatively selective process of interpretation of the foot shape and the definition of locations and orientations of segment boundaries. Fortunately, for this particular model, when applied to a healthy population, the motion segments defined matched well with pressure areas, which were easily identifiable because of the large gradients demarcating the boundaries of interest. In pathological feet, however, these boundaries may not be present, and thus error could be introduced to the model due to the subjective interpretation of matching pressure areas to contact areas.

This problem of introducing subjective interpretation into the partitioning of the pressure continuum is easily overcome. Knowledge of reflective marker locations could potentially be used to automatically partition the pressure data using accurate positional data, which could be mapped directly onto the pressure matrix. This could further be enhanced by the use of virtual markers, marker points determined during static trials, which are used to relate anatomical points to physical marker points. These virtual markers could be used to specify the boundaries of the pressure map using anatomical references. This would require integration of the video and pressure systems, which, to date, has not been accomplished commercially, but could be overcome with custom software.

Once "masks" are applied to the pressure continuum, the problem then shifts to one of how to utilize the data contained within these areas of interest. How this is performed is of course dependent both upon the system and software utilized to collect and process the pressure data and upon the application, which will then utilize these data. In our work, this process required the following cumbersome procedure. The entire pressure continuum file reflecting stance phase of the whole foot was opened, then one mask at a time was hand drawn using a software application to outline the contact segment of interest (in our model there were six such contact segments). All pressures outside this mask were then deleted and a new file was created, which contained only the pressures within the masked area. An additional step was required using another program to override automated side and orientation manipulation as the software attempted to interpret each mask as an entire left or right foot oriented in a forward or backward direction. Once corrected to specify the correct side and orientation of the segment, yet another application was needed to export the data to an ASCII file format, which could then be read by subsequent software, which extrapolated the normal force and center of pressure within the mask. This process was then repeated for each contact segment. The remaining shear terms were then added using the force plate data according to the process described previously. This resulted in a full complement of force components for each individual contact segment. The following discussion covers utilization of this force information.

34.2.5 Force Input File Specifications

While custom software may be developed to perform inverse dynamic computations, most users would likely prefer to use the same software utilized for clinical gait analysis or another commercial package, which interfaces with the hardware, database, and file formats used for motion capture. One obstacle caused by using these commercial products is their reliance on standard file formats (e.g., the C3D or TRC file format) for input. The commercial software packages are set up to handle various force information stored in the standard file format by reading information contained within the file, which specifies the type of commercial force plate used to generate the data. Appropriate gains, scales, and offsets are applied to translate analog voltage data into force values. Plantar pressure systems are not recognized as valid devices. To utilize information from a pressure mat or platform, pressure data must be converted and written to the standard file format in a format that mimics one of the commercial force plate types. Appropriate gains, scales, and offsets must also be stored so that translation of the force data occurs appropriately. To achieve this in our study, each of the segments of the foot that contacts the ground was treated as a virtual individual force plate.[10] Each of the virtual force plates was specified to have the same dimensions as the active surface of the plantar pressure mat and was located appropriately with respect to the laboratory coordinate system to match the location during calibration. In this arrangement, each of the force plates, which is used to express the segment force data, occupies exactly the same space as far as the software reading the standard file format (in our case, the C3D file format) is concerned. Each of the ground reaction force vectors associated with the various contact segments is then written as data corresponding to one of the virtual force plates (Figure 34.3).

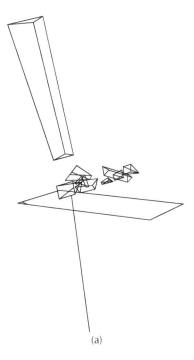

(a)

FIGURE 34.3 Sequence depicting segmental force application, which represents the culmination of the integration of the pressure and force measurement systems. Foot segments are shown as geometrical shapes; ground reaction force vectors are indicated by line segments. Force data are stored as separate overlapping force plates for each contact segment. At initial contact (a) only the heel segment contacts the ground. During mid-stance (b), heel and midfoot segments contribute to the ground reaction force. During push off (c) the toe segments and the medial forefoot contribute. Shear force contributions are clearly evident by the angle of the force vectors during contact and push off.

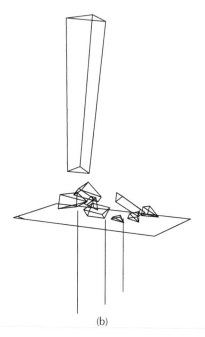

(b)

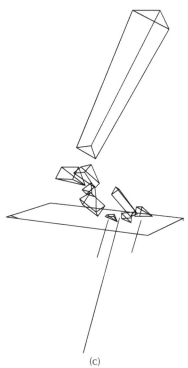

(c)

FIGURE 34.3 (Continued).

34.2.6 Specification of Inertial Components

The external forces acting on the foot during gait include the ground reaction force, gravitational forces of the foot segments and the body segments proximal to the foot, and inertial forces. To accurately compute inertial forces, both the motions of the segments and the properties of the segmental masses must be known. These mass properties include the segment mass, the location of the mass centroid, and mass moments of inertia or, equivalently, the radii of gyration. While these quantities are readily available for more standard segments such as the pelvis, femur, or shank, and even for the foot as a whole, properties of individual segments of the foot are unknown. To estimate these values in our work, we employed a solid modeling package to partition a solid three-dimensional bone model reconstructed from a computed tomography (CT) scan into segments matching the kinematic model.[10] The masses, center of mass locations, and radii of gyration were computed on the basis of a percentage of the mass of the total foot. Total foot mass was estimated by scaling published data for adult feet to the subject-specific foot based on foot length. This process could be improved by using a more complete model of the foot, which would include muscles, ligaments, skin, and the appropriate densities for these various structures. However, given the relatively small contribution of inertial forces, particularly during stance phase, to the overall force components, such detailed analysis may not significantly improve the overall model.

34.2.7 Inverse Dynamic Computation

The remaining steps toward computing kinetics are to first specify the locations of the model's motion segments (and correspondingly express the intersegmental angles, though this is only integral to the kinematic process), and then to use the measured ground reaction forces on each of the segments contacting the ground to compute the joint moments. The process of combining inertial forces, gravitational forces, and ground reaction forces to compute net joint moments through a kinematic chain is generally termed "inverse dynamics." The Euler equations of motion for this process are well defined, but somewhat complex due to the many terms. Hence most users prefer to take advantage of existing software to perform these computations. In the referenced publication, we utilized one such package, Vicon Body-Builder (Vicon Motion Systems, Lake Forest, CA).[10] We chose this modeling package for several reasons. First, it interfaced with the motion capture data format; second, the kinematic model could be defined and evaluated; third, the inverse dynamics computations could be carried out; and finally, the resulting code could easily be shared with other laboratories for their own use and further enhancements. Computation of inverse dynamics within this package necessitated the ground reaction force data formatting as previously addressed. Aside from this formatting and the associated manipulation of the C3D file, the remainder of the process was straightforward. One nonstandard process that was required, however, was to manually associate each contact segment with the specific force plate, which held its data. Because each of these virtual force plates occupied the same space, the default automatic association between segments and force plates failed to function appropriately.

34.3 DISCUSSION

The detailed methods presented here demonstrate that kinetic measures of the foot are possible with current technology. However, the procedures necessary for computation are too cumbersome and time intensive for most clinical applications; we are aware of only two efforts that have attempted to determine kinetics within the foot.[10–13] This is largely because the necessary hardware and software have not been integrated with commercial motion capture systems. Currently, with some software packages, it is not even possible to collect marker and pressure data simultaneously from a single work-station. Proprietary file formats embedded with pedobarograph systems are an additional hurdle to integration. While commercially available software was used to develop a model that could be shared for future development, there are currently no software packages capable of automating the process for integration of pressure data within any standard motion file format. Additionally, the pressure-masking process and other steps necessary to separate out the normal force and center of pressure data for individual contact segments from the pressure continuum are time intensive. These hurdles make the kinetic portion of the model difficult to attain. Such difficulties highlight the need for manufacturers to work together to create an integrated system, as has been done with motion capture and electromyography (EMG) and force plate technologies. Pedobarograph systems present a special challenge because they cannot be simply channeled through a standard analog to digital (A/D) collection unit as force plate and EMG data are. Reading the data stream from such a device would necessitate a multiplexor that may be incorporated into the standard A/D board or as a separate unit generating a separate data file. This type of development, however, will not occur until user demands drive the development and give such a system an advantage in the marketplace.

REFERENCES

1. Carson, M.C., Harrington, M.E., Thompson, N., O'Connor, J.J., Kinenatic analysis of a multi-segment foot model for research an clinical applications: a repeatability analysis, Theologis, T.N., *J. Biomech.*, 2001, 34, 1299.
2. Hunt, A.E., Smith, R.M., Torode, M., Keenan, A.M., Extrinsic muscle activity, foot motion and ankle joint movements during stance phase of walking, *Clin. Biomech. (Bristol, Avon)*, 2001, 16, 592.
3. Kidder, S.M., Abuzzahab-FS, J., Harris, G.F., Johnson, J.E., A system for the analysis of foot and ankle kinematics during gait, *IEEE Trans. Rehabil. Eng.*, 1996, 4, 25.
4. Leardini, A., Benedetti, M.G., Catani, F., Simoncini, L., Giannini, S., An anatomically based protocol for the description of foot segments during gait, *Clin. Biomech. (Bristol, Avon)*, 1999, 14, 528.
5. Rattanaprasert, U., Smith, R., Sullivan, M., Gilleard, W., Three-dimensional kinematics of the forefoot, rearfoot, and leg without the function of tibralis posterior in comparison with normals during the stance phase of walking, *Clin. Biomech. (Bristol, Avon)*, 1999, 14, 14.

6. Sampath, G., Abu-Faraj, O., Smith, P.A., Harris, G.F., Preliminary clinical application of an active marker based pediatric foot and ankle motion analysis system. *Gait Posture*, 1998, 7(2), 176.

7. Simon, J., Metaxiotis, D., Siebal, A., Bock, H.G., Döderlein, L., A model of the human foot with seven segments. *Gait Posture*, 2005, 12, 63–64.

8. Woodburn, J., Nelson, K.M., Siegel, K.L., Kepple, T.M., Gerber, L.H., *J. Rheumatol.*, 2004, 31, 1918.

9. Wu, W.L., Su, F.C., Cheng, Y.M., Huang, P.J., Chou, Y.L., Chou, C.K., *Gait Posture*, 2000, 11, 54.

10. MacWilliams, B.A., Cowley, M., Nicholson, D.E., *Gait Posture*, 2003, 17, 214.

11. Abuzzahab, F.S. Jr, Harris, G.F., Kidder, S.M., *Gait Posture,* 1997, 5(2), 148.

12. Cowley, M.S., MacWilliams, B.A., Armstrong, P.F., *Gait Posture* 2001, 13(3), 297.

13. MacWilliams, B.A., Cowley, M.S., *Proceedings of the 2001 International Society of Biomechanics,* 2001, 28.

35 Triaxial Plantar Force Sensor: Design, Calibration, Characterization, and Subject Testing

Emily J. Miller, Dean C. Jeutter, Robert J. Stango, and Gerald F. Harris

CONTENTS

35.1 INTRODUCTION

The reaction forces exerted on the plantar surface of the foot can be resolved into vertical, anterior–posterior (A–P), and medial–lateral (M–L) components. Knowledge of these forces and the corresponding pressure distributions has both research and clinical applications. For example, plantar pressure measurements are incorporated into kinetic foot models. Existing commercial pressure mats measure vertical plantar pressure, and this information is used to determine the contribution of each foot segment to the total vertical ground reaction force. Because there is no device that measures the shear pressure distribution, assumptions are necessary to complete kinetic foot models, and shear loads are often distributed on the basis of the segmental contribution to the vertical ground reaction force.[1] Plantar pressure measurements also provide information regarding the effect of footwear on gait, the diagnosis of foot pathology, and the effectiveness of clinical intervention. For example, research has shown that prolonged application of large mechanical forces acting on the skin lead to cell necrosis and ulceration.[2] A number of studies have shown that the largest vertical pressures caused ulceration,[3] whereas other studies have shown that ulceration occurs where the shear stress is maximum.[4] Force plates are used to simultaneously measure all three force components on the plantar surface of the foot, but force plates permit only a single determination of the aggregate force and do not allow the measurement of the loading in the individual segments of the foot.[2] The Emed System® (Novel Electronics, Inc., St. Paul, MN) and the F-Scan®/F-Mat System (Tekscan, Inc., South Boston, MA) are the most widely used commercial technologies for measuring vertical, static, and dynamic pressure distributions beneath the plantar surface of the foot.

A limited number of experimental sensors have been developed to measure the shear stresses on the sole of the foot.[5–11] These sensors are embedded in shoe insoles and are only used by the investigators to measure shear stress at discrete locations on the plantar surface of the foot. These experimental shear sensors have been tested clinically, but only the sensors developed by Lebar et al.[10] and Hosein and Lord[11] have been fully characterized. Additionally, a pressure plate, utilizing strain gauge technology, has been designed by Davis et al. to measure vertical, A–P, and M–L shear forefoot pressures.[12] However, design limitations included fabrication, maintenance, and size restrictions. Therefore, in order to accurately complete the kinetic foot model, continued development of a sensor that simultaneously measures vertical and shear pressures at multiple discrete locations on the plantar surface of the foot is necessary.

35.2 METHODOLOGY

35.2.1 SENSOR DESIGN

The active shear components of the triaxial plantar force sensor were a central post surrounded by four parallel plates. These components were clearly visible in the first prototype, as shown in Figure 35.1. The active vertical components of the sensor were the central post and a load cell. As shown in Figure 35.2, the shear and vertical

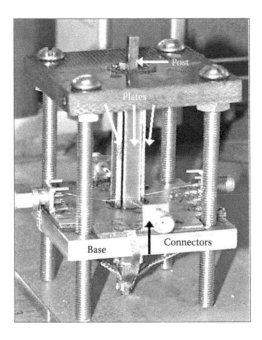

FIGURE 35.1 Triaxial plantar force sensor: shear components.

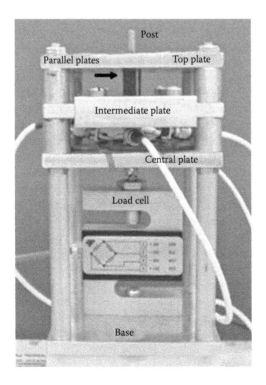

FIGURE 35.2 Triaxial plantar force sensor: shear and vertical components.

TABLE 35.1
Triaxial Plantar Force Transducer: Specifications

Component		Specification
Post	Material	Brass
	Height	60 mm
	Cross-section	3.0 × 3.0 mm
Parallel plates	Material	1/16 in. double-sided FR10 glass epoxy PCB with 1 mil copper (one side)
	Height	45 mm
	Width	5.0 mm
	Distance from post	1.0 mm
Load cell	Height	6.35 cm
	Cross-section	5.1 × 1.9 cm
	Maximum load	222 N
Support structure	Material	Aluminum

components were housed in a structure consisting of a top, intermediate, central, and base plates. This design, which included the shear and vertical components, was used to characterize the sensor and conduct subject testing. When conducting subject testing, this sensor was designed to be an in-ground array embedded in a walkway surface instead of being inserted into footwear. The sensor's specifications are listed in Table 35.1.

A novel differential capacitive sensing technique was developed to measure the A–P and M–L plantar shear forces. The central post and parallel plate configuration made it possible to clearly distinguish the A–P direction from the M–L direction, and a square post was selected instead of a circular post to ensure that the applied forces were resolved into discrete A–P and M–L components. Capacitive sensing was preferred over strain gauge approaches due to the fabrication, maintenance, and size limitations associated with using strain gauges. The arrangement of the central post and the four parallel plates created a capacitor between each face of the post and the parallel plate that it opposed. The bottom of the post was tightly secured to the top of a compression load cell and the top of the post extended 1.5 cm beyond the top of each of the plates. When a subject exerted force on the post, the forces on the plantar surface of the foot caused the post to be deflected. As the post was deflected, it bent like a vertical cantilever beam. The distance between the post and each of the plates changed and this altered the capacitance. Calibration data were used to determine the applied force. In the current application, the pressure was calculated by dividing the applied pressure by the surface area of the post (SA = 9.0 mm^2).

A commercial load cell was used in conjunction with the central square post to simultaneously measure the vertical plantar force. The bottom of the central post was secured tightly in a square hole in a bolt that was screwed into a hole in the sensing arm of the load cell (Model SBO-50, Transducer Techniques, Temecula, CA).

This transducer utilized strain gauge technology, and the load cell's specifications are listed in Table 35.1. As the subject's foot applied force to the post, the post was loaded vertically and the applied vertical force was measured.

35.2.2 SIGNAL CONDITIONING CIRCUITS

A signal conditioning circuit was designed to convert the capacitance signal of the transducer to a proportional voltage signal. The shear components of triaxial plantar force sensor were a spacing variation sensor, meaning the capacitance changed as the distance between the post and plate changed. The capacitance was nonlinear with the spacing, so an appropriate circuit design helped linearize the sensor.[13] Prior to designing an appropriate signal conditioning circuit, a Vector Network Analyzer (Model 8753A, Hewlett-Packard, Houston, TX) was used to measure the capacitance between the post and each of the four plates. The average capacitance of the sensor when the post was not deflected was 4.9 pF, and the average capacitance of the sensor when the post was in maximum deflection was 7.6 pF.

The parallel plate arrangement of the triaxial sensor created a differential pair transducer for each shear direction. A separate signal conditioning circuit was necessary for each shear direction, so the parallel plate configuration for each direction was placed in a separate bridge circuit. However, both shear signal conditioning circuits were implemented on the same printed circuit board and the board was enclosed in a solid plastic case for shielding purposes. Each parallel plate was connected to an SubMiniature version A (SMA) connector on the base of the transducer. A voltage regulator (78L06) and voltage converter (MAX660, Maxim Integrated Products, Inc., Sunnyvale, CA) were used in the circuit to provide the correct voltage to the op amps and the potentiometers. A crystal oscillator (HSC-2E, Fox Electronics, Fort Myers, FL) was used to provide a 1 MHz sine wave excitation signal. The high bridge power supply frequency, provided by the 1 MHz crystal oscillator, was also used to reduce the sensor's capacitive reactance to reasonable levels, which increased the sensitivity of the system to small deflections. When the post was deflected, the bridge was unbalanced and the differential signal was amplified. The signal was then converted from an AC signal to a DC signal and the signal was amplified again.

In the circuit for the shear force system, as shown in Figure 35.3, the parallel plates for each shear direction (C1, C2) made up two arms of the bridge and were connected to the circuit via SMA connectors and coaxial cables. The bridge was completed with two capacitors (C3 = C4 = 7.5 pF). As the post was deflected, there was a change in capacitance between the post and the parallel plates. This unbalanced the bridge and altered the amplitude of the excitation wave. The parallel plate arrangement of the transducer created a differential pair transducer for each shear direction, which was beneficial because differential measurements improve the linearity of a sensor by canceling out or removing even harmonics and doubling the sensor's sensitivity. After the bridge was unbalanced, the output was amplified (U1 = LT®1722) (Linear Technology Corporation, Milpitas, CA); R1 = R2 = 10 kΩ, R3 = R4 = 100 kΩ; C5 = C6 = 1.0 nF), filtered (C8 = 10 nF, R5 = 1.0 kΩ, fc = 16 kHz), and rectified (D1 = Schottky common anode; C9 = 10 nF, R6 = 10 kΩ, fc = 1.6 Hz).

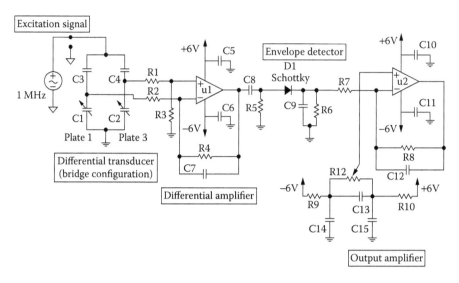

FIGURE 35.3 Shear force signal conditioning circuit.

The signal passed through a final amplification stage before it was acquired (U2 = LT1722; R7 = 10 kΩ, R8 = 6.8 MΩ; R12 = 1 k, R9 = R10 = 13 kΩ; C10 = C11 = C13 = C14 = C15 = 1 nF).

As shown in Figure 35.4, a separate signal conditioning circuit was designed for the sensor's vertical components. When the post was loaded vertically, the applied vertical load was transferred directly to the load cell and the load cell's internal strain gauge was unbalanced. The differential signal was then amplified using two amplification stages. The amplifier used in both gain stages was a single-supply instrumentation amplifier (LT1167).

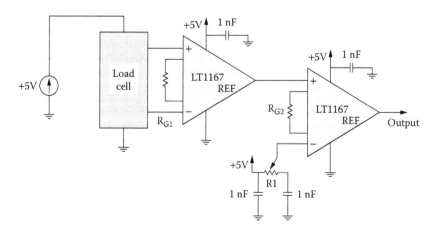

FIGURE 35.4 Vertical force signal conditioning circuit.

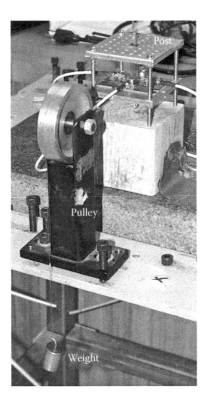

FIGURE 35.5 Shear force calibration technique.

35.2.3 Sensor Calibration

To perform a static calibration of the shear components, a piece of nylon line was tied to the top of the central post and suspended over the top of a pulley, as shown in Figure 35.5. The shear components were calibrated using a series of loads ranging from 0 to 1400 g, applied in 100 g increments. To perform a static calibration of the vertical components, the weights were applied directly to the top of the post. The calibration was done using vertical loads of 11 N, 22 N, 33 N, and 44 N. For both the shear and vertical static calibrations, the sensor was loaded and unloaded incrementally with the applied loads and the corresponding voltage output was measured for each load. The data were then used to generate a calibration curve to characterize the sensitivity and linearity of the sensor. The hysteresis was also determined from the loading and unloading data, and the cross-talk matrix was generated by monitoring the output in all three directions simultaneously (A–P shear, M–L shear, and vertical) during the loading and unloading routines. The rise time and the natural frequency of the post were also determined using a step impulse. The step impulse was applied by placing the post in maximum deflection in each direction. The post was then released and allowed to return to its original position.

35.2.4 SUBJECT TESTING

Subject testing was conducted to evaluate the response of the sensor to forces applied by the plantar surface of the foot. The sensor was placed on the floor and a platform (length: 2.4 m, width: 1.0 m, height: 17 cm) was built around the sensor to provide a walkway surface that was level with the top of the sensor. Data from each of the three channels of the triaxial sensor were collected at a sampling rate of 1000 Hz using a LabView data acquisition program. One subject (age: 26, body weight: 66 kg, height: 1.68 m) was tested barefoot to evaluate the sensor's performance. The volunteer was a normal, healthy adult with no history of foot and ankle surgery or pathology. Testing was completed when the subject made direct contact with the triaxial plantar force sensor five times with each foot during heel strike. The subject was instructed to walk at a comfortable pace, but unfortunately, due to the sensor's small surface area, targeting was not avoided. The sensor's axis system followed the lab's axis system. Deflection of the central post in the direction of the walkway occurred in the $\pm x$-direction, which corresponded to A–P shear and deflection of the central post perpendicular to the direction walkway occurred in the $\pm y$-direction, which corresponded to M–L shear. Lastly, deflection of the post vertically occurred in the $-z$-direction. The forces in each direction were computed using the calibration data.

35.3 RESULTS

35.3.1 STATIC CALIBRATION

The sensor was calibrated in each direction and each plate was characterized individually to simulate forward and reverse shear forces in both the A–P and M–L directions. The results of the calibration and sensor characterization are summarized in Table 35.2. The calibration curve for plate three is shown in Figure 35.6. A linear regression for each of the calibration plots was calculated to generate the calibration curves and determine the sensor's sensitivity. Because the shape and orientation of the plates with respect to the post was the same for all four plates, it was not unexpected that the performance (sensitivity) of each of the four plates during shear force calibration was similar. Therefore, the linear regressions of the calibration curves were averaged to generate a single shear force calibration curve with a mean sensitivity of 133 mV/N. The post and load cell were also calibrated to generate a vertical calibration curve, as shown in Figure 35.7. An average linear regression was calculated using the loading and the unloading curves with a mean vertical sensitivity of 25 mV/N.

35.3.2 CROSS-TALK SENSITIVITY

The cross-talk sensitivities were determined for both shear and normal loading. The output was graphed for each of the unloaded (off-axis) channels and the slopes of the regression lines were used to determine the cross-talk sensitivities. The average sensitivity of the shear components of the sensor to off-axis shear loads was 2.8 mV/N. The shear cross-talk due to the vertical loading was also minimal. The average

TABLE 35.2
Triaxial Plantar Force Transducer: Calibration and Characterization Results

	Shear Components	Vertical Components
Force range	0–14 N	0–44 N
Sensitivity	133 mV/N	25 mV/N
Nonlinearity	6.6%	15%
Hysteresis	0.33%	2.5%
Cross-talk sensitivity (off-axis shear loads)	2.8 mV/N	0%
Cross-talk sensitivity (normal loads)	45 mV/N	—
Response time	5 msec	
Natural frequency	Overdamped system	

sensitivity of the shear components of the sensor to vertical loads was 45 mV/N. The vertical components did not experience any cross-talk during shear loading.

35.3.3 NONLINEARITY

The nonlinearity was described as the percentage of maximum deviation of the input from a best-fit straight line with respect to the full-scale input (shear calibration: 1400 g; vertical calibration: 44 N). The overall (average) nonlinearity of the shear components was 6.6 ± 0.5%. The nonlinearity of the vertical components of the sensor was 15%.

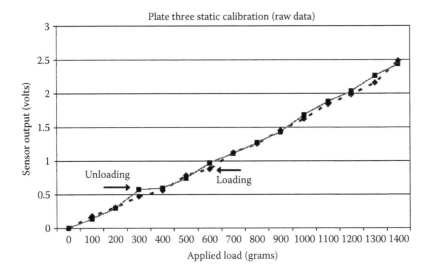

FIGURE 35.6 Shear force calibration curve.

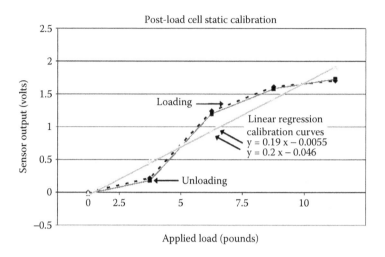

FIGURE 35.7 Vertical force calibration curve.

35.3.4 HYSTERESIS

The hysteresis of the transducer was computed by calculating the maximum difference between the loading and unloading curves and then dividing the difference by the full-scale output. The overall mean hysteresis of the shear components was 0.33% ± 0.35% and the hysteresis of the sensor's normal components was 2.5%.

35.3.5 RISE TIME AND NATURAL FREQUENCY

A step impulse was manually applied to the sensor to test the rise time and natural frequency of the post. The rise time was described as the time in seconds for the amplitude of the signal to rise from 10 to 90% of its final value. The rise time of the sensor was 5 msec. After the application of the step impulse, the post returned to its equilibrium position without overshoot, which demonstrated that the system was overdamped.

35.4 SUBJECT TESTING RESULTS

35.4.1 PEAK SHEAR AND VERTICAL FORCES

A single triaxial plantar force sensor was used to collect preliminary triaxial plantar force data from one subject during the initial contact phase of gait. Even though the subject contacted the sensor during initial contact five times with each heel, due to targeting and deviations in heel placement, only four of the ten trials with heel contact produced a measurable signal in all three directions. The results from one of the four successful trials are shown in Figure 35.8. Based on these four successful trials, peak A–P, M–L, and vertical forces were calculated. The average peak forces were 6.0 N ± 1.0 N in the A–P direction, 3.3 N ± 1.0 N in the M–L direction, and 33.5 N ± 2.4 N in the vertical direction.

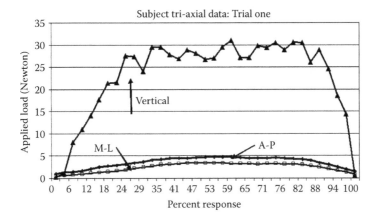

FIGURE 35.8 Triaxial subject force data.

35.4.2 INITIAL HEEL CONTACT DURATION

The initial contact durations were calculated for each trial and the results were extremely variable. Contact time between the heel and the sensor during the initial contact phase of gait ranged from 41 to 67 msec. For the four successful trials, the average contact time between the heel and the sensor was 58 ± 12 msec.

35.5 DISCUSSION

35.5.1 SENSOR CHARACTERISTICS

The novel triaxial plantar pressure sensor was calibrated and extensively characterized, as shown in Table 35.2, to understand the sensor's performance characteristics and to allow an evaluation of the data collected during subject testing. The measurable shear (0 to 14 N) range designed for this sensor was appropriate for the subject evaluated in this study and it fell within the range of the measured shear forces at the heel, 1.2 N[10] to 15 N,[9] as reported in the literature for previous in-shoe shear sensors. Altering the post dimensions, materials, and the post/parallel plate spacing would allow for a change in the full-scale shear force input. However, it may not be necessary to increase the full-scale capabilities of this sensor. The previous shear sensors were discrete in-shoe sensors, and these sensors may have measured artificial shear forces as the shoe insole interacted with the foot and the shoe. The sensor developed in this chapter was a surface mount sensor mounted on a stable surface. The only forces acting on this sensor were the applied loads.

The calibration data demonstrated that the triaxial plantar force transducer was extremely sensitive (133 mV/N) in the shear direction, even though the capacitance values were very small and the post experienced minimal deflection. The sensitivity was predicted by the initial capacitance measurements. The difference between the initial and maximum capacitance measurements was a large percentage of the initial measurements, which indicated that the transducer was capable of detecting small changes.

Therefore, this sensor was appropriate for measuring small shear forces, which was beneficial considering shear forces were typically less than 20% of a human subject's total body weight. This sensor exhibited nearly linear behavior and it experienced minimal cross-talk and hysteresis, as shown in Table 35.2. The major sources of non-linearity with the shear components were due to the mechanisms of attachment between the post and the load cell and the nonlinearity associated with capacitive sensing when a distance change occurred between the capacitive plates. The source of nonlinearity with the vertical components was also due to the fixation of the post within the sensor. The post was designed to only be attached to the load cell for a pure transfer of the vertical load through the post to the load cell. Although, in order to constrain the deflection of the post, it passed through a snug hole in the central base and a percentage of the vertical load was also transferred to the central base. The post–load cell combination will need improvement to increase the linearity of the vertical components.

35.5.2 Subject Application

The evaluation of a healthy, normal subject demonstrated that the triaxial plantar force sensor could measure and withstand the shear and normal forces of repetitive gait. The peak shear and normal forces at heel strike and their corresponding heel contact intervals were calculated. The mean peak forces were 6.0 N ± 1.0 N in the A–P direction, 3.3 N ± 1.0 N in the M–L direction, and 33.5 N ± 2.4 N in the vertical direction. (Pressure can be calculated by dividing the measured force by the surface area of the post.) Few authors have collected hindfoot pressures, and the shear and vertical pressures reported by these authors varied greatly from study to study. In order to compare the different hindfoot pressures and the data collected in this study, the applied forces were calculated using the sensor's surface area. With regards to shear forces, Lebar et al.[10] used a discrete optoelectric insole sensor and reported a mean peak value of 6.7 kPa (1.2 N) A–P shear at the posterior heel. Laing et al.[7] developed a magnetoresistive insole sensor and reported mean pressures of 80 kPa (6.3 N) at the medial heel and 120 kPa (9.4 N) at the lateral heel. Akhlaghi and Pepper[9] tested with a biaxial insole shear sensor and reported peak pressure values of 150 kPa (15 N) in the A–P direction and 60 kPa (6 N) in the M–L direction at the heel. Finally, Hosein et al.[11] used an insole magnetoresistive sensor at the heel and noted a peak shear pressure of 48.5 kPa (9.7 N). The results of these studies indicated that applied shear forces at the heel ranged from 1.2 N[10] to 15 N[9]. Additional studies have been reviewed to examine vertical hindfoot pressures. Bryant et al.[14] tested with an EMED-SF-4 pressure mat and noted a peak vertical heel pressure of 350 kPa (8.75 N) and a mean vertical heel pressure of 167 kPa (4.2 N). Kanatli et al.[15] also tested with an EMED-SF pressure mat and reported a peak vertical pressure value of 317 kPa (15.85 N) at the heel. The results of these studies indicated that applied peak vertical forces at the heel ranged from 8.75 N[14] to 15.85 N[15]. The differences noted among these studies may be attributed to the different sensors (sensor dimensions and sensing technology), variations among subject populations, different test protocols, calibration procedures, and other sensor characteristics.

The shear force values measured using the triaxial plantar force sensor fell within the range of values reported by other authors. Therefore, the results of this study demonstrate that the allowable maximum deflection of the post, which determined the full-scale input, was sufficient for measuring shear plantar forces. Additionally, at initial contact, the A–P shear was typically greater than the M–L shear and the results collected with the triaxial plantar force sensor reflect this. The relative magnitudes of the forces were also consistent with traditional findings. The average A–P force was about 20% of the average vertical force and the average M–L was about 10% of the average vertical force. The vertical forces measured, using the triaxial plantar force sensor, were significantly smaller than the values reported by the authors. Again though, the relative magnitudes of the three forces were consistent with traditional findings. When analyzing the shear and vertical forces, it was necessary to remember that only one active sensor was utilized during subject testing. Also, the surface area of the triaxial plantar force sensor was small and the subject employed minimal targeting to ensure solid contact between the heel and a single post during the initial contact phase of gait. This extra awareness to foot placement and adjustment of the gait pattern may have impacted the force measurements.

35.6 CONCLUSION

A unique sensor was successfully designed to simultaneously measure A–P and M–L shear plantar forces and vertical plantar force in human subjects. Future projects involve optimizing the post design, modifying the vertical sensing components, and incorporating the individual triaxial plantar force sensor into an array containing multiple sensors to measure plantar pressure. In order to successfully improve the triaxial plantar force sensor and develop a matrix of triaxial force sensors, it is necessary to implement a smaller vertical sensing component. The current commercial load cell is too large to develop an appropriate array of sensors. These steps are necessary for developing a functional matrix of triaxial force sensors. The data collected with this sensor may greatly aid in the final development of a complete kinetic foot model. Additionally, triaxial plantar force data from this transducer will provide a greater understanding of foot function and foot kinetics, and they have the potential to advance both clinical and research projects.

ACKNOWLEDGMENT

E.J. Miller wishes to acknowledge the support of the Orthopaedic and Rehabilitation Engineering Center, OREC (Marquette University/Medical College of Wisconsin) and the Biomedical Telemetry Laboratory (Marquette University) in the completion of this project.

REFERENCES

1. Abuzzahab, F.S., Harris, G.F., Kidder, S.M., Johnson, J.E., A kinetic biomechanical model of the foot and ankle, *IEEE-EMBC and CMBEC Theme 5: Neuromuscular Systems/Biomechanics*, IEEE Press, 1995, 1271–1272.
2. Koulaxouzidis, A.V., Homes, M.J., Roberts, C.V., Handerek, V.A., A shear and vertical stress sensor for physiological measurements using Fibre Bragg Gratings, *22nd Annual EMBS International Conference*, Chicago, IL, 2000.

3. Pollard, J.P., Le Quesne, L.P., Method of healing diabetic forefoot ulcers, *BMJ*, 286, 436–437, 1983.

4. Ctercteko, C.G., Dhanendran, M., Hutton, W.C., Le Quesne, L.P., Vertical forces acting on the feet of diabetic patients with neuropathic ulceration, *Br J Surg*, 68, 608–614, 1981.

5. Tappin, J.W., Pollard, J., Beckett, E.A., Method of measuring 'shearing' forces on the sole of the foot, *Clin Phys Physiol Meas*, 1, 1, 83–85, 1980.

6. Pollard, J.P., Le Quesne, L.P., Tappin, J.W., Forces under the foot, *J Biomed Eng*, 5, 37–40, 1983.

7. Laing, P., Deogan, H., Cogley, D., Crerand, S., Hammond, P., Klenerman, L., The development of the low profile Liverpool shear transducer, *Clin Phys Physiol Meas*, 13, 2, 115–124, 1992.

8. Lord, M., Hosein, R., Williams, R.B., Method for in-shoe shear stress management, *J Biomed Eng*, 14, 181–186, 1992.

9. Akhlaghi, F., Pepper, M.G., In-shoe biaxial shear force measurement: the Kent shear system, *Med Biol Eng Comput*, 34, 315–317, 1996.

10. Lebar, A.M., Harris, G.F., Wertsch, J.J., Zhu, H., An optoelectric plantar "shear" sensing transducer: design, validation, and preliminary subject tests, *IEEE Trans Rehabil Eng*, 4, 4, 310–319, 1996.

11. Hosein, R., Lord, M., A study of in-shoe plantar shear in normals, *Clin Biomech*, 15, 46–53, 2000.

12. Davis, B.L., Perry, J.E., Neth, D.C., Waters, K.C., A device for simultaneous measurement of pressure and shear force distribution on the plantar surface of the foot, *J Appl Biomech*, 14, 93–104, 1998.

13. Baxter, L.K., *Capacitive Sensors: Design and Applications*. Piscataway, NJ: IEEE Press 1997, 1, 57–59.

14. Bryant, A.R., Tinley, P., Singer, K.P., Normal values of plantar pressure measurements determined using the EMED-SF system, *J Am Podiatr Med Assoc*, 90, 6, 295–299, 2000.

15. Kanatli, U., Yetkin, H., Simsek, A., Besli, K., Ozturk, A., The relationship of the heel pad compressibility and plantar pressure distribution, *Foot Ankle Int*, 22, 8, 662–665, 2001.

36 Quasi-Stiffness of the Ankle during Able-Bodied Walking at Different Speeds: Implications for Design of Prostheses

Andrew H. Hansen, Steven A. Gard, and Dudley S. Childress

CONTENTS

36.1   INTRODUCTION

Muscles within and surrounding the ankle–foot complex contain active and passive elements that are important during walking. However, the net effect of these active and passive muscular elements could create a system that can be mimicked by a prosthesis using purely passive elastic elements under appropriate conditions. Davis and DeLuca[1] and Mesplay[9] have examined the *quasi-stiffness* of the ankle during walking by creating and analyzing ankle moment vs. ankle dorsiflexion curves. Davis and DeLuca[1] did not report on the effects of speed on *quasi-stiffness* properties and Mesplay[9] examined the effects of changing cadence on the ankle moment-angle curve with one subject. The term *quasi-stiffness* used here, as suggested by Latash and Zatsiorsky,[8] refers to the slope of the ankle moment vs. ankle dorsiflexion curve and is used because measurements are not performed at equilibrium and because the exact

599

nature of the moments are not known. Palmer [10] studied sagittal plane ankle moment vs. ankle dorsiflexion curves during various stages of the gait cycle and concluded that an augmented system would be needed to replicate the behavior of the able-bodied ankle at most walking speeds. The work described in this chapter aims at examining the behavior of the able-bodied ankle joint during walking at various speeds. Understanding the quasi-stiffness of the able-bodied ankle during walking could help in the development of biomimetic ankle-foot prostheses, i.e., artificial limbs that mimic the biological human ankle and foot complex. Knowledge of quasi-stiffness behavior at different speeds could assist in creating prostheses that can adapt as prosthesis users change their walking speed.

The purpose of this study was to examine the ankle moment vs. ankle dorsiflexion relationship for able-bodied persons walking over a range of speeds. We hypothesized that quasi-stiffness properties would change with walking speed. This hypothesis was based on our previous findings that the effective rocker shapes created by the ankle-foot system from heel contact to opposite heel contact (OHC) did not change appreciably with changes in speed.[6] These effective rockers—the ankle–foot roll-over shapes—did not change with speed although forces experienced by the ankle–foot system clearly increase with walking speed. The combination of increased forces and similar deflections (similar ankle flexion angles and ankle–foot roll-over shapes) suggested a stiffening of the ankle as walking speed was increased.

36.2 METHODOLOGY

36.2.1 EXPERIMENTAL PROTOCOL

Data were collected from gait analyses that were performed on 24 able-bodied subjects (10 male, 14 female). Each of the subjects signed a consent form approved by Northwestern University's Institutional Review Board. The age, height, and weight of each subject were recorded directly before or after the gait analysis sessions. Subjects walked at either three (slow, normal, and fast) or five (very slow, slow, normal, fast, and very fast) self-selected walking speeds ranging from 0.4 to 2.4 m/sec. All subjects walked using soft-soled gym shoes. Markers were placed on the subjects according to a modified Helen Hayes marker set [7]. This marker set included the following markers that were used in the analysis: ANKLE (lateral malleolus), TOE (dorsum of foot, near the midline of the foot), HEEL (posterior to the calcaneus), and KNEE (lateral femoral condyle). Data were acquired at the VA Chicago Motion Analysis Research Laboratory, which has eight motion analysis cameras (Motion Analysis Corporation, Santa Rosa, CA, U.S.) and six force platforms (Advanced Mechanical Technology, Incorporated, Watertown, MA, U.S.). Trials were repeated at a given walking speed until three "clean" force platform hits had been performed by each foot. "Clean" force plate hits were ones in which only one foot contacted a force platform, without stepping over the edges of the platform. Ankle dorsiflexion angles were computed in the plane of progression by finding the angle between a line connecting a heel and toe marker and a perpendicular line to the line through the ankle and knee markers (Figure 36.1, left). The ankle moment for each sample was computed assuming a static equilibrium in the plane of progression, i.e., it was found by multiplying

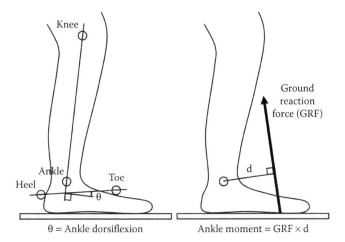

FIGURE 36.1 (Left) Ankle dorsiflexion was measured in the sagittal plane as the angle between a line connecting the heel and toe markers and a perpendicular to the line connecting the ankle and knee markers. (Right) Ankle moments were found as the product of the GRF and the perpendicular distance from the ankle to the GRF.

the ground reaction force (GRF) by the perpendicular line connecting it and the ankle marker (Figure 36.1, right). Ankle moments found using this approach were found to have negligible differences when compared with ankle moments found using the inverse dynamics approach.[12] Ankle powers were estimated by multiplying the normalized ankle moments by the angular velocities of the ankle joint. Ankle angular velocities were found by numerical differentiation of the ankle angular position data.

36.2.1.1 Data Processing

Walking speed for each trial was estimated by dividing the total displacement of the sacral marker in the direction of forward progression during the trial (approximately 5 m) by the length of time taken for the sacral marker to move this distance. Ankle moments from all subjects were first normalized by the mass of the subjects (in kg) and then the moments and angles were sorted into five ranges of walking speeds: 0.4 to 0.8 m/sec, 0.8 to 1.2 m/sec, 1.2 to 1.6 m/sec, 1.6 to 2.0 m/sec, and 2.0 to 2.4 m/sec. A cubic spline interpolation was used to convert the moments and angles from individual trials into equal length arrays (length equal to 101 samples). The mean ankle moments and angles at each of the equal length arrays' points in each walking speed range were calculated. The standard deviations of ankle dorsiflexion and ankle moment were also calculated and were represented at each point as lines extending from the mean values.

Ankle powers were treated in a similar fashion as ankle moment data. After each trial was sorted into the appropriate speed range, the ankle power data were converted into equal length arrays (using a cubic spline interpolation), and the means and standard deviations at each normalized time sample were found.

TABLE 36.1
Number of Trials Included in the Calculation for Each Walking Speed Range

Walking Speed Range (m/sec)	Number of Trials Included[a]
0.4–0.8	61
0.8–1.2	244
1.2–1.6	337
1.6–2.0	341
2.0–2.4	103

[a]Trials were pooled from 24 able-bodied participants.

36.3 RESULTS

The mean age of the subjects was 27 yr (standard deviation of 5 yr), their mean height was 172 cm (standard deviation of 10 cm), and their mean mass was 74 kg (standard deviation of 18 kg). The numbers of trials sorted into each walking speed range are shown in Table 36.1. The ankle moment vs. ankle dorsiflexion angle curves are shown in Figure 36.2 for the five ranges of walking speed. Dots are shown on

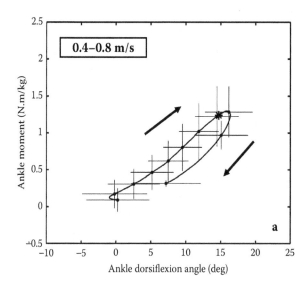

FIGURE 36.2 Ankle moment vs. ankle dorsiflexion angle curves during stance phase for various walking speed ranges: (a) 0.4 to 0.8 m/sec, (b) 0.8 to 1.2 m/sec, (c) 1.2 to 1.6 m/sec, (d) 1.6 to 2.0 m/sec, and (e) 2.0 to 2.4 m/sec. Dark solid curves indicate the mean moments and angles for all trials from the 24 subjects that were in the particular range of walking speeds. Lighter lines appear at every 10% of the stance phase (with respect to time) and indicate standard deviations of the moments and the angles. An asterisk is shown in each plot to indicate the time of OHC. Arrows indicate the direction of the trace with time.

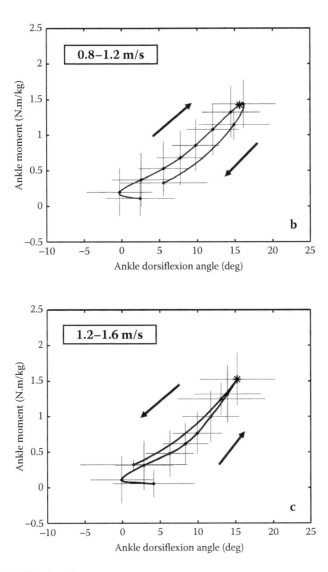

FIGURE 36.2 (Continued).

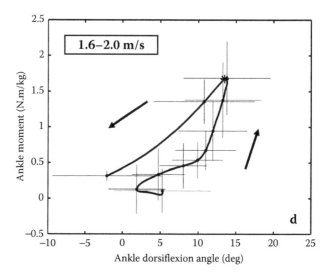

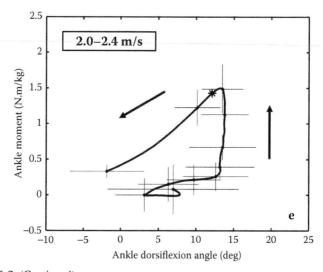

FIGURE 36.2 (Continued).

the curves at each 10% increment of time within the period of heel contact to toe-off to help show the timing of these curves during stance. Asterisks are shown at the time of OHC. Arrows are shown to indicate the direction of these curves during loading and unloading. The moment vs. angle characteristics of the anatomical ankle joint changes as walking speed is increased, supporting the hypothesis.

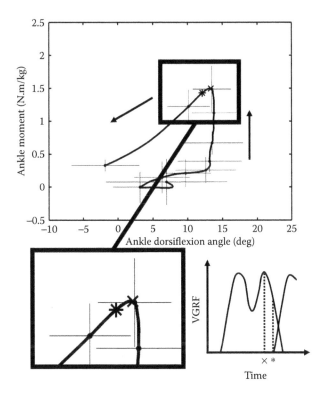

FIGURE 36.3 Closeup of the ankle moment vs. ankle dorsiflexion angle curve for the fastest walking speed range (2.0 to 2.4 meters/second). The asterisk shows where OHC occurs and an "X" has been added to show the time of the second peak of the VGRF. The ankle plantarflexes only slightly before the second peak in VGRF. The main plantarflexion of the ankle occurs after the second peak in VGRF and the OHC also occurs after this second peak. The differences in timing of these events for the other speed ranges were much smaller than the difference shown for this range of speeds.

For the fastest speed range, the second peak in the vertical GRF (VGRF) occurs prior to the OHC, illustrating a short period of descending force just prior to the complete unloading of the foot to the contralateral side (Figure 36.3). The timing of the second peak of the VGRF was found to be at nearly the same point in time as the time of OHC for the other four walking speed ranges.

The mean loading and unloading portions of the ankle moment vs. ankle dorsi-flexion angle curves (Figure 36.2) are plotted in separate graphs in Figure 36.4. The loading and unloading curves in Figure 36.4 are shown without standard deviation lines and are superimposed onto the same graph to facilitate comparison of the curves at different speeds.

The ankle power curves for increasing walking speed are shown in Figure 36.5. Large vertical lines in each of the graphs indicate the timing of OHC. Smaller lines extending from each point of the curve indicate one standard deviation from the mean ankle power at each point in time.

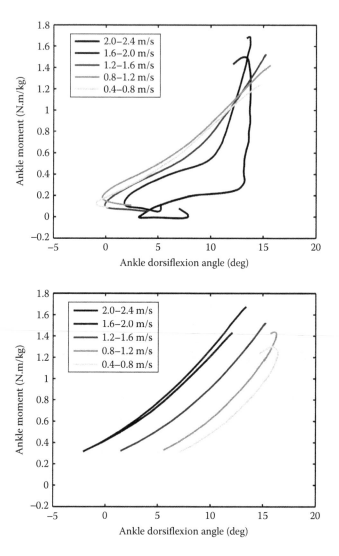

FIGURE 36.4 Loading (top) and unloading (bottom) curves of ankle moment vs. ankle dorsiflexion angle for five walking speed ranges. Loading curves illustrate quasi-stiffness behavior between the time of heel contact to OHC and unloading curves show quasi-stiffness of the ankle between OHC and toe-off events. The quasi-stiffness of the ankle in loading changes as speed is changed, becoming more nonlinear as persons walk faster. The unloading curves have similar slopes but tend to shift toward plantarflexion, suggesting a change in the ankle's resting position, or zero torque position.

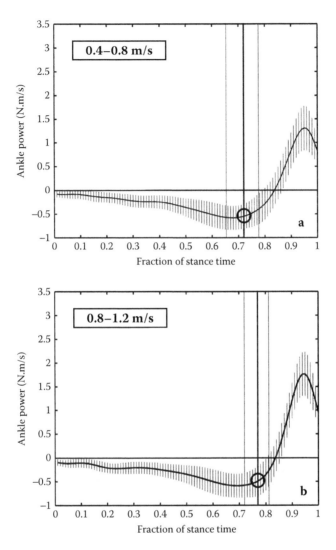

FIGURE 36.5 Ankle power vs. fraction of stance time for various walking speed ranges: (a) 0.4 to 0.8 m/sec, (b) 0.8 to 1.2 m/sec, (c) 1.2 to 1.6 m/sec, (d) 1.6 to 2.0 m/sec, and (e) 2.0 to 2.4 m/sec. Dark solid curves indicate the mean ankle powers for all trials from the 24 subjects that were in the particular range of walking speeds. Lighter lines appear at every hundredth of the stance phase and indicate standard deviations of the ankle powers. A long dark vertical line is drawn in each plot to indicate the mean time of OHC. The lighter vertical lines on each side of the dark line indicate one standard deviation in each direction of the time of OHC. A circle is drawn in each plot to indicate the mean ankle power at the time of OHC.

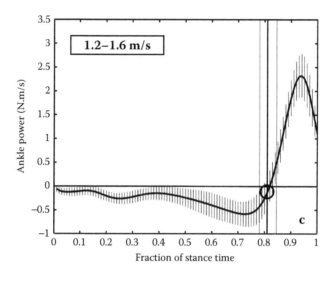

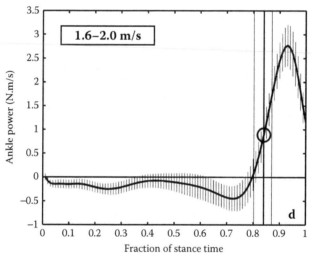

FIGURE 36.5 (Continued).

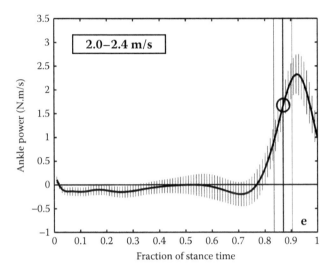

FIGURE 36.5 (Continued).

36.4 DISCUSSION

While the overall system appearance of the ankle in the sagittal plane may be approximated using this methodology, it is important to remember that complex active and passive components are involved inside the system to create the kinematics and kinetics involved in the analysis. Also, the precise physical nature of the resistive torques measured is disregarded in the analysis.[8] However, for use in the field of prosthetics, the information gathered about the overall system appearance may have value for use in the design of simple and effective devices because the entire physiologic systems are frequently being replaced in these cases.

The ankle moment vs. dorsiflexion angle curves show clockwise hysteresis loops for the two slowest walking speed ranges (0.4 to 1.2 m/sec). The area between the loading and unloading phases of the curves appears to be reduced as the speed nears the normal range (1.2 to 1.6 m/sec). At the normal range of speeds, the loading and unloading curves are nearly the same. As the speed is increased above the normal range of speeds (1.6 to 2.4 m/sec), the hysteresis loops start traversing a counterclockwise pattern. The direction of the hysteresis loops indicates whether net work is lost in the cycle (clockwise) or whether net work is generated by the system (counterclockwise). Therefore, the results indicate that at slow speeds, the ankle has an overall system appearance that is passive. The passive system appearance continues up to the typically normal range of walking speeds (1.2 to 1.6 m/sec). Above the normal range of walking speeds, the ankle begins to have an active system appearance. The curves at speeds in the 1.6 to 2.0 m/sec range are similar to the curves shown by Mesplay[9] and by Davis and DeLuca.[1] The area within the hysteresis loops indicates the amount of net work that is lost or generated by the system. At slow speeds, energy is lost, and as the speed is increased less energy is lost. Near the normal range of speeds, almost no energy is lost. As the speed is increased above the normal range of speeds, energy appears to be generated by the system and the amount generated seems to increase with the speed. This finding is consistent with the work of Fujita et al. [3] who also suggested a passive-to-active function of the ankle plantar flexors as walking speed is increased.

Because the biologic ankle plantarflexes prior to OHC when walking at very high speeds (2.0 to 2.4 m/sec), the question arose as to whether or not this behavior was the ankle "pushing" against the weight of the body at this speed or whether this could possibly be attributed to effects of the GRF. For this reason, the timing of the second peak of the GRF was found on all moment vs. angle curves shown in Figure 36.3. All curves except for the fastest walking speed range showed second peaks in the GRF that occurred at nearly the same time as the OHC event. Only in the fastest speed range was there a large shift in these timings (this is why these times are shown only for the fastest speed in Figure 36.3). As Figure 36.3 shows, the second peak in the GRF happens near the time at which the ankle begins to plantarflex. The ankle then plantarflexes up until and beyond the time of OHC. This implies that the plantarflexion may come from the rapid reduction in the force that is acting on the system. Regardless of the nature of the plantarflexion, this analysis cannot determine where energy from the ankle goes (i.e., whether it is used to push the body forward, help initiate swing of the leg, or do something else).

The moment vs. angle loading curves [as shown in Figure 36.4 (top)] show that as the walking speed is increased, the ankle's moment vs. angle relationship becomes more and more nonlinear. It would probably be possible, however, to approximate the loading moment vs. angle characteristics of the biologic ankle closely with a passive mechanical device for speeds up to 1.2–1.6 m/s. The moment vs. angle unloading curves [Figure 36.4 (bottom)] all seem to have a similar slope but appear to be offset with respect to the dorsiflexion angle. There appears to be a shift of the zero torque angle (i.e., the angle at which there is no torque). Mesplay [9] suggested this explanation based on moment–angle curves of one subject walking at various cadences. This shifting behavior is a characteristic that may be explained by Feldman's [2] equilibrium point theory. [9] This changing behavior during unloading may be difficult to replicate in a prosthetic device without the use of active or biarticular components.

Figure 36.5 shows the mean ankle power for the five different walking speed ranges. At speeds less than 1.2 m/s the mean ankle power at OHC is negative, indicating that the ankle is absorbing energy (i.e., is being "worked" on). As speeds approach the normal range (1.2 to 1.6 m/sec), the power at the ankle at OHC is nearly zero. At higher walking speeds (1.6 to 2.4 m/sec), the power at the ankle at OHC becomes positive, indicating that the ankle is actively generating work. These characteristics support the idea that the ankle has a passive system appearance at slow walking speeds and an active appearance at high speeds. The characteristics also suggest that persons may choose to walk at speeds that minimize the amount of hysteresis in the moment–angle relationship, i.e., at the maximum speed that still appears passive.

The total amount of work done on or by the ankle system over the walking cycle can be found by examining either the area under the ankle power vs. time curve or the area under the moment vs. angle curve. These two approaches, in theory, should give identical results because:

$$\int M d\theta = \int M \frac{d\theta}{dt} dt = \int P dt \tag{36.1}$$

where M is moment, θ is angle, t is time, and P is power. However, examining the work using the moment vs. angle plots may be a superior method because a numerical differentiation of the angle data is not needed.[5]

Another approach for examination of the ankle-foot system in walking is the roll-over shape.[4] The ankle–foot roll-over shape is the effective rocker shape that the foot and ankle combine to create during the period of heel contact to OHC and is found by transforming the center of pressure of the GRF into a shank-based coordinate system. The roll-over shapes of the able-bodied ankle–foot system do not appear to change as drastically as ankle quasi-stiffness as walking speeds are increased.[6] In fact, the ankle quasi-stiffness may become more nonlinear as speeds increase to maintain the same general roll-over shape of the combined foot-ankle system. With increased speeds, the forces on the ankle increase. Without modifying the quasi-stiffness, the displacement of the ankle would increase and produce changes in the roll-over shape radius. In particular, the radius of the roll-over shape could be expected to decrease with increased walking speed if changes were not made with regard to quasi-stiffness. However, the radius stays relatively constant for most speeds and actually increases somewhat as walking speed reaches the higher levels.[6] This behavior may serve to physically push the leg into swing near the end of stance phase, or could be overcompensation of the system trying to obtain a target roll-over shape.

Because of its more invariant nature, roll-over shape has been used as a constraint in the design of a low-cost prosthetic ankle-foot mechanism.[11] Designing new prosthetic ankle–foot mechanisms based on able-bodied roll-over shape and quasi-stiffness characteristics simultaneously may provide the most biomimetic function for prosthesis users.

36.5 CONCLUSIONS

The biologic ankle appears to change quasi-stiffness characteristics as walking speed is increased, perhaps to keep a similar roll-over shape at all speeds. The ankle also appears to have a passive system appearance at slow walking speeds and an active system appearance at high walking speeds with a crossover near the normal walking speed range (1.2 to 1.6 m/sec).

ACKNOWLEDGMENTS

The authors would like to acknowledge the use of the VA Chicago Motion Analysis Research Laboratory of the Jesse Brown VA Medical Center, Lakeside CBOC, Chicago, Illinois.

The work described in the paper was supported by the Department of Veterans Affairs, Rehabilitation Research and Development Service and is administered through the Jesse Brown VA Medical Center, Lakeside CBOC, Chicago, Illinois.

This work was also funded by the National Institute on Disability and Rehabilitation Research (NIDRR) of the U.S. Department of Education under grant Nos. H133E980023 and H133E030030. The opinions contained in this publication are those of the grantee and do not necessarily reflect those of the Department of Education.

REFERENCES

1. Davis R., DeLuca P., 1996. Gait characterization via dynamic joint stiffness. *Gait Posture,* 4(3), 224–231.
2. Feldman, A., 1986. Once more on the equilibrium-point hypothesis (lambda model) for motor control. *J Mot Behav,* 18(1), 17–54.
3. Fujita M., Matsusaka N., Norimatsu T., Suzuki R., 1983. The role of the ankle plantar flexors in level walking. In: Winter, D. et al., eds. *Biomechanics* IX-A, 484–488.
4. Hansen A., 2002. Roll-Over Characteristics of Human Walking with Applications for Artificial Limbs. PhD thesis, Northwestern University, Evanston.
5. Hansen, A., Childress, D., Miff, S., Gard, S., Mesplay, K., 2004A. The human ankle during walking: implications for design of biomimetic ankle prostheses and orthoses. *J Biomech,* 37(10), 1467–1474.
6. Hansen, A., Childress, D., Knox, E., 2004B. Roll-over shapes of human locomotor systems: effects of walking speed. *Clin Biomech,* 19(4), 407–414.
7. Kadaba M., Ramakrishnan H., Wootten M., 1990. Measurement of lower extremity kinematics during level walking. *J Orthop Res,* 8, 383–392.
8. Latash M., Zatsiorsky V., 1993. Joint stiffness: myth or reality? *Hum Mov Sci,* 12, 653–692.
9. Mesplay K., 1993. Mechanical Impedance of the Human Lower Limb During Walking. PhD thesis, Northwestern University, Evanston.
10. Palmer M., 2002. Sagittal Plane Characterization of Normal Human Ankle Function Across a Range of Walking Gait Speeds. MS thesis, Massachusetts Institute of Technology, Cambridge.
11. Sam, M., Childress, D., Hansen, A., Meier, M., Lambla, S., Grahn, E., Rolock, J., 2004. The *shape&roll* prosthetic foot (Part I): design and development of appropriate technology for low-income countries. *Med Confl Surviv,* 20(4), 294–306.
12. Wells R., 1981. The projection of the ground reaction force as a predictor of internal joint moments. *Bull Prosthet Res,* 18(1), 15–19.

37 Development of an Advanced Biofidelic Lower Extremity Prosthesis*

Moreno White, Brian J. Hafner, and Walter J. Whatley

CONTENTS

37.1 INTRODUCTION

Loss of a limb is a traumatic and life-altering event. For many amputees, recovery and rehabilitation after limb loss include the use of a prosthetic limb to replace the lost extremity. In the case of a lower-extremity amputation such as a transtibial, or below-knee (BK) amputation, the prosthesis typically includes a socket, pylon, and prosthetic foot. The design of the prosthetic foot is critical because it functionally replaces the intact foot–ankle complex. This sophisticated collection of bones, tendons, ligaments, and muscles supports the body's weight, accommodates the ground surface, and propels the body forward.

---

* This research is funded by a grant from the National Institute of Child Health and Human Development (NICHHD), National Institutes of Health; Grant No. 5 R01 HD 038933–04.

The objective of this research was to develop a lower-extremity prosthesis capable of mimicking a natural, nonamputee gait. To meet this ambitious objective, the researchers combined clinical data from both nonamputees and lower-extremity amputees to develop gait and force data during ambulation. These data were used as inputs to a three-dimensional (3D), dynamic, nonlinear finite element model (FEM) of a transtibial prosthesis. The results of these analyses were used to design the advanced biofidelic lower extremity (ABLE) prosthetic ankle. This device uses novel, patented,[1] advanced composite architecture tension bands, which provide the nonlinear, unidirectional rotational or bending moments (sagittal and coronal) for the ankle.

This chapter gives an overview of ongoing research[2] to develop and validate the function of a flexible, multiaxial, lower-limb ABLE prosthetic ankle with dynamic properties that allow the amputee to mimic a nonamputee gait. As outlined above, the ABLE prosthesis concept utilizes functional gait analysis, including both amputee and nonamputee clinical data to define inputs and boundary conditions for a dynamic finite element analysis (FEA) of the ABLE prosthetic limb. Data from the analytical models are used to develop a biofidelic prosthesis that will be clinically evaluated by amputees. Functionally, the unique multiphase response of the ABLE elastic elements closely mimics the function of the triceps surae and tibialis anterior muscles. This enhances mid-stance stability while providing a natural dynamic response for all phases of gait (from heel strike, to foot-flat, through mid-stance, to toe-off). The ABLE prosthesis design was developed using nonlinear, unidirectional (tension-only) springs (tension bands) to control the angular rotation of the prosthetic ankle during the gait cycle. The ability to partially or totally decouple the anterior/posterior (A/P) and medial/lateral (M/L) response allows the prosthetist to select a customized set of tension bands for specific amputees.

The intact foot–ankle complex provides a number of important functions throughout gait, including positioning the foot, accommodating to the ground, controlling the motion of the leg, and propelling the leg forward. When the heel of the foot first contacts the ground in the walking gait, the ankle functions to position the foot to accept weight and serve as a pivot point throughout stance. The pretibial muscles eccentrically contract to provide controlled plantarflexion of the foot down to the ground in order to provide a solid and stable base of support for the stance limb. This controlled plantarflexion also serves to promote knee flexion and the forward rotation of the tibia. This important mechanism, often referred to as "heel rocker," converts some downward momentum into useful forward momentum.[3] Current prosthetic foot designs are limited in their ability to replicate this function in the ambulatory amputee. Single-axis prosthetic feet rapidly plantarflex after initial contact, but do not promote motion of the tibia over the stance foot. Conversely, rigid-ankle feet pivot on the heel and advance the tibia quickly, often pitching the amputee forward and requiring excessive action of the knee muscles. This demand on the knee is even more apparent when descending an incline. Although not ideal, the cushioned heel of the foot can absorb shock and simulate the plantarflexion motion, but it still requires excessive muscular effort from the amputee.

Once the foot is flat on the ground, the contralateral, or opposing limb, lifts off the ground. The ankle then dorsiflexes throughout stance phase as the body passes over the limb. During this time, the foot must be stable and provide a smooth "rollover" motion of the tibia. While many prosthetic feet have a suitable rollover

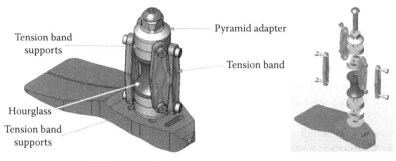

Cosmetic "flesh" removed for clarity

FIGURE 37.1 Assembled and exploded views of the baseline ABLE prosthesis.

behavior on level ground, most do not accommodate well to uneven terrain. In this situation, the foot must invert or evert and sometimes rotate in the transverse plane to achieve a stable position. Clinical feedback from patients and prosthetists suggests that lower-limb prostheses function could be greatly improved if the prosthetic foot and ankle were better able to accommodate to the individual and to the various terrains that a patient encounters on a daily basis. Some prosthetic feet available to patients today offer a small degree of customization, such as the selection of compression "bumpers" that are inserted in the foot to control plantar and dorsiflexion. These designs do not, however, allow for customization of the M/L or rotational components of the foot.

The ABLE prosthesis is an advanced design that can provide greater customization, improved accommodation, and a more natural motion than current prosthetic designs. Such a design requires nonlinear rotational stiffness at the ankle; a decoupling of rotations in the three planes of motion; and the use of novel advanced composite materials to provide controlled plantarflexion in early stance, multidimensional stability in mid-stance, and energy response to promote swing phase in late stance. Figure 37.1 shows an assembled and exploded view of the initial ABLE prosthetic ankle baseline design concept. In the initial design, the center "hourglass" component (so named due to its shape) would carry the axial load while allowing relatively free rotation in both the sagittal and lateral planes. The tension bands provide the nonlinear bending load resistance, and the tension band support allows angular adjustment of each tension band. The tension bands incorporate SPARTA's *In situ* Dynamic Engineered Compliance (IDEC) technology to achieve the nonlinear response needed to mimic nonamputee gait.

37.2 ESTABLISHING DESIGN PARAMETERS

The preliminary design requirements for the ABLE prosthesis were derived from the clinical trials of able-bodied subjects and unilateral, transtibial amputees conducted by the Prosthetics Research Study (PRS, Seattle, WA). Although kinetic (force) and kinematic (motion) data for able-bodied subjects and transtibial amputees have been reported in literature,[4–9] variations in study design, anatomical modeling, and capture methods limit the usefulness of these data for establishing the rigid design requirements of the ABLE prosthesis.

Because the goal of the ABLE project is to replicate the motion of the able-bodied ankle joint in a prosthetic ankle, the clinical trial was designed first to assess the kinematics of able-bodied gait, and then to assess the gait of transtibial amputee subjects. Twenty-four able-bodied subjects (11 males and 13 females with a mean age of 35 yr) were first recruited to establish a baseline for walking function. All subjects were required to be physically healthy and possess no abnormal gait deviations. Kinematic analysis of the foot and ankle was performed (see "Kinematic Analysis" section below) to assess able-bodied function of the ankle joint.

Ten unilateral, transtibial amputees (six males and four females with a mean age of 51 yr) were recruited from the local-area amputee population to assess kinetics and kinematics of amputee gait (see section "Kinetic Analysis" and "Kinematic Analysis" section below). Inclusion criteria required subjects to be Medicare Functional Classification Level (MFCL) 3 (i.e., community ambulators), physically healthy, and at least 3 yr postamputation. Subjects were excluded if they exhibited gross ambulatory problems or residual limb problems, such as sores, or if they experienced significant pain while walking. Experimental procedures for both able-bodied and amputee subjects were approved by the University of Washington's Human Subject Division, and informed consent was obtained from all subjects.

37.2.1 KINEMATIC ANALYSIS

Three-dimensional kinematic data of both able-bodied and amputee subjects were collected using a two-camera motion analysis system and Spica DMAS 5.0 motion capture software (Spica Technology, Kihei, HI). Reflective markers were placed on the toe, heel, ankle, knee, hip, mid-leg, and mid-thigh to define foot, leg, and thigh segments of a kinematic model (Figure 37.2).

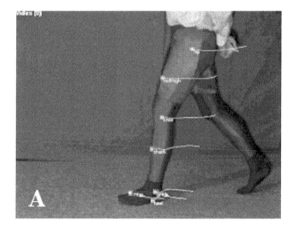

FIGURE 37.2 Kinematic markers placed on the (A) able-bodied and (B) transtibial amputee subjects.

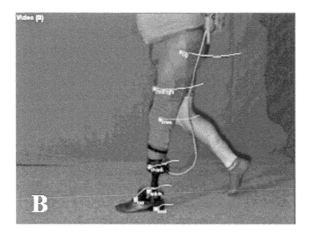

FIGURE 37.2 (Continued).

Kinematic (able-bodied and amputee subjects) and kinetic (amputee subjects only) data were collected during level-ground walking at self-selected walking velocities (SSWV), level-ground walking at slow-walking velocity (80% of SSWV), level-ground walking at fast-walking velocity (130% of SSWV), incline (10°) walking at SSWV, and decline (10°) walking at SSWV. These data represent the predominant activities that a K3-level amputee would experience during daily use of a prosthesis.

All subjects were tested walking indoors on a carpeted floor or plywood ramps without the use of shoes. Amputee subjects were fitted with a specialized Dynamic Prosthesis designed by PRS (Figure 37.3).

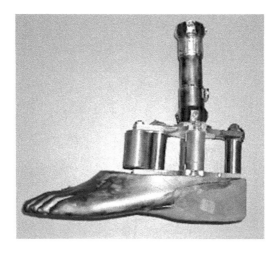

FIGURE 37.3 PRS dynamic prosthesis prototype.

The stiffness of the Dynamic Prosthesis ankle is controlled by the selection of four compression bumpers located anterior, posterior, medial, and lateral to a universal joint hinge. Subjects were allowed to walk, as desired, in the laboratory while bumpers of varying stiffness were interchanged in the test prosthesis. Each subject was allowed to select the bumpers he or she found most comfortable during normal gait. These selected bumpers were then used in the initial clinical study for the ABLE ankle.

37.2.2 KINETIC ANALYSIS

Preliminary kinetic analysis of the amputee subjects was acquired using a novel pylon-mounted force transducer. The prosthesis force transducer (PFT) was developed at PRS for the remote monitoring of forces and moments imposed at the socket–pylon interface. The system includes a customized six-degree-of-freedom load cell, power supply, 12-bit digital signal processing board, and RS232 wireless data transmission system (Figure 37.4).

Unlike traditional force platforms, which are typically mounted in the floor of a gait laboratory, the PFT is contained within the prosthesis. This allows the research team to collect kinetic data over multiple steps in sequence or along a nonlevel surface, such as stairs or ramps, where placement of a force platform would be difficult, if not impossible.

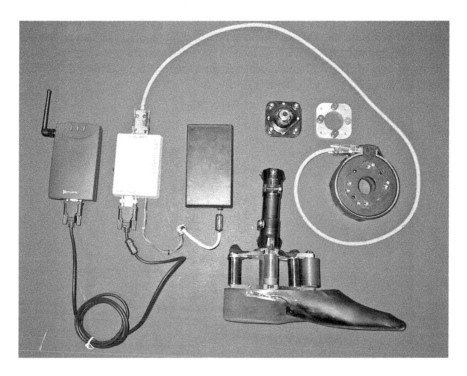

FIGURE 37.4 PRS PFT system.

Marker coordinates were sampled at 120 Hz and exported to tab-delimited ASCII files. A minimum of five samples per walking speed and incline were collected for each amputee subject. The exported kinematic data were digitally filtered with a fourth-order Butterworth low-pass filter and fit with a B-Spline using custom-written MatLab (MathWorks, Natick, MA) software. The splined data were evaluated at 200 data points between initial contact and terminal stance, as defined by the motion of the heel marker. The 3D marker coordinates were used to define the kinematic model and determine the position of the foot and leg segments in the coronal and sagittal planes with respect to the ground plane. The relative positions of the model segments were then used to assess ankle flexion and angular velocity during stance, and reported as a function of mean stance time. The leg (or shank) angle, with respect to the ground and the foot segment, was reported in both the sagittal and coronal planes. Additionally, temporal data such as the mean stance time and time to foot-flat were obtained from the kinematic records. Each trial as well as each individual- and population-specific minimum, maximum, and mean data were presented in graphical and tabular formats for both the able-bodied and amputee populations. Figure 37.5 illustrates an example of the angular motion and forward velocity derived from the PRS video image laboratory. These data were used to develop the inputs and boundary conditions of the 3D FEM.

The axial force, M/L force, A/P force, and moments about all three axes were collected at 100 Hz using a customized LabVIEW (National Instruments, Austin, TX) interface. The data were collected in binary format and exported for postprocessing with the kinematic data. The kinetic data were similarly filtered, splined, and sampled at 200 data points over the stance period, as defined by the vertical force channel. Axial force, M/L force, A/P force, axial torque, and A/P and M/L bending data were obtained in this manner. The coronal and sagittal ankle moments were calculated from

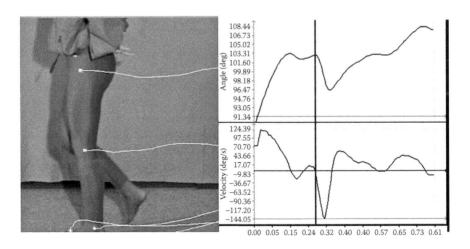

FIGURE 37.5 Video image of camera 1 motion tracing with sample output curve of shank-foot angle and angular velocity as a function of gait.

TABLE 37.1
Basic Data Set from Initial Clinical Trials

Force/Moment Data		
Force (lb)	Axial A/P M/L	
Moment (lb)	Torsion A/P M/L	

Angular Data		
Component	**Plane**	**Value**
Foot	Sagittal	Minimum
	Lateral	Maximum
		Average
Shank	Frontal	Minimum
		Maximum
		Average
Ankle	Anterior/posterior	Minimum
		Maximum
		Average
Ankle	Medial/lateral	Minimum
		Maximum
		Average
Ankle	Angular velocity	Minimum
		Maximum
		Average
Shank	Angular velocity	Minimum
		Maximum
		Average

a combined analysis of the kinetic and kinematic data using MatLab software, as shown in Figure 37.5.

The results of this clinical trial served as the preliminary design parameters for the ABLE prosthesis. Approximately 1800 data files from the PRS clinical results were normalized to percent of gait. To bound the design space, shown in Table 37.1, the minimum, maximum, and average parameters were calculated throughout the gait cycle, as shown in Figure 37.6.

Results from the able-bodied gait trails were used to determine the motion of the foot and shank with respect to ground. Specifically noted were the time from heel strike to foot-flat, the time from foot-flat to heel rise, the time from heel rise to toe-off, and the angular velocity of the shank throughout stance. Minimum, maximum, and mean values of these parameters were calculated, recorded, and normalized to the mean stance phase period. These data were used to determine the able-bodied baseline linear and angular motion. Figure 37.6 shows an example of the data for the A/P response. In this example, foot-flat occurs at approximately 18% of the stance phase period (~0.08 sec).

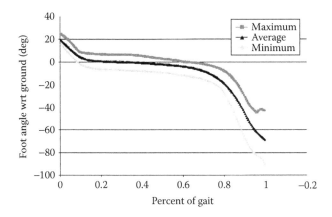

FIGURE 37.6 Example of gait data used to develop the ABLE tension band design.

Using kinetic and kinematic data collected on amputee subjects in the clinical trial, kinetic and kinematic baseline data for amputee subjects were also developed, and ankle loads during gait were determined using the Dynamic Prosthesis. Load data were used as a guide to develop the initial response of the IDEC tension bands. Baseline ABLE prosthetic kinematic design goals from the PRS clinical data are shown in Table 37.2.

37.2.3 Analysis and Design of the ABLE Prosthetic Ankle

The primary load-bearing members of the ABLE prosthetic ankle design (Figure 37.1) are the hourglass center compression member and tension bands. Ideally, the hourglass is designed to take all the axial compression loads, while allowing free rotation of the ankle in both the sagittal and coronal planes. The tension bands (unidirectional, tension-only springs) provide most of the ABLE ankle assembly's resistance to bending, planterflexion/dorsiflection, and inversion/eversion.

The analysis and design effort focused on developing a full 3D, nonlinear ABLE prosthesis ankle FEM to investigate system-level, macroresponse of a BK ABLE

TABLE 37.2
Baseline Kinematic Design Goals

	Time (sec) to		
	Foot-Flat	Heel-Off	Toe-Off
Average	0.08	0.49	0.79
Maximum	0.12	0.60	0.91
Minimum	0.04	0.37	0.66

Time is from heel strike to gait position

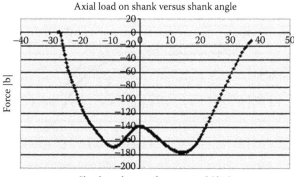

FEA tibial load

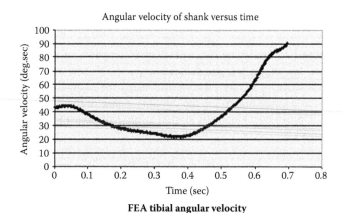

FEA tibial angular velocity

FIGURE 37.7 ABLE FEA baseline input loads and boundary conditions.

prosthesis. The FEM included a pylon, Seattle Carbon Lightfoot (Seattle Systems, Poulsbo, WA) prosthetic foot, and the dynamic ABLE prosthesis ankle model. The FEM foot included polymer "flesh" on the bottom of the foot to account for the compliance of the foot cosmesis and the composite keel structure in the foot. This model was used to define the tension band and hourglass load-deflection and strength requirements that would mimic the able-bodied gait data (load time histories and ankle rotational dynamics) obtained from PRS.

The figures of merit* for the results are matching the able-bodied gait time history for (1) time from heel strike to foot-flat, (2) time from foot-flat to heel-off, and (3) time from heel-off to toe-off. The primary loading, shown in Figure 37.7, was the nominal time-history of the "tibial" axial load measured on amputees, and tibial rotation measured on able-bodied subjects. A sophisticated, detailed, 3D, dynamic nonlinear FEA[12] was used to determine the properties of the tension bands and center support needed to enable the amputee to have a gait pattern consistent with that of

---

* Figure of merit is the measure of specific parameters that govern overall performance or design goals.

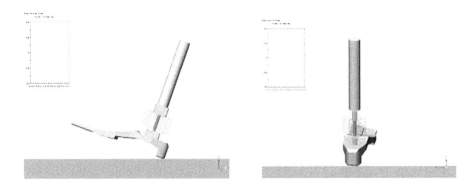

FIGURE 37.8 ABLE prosthesis finite element model.

able-bodied subjects. Once the nominal gait parameters were achieved, additional tension bands were developed to bracket, softer and stiffer, the nominal design. This allowed the clinician to closely match individual preferences during the clinical trials.

In the FEM analyses, the weight of the patient was approximated by a sagittally unrestrained inertial mass located on the proximal pylon. The pylon also had a defined angular velocity corresponding to the nominal able-bodied ambulatory speed. Figure 37.7 illustrates the FEM input loads and angular forcing function. The analysis commenced just prior to heel strike and ended at toe-off. The ambulatory 3D, dynamic, nonlinear finite element ABLE model was developed, as shown in Figure 37.8, and included the tension band response; foot, keel, and flesh geometries; and directional mechanical properties of each specific material. The model consisted of a composite pylon; proximal and distal composite tension band attachment supports; four unidirectional tension bands; and a 27-cm Seattle Carbon Lightfoot prosthetic foot with the "flesh" polymer and composite keel. The prosthetic foot was rigidly attached to the distal tension band support. The FEA was performed with the foot externally rotated 7° with respect to the direction of travel, shown in Figure 37.9.

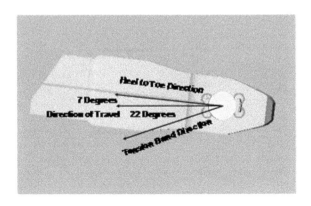

FIGURE 37.9 Coordinate map for the ABLE prosthesis analysis.

To provide realistic results with the clinical tests, the ABLE ankle assembly had to fit within the cosmesis of a 27-cm Seattle Carbon Lightfoot. This required the outside diameter of the ABLE ankle to be less than or equal to 1.75×2.50 in., which limited the tension bands' resisting moment arm to approximately 0.75 in. As a result, the tension bands had to carry high loads, in some cases up to 1000 lb, while allowing less than 0.10 in. of deflection. The 27-cm Lightfoot was selected by PRS as representative of most patients who would be involved in the clinical trials.

37.2.4 DETAILED ANALYSIS AND DESIGN

The primary load-bearing members of the ABLE assembly are the center support, also referred to as the "hourglass" due to its shape, and tension bands. The center support was designed to take all the axial compression loading while allowing free rotation of the ankle. The tension bands provide almost all rotational loading resistance and all the customizable bending properties of the ABLE assembly. They are the primary tools used to "tune" the deformation vs. load-bending curve to provide the correct rotational/bending dynamics of the ABLE ankle.

37.2.5 E. CENTER SUPPORT DESIGN

The hourglass center compression member must react the high compressive loads with little or no axial deflection and have minimal resistance to A/P and M/L bending forces. Polyurethane hourglasses were fabricated using durometers ranging from 35 to 85D shore hardness to give low bending resistance. This did achieve low bending resistance; however, it did not provide sufficient resistance to axial compression. The ABLE prosthetic analysis showed that a small axial deflection in the hourglass could release the tension in the bands, which would lead to a significant degradation of the ankle's stability. To strengthen the hourglass axial stiffness, a flat lands (coils) spring was incorporated. The lands were touching when the spring was not loaded (Figure 37.10), satisfying the requirement for a stiff compressive center support (the spring cannot deform axially under a compressive load). However, the spring could accommodate bending by pivoting about the inside lands while having the outside lands open up to allow the required ankle rotations with minimal resistance. Each

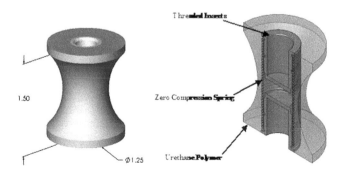

FIGURE 37.10 Solid model of the center support "hourglass" design.

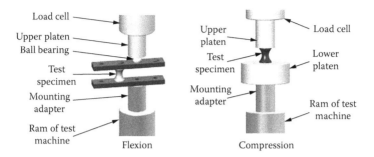

FIGURE 37.11 Hourglass mechanical test setups.

center support hourglass also contained threaded brass inserts that fit inside the coil spring, comolded into the proximal and distal ends of the hourglass and spring. The brass inserts provide the attachments to the prosthetic pylon via a pyramid adapter and the prosthetic foot via M10 bolts. Various durometer center support hourglass polymers were tested in compression and flexion to obtain macroproperties to use in the analysis, as shown in the test setup in Figure 37.11. Mechanical test loads were taken from the clinical test data, shown in Figure 37.7. The tests were performed on SPARTA's MTS (MTS Systems Corporation, Eden Prairie, MN) static and fatigue testing machine. The tests were performed in "displacement control mode" at 0.10 in/min. Loading was from 0 to ~50 lb in flexion and 0 to 200 lb in axial compression. Hourglasses of the same durometer polymer had very similar load-deflection characteristics and no failures were observed.

37.2.6 PRECLINICAL TRIALS

Preclinical tests were performed by PRS personnel to evaluate the safety and stability of the ABLE construct prior to clinical tests with amputees. This prescreening was accomplished by attaching the ABLE ankle to customized ski boots as shown in Figure 37.12. The boots were designed as a way for an able-bodied individual to

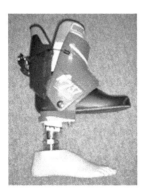 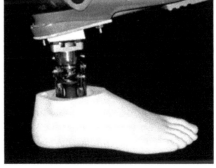

FIGURE 37.12 Preclinical tests using ski boots to simulate prosthetic function.

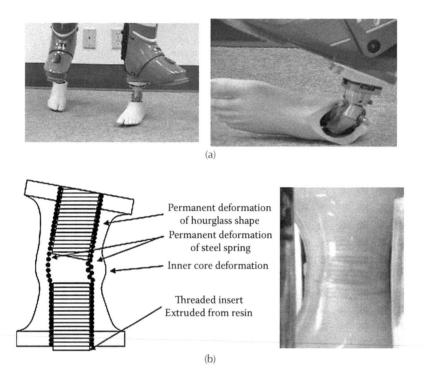

(a)

(b)

Permanent deformation
of hourglass shape

Permanent deformation
of steel spring

Inner core deformation

Threaded insert
Extruded from resin

FIGURE 37.13 (a) Hourglass had insufficient torsional rigidity. (b) Ankle instability due to excess torsional and lateral deformation in the co-molded flat land spring.

test the basic function, feel, and safety of a prosthetic foot. PRS researchers have used these boots to assess a number of prosthetic feet (single-axis composite heel [SACH], single-axis, and energy-storing). Initial evaluations of the ABLE P1 prototype in the walking boots revealed a significant torsional instability in the hourglass. This overloaded the tension bands and caused catastrophic failure of the center support and bands (Figure 37.13a and b). The flat-coiled springs had high compressive strength and stiffness but minimal torsional or lateral rigidity. The low torsional stiffness of the polymer-flat spring center support leads to excessive rotation of the tibia with respect to the foot during ambulation. This was clearly visible as the tibia was rotated while the prosthetic foot was planted on the floor. In the center support failure mode analysis and evaluation (FMAE), the deformation of the flat lands coil springs was apparent through the hourglass resin. Although it is difficult to be definitive, the most likely failure scenario was that the rotational instability of the hourglass center support induced an overextension and out-of-plane loading of the tension bands, leading to failures in both the hourglass and tension bands (Figure 37.13b).

To address this failure mode, the center support of the ABLE construct was redesigned using a steel "U-joint" design shown in Figure 37.14. The steel U-joint, while considerably heavier than the reinforced polymer hourglass design, provided

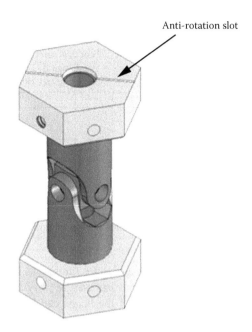

FIGURE 37.14 Revised ABLE center support U-joint.

the axial, lateral, and torsional stiffness and strength required to react to the large and complex loads experienced by the ankle during ambulation. The U-joint also provided negligible bending resistance. Axial rotation was restrained by mechanical locks as also shown in Figure 37.14. The facets on the proximal and distal caps provide the ability to attach the four tension bands at 0-, ±60-, and ±120-degree positions around the ABLE ankle. Ski boot tests of the U-joint center support showed no failures while allowing bend freedom in the ankle.

37.3 TENSION BAND DESIGN

As noted above, the tension bands are used to define the A/P and M/L bending characteristics/response of the ankle. The tension bands are essentially uncoupled, nonlinear, unidirectional springs. Uncoupled, unidirectional tension bands allow the prosthetist to control the ankle sagittal and coronal bending response on the basis of patient-specific attributes such as weight, activity level, terrain, etc. Initial analyses used linear load-deformation tension bands. However, as shown in Figure 37.15, linear tension bands could not meet the correct load deflection criteria necessary for "normal" gait.

To achieve the dynamics of the ABLE assembly and provide adequate stability, the tension bands must exhibit relatively little resistance upon initial loading, but increase exponentially as foot–tibia rotation increases. Stability can be maintained throughout gait because there is always at least one band in tension that opposes the

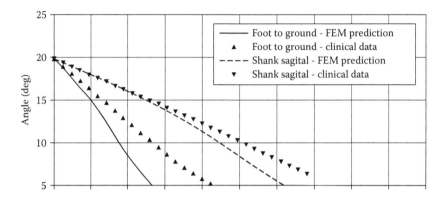

FIGURE 37.15 Comparison of analysis to clinical results using linear tension bands.

direction of motion. As noted above, the geometry limitations imposed by cosmetic concerns require that the maximum ankle diameter be very small. Therefore, the required instantaneous "spring constant" of the bands can be quite large. The A/P bands need to react to a moment induced by a load generated over 5 to 6 in. with a moment arm of about 0.5 to 1.0 in. In other words, the load on the bands could be up to 10× to 15× of the actual force on the foot. The maximum tension band deflection was calculated to be approximately 0.10 in. due to the very short moment arm allowed by the Seattle Lightfoot ankle geometry.

37.3.1 NONLINEAR TENSION BAND

The results also showed that a linear tension band could not meet the desired nonamputee gait parameters, and developing a nonlinear stiffness tension band became a major focus in the research program. This development effort relied heavily on SPARTA's IDEC technology.[1] IDEC allows the designer to engineer nonlinear compliance over a broad range by controlling the micromechanics and local *in situ* geometry of the load-bearing fiber component. IDEC technology can also produce a specific nonlinear response while keeping the constituent fiber or matrix below their elastic limits, thus extending the fatigue endurance of an IDEC component such as the ABLE ankle. Several fiber architectures for the new IDEC tension bands were evaluated using FEA models (Figure 37.16). Each of the fiber bundle architectures provides different specific load-deflection characteristics. Stiffer fibers required more "waviness" in the bundle geometry to generate similar nonlinear responses than less stiff fiber bundles. The tension band analyses incorporated various fiber architectures, fiber tow sizes, fiber types, and matrix polymers. The fiber tow bundles were modeled as discrete beams. However, because of the unique fiber volume architecture of the tension bands, a separate 3D FEM, shown as a "fiber tow bundle" cross section in Figure 37.17, was required to predict the discrete tow bundle mechanical properties for a variety of fiber types and polymers matrixes. The FEA fiber tow model was validated by comparing

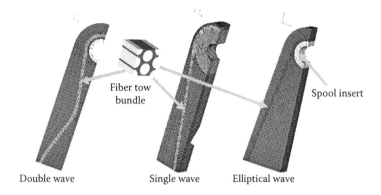

FIGURE 37.16 Quarter symmetry FEA models of IDEC tension band baseline architectures.

the analysis load-deformation results of a specific tow bundle incorporated in a tension band to empirical load-deformation test data of a tension band fabricated with the same fiber, matrix, and architecture as the analytical model (see the 60% fiber volume fraction plot in Figure 37.17). The tow bundle data were input into the ABLE tension band FEA shown in Figure 37.18.

Figure 37.18 shows a double-wave tension band model depicted at zero load and at the maximum deflection of 0.10 in. (0.925 of the design load). Figure 37.18 also shows movement of the fiber and the mechanical response of the tension band transitions from a polymer-dominated to a fiber-dominated response. The FEA results in Figure 37.19 show that high strains can occur at the interface between the reinforcing fibers and the matrix. These results suggested that a high-strength carbon fiber was required to take the load, and that a very low-stiffness polymer was needed to allow the fibers to align to the load path after a moderate axial deformation.

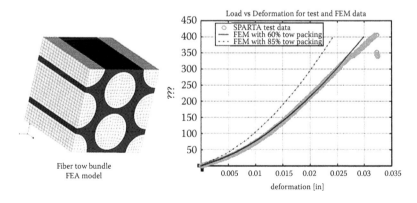

FIGURE 37.17 Analytical model of the *in situ* fiber tow and validation of the analytical predictions with test data.

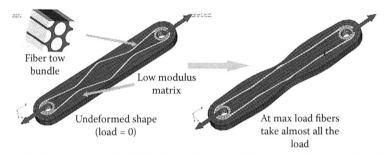

Material	E1 (psi)	E2 (psi)	E3 (psi)	G12 (psi)	G23 (psi)	G13 (psi)	nu12	nu23	nu13
Carbon fiber	29000000	960000	960000	437900	437900	437900	0.1	0.003	0.003
Matrix material	150	150	150	NA	NA	NA	0.4	0.4	0.4
Fiber bundle	24279958	1313.757	1313.757	280000	285.6	280000	0.1	0.4	0.1

FIGURE 37.18 IDEC *in situ* geometry of the baseline able tension bands from the unloaded state to near maximum load.

This, however, resulted in a high polymer tensile strain in the area where one fiber bundle was pulling away from the adjacent, mirror image fiber bundle. A high strain-to-failure (~400%) polyurethane resin and high-modulus carbon fiber reinforcement generate an exponential load-deflection curve close to the required baseline load-deflection response. There was almost five orders of magnitude difference between the fiber and matrix modulus. The double-wave design provided both nonlinear

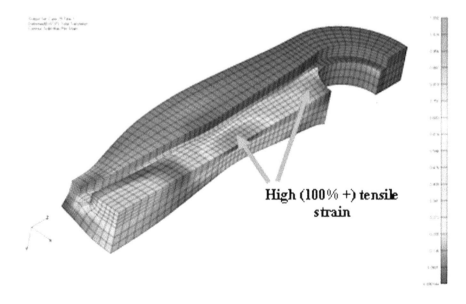

FIGURE 37.19 FEA principal strain contours in a typical tension band model under moderate to high loading.

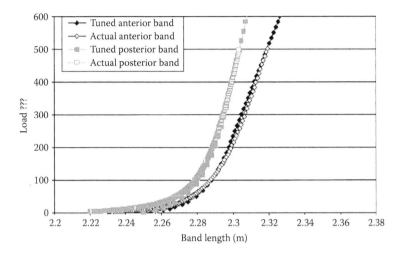

FIGURE 37.20 Mechanical tests verify the nonlinear FEA analysis.

results and the required strength and stiffness at a deflection of 0.10 in. However, the high-stiffness carbon fiber required a significant high-amplitude waviness in the tow bundle to achieve an initial low-stiffness response in the tension band. When the baseline tow bundle data were input into the ABLE tension band FEA, as anticipated, there was a high but manageable tensile strain where the fiber bundles that are close together pull away from the centerline, shown in Figure 37.19. There was also a very local, moderate-to-high tensile strain at the spool/fiber tangent area. While the polymer could theoretically absorb this strain, microscopic flaws such as an entrapped air bubble or unconsolidated fiber could significantly increase the apparent strain the polymer senses, thereby causing failure.

The tension band FEA closely predicted the load-deflection response obtained in the mechanical tests, as presented in Figure 37.20. Analytical results, in the figure, are the "tuned" curves and these data show a close correlation between the predicted and actual test data, validating the analytical approach and the FEM.

The full ABLE analysis was performed parametrically using the DYNA 3D FEA hydrocode* to determine the timing from heel strike to foot-flat, mid-stance, and heel-off to toe-off for a variety of nonlinear spring load/deflection curves. Figure 37.21 shows selected frames from a full 3D ambulatory (walking) FEA. The output from the ambulatory model provided the nonlinear tension band parameters required to simulate the baseline able-bodied gait.

The baseline tension band, shown in Figure 37.18, used a carbon fiber tow bundle and a low durometer polymer (see the material property data in Figure 37.18). The band design incorporated a metal "spool" insert to address end-effects issues of tow-bundle spreading during fabrication, fibers shearing through the polymer matrix under load, and providing a uniform loading of the *in situ* fiber bundle tows. Carbon

---

* Hydrocodes are specialized finite element codes that can solve problems involving large deformations, as well as highly nonlinear materials and loading conditions.

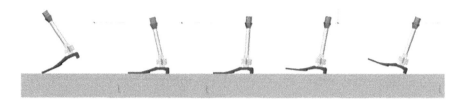

FIGURE 37.21 Stop action of ABLE gait analysis sequence.

fiber was selected for the tow bundle because of its high strength and stiffness. The double-wave geometry was selected because it provided the large deformations needed for the ABLE assembly while not overstraining the high-stiffness carbon fiber bundle. As shown in Figure 37.18, the fibers are initially aligned off-axis with respect to the load direction. As the load increases, the fibers begin to straighten out, taking more of the load and providing more resistance to the applied load.

Specific band performance parameters were determined by running the FEA model through the gait cycle from heel strike to toe-off. Using these data to bound the band load/deflection characteristics, over 150 tension bands were fabricated and characterized through mechanical testing. This large number of bands provided the clinician a wide variety of bands to select for each patient. Each band was mechanically tested from zero load to 450 lb (maximum stiffness). Initial testing of the bands was conducted to 950 lb to insure the band design integrity. A spreadsheet was developed, which had the actual load-deflection characteristics of each band from 0 to 450 lb. Each band's stiffness was presented in linear 50-lb increments and could be compared to another arbitrary band using color-coded cells in the spreadsheet database. The spreadsheet allowed the clinician to determine the relative stiffness of a specific band at each load, compared to either the reference tension band or another selected band.

37.3.2 Tension Band Fabrication and Mechanical Validation Tests

Tension bands were fabricated using a closed mold process applicable to a variety of fibers, matrixes, and *in situ* geometries. As noted earlier, the tension band fibers were wrapped around a spool-shaped insert, which provided a uniform loading of the fibers and also maintained the fiber bundle integrity. This spool also provided a robust method of attaching the band to the prosthetic ankle body. The nonlinear tension bands went through multiple design and experimental validation iterations. IDEC tension band development also required a significant research effort to develop a repeatable, stable fabrication technology. Figure 37.22 shows an "as-fabricated" tension band and the tension band mechanical test setup. The tag on the tension band is a resin overflow feature and is removed before use.

37.3.3 Preclinical Evaluation

As noted earlier, preclinical tests were performed by PRS personnel to evaluate the ABLE ankle construct prior to clinical tests with amputees. These tests were conducted

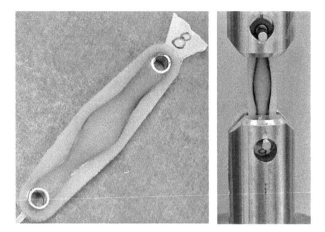

FIGURE 37.22 As-fabricated double wave tension band and tension band test setup.

using the modified ski boots (Figure 37.23) and revealed that the torsional stiffness of the center support was insufficient. A redesign of the center support to a steel U-joint solved the problem of lack of torsional stiffness in the center support, but revealed another problem. Preclinical assessment by PRS personnel found that the posterior tension bands failed after only a few steps. Band failure occurred at the high-strain regions noted in the FEA (Figure 37.24). These regions occurred where the fiber tension put the polymer in high transverse tension over a small distance. This produced very large strain gradients and, eventually, fiber/matrix separation.

Because the posterior bands failed before the anterior bands, there was concern that the walking boots used in the preclinical evaluation may have applied excessive forces to the ABLE ankle joint in terminal stance because of the rigid boot design. Weight bearing on the toe of the boot in terminal stance would likely induce significantly larger moments about the ankle in the sagittal plane than would be induced by a transtibial amputee. The boot design was modified by PRS to remove the rigid toe, thereby minimizing any additional moment induced by the boot in terminal stance (Figure 37.25). The effect of this modification was immediately seen

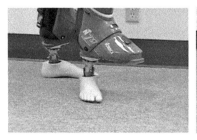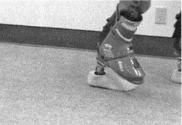

FIGURE 37.23 Preclinical walking trials with the ABLE ankle attached to the ski boot and a Seattle Carbon LightFoot.

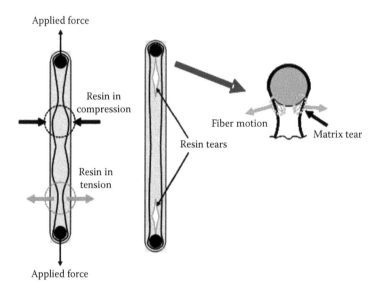

FIGURE 37.24 Schematic of double-wave tension band failure.

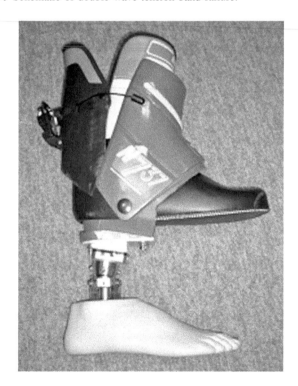

FIGURE 37.25 Ski boot test bed with hard-shell toe removed to minimize the effect of "toe walking" and reduce the additional moment caused by the user putting pressure on the ball of his foot inside the boot.

in that the posterior tension band could take significantly more cycles (number of steps) before another incident; however, continued preclinical evaluation eventually elicited failure in the high-strain areas of the posterior bands.

More research is needed to fully characterize the increase in loading, which may be associated with the use of rigid boots for prosthetic evaluation. The use of the boots in the preclinical trial to simulate the "feel" of a prosthetic limb for an able-bodied individual offers many advantages, including simple, qualitative assessment and safety testing prior to subject use of a prototype device. It should be noted that the boots may apply forces and moments in excess of those experienced by an amputee subject because of the increased limb length and/or rigid construction of the boot itself. However, PRS personnel anticipated that the increased forces for a lightweight, able-bodied individual walking slowly in the boots would not exceed those induced by an amputee ambulating at normal and high walking speeds or walking up and down inclines. Every attempt was made to match loading patterns in the boots with those that could be seen in the clinical trial. Because the ABLE ankle becomes unstable when one or more bands fail, this preclinical evaluation was necessary to assess the safety of the ABLE ankle prior to use by amputee subjects.

The analysis and empirical data showed that the IDEC technology would carry less risk if the fiber bundle put the matrix in compression rather than tension; however, the high stiffness of the carbon fiber bundles would require a significant amount of time to redesign the tension bands to eliminate the localized high-tension areas. An elliptical single-wave geometry was developed as the new tension band *in situ* architecture. This architecture, shown in Figure 37.26, would put the polymer

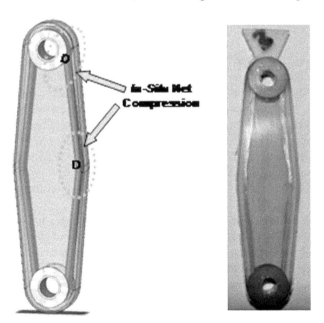

FIGURE 37.26 Elliptical wave *in situ* fiber bundle architecture — critical areas in net matrix compression.

matrix in compression during loading; however, the single-wave design did not allow sufficient *in situ* lateral fiber bundle displacement using high-stiffness carbon tow bundle. To compensate for this, Kevlar® (E.I. duPont de Nemours & Company, Inc., Wilmington, DE) fiber was used as the fiber tow bundle. Kevlar has about half the stiffness of carbon, which allowed the correct load deformation response without having to increase the external geometry of the existing tension band or use *in situ*, multiwave bundle architecture with its inherent lateral tensile strains in the polymer.

By changing the cross-sectional area of the Kevlar tow bundle and the tow bundle wave shape, the design load/deformation response could be engineered to accommodate the design strength and stiffness. Over 45 Kevlar tension bands were fabricated and mechanically tested, with no failures or internal delamination. SPARTA also subjected these bands to "preclinical" modified-toe ski boot walking with no failures. The Kevlar tension bands were delivered to PRS for clinical evaluation. This redesign demonstrates the flexibility of the IDEC technology, which can be quickly modified and adapted to accommodate unanticipated events.

The modified tension bands were again tested by PRS in a preclinical trial to evaluate their strength and resiliency in walking gait. Initial laboratory testing in the walking boots revealed no failures within a minimum of 500 steps. Qualitative analysis revealed that the ABLE ankle responded as anticipated with controlled plantarflexion, stable but flexible midstance, and propulsive energy return in late stance. These results were sufficient to convince PRS personnel that the ABLE device was ready for a clinical evaluation of transtibial amputee subjects. An ongoing three-person clinical trial is in progress to assess the efficacy of the ABLE design with Kevlar tension bands.

37.4 CONCLUSION

The objective of this research was to develop an ABLE prosthetic ankle capable of mimicking a natural, nonamputee gait. A major step in achieving this objective was developing complex, dynamic, nonlinear FEMs that could approximate the human ankle function. These models were developed based on extensive clinical data from both able-bodied and amputee subjects. Able-bodied data were used to develop the FEA geometric and dynamic functions. Amputee data were used to provide guidance for the input parameters and boundary conditions of the analytical models. The output of these analyses was used to design prototype ankle components and full-scale ankle assemblies. The validity of this approach was demonstrated through both mechanical and limited, to-date, clinical testing.

The ABLE ankle design offers many theoretical advantages to an amputee. The ABLE design includes some of the best features from a variety of prosthetic foot types, including rapid plantarflexion in early stance, accommodation to uneven terrain, and energy response to assist in forward propulsion of the amputated limb. While the final design has not yet been achieved, the interim results show promise for an adaptable and customizable prosthesis that will address an unmet need for a device that provides able-bodied motion, as well as the safety and stability required by amputees. This research has also demonstrated the ability to design and fabricate IDEC nonlinear springs that provide the required properties to tailor prosthesis performance to the individual's needs. Preliminary input from the ongoing clinical trial indicates that the

ABLE concept is sound and holds the potential for a novel prosthetic biofidelic device. The clinicians have been impressed by the smooth action and lifelike behavior of the ABLE ankle. The original belief that amputees are in need of a device which can provide safety and stability in stance, accommodate to uneven terrian, and provide energy return in gait is still valid. The initial feedback from the clinical tests indicate that the ABLE concept is a solid step toward that goal.

ACKNOWLEDGMENTS

The authors wish to acknowledge the support and help of the National Institutes of Health, National Institute of Child Health and Human Development (NICHHD) under Grant No. 5 R01 HD038933-04, and NICHHD's willingness to accommodate the various nuances of this research effort. We would also like to thank Andrew Kostuch of Quartus Engineering Incorporated, San Diego, CA, and Larry Foster of Foster Engineering, San Diego, CA, for their development of the highly complex FEMs and FEAs, as well as their contribution to the overall design of the ABLE prosthesis. We also wish to thank Jim Beck for his design and work on the initial clinical trials, and his compilation of the massive amount of data from these trials. These data were used to define the design requirements for the ABLE ankle prosthesis.

REFERENCES

1. In-situ Dynamic Engineered Compliance (IDEC); White, M., SPARTA, Inc. Patent Pending No. 10/976,556; entitled "Non-Linear Fiber Matrix Architecture," Oct 29, 2004.
2. White, M., Whatley, W., Smith, D., Beck, J., Kostuch, A.; "Development of an Advanced Biofidelic Lower Extremity (ABLE) Prosthesis," *Pediatric and Foot and Ankle: New Horizons in Clinical Treatment and Innovative Technology,* November 15, 2003; National Institutes of Health, Bethesda, MD.
3. Perry, J., *Gait Analysis: Normal and Pathological Function,* Slack Incorporated, Thorofare, 1992.
4. Bresler, B. and Frankel, J.P., The forces and moments in the leg during level walking, *Trans. ASME,* 72, 27–36, 1950.
5. Czerniecki, J.M., Foot and ankle biomechanics in walking and running. A review, *Am. J. Phys. Med. Rehabil.,* 67(6), 246–252, 1988.
6. Mann, R.A. and Hagy, J., Biomechanics of walking, running, and sprinting, *Am. J Sports Med.,* 8(5), 345–350, 1980.
7. Breakey, J, Gait of unilateral below-knee amputees, *Orth. Prosth.,* 30(3), 17–24, 1976.
8. Gitter, A., Biomechanical analysis of the influence of prosthetic feet on below-knee amputee walking, *Am. J. Phys. Med. Rehabil.,* 70(3), 142–148, 1991.
9. Winter, D.A. and Sienko, S.E., Biomechanics of below-knee amputee gait, *J. Biomech.,* 21(5), 361–367, 1988.
10. NASTRAN (MSC Software, Santa Ana, CA): Dynamic and non-linear Eulerin Code; and DYNA 3-D (Livermore Software Technology, Livermore, CA): Dynamic, non-linear Lagrangean hydro code.

38 The Role of Robotic Technology in Gait Simulation and Foot Mechanics

James C. Otis

CONTENTS

38.1 INTRODUCTION

Historically, foot biomechanics has not received the attention that has been received by hip and knee biomechanics. This is due, in large part, to two factors: the hindfoot and midfoot are structures that must be analyzed in three dimensions whereas the hip and knee are amenable to two-dimensional analyses, e.g., in the sagittal and frontal planes; and, unlike the hip and knee joints, painful disorders of the hindfoot and midfoot joints can be often be treated with fusions without the functional limitations associated with a hip or knee fusion. The foot with its many joints can more readily compensate for the loss of motion of some of its joints. Adequate models to study the mechanical and functional properties of the foot are necessary in order to understand normal and pathological mechanics and to develop more effective treatments for foot disorders.

This chapter will discuss methods used for characterizing the mechanical properties of joints and the need for and implementation of cadaver models and sophisticated gait simulators to understand the intrinsic kinematics and kinetics of the foot during gait. It will further discuss the potential for extending the use of robotic technology that has been applied to quantify mechanical properties of the knee joint, glenohumeral joint, and intervertebral joints of the spine to quantify mechanical properties and simulate external loading conditions of the foot during functional activities. The discussion will center on a foot disorder, posterior tibial tendon dysfunction (PTTD), which has particularly benefited from the use of cadaver models and gait simulators.

In the 1990s, the Research Committee of the American Orthopaedic Foot and Ankle Society ranked PTTD as the foot disorder with the highest research priority.[1] The disorder results in a functional deficit, the loss of a muscle/tendon unit, which leads to progressive structural changes over the long term and eventually an acquired flatfoot deformity. The acquired flatfoot deformity can become extreme when the medial arch structures that normally span the ground have collapsed to the point where they are in contact with the ground and the forefoot becomes abducted, as illustrated by the model in Figure 38.1. Restoration of alignment without fusing joints of the hindfoot was in need to improve operative treatments for PTTD. Historically, studies to understand the biomechanics of acquired flatfoot deformity and investigate potential operative treatments were performed on mid-tibia–amputated specimens with only a vertical load applied through a weight placed on the top of the tibia. Such studies were limited in their relevance to foot during stance

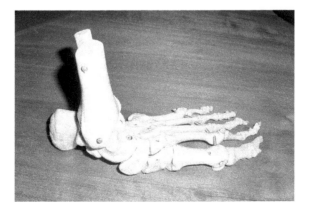

FIGURE 38.1 Skeleton model of foot illustrating the failure of the medial arch and abduction of the forefoot associated with acquired flatfoot deformity.

conditions with little or no muscle action. Given the structural complexity of the foot and a disorder that involves structural and muscle/tendon components, it was readily apparent that experimental studies were needed to account for the role of the posterior tibial muscle and other muscles in order to understand the mechanisms by which the medial arch is stabilized throughout the stance phase of gait. It was also apparent that it was not practical to perform the necessary studies on human subjects, and that the mechanical complexities of the foot were not sufficiently documented to permit the development of a mathematical model. The direction chosen was to develop a cadaver model for PTTD that could be implemented for testing new operative procedures to determine whether procedures result in clinically relevant improvements.[2]

Early biomechanical studies of the hip and knee joints have been performed on closed-loop hydraulic test systems. Studies employing these closed-loop control systems, even when using the biaxial models that allow control of one linear axis and one rotational axis, often required augmentation with custom-made test jigs to provide the necessary degrees-of-freedom. This had been of particular importance when studying the knee joint, as it is inherently a less constrained joint than is the hip joint. These custom test jigs can require as much, or more, time and effort than is required to perform the experimental work. Furthermore, the jigs require considerable time and expense, and are often limited in the types of applications for which they may be used. This approach is less attractive for understanding the mechanics of the foot, both because of its three-dimensional (3D) behavior and the fact that multiple articulations exist between the input and output of the test, unlike the knee where the femur is attached on one side of the test apparatus and the tibia on the other with a single articulation between the two bones.

38.2 METHODOLOGY

38.2.1 PTTD MODEL REQUIREMENTS

Our requirements for the PTTD model were that loss of the posterior tibial muscle action result in (a) a deformity consistent with that occurring clinically and (b) an increased strain on the spring ligament at the medial arch consistent with the ligament's observed clinical failure.[3] A cadaver foot testing system was designed to simulate external force and position conditions at a specific time during the gait cycle, i.e., when loss of the posterior tibial muscle would have its greatest effect. An experimental condition was established which reflected the posterior tibial muscle's most demanding role during gait. Electromyographic (EMG) patterns presented by Perry[4] illustrate that maximal EMG activity for the posterior tibial muscle occurs at approximately 40% of the gait cycle, corresponding to early heel rise. To appreciate the role of the posterior tibial muscle, it is, therefore, important to document the response of the foot to loss of this muscle force at this most demanding time. The EMG patterns[4] also illustrate that the other extrinsic muscles of the foot, i.e., the soleus, gastrocnemius, flexor digitorum longus, flexor hallucis longus, peroneus brevis, and peroneus longus, all demonstrate their peak activity at approximately 40% of the gait cycle. Therefore, with respect to PTTD, consideration should be given to all of these muscles when simulating gait performance at 40% of the gait cycle.

38.2.2 CADAVER MODEL

38.2.2.1 Requirements

It was necessary to determine whether the proposed cadaveric foot model simulating gait at 40% of the gait cycle would be sensitive to the loss of the posterior tibial muscle/tendon force in a manner that was consistent with the development of an acquired flatfoot deformity that is observed clinically. Clinical evidence suggested that loss of tendon function causes failure of the spring ligament in the arch[3] in association with the acquired deformity. However, it was not likely that a loaded cadaver model could produce failure of the spring ligament of the medial arch during a single experimental event consistent with loss of the muscle/tendon force at 40% of the gait cycle. Furthermore, it was not likely that spring ligament failure could be generated in a cadaver model simulating gait because it would require cyclic testing with external loads and muscle loads that the cadaveric specimen would not tolerate in areas other than the spring ligament, e.g., failure of the cemented fixation interface between the tibia and the apparatus or failure of the tendon attachments to their respective transducers and cables. Given these limitations, it was decided that the best indicator of potential injury to the spring ligament was to measure the strain of the ligament.

38.2.2.2 Instrumentation

We had used liquid metal strain gages in prior studies to measure strain in the medial longitudinal arch in the loaded plantigrade foot with no tendon loads. Each displacement gage consisted of mercury-filled Silastic tubing, which, when incorporated into a Wheatstone bridge circuit, yielded a voltage related to the length of the gage. The gage location of primary concern was below the track of the posterior tibial tendon and was subjected to compressive loads, which can introduce artifact into the liquid strain gage measurement when the tendon is loaded. We examined the behavior of this type of gage in a prototype system, which employed a plantar flexion angle sensor and a pneumatic actuator attached to the Achilles tendon, which automatically responded to maintain a target plantar flexion angle. Removal of the posterior tibial tendon load, while maintaining plantar flexion via the Achilles, resulted in eversion; however, we detected artifact in the strain readings. Our preliminary data demonstrated strain readings with artifact as a result of the posterior tibial tendon compressing it. We realized from this exercise that the liquid metal strain gages would not meet the needs of the current proposal and, secondly, that a pneumatic actuator to generate tendon force was not sufficiently responsive for our experimental demands. To deal with the strain measurement problem, differential variable reluctance transducers (DVRTs, Microstrain, Inc., Burlington, VT) were used to measure ligament strain. These devices eliminated the compression artifact.

In addition to changes in strain of the spring ligament, it was necessary for the cadaver model to displace in a manner consistent with the deformity, i.e., forefoot dorsiflexion, eversion, and abduction. However, it is not possible to generate in a cadaver foot model the degree of deformity that occurs over an extended period of time and is observed clinically. Even cyclic testing with external loading and muscle loads could not produce the soft tissue failures necessary to create the degree of deformity observed clinically because the test setup would prove to be the weaker link. Creating the deformity is only possible if the appropriate soft tissue structures are compromised[5] and may include cyclic loading, a technique that has been used to develop a cadaver flatfoot model to study treatments for cases of advanced acquired flatfoot deformity. Thus, the model described in this chapter will be appropriate to test operative treatments to be used in the early stages of PTTD.

To measure deformity, joint kinematics was monitored using electromagnetic tracking sensors (Polhemus FASTRAK, Colchester, VT). The 3D motion sensors were rigidly attached to the talus, cuboid, calcaneus, and navicular to monitor the motion of each of these bones. Of particular interest was the displacement of the navicular with respect to the talus because the talonavicular joint is the primary joint of the medial arch. In the acquired flatfoot, the displacement of the navicular with respect to the talus in the sagittal, transverse, and frontal planes is dorsiflexion, abduction, and eversion, respectively.

38.2.3 HYPOTHESIS

The likely mechanism for the resulting deformity is that the loss of tendon function leads to progressive deformity and increases the strain in the ligaments in the medial longitudinal arch. Although ligaments in addition to the spring ligament undoubtedly fail, the spring ligament is the only ligament at present, which has been documented to fail in PTTD (with the exception of the deltoid ligament, which fails in end-stage disease). Therefore, for the cadaver model, it was hypothesized that loss of the posterior tibial tendon force during the early heel rise portion of the gait cycle would result in dorsiflexion, abduction, and eversion of the navicular with respect to the talus and there would be an associated increase in strain in the spring ligament of the medial longitudinal arch.

38.2.4 SIMULATION OF EARLY HEEL RISE

38.2.4.1 Loading Apparatus

A cadaveric loading apparatus was developed, which allows the application of external loads (which simulate three components of ground reaction force) provides for the simulation of muscle forces for up to five tendons, monitors and provides feedback of two foot angular positions, monitors the 3D positions of up to four joints, and permits the measurement of soft tissue strain. The system is operated using a LabVIEW for Windows virtual instrument. The ground reaction force components are applied through three stepper motors in series with force transducers. The apparatus, shown schematically in Figure 38.2, is an epoxy-coated wooden frame with three platforms at different levels for mounting the stepper motors, supporting the cadaver foot, and applying the ground reaction forces. The frame measures 8 ft. tall by 3 ft. wide by 2.5 ft. deep. A Garolite sheet is used to rigidly mount the stepper motors. Wood and Garolite

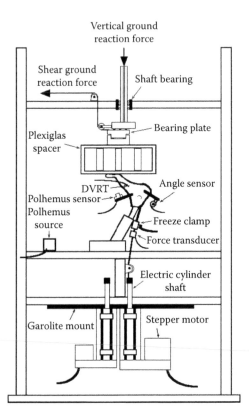

FIGURE 38.2 Cadaveric foot-loading apparatus with tibia fixed to frame; ground reaction force components applied from above; muscle loads applied from stepper motors at bottom; freeze clamps and force transducers connecting tendons to cables from motors; DVRT location; Polhemus source and sensors to measure displacements of four bones; and angle sensor to monitor tilt in sagittal and coronal planes.

were chosen as structural materials because they do not interfere with the Polhemus 3Space FASTRAK system.

The experimental arrangement simulates conditions at the foot as they occur during gait. We have taken the approach that the muscles of the lower extremity will respond to the external forces as necessary to achieve and maintain the desired foot position. Thus, the two muscles controlling the plantar flexion and inversion angles are adjusted to achieve the desired position. The development of these capabilities permits us to ask and seek answers to clinically relevant research questions about PTTD and its treatment at a level of sophistication that had not been possible in the past. The system developed and used by Sharkey et al.[6] to measure strain in the second metatarsal provided invaluable direction for us in the development of this system. Our system, however, differs in that we simulate external ground reaction forces so that the muscle forces generated are in response to these loads and the need to achieve the target positions. An alternate approach is to fix the distance from the tibia to the ground, fixed to allow the heel rise position and generate muscle forces based upon EMG data until achieved. With this approach, the generated ground reaction force is arbitrarily found by estimating all of the muscle forces. Also, we have designed our system to allow us to use the magnetic space tracker and measure ligament strain.

38.2.4.2 Tendon Clamps

The ability to grasp tendons and apply high loads was a problem early on. This was solved by implementing a method of freeze clamping to couple the tendons to the cables. This method was used by Sharkey et al.[7] to study the rotator cuff in abduction and also to load the Achilles tendon and other muscles of the calf in a study of second metatarsal strain and loading during heel lift.[6] A modification of their technique was implemented. The tendon was fed through a hole into a chamber, the end was knotted, and the chamber perfused by liquid nitrogen coolant to solidify the knot. The tendon freezes in three to five minutes and is maintained by perfusing liquid nitrogen, as needed, such that the tissue is frozen 1 cm distal to the clamp as evidenced from the tidemark. The tendons can be thawed and used again at a later time. This method was implemented for up to five tendons.

38.2.4.3 Internal Forces

The experimental method chosen was to apply the tendon forces in order to control plantar flexion and inversion/eversion, i.e., the experiment is performed in a position feedback mode. Plantar flexion was controlled primarily by pulling on the Achilles tendon to counter the dorsiflexion moment created by the ground reaction force at the forefoot. Version was controlled by pulling on the posterior tibial tendon to counter not only any eversion moment created by the ground reaction force, but also the moment created by the peroneus longus and peroneus brevis tendons. The peroneal tendon loads were included because these muscles have their peak activity during early heel rise of the gait cycle. Based on the muscle architecture studies by Wickiewicz et al.[8] and Silver et al.,[9] the relative physiologic cross-sectional areas for the gastrocnemius/soleus muscle group, the posterior tibial muscle, the peroneus brevis, and peroneus longus as a percent of the gastrocnemius/soleus muscle group are 100, 17.2, 5.7, and 11.7%, respectively. Using a conservative estimate of 40 N/cm^2 for muscle force generating potential[10] and cross-sectional areas of 6 and 12 cm^2, respectively, the peroneus brevis and peroneus longus are capable of generating 240 and 480 N of force. Because muscle fatigues when utilizing greater than 50% of maximum strength, initially the muscles were assumed to operate at one-fourth of their capacities, i.e., 60 and 120 N, respectively, when conducting experiments at 100% body weight. This is a reasonable level at which repetitively loaded muscles can be expected to function during a routine daily activity. Motion analysis data obtained for knee extensors during gait support a level of 25% of maximum capability during repetitive loading.[11]

For the intact condition, an external force equivalent to the average ground reaction force at 40% of the gait cycle (GC) for 15 normal subjects is applied to the plantar surface of the foot, and the Achilles and posterior tibial tendon forces are increased to achieve the desired amounts of plantar flexion and inversion, respectively. Prior to loading these tendons, the peroneus brevis and longus force levels were assigned based upon cross-sectional area. For the PTTD condition, the posterior tibial tendon force is removed and the angular displacements of the talus with respect to the navicular and the change in strain at the spring ligament are monitored to see if the changes are consistent with clinical observations of PTTD.

In early pilot work, the above method of estimating a combined peroneal force in achieving our equilibrium position was used, and the Achilles and posterior tibial tendon forces were within acceptable limits; however, for some specimens it was necessary to increase the peroneal forces beyond our initial estimates in order to achieve the desired inversion position in the intact foot at equilibrium. The need to increase the peroneal forces was not surprising because initial estimates were conservative, i.e., using factors of 40 N/cm^2 and 25% of maximum force. The calculated estimates were a starting point, whereas our loading model, which appropriately accounts for external loads, provided more functional estimates of the forces required of these muscles in order to meet the demands placed on the foot. As a result of this experience, the force required of these muscles to achieve 3° of eversion for each specimen was determined with the posterior tibial muscle force set to zero.

38.2.4.4 External Load

Experiments were conducted using external loads of 50, 75, and 100% body weight. This served two purposes. If any cadaveric specimens were unable to tolerate the 100% body weight load without failure, data would have been collected at the partial body weights. Furthermore, collecting performance data for the model over the range of loads allows the comparison of outcomes as a function of external loads. If the 50 or 75% body weight loads resulted in a behavior that was the same as for 100%, with the exception of being scaled down, then the model outcome at the lesser loads would have validity.

38.2.5 Model Outcome

The displacements that resulted when the posterior tibial tendon force was removed at the early heel rise position for four specimens are illustrated in Figure 38.3. When the posterior tibial tendon force was removed, the navicular dorsiflexed 2.5 ± 1.1°, everted 5.3 ± 0.4°, and abducted 2.1 ± 0.6°. Each is the mean and one standard deviation over the 50, 75, and 100% body weight loads. As a result of releasing the posterior tibial tendon force, strain increases ranged from 2.0 to 3.5%. The strain change and the associated displacement change for each of the three axes are plotted in Figure 38.4 for a typical specimen. Each data point represents the average displacement of the specimen about the respective axis and the associated average change in strain, e.g., the smallest change in strain was associated with the smallest displacement about each of the three axes. The lesser changes in strain were

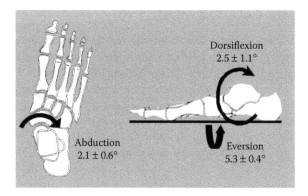

FIGURE 38.3 Schematic of foot illustrating the rotational changes of the navicular in the sagittal, frontal, and transverse planes relative to the talus following release of the posterior tibial tendon force.

associated with the 50% body weight trials, and the greater changes in strain and displacement were associated with the 100% body weight trials.

Thus, the cadaver model, when subjected to the simulated loss of posterior tibial tendon force at heel rise, responded with (1) a displacement of the talonavicular joint that was consistent with the direction of the acquired flatfoot deformity and (2) an associated increase in strain of the spring ligament consistent with its observed clinical failure. Note that the strain increases observed do not reflect absolute strain, but increases beyond that which existed at the heel rise position prior to release of the posterior tibial tendon force.

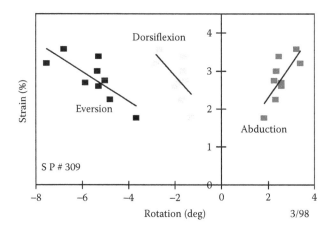

FIGURE 38.4 Plot of the strain changes associated with the rotational change of the navicular relative to the talus following release of the posterior tibial tendon force.

38.3 DYNAMIC CADAVER MODELING

Currently in place are systems more sophisticated than that described here, which simulate the stance phase of gait rather a single event during the stance phase.[12,13] Sharkey and coworkers[14] developed the system shown in Figure 38.5 that allows the tibia to advance with its proximal portion constrained to move along a cam profile such that, as the tibia advances, its proximal portion maintains the same distance from the ground as during normal gait. This distance defines ankle plantar flexion as the tibia advances. The muscle actuators are attached to and advance with the tibia. They are activated to generate tendon forces in accordance with the criteria selected, e.g., to initially match the EMG levels throughout the stance phase. The force plate and pedobarograph allow the investigator to monitor the ground reaction force and foot pressure pattern throughout the stance phase. This is a valuable feedback that allows the muscle forces to be adjusted as necessary to achieve agreement between these outputs and the force and pressure measurements that occur for the normal or pathologic gait being studied.

An alternative approach to dynamic cadaver foot modeling, an extension of the static model described above, is to apply the ground reaction force to match that which occurs during the stance phase and to generate the muscle forces necessary to match the foot kinematics to the kinematics of the normal or pathologic gait being studied. In such a system, the proximal tibia would translate forward along a horizontal line. The changing effective length of the lower leg segment with plantar flexion and dorsiflexion would be accommodated by the platform generating the ground reaction

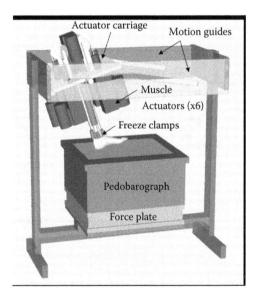

FIGURE 38.5 Apparatus for dynamic cadaver modeling of the stance phase of gait. (With permission from Neil A. Sharkey, Ph.D., Professor, Penn State University.)

force components. The ability to accommodate the effective length of the lower leg segment more readily allows for the simulation of abnormal gait patterns, e.g., an equinus gait or a heel rise deficient gait. The choice of the method for simulating the gait of the lower segment is often based upon the types of studies that need to be performed.

38.4 ROBOTIC TECHNOLOGY

38.4.1 JOINT STUDIES

The use of robotic technology to characterize the mechanical characteristics of diarthrodial joints has become popular in recent years.[15] In addition, the potential for extending modeling capabilities for functional activities beyond current capabilities exists through the versatility of robotic technology. Figure 38.6 shows a robot with six degrees-of-freedom and a payload capability of 165 kg. Thus, when used in joint mechanics, it can generate a compressive load of 165 kg, one body weight, across the joint. The robot is combined with a universal force-moment sensor. The six degree-of-freedom universal force-moment sensor monitors the three forces and three moments generated at the effector end of the robot arm as it moves through its trajectory. The sensor provides the feedback necessary to operate in force mode.

The extension of robotic technology to investigate biomechanics of the foot has potential benefits at two levels of investigation: at a basic level to study individual joints, and at a more sophisticated level as part of a gait simulation system. In the former, it can characterize the mechanical properties of ligaments and retinacular structures that are felt to be critical to the stability of diarthrodial joints. To date, studies have been performed that characterize the mechanical properties of several joints. Beyond that, the ability to characterize loads during functional activities will be possible when kinematics and kinetics are established through motion analysis studies.

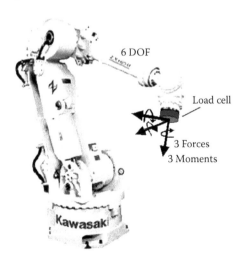

FIGURE 38.6 Six degree-of-freedom, 165-kg payload robot with load cell attached.

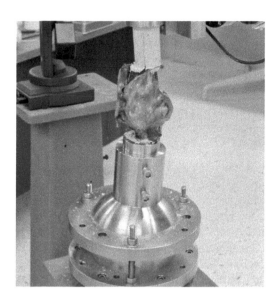

FIGURE 38.7 Cadaveric knee specimen installed for testing by robotic system. The shaft of the tibia, previously potted in cement, is rigidly secured to a cylindrical clamp (partially shown at top) that is mounted on the universal force-moment sensor on the robot. The femur is clamped to a pedestal that is rigidly attached to the floor.

Robotic testing of diarthrodial joints utilizes the principle of superposition. Figure 38.7, showing a cadaver knee specimen ready for testing, provides an appreciation of the mounting requirements. The shaft of the proximal half of the tibia, which has been previously potted in cement in cylindrical form, is rigidly secured to a cylindrical clamp (partially shown) that is mounted on the universal force-moment sensor on the robot. The femur is attached in a similar manner to a clamp on a pedestal that is securely attached to the floor. Thus, the tibia moves relative to the femur through a pathway that meets specific criteria. The ability to measure the ligament force with such a system is illustrated schematically in Figure 38.8. The generic joint shown in Figure 38.8a has the concave side secured to the ground and the convex side secured to the universal force-moment sensor mounted on the robot. To keep with the theme of foot mechanics, one could imagine this as representing a talonavicular joint.

It is desired to determine the contribution of ligament A to the stability of the joint when the joint has an upward force of 100 N applied as shown in Figure 38.8b. The pathway is defined by incrementally increasing the vertical force, while maintaining the remaining forces and moments at zero, until the equilibrium position is achieved with the 100 N vertical load (Figure 38.8b). The equilibrium position is recorded as are the force and moment data, and the joint is returned to its unloaded position (Figure 38.8c). At this time, a different force and/or moment can be applied, e.g., a 100 N load to the right and a second equilibrium position (not shown) can be recorded in the same manner as was conducted for the 100 N vertical force.

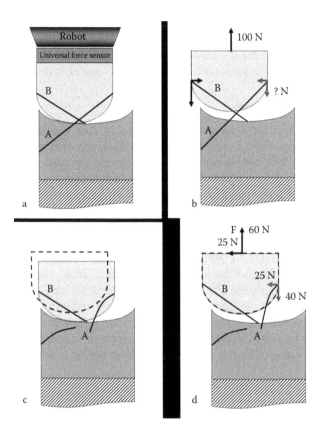

FIGURE 38.8 Schematic of joint during robotic testing: (a) initial position; (b) equilibrium position with 100 N force applied; (c) return to initial position and resection of ligament; and (d) return to equilibrium using displacement mode.

The joint is again returned to its unloaded position. This can be done for as many loading conditions as desired. Once the loading scenarios are completed and the joint is returned to its unloaded position, ligament A is cut (Figure 38.8c). With the robotic system operating in displacement control mode, the joint is restored to the equilibrium position (Figure 38.8d). The universal force-moment sensor data show that, instead of a 100 N vertical component, the force to maintain this position without ligament A consists of a 60 N vertical component and a 25 N horizontal component to the left. Applying the principle of superposition, the intact ligament A would have exerted force components on the bone segment of 40 N downward and 25 N to the left. If other load conditions were investigated, the joint would be moved to each of those equilibrium positions under displacement control and the contribution of ligament A when intact at each of the positions could be similarly determined using the superposition principle.

The joints of the foot that are more amenable to being studied using a robotic system are the freely moving joints, such as the ankle, subtalar, and talonavicular joints. Joints like those between the tarsal bones of the midfoot and the calcaneocuboid joint, which are extremely limited in their motion, are unlikely candidates for robotic studies with the system described in this chapter. Studies of the phalangeal joints may be amenable for robotic studies using a smaller scale robotic system.

38.4.2 GAIT SIMULATION

The utilization of a robot for simulation of gait in foot and ankle studies offers several advantages. From a cost standpoint, the robotic system would minimize the need for custom-built testing capabilities by allowing the control of load and displacement parameters through software programming rather than through the design and fabrication of custom hardware. From a utilization standpoint, the robotic system can be used for testing of lower and upper extremity joints and joints of the spine, both natural and artificial, such that the costs to purchase and to maintain the robotic capability can be shared by several investigative groups.

The upper portion of Figure 38.9 shows a more traditional arrangement for dynamic testing of the foot during a simulated stance phase. The tibia is advanced with muscle loads consistent with the geometry and external loads applied to the foot. This generally requires the advancement of the muscle actuators with the tibia. Note the relationship of the ground reaction force and force plate with respect to the lower leg segment and the foot. Implementation of the robot as shown in the lower portion of Figure 38.9 can provide this relationship without having to advance the tibia and

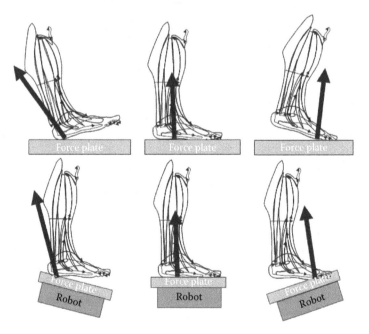

FIGURE 38.9 Upper figures show relationship of external force vector to foot with tibial advancement during stance phase. Lower figures show how relationship can be preserved with the tibia stationary and robotic control of the force platform.

its muscle actuators. This is not a simple task, but can be accomplished by programming the advancement of the force plate in a pattern that is coordinated to maintain the distance from the knee, similar to the goal of the cam profile in the dynamic simulator described above. The muscle actuators can be tweaked and programmed to generate the appropriate ground reaction force pattern. As an alternative, the ground reaction force vector can be applied and the muscle actuators adjusted until the target angles for plantar flexion and inversion are achieved. Whether one prefers the former or latter method of control, implementing a robot or not, it must be appreciated that these are tedious, time-consuming, and demanding experiments to conduct. Clearly, there are more options available than there have been in the past.

REFERENCES

1. Saltzman C.L. et al., Foot and ankle research priority: report from the Research Council of the American Orthopaedic Foot and Ankle Society, *Foot Ankle,* 18, 447, 1997.
2. Hansen M.L. et al., A closed-loop cadaveric foot and ankle loading model, *J Biomech,* 34, 551, 2001.
3. Gazdag A.R. and Cracchiolo A., Rupture of the posterior tibial tendon, *J Bone Joint Surg,* 79A, 675–681, 1997.
4. Perry J., *Gait Analysis: Normal and Pathological Function,* Slack Inc., Thorofare, 1992, 59.
5. Choi K. et al., Anatomical reconstruction of the spring ligament using peroneus longus tendon graft, *Foot Ankle Int,* 24, 430, 2003.
6. Sharkey N.A. et al., Strain and loading of the second metatarsal during heel-lift, *J Bone Joint Surg,* 77A, 1050–1057, 1995.
7. Sharkey N.A., Marder R.A., and Hanson P.B., The entire rotator cuff contributes to elevation of the arm, *J Orthop Res,* 12, 699, 1994.
8. Wickiewicz T.L. et al., Muscle architecture of the lower limb, *Clin Orthop Relat Res,* 179, 275, 1983.
9. Silver R.L., Garza J., and Rang M., The myth of muscle balance: a study of relative strengths and excursions of normal muscles about the foot and ankle, *J Bone Joint Surg,* 67A, 432, 1985.
10. Maughan R.J., Watson J.S., and Weir J., Strength and cross-sectional area of human skeletal muscle, *J Physiol,* 338, 37, 1983.
11. Otis J.C. et al., Quantitative assessment of patient performance after major limb reconstruction, In: Brown K.L.B., ed., *Complications of Limb Salvage,* Isols, Montreal, 1991, 25–31.
12. Sharkey N.A. and Hamel A.J., A dynamic cadaver model of the stance phase of gait: performance characteristics and kinetic validation, *Clin Biomech (Bristol, Avon),* 13, 420, 1998.
13. Kim K.J. et al., An in vitro study of individual ankle muscle actions on the center of pressure, *Gait Posture,* 17,125, 2003.
14. Hamel A.J., Donahue S.W., and Sharkey N.A., Contributions of active and passive toe flexion to forefoot loading. *Clin Orthop Relat Res,* 393, 326, 2001.
15. Woo S.L. et al., Use of robotic technology for diarthrodial joint research, *J Sci Med Sport,* 2, 283, 1999.

Section E

Research Support

39 Supporting Rehabilitation Research on Foot and Ankle Motion Analysis

Louis A. Quatrano and Hameed Khan

CONTENTS

39.1 INTRODUCTION

While a large number of rehabilitation interventions involve the foot and ankle, the contributions of the foot and ankle to normal gait are not well understood.[1] More specifically, understanding the effects of congenital defects, injuries, or other alterations in the lower limb and particularly the foot and ankle on mobility in children and adults is a continuing challenge to medical rehabilitation researchers. Among the factors contributing to this are the complex structures of the musculoskeletal system in the foot and ankle, the interrelationship with other structures of the lower limb and trunk, the neurological control for activating movement, and developmental aspects of children. Nonetheless, because unassisted or assisted walking/mobility is associated with independence, it is highly valued by children and adults. Providing a scientific basis for movement remains a goal of medical rehabilitation researchers, in order to inform surgical or other rehabilitation interventions that aim to restore mobility in children and adults.

Fortunately, a number of scientific advances in other fields such as computer science, neuroscience, orthopedics, imaging, and bioengineering are beginning to elucidate how the musculoskeletal system functions and are providing new or improved research tools for exploring physiological systems dynamically. Some of these advances can be employed to begin developing paradigms for examining individual relationships between specific impairments, limitations, and disabilities in the gait of children and adults. In some instances, interdisciplinary teams of researchers will be needed. One of the challenges will be to explore the links between pathophysiology, impairment, and functional limitation.[1] Some areas for potential research include development of models to predict surgical outcome, construction of supportive structures such as orthotics or exoskeletons, therapeutic interventions to improve performance of the foot and ankle, organizing interdisciplinary teams to review the role of the foot and ankle in mobility, and more.

39.2 THE NATIONAL INSTITUTES OF HEALTH

39.2.1 BACKGROUND

The National Institutes of Health (NIH) is the principal government agency dedicated to conducting medical and behavioral research and developing and increasing medical understanding throughout the U.S. The NIH is a large organization with 20 Institutes and seven Centers. Of the Institutes at NIH, the National Institute of Child Health and Human Development (NICHD) has a budget exceeding one billion dollars per year. Although less than 12% of the budget is spent on in-house research, more than 88% of the budget is made available to investigators outside NIH. One of the Centers at the NICHD is the National Center for Medical Rehabilitation Research (NCMRR), which promotes musculoskeletal research for treatment of persons with disabilities.

The NCMRR invites novel ideas to treat gait and function in patients with disabilities, encouraging investigators whose work ranges from the robotic to the genetic revolution. Some research initiatives indicative of NCMRR's mission are the use of nanotechnology to construct miniaturized devices for dynamic coupling and the use of stem cells to strengthen muscle in experimental animals without increasing spasticity or tightness. Recent work on zebra fish and amphibians has shown that these species carry genes that tend to regenerate organs on removal. Investigators are working to demonstrate not only the usefulness of these genes, but also to identify, sequence, and splice these genes in experimental animals with cerebral palsy. The National Institute of Arthritis and Musculoskeletal and Skin Disease also funds research on musculoskeletal disorders and treatments. The National Institute on Aging funds research on skeletal problems associated with aging. Resources to pursue this research can be sought from a combination of public and private funds.

The NIH budget was doubled between financial year (FY) 1999 and FY 2003. The 2004 budget was 28 billion dollars with 82% of this supporting research grants, training and research, and development contracts (Figure 39.1). The number of

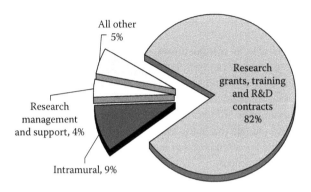

FIGURE 39.1 Distribution of NIH budget, FY 2004: $28 billion.

applications received by the Center for Scientific Review at NIH, which receives approximately 70% of the research grant applications submitted to NIH, from 2002 to 2003 increased from 55,030 to 68,478 or 24%. In summary, the resources available for research have increased, but the number of new and renewal applications submitted by investigators has also increased.[3]

In preparing to submit an application, two initial steps should be considered. First, applicants should contact a program official at one of the Institutes interested in their research topic. This program person can inform the applicant of any specific Institute requirements beyond the general announcement that must be taken into consideration. Second, the applicant should review the list of study sections in the Center for Scientific Review (CSR) (www.csr.nih.gov) to identify a potential review group for the application. Two of the most frequently visited CSR Web sites that applicants might find useful are the Roster Index (www.csr.nih.gov/committees/rosterindex.asp) and the IRG Index (www.csr.nih.gov/review/irgdesc.htm). Other helpful information describing the process is available at the CSR Web site. If the Web addresses change, use the general address (www.nih.gov) for information.

Advances in computer handling of administrative information have stimulated administrative changes in government. In response to a congressional mandate, the NIH created the electronic research administration (eRA) project to transform all federal agencies into paperless, electronic systems. The eRA is a division of the NIH that conducts interactive, electronic transactions for the receipt, review, and administration of grant awards to biomedical investigators worldwide. The Web site grants.gov (www.grants.gov/CustomerSupport) allows organizations to electronically find and apply for competitive grant opportunities from all federal grant making agencies. New procedures are required to submit a grant application using the SF424 Research and Related Areas (R&R) form to the NIH: (a) Register your organization at grants.gov; (b) register your organization and principal investigator (PI) in the NIH eRA Commons; (c) submit the application and receive the grants.gov tracking number; (d) after agency validation, receive the agency tracking number; and (e) verify in the eRA Commons. One the great advantages of eRA submission is that incomplete applications will not be accepted and the PI will immediately learn about the missing information. Another advantage is that colored photos and diagrams are reproduced clearly.

Given the variations in administrative support where potential applicants reside and the changing guidelines and reorganization at the NIH, applicants are encouraged to learn about the current administrative process of completing, submitting, and following up on a grant application through grants.gov. As mentioned earlier, to facilitate application submission, the NIH is moving toward a common application form (SF424 R&R) and eRA. Individuals can learn about these new procedures by reading material on the NIH Web site or attending seminars sponsored by NIH staff at national or regional scientific conferences.

39.2.2 PURSUING A RESEARCH CAREER

Building a research career can be a formidable task. A number of personal factors should be considered such as intriguing areas of science or special techniques used in a field that are of interest, as well as the status of this topic of interest. Namely, is it a new area of science, or, is there a specific location with a particular mentor, who is recognized as a leader in the field? Once started in a particular direction of scientific research, one should consider long- and short-term projects or a balance of low- and high-risk projects that are different from those of their mentor.

The ingredients for constructing a research application involve reviewing the current literature and discussing the topic with colleagues; defining and refining the problem to be studied; developing hypotheses and likely outcomes; identifying research methods, approaches, and alternative approaches to address the problem; and considering how the findings of the research will impact on the field of science. As part of this preliminary approach, consideration of the resources, equipment, or reagents, your needs should be considered. Assembling a team of collaborators may be required to have access to research subjects or animals. Pilot results may be required to demonstrate the feasibility of the idea, commitment to research, competence to handle potentially highly specialized techniques, and ability to gather and publish data.

In preparing the application for submission, a number of considerations should be included such as a focused application with explicit goals, sufficient technical information on outcome measures and plans for analysis, details of collaborations, defined subject population and/or range of disabilities, and material regarding human subjects. Finally, the application must be reviewed to ensure that it is neat, accurate, and complete before submission.

39.2.3 CAREER DEVELOPMENT SUPPORT

A variety of research resources are available to pursue one's research interests, and, depending on research career status, one particular mechanism may be more appropriate than another (www.nichd.nih.gov/training/training.htm). If eligible, students at a number of academic levels, starting with high school, interested in health-related research can apply for a Research Supplement to Promote Diversity in Health-Related Research (Grants2.nih.gov/grants/guide/pa-files/PA-05-015.html).

At the college level, students may be eligible for Minority Access to Research Careers (MARC), Minority Biomedical Research Support (MBRS) programs, or the National Institute of Mental Health Career opportunities in research education and training (COR) honors undergraduate Research Training Grant (T34). A student in a graduate school or pursuing a postdoctoral training might consider submitting an Individual Predoctoral Fellowship (F31), an Institutional Training Grant (T32), or Postdoctoral fellowship (F32). At the investigator level, the Mentored Research Development award (K01), Independent Scientist Award (K02), and the Senior Fellowship (F33) are possible options. For medical students, the career path can begin with the Short-Term Training Grant (T35) that is available upon acceptance to medical school. During the internship, residency, and specialty training, Institutional Training Grants (T32), Individual Postdoctoral Fellowships (F32), Scientist Development Program (K12), and Mentored Clinical Scientist Award (K08) are potential support mechanisms.

For a new clinical scientist, opportunities for support such as the Mentored Patient-Oriented Research K23, Mid-Career Investigator in Patient-Oriented Research (K24), or a Senior Fellowship (F33) are available.

39.2.4 RESEARCH SUPPORT

A Research Project grant is awarded to an institution on behalf of a PI to facilitate pursuit of a scientific focus or objective in the area of the investigator's interest and competence. Institutional sponsorship assures the NIH that the institution will provide facilities necessary to accomplish the research and will be accountable for the grant funds. Applications are accepted for health-related research and development in all areas within the scope of NICHD's mission.

In general, any organization is eligible to apply for regular NIH research grants, and unsolicited applications are welcome. The applicant is the research organization, although a PI writes the research proposal, and if a grant is awarded, the grantee is the applicant organization. Applications may be submitted by domestic or foreign, profit and nonprofit organizations, public and private, such as universities, colleges, hospitals, laboratories, units of state and local governments, and eligible agencies of the federal government. The NCMRR encourages applications from new investigators.

39.2.5 SPECIFIC ANNOUNCEMENTS

Many applicants wait for research topics to be announced by the Institutes; however, the overwhelming majority of NIH grants are made available to investigator-initiated applications. Two of the common approaches that the NIH employs to announce research opportunities are Requests for Applications (RFAs) or Program Announcements (PAs). RFAs are solicitations for grant applications addressing a defined research topic. Each RFA specifies the scope and objectives of the research to be proposed, application requirements and procedures, and the review criteria to be applied in the evaluation of applications submitted in response to the RFA.

A PA is used by the Institute to announce its interest in building or enhancing its research program in a particular area. The PA typically is an ongoing solicitation, accepting applications for multiple receipt dates, for up to 3 yr. The PA specifies the scope and objectives of the research of interest, application requirements and procedures, and review criteria to be applied.

Cooperative agreements are grants that are awarded to assist and support research and related activities. They differ from other grants, however, in that while other grant mechanisms require minimal or no involvement of the NIH during the performance of project activities, cooperative agreements involve a substantial NIH programmatic (i.e., scientific-technical) role. This role may involve cooperation and/or coordination to assist awardees in carrying out the project or review and approval of certain processes/phases in the scientific management of the project.

Policies and procedures for the application, review, and administration of cooperative agreements are similar to those for other grants. An important difference, however, is that the NICHD issues a specific RFA describing the program, functions, or activities that it proposes to support by cooperative agreement and the nature of the proposed NICHD staff involvement. Terms and conditions of awards are outlined in the RFA, above and beyond those required for the usual stewardship of grants, to establish the rights, responsibilities, and authorities of the prospective awardees and the NICHD.

39.2.6 INVESTIGATOR-INITIATED APPLICATIONS

Applicants do not have to wait until an announcement appears on a research topic of interest. They may submit an investigator-initiated application on any of the appropriate submission dates. At the investigator level, there are a variety of support mechanisms to pursue investigator-initiated research (nichd.nih.gov/funding/applying.htm#nih_forms). When submitting applications, investigators are required to respond to the following five standard criteria: (1) significance, (2) approach, (3) innovation, (4) investigators, and (5) environment.

39.2.6.1 Significance

Does this study address an important problem? If the aims of the application are achieved, how will scientific knowledge or clinical practice be advanced? What will be the effect of these studies on the concepts, methods, technologies, treatments, services, or preventative interventions that drive this field?

39.2.6.2 Approach

Are the conceptual or clinical framework, design, methods, and analyses adequately developed, well integrated, well reasoned, and appropriate to the aims of the project? Does the applicant acknowledge potential problem areas and consider alternative tactics?

39.2.6.3 Innovation

Is the project original and innovative? For example: Does the project challenge existing paradigms or clinical practice or address an innovative hypothesis or critical barrier to progress in the field? Does the project develop or employ novel concepts, approaches, methodologies, tools, or technologies for this area?

39.2.6.4 Investigators

Are the investigators appropriately trained and well suited to carry out this work? Is the work proposed appropriate to the experience level of the PI and other researchers? Does the investigative team bring complementary and integrated expertise to the project (if applicable)?

39.2.6.5 Environment

Does the scientific environment in which the work will be done contribute to the probability of success? Do the proposed studies benefit from unique features of the scientific environment or subject populations, or employ useful collaborative arrangements? Is there evidence of institutional support?

Most of the grants vary in resources available, time, and purpose. Identifying the right grant type for your research is a first step. For example, the Academic Research Enhancement Award (AREA) grants (R15) support individual research projects in the biomedical and behavioral sciences conducted by faculty, and involving their undergraduate students, who are located in health professional schools and other academic components that have not been major recipients of NIH research grant funds. There are other grants for doing exploratory research, such as the R03 and R21, and grants available to independent researchers with more research experience that are initiating large projects such as program projects (P01) or cooperative agreements (U01) (www.nichd.nih.gov/funding/mech research.htm).

The NIH R03 award supports small research projects that can be carried out in a short period of time with limited resources. The NCMRR uses the Small Grant to support new biomedical and behavioral research projects relevant to the NCMRR mission in medical rehabilitation research (www.nichd.nih.gov/funding/mech_research.htm#r03). The Exploratory/Developmental Grant (R21) is used to encourage the development of new research activities in categorical program areas. Applications submitted under this mechanism should be exploratory and novel. These studies should break new ground or extend previous discoveries toward new directions or applications. Support is generally restricted in level of support and in time. Complete descriptions of eligibility requirements, scope, and application procedures would be presented in a Request for Applications (RFA) utilizing this mechanism or can be accessed by the NIH R21 PA at grants2.nih.gov/grants/guide/pa-files/PA-03-107.html.

The purpose of the P01 mechanism is to encourage multidisciplinary approaches to the investigation of complex problems relevant to NCMRR's mission and to facilitate economy of effort, space, and equipment. The program project grant is an institutional award made in the name of a program director for the support of a broadly based, long-term, multidisciplinary research program that has a well-defined central theme, research focus, or objective. The grant funds at least three interrelated projects and, often, core resources. Interrelationships and synergism among component research projects should result in greater scientific contributions than if each project were supported through a separate mechanism. The grant is based on the concept that projects closely related to a central theme can be conducted more effectively and efficiently through a coordinated, collaborative, multidisciplinary approach.

TABLE 39.1
Comparison of SBIR and STTR Programs

SBIR (R43/R44)	STTR (R41/R42)
Purpose — to increase private sector commercialization of innovations derived from federal research and development.	Purpose — to increase private sector commercialization of innovations derived from federal research and development.
The SBC may conduct the entire SBIR project without outside collaboration.	The STTR program requires that an SBC (applicant organization) "team" with a research institution in the collaborative conduct of a project that has potential for commercialization.
The SBIR program requires that the PI have his/her primary employment (>50%) with the SBC at the time of award and during the conduct of the project.	The PI may have his/her primary employment with an organization other than the SBC, including the research institution. However, there must be an official relationship between the PI and the SBC. PI must devote not less than 10% effort to the project.
The total amount of all contractual costs and consultant fees normally may not exceed 33% for Phase I, or 50% for Phase II, of the total costs requested.	At least 40% of the work is performed by the SBC, and at least the research institution performs 30% of the work. (% based on costs in award)
Research space must be occupied by the small business, generally not shared with another organization, and is under the exclusive control of the awardee.	Research space must be occupied by the small business, generally not shared with another organization, and is under the exclusive control of the awardee.
At least 51% of the SBC owned by a U.S. citizen or lawfully admitted resident alien.	At least 51% of the SBC owned by a U.S. Citizen or lawfully admitted resident alien.
Phase I normally not to exceed $100,000 DC, Facilities and Administration (F&A), and fee for a period normally not to exceed 6 months. May exceed this level (recommend 12 months, no additional $)	Phase I normally not to exceed $100,000 for DC, F&A, and fee for a period normally not to exceed 1 yr. May exceed this level.
Phase II: Awards normally may not exceed $750,000/- for DC, F&A, and fee for a period normally not to exceed 2 yr. May exceed this level	Phase II: Awards normally may not exceed $750,000 for DC, F&A, and fee for a period normally not to exceed 2 yr. May exceed this level.
Phase III: The objective of this phase is for the SBC to pursue with non-SBIR funds the commercialization of the results of the research or R&D funded in Phases I and II.	Phase III: Same objective. In some federal agencies, Phase III may involve follow-on non-STTR funded R&D or production contracts for products or processes intended for use by the U. S. government.
Receipt dates August 1, December 1, April 1	Receipt dates August 1, December 1, April 1.

Small businesses that are interested in health-related research can apply for grants. Check the eligibility section of the announcement. Usually, the individuals in business partner with academic groups in submitting applications. Small Business Innovation Research Grants (SBIR) and Small Business Technology Transfer Grants (STTR) are two mechanisms that are available to interested applicants (Grants1.nih.gov/grants/funding/sbir.htm). Table 39.1 contrasts the two programs.

Small Business grants are not small. The set-aside budget for all government agencies for Small Business grants exceeds $2.2 billion dollars. The Department of Health and Human Services (DHHSs) provides under Small Business for both SBIR and STTR. The budget is approximately $71 millions for SBIR and $69 millions for STTR. Under SBIR or STTR programs, junior investigators could benefit from this funding mechanism because if they are in a university research environment, they could have experience in research on ankle and foot injuries and they could work in collaboration with investigators in other universities or small businesses, for example a robotic firm developing devices for dynamic coupling for acceleration of the knee toward flexion during normal walking. Under Phase I of SBIR, junior investigators could receive up to $100,000, by collaborating with a small business concern (SBC) and complete the project within six months. The same amount of funds are available to junior investigators under STTR if they could finish the project within a year. STTR programs require that small business and academic institutions work together. At least 40% contribution by the small business and at least 30% support is provided by the academic institutions. If the investigators can reach the milestones (Specific Aims) they proposed in Phase I, larger funds and more time are made available under Phase II. Under SBIR Phase II, a sum of $750,000 is made available for up to 2 yr (additional funds and times are provided upon accomplishing milestones). Commercialization of the product is expected under Phase III, therefore no government funds are provided. However, some Institutes have SBIR/STTR programs available to meet the Food and Drug Administration requirements for devices or drugs.

39.3 DISCUSSION

Initiating, establishing, and maintaining a research career is difficult work, writing grant applications is time-consuming, and finding adequate resources can be difficult. However, the reward of adding new knowledge to the field or providing effective interventions to individuals with disabilities can be very satisfying. For those seeking the challenge, there are a number of research questions concerning the role of the foot and ankle in ambulation that remain to be resolved.

REFERENCES

1. Rose, J and Gamble, JG. *Human Walking*. Williams and Wilkins, 1994.
2. Research Plan for the National Center for Medical Rehabilitation Research, National Institute of Child Health and Human Development, National Center for Medical Rehabilitation Research, 35, 1993.
3. Peer Review Notes, National Institutes of Health, Jan 2004.

Index

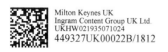

9 780367 388737